Advanced Nutrition and Dietetics in Gastroenterology

Editor

Miranda Lomer PhD RD

Series Editor

Kevin Whelan PhD RD

T0256835

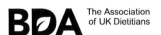

WILEY Blackwell

Registered Office
John Wiley & Sons, Ltd, The Atrium, Southern Gate, Chichester, West Sussex, PO19 8SQ, UK

Editorial Offices
9600 Garsington Road, Oxford, OX4 2DQ, UK
111 River Street, Hoboken, NJ 07030–5774, USA

For details of our global editorial offices, for customer services and for information about how to apply for permission to reuse the copyright material in this book please see our website at www.wiley.com/wiley-blackwell

Library of Congress Cataloging-in-Publication Data

Advanced nutrition and dietetics in gastroenterology / editor, Miranda Lomer.
    1 online resource.
  Includes bibliographical references and index.
  Description based on print version record and CIP data provided by publisher; resource not viewed.
  ISBN 978-1-118-87289-5 (ePub) – ISBN 978-1-118-87291-8 (Adobe PDF) – ISBN 978-0-470-67132-0
  I. Lomer, Miranda, editor.
  [DNLM: 1. Digestive System Diseases. 2. Dietetics. 3. Digestive System Physiological Phenomena.
4. Nutrition Therapy. 5. Nutritional Status. WI 140]
  RC801
  616.3′3–dc23

                    2014006436

A catalogue record for this book is available from the British Library.

Set in 9/11.5pt Times by SPi Publisher Services, Pondicherry, India

Printed in the UK

ADVANCED NUTRITION AND DIETETICS BOOK SERIES

Dietary recommendations need to be based on solid evidence, but where can you find this information? The British Dietetic Association and the publishers of the *Manual of Dietetic Practice* present an essential and authoritative reference series on the evidence base relating to advanced aspects of nutrition and dietetics in selected clinical specialties. Each book provides a comprehensive and critical review of key literature in the area. Each covers established areas of understanding, current controversies and areas of future development and investigation, and is oriented around six key themes:

- Disease processes, including metabolism, physiology and genetics
- Disease consequences, including morbidity, mortality and patient perspectives
- Clinical investigation and management
- Nutritional consequences of disease
- Nutritional assessment, including anthropometric, biochemical, clinical, dietary, economic and social approaches
- Nutritional and dietary management of disease

Contents

Preface

In recent years there has been an overwhelming interest in the role of diet and nutrition in gastrointestinal health and disease. There are a number of general books that focus on combining these topics but not specifically at an advanced level. The aim of this book is to be an essential and authoritative reference and review for an international audience of health professionals involved in the management or research of patients with gastrointestinal disorders.

The book is divided into four main sections:

- The first section is devoted to the physiology and function of the gastrointestinal and hepatobiliary tract including all the major organs, the gastrointestinal microbiota and the role of the gut neuroendocrine system in appetite regulation.
- The second section covers specific dietary components including fibre, short-chain fermentable carbohydrates, probiotics and the gastrointestinal microbiota and prebiotics in relation to gastrointestinal health.
- The third and fourth sections focus on gastrointestinal and hepatobiliary disorders respectively. These are comprehensive sections reviewing the evidence base relating to the pathogenesis, nutritional consequences and dietary management of disease.

The book provides a cutting-edge review of the evidence base relating to the basic aspects (for example, mechanistic aspects of physiology, immunology, microbiology, etc.) and applied aspects (for example, dietary impact and intervention) of diet and nutrition in gastrointestinal health and extensive focus on diet in the causation and treatment of gastrointestinal disease.

Each chapter provides a critical review of the key literature in each area, focussing on established areas of understanding and also on current controversies and areas of current and future development and investigation. The chapters extensively draw upon the literature with a focus on mechanisms as well as critical reviews of the efficacy of interventions and, where available, reference systematic reviews and meta-analyses.

The book is pitched at an advanced level to reflect the expertise of the readership. The intended readership is practitioners, researchers and educators in the area of gastrointestinal health and disease. This will include an interprofessional mix of dietitians, gastroenterologists, hepatologists, nutritionists, specialist nurses and surgeons. Due to the advanced level of the book, it may also be an invaluable resource for students in the final year of a Bachelors or Masters Degree in dietetics, nutrition, medicine or nursing, especially those undertaking relevant course units or research projects. It will also be of interest to those doing applied research in the areas of gastrointestinal immunology or microbiology. The book will also be of use for university educators preparing teaching materials in the above areas.

Miranda Lomer PhD RD
Senior Consultant Dietitian
Guy's and St Thomas' NHS Foundation Trust

Honorary Senior Lecturer
King's College London
Editor
Advanced Nutrition and Dietetics in
Gastroenterology

This book is the first title in a series commissioned as part of a major initiative between the British Dietetic Association and the publisher, Wiley. Each book in the series provides a comprehensive and critical review of the key literature in each clinical area. Each book is edited by one or more experts who have themselves undertaken extensive research and published widely in the relevant topic area. Each book chapter is written by experts drawn from an international audience and from a variety of disciplines as required of the relevant chapter (for example, dietetics, medicine, public health, basic sciences). We are proud to present the first title in the series: *Advanced Nutrition and Dietetics in Gastroenterology*. We hope that it impacts on health professionals' understanding and application of nutrition and dietetics in the management of people with gastrointestinal disease and improves outcomes for such patients.

Kevin Whelan PhD RD
Professor of Dietetics
King's College London
Series Editor
Advanced Nutrition and Dietetics Book Series

Foreword

It is an honour and a privilege to write a foreword for this exceptional book devoted to nutrition and dietetics in gastrointestinal health and disease. Nutrition is a major discipline in gastroenterology and is often overlooked.

The first question a patient asks when faced with gastrointestinal problems is regarding diet. Up to now gastroenterologists have been poorly informed in answering this question. Nutrition should be an integral part of the undergraduate curriculum. It should also be included as a module for trainees in gastroenterology. This is largely ignored. Dietitians have a key role in the multidisciplinary team that cares for patients with gastrointestinal conditions and are experts in food and nutrition.

This book is very welcome as it has contributions from key opinion leaders in gastroenterology who have contributed significantly to the field of nutrition. *Advanced Nutrition and Dietetics in Gastroenterology* is edited by Miranda Lomer who has extensive knowledge and an enviable Curriculum Vitae in both research and clinical management of dietary challenges.

This book is a comprehensive text, and reviews concisely and succinctly, carefully annotated sections relating to the physiology and function of the gastrointestinal and hepatobiliary tract; dietary components relevant to gastrointestinal health; and the role diet plays in gastrointestinal and hepatology disorders. It is logical that diet has an effect on the microenvironment of the gut. Diet can affect the gastrointestinal mucosa directly and indirectly by altering the gastrointestinal microbiota. Nutrition in gastroenterology is a vast area to cover and in addition to practical aspects, this book thoroughly reviews the evidence base and proposes new areas for research.

This book is the result of close collaboration between dietitians, gastroenterologists and scientists dedicated to gastroenterology. It highlights the importance of diet in the multidisciplinary management of patients with gastrointestinal and hepatobiliary disease. It explores the therapeutic dietary strategies required and will improve patient care.

I would recommend *Advanced Nutrition and Dietetics in Gastroenterology* as essential reading for dietitians, physicians, surgeons and scientists with an enquiring mind on the role of diet in health and disease, and it should be mandatory for trainees in gastroenterology.

Professor Colm O'Morain
Emeritus Professor of Medicine
Trinity College Dublin
President of the United European
Gastroenterology Federation 2011–2013

Editor biographies

Miranda Lomer PhD RD

Miranda Lomer is a Senior Consultant Dietitian for Gastroenterology at Guy's and St Thomas' NHS Foundation Trust and an Honorary Senior Lecturer in the Diabetes and Nutritional Sciences Division at King's College London. Her clinical speciality and research interests include the dietary management of functional gastrointestinal disorders and inflammatory bowel diseases. Dr Lomer was formerly chairperson of the Gastroenterology Specialist Group of the British Dietetic Association and led the writing of the British Dietetic Association evidence-based guidelines for the dietary management of irritable bowel syndrome in adults and the British Dietetic Association evidence-based guidelines for the dietary management of Crohn's disease in adults. Dr Lomer is on the panel of the National IBD Standards Group and represented the British Dietetic Association on a National Institute for Health and Clinical Excellence guideline for the diagnosis and management of irritable bowel syndrome in primary care. For her contribution to clinical practice, education and research, Dr Lomer was awarded the British Dietetic Association Elsie Widdowson prestigious annual lecture in 2014.

Kevin Whelan PhD RD

Kevin Whelan is the Professor of Dietetics in the Diabetes and Nutritional Sciences Division at King's College London. He is a Principal Investigator leading a research programme exploring the interaction between the gastrointestinal microbiota, diet and health and disease. Professor Whelan undertakes clinical trials of probiotics, prebiotics, fibre and fermentable carbohydrates, together with molecular microbiology to measure their impact on the microbiota. In 2012 he was awarded the Nutrition Society Cuthbertson Medal for research in clinical nutrition. Professor Whelan is the Associate Editor-in-Chief for the *Journal of Human Nutrition and Dietetics* and is on the International Editorial Board for *Alimentary Pharmacology and Therapeutics*.

Contributors

Stuart Allan MBBS MRCS
Northumbria NHS Trust
North Shields, UK

Simran Arora MSc RD
Specialist Hepatology and Liver Transplant Dietitian
Royal Free London NHS Foundation Trust
London, UK

Stephen E. Attwood MD FRCS
Consultant Surgeon
Northumbria NHS Trust
North Shields, UK

Imran Aziz MBChB MRCP
Gastroenterology Clinical Research Fellow
Royal Hallamshire Hospital
Sheffield, UK

Qasim Aziz PhD FRCP
Professor of Neurogastroenterology
Wingate Institute of Neurogastroenterology
Queen Mary University of London
London, UK

Paul A. Blaker BSc MRCP
Clinical Fellow in Gastroenterology
Guy's and St Thomas' NHS Foundation Trust
London, UK

Stephen R. Bloom FRS
Head of Division of Diabetes, Endocrinology
and Metabolism
Imperial College London
London, UK

Gudrun De Boeck PhD
Professor
University of Antwerp
Antwerp, Belgium

Sorrel Burden PhD RD
Lead Dietitian
Central Manchester NHS Foundation Trust
Manchester, UK

Helen Campbell PhD RD
Research Dietitian
Guy's and St Thomas' NHS Foundation Trust
and King's College London
London, UK

Emma V. Carrington MSc MRCS
Clinical Research Fellow
Wingate Institute of Neurogastroenterology,
Queen Mary University of London
London, UK

Yolande M. Causebrook BSc RNutr
Nutritionist
Newcastle University
Newcastle upon Tyne, UK

Jaimini Cegla MSc MRCP
Wellcome Trust Clinical Research Fellow
Imperial College London
London, UK

Saira Chowdhury BSc RD
Highly Specialist Upper Gastrointestinal GI Surgery
Dietitian
Guy's and St Thomas' NHS Foundation Trust
London, UK

Alison Culkin PhD RD
Research Dietitian
St Mark's Hospital
Harrow, UK

Emma Currie MSc RD
Specialist Gastroenterology Dietitian
Addenbrooke's Hospital
Cambridge, UK

Barbara Davidson RD
Lead Specialist Dietitian Nutrition Support
Freeman Hospital
Newcastle upon Tyne, UK

Ashish P. Desai FRCS
Consultant Paediatric Surgeon
King's College Hospital NHS Foundation Trust
London, UK

Frances Dorman BSc RD
Specialist Hepatology Dietitian
King's College Hospital NHS Foundation Trust
London, UK

Michael P. Escudier MD FDSRCS
Reader and Consultant in Oral Medicine
King's College London and Guy's and
St Thomas' NHS Foundation Trust
London, UK

Adam D. Farmer PhD MRCP
Clinical Research Fellow
Wingate Institute of Neurogastroenterology,
Queen Mary University of London
London, UK

Lynnette R. Ferguson DPhil DSc
Professor and Head of Department of Nutrition
University of Auckland
Auckland, New Zealand

Mark Fox MD MRCP
Professor of Gastroenterology
University Hospital Zürich
Zürich, Switzerland
University of Nottingham
Nottingham, UK

Gillian Gatiss MSc RD
Specialist Hepatology and Liver Transplant Dietitian
Cambridge University Hospitals NHS Trust
Cambridge, UK

Liljana Gentschew MSc
Genetic Scientist
University of Kiel
Kiel, Germany

Konstantinos Gerasimidis PhD APHNutr
Lecturer in Clinical Nutrition
University of Glasgow and Glasgow Royal
Hospital for Sick Children
Glasgow, UK

Pascale Gerbault PhD
Research Associate
University College London
London, UK

Glenn R. Gibson PhD
Professor of Food Microbiology
University of Reading
Reading, UK

Henriette Heinrich MD
Clinical Research Fellow
University Hospital Zürich
Zürich, Switzerland

Mary Hickson PhD RD
Research Dietitian and Honorary Senior Lecturer
Imperial College Healthcare NHS Trust and
Imperial College London,
London, UK

Orla Hynes BSc RD
Highly Specialist Upper GI Surgery Dietitian
Guy's and St Thomas' NHS Foundation Trust
London, UK

Peter Irving MD FRCP
Consultant Gastroenterologist
Guy's and St Thomas' NHS Foundation Trust and
King's College London
London, UK

Santhini Jeyarajah MD FRCS
Clinical Research Fellow
King's College Hospital NHS Foundation Trust
London, UK

Yiannis N. Kallis PhD MRCP
Consultant Heptalogist
Barts Health NHS Trust, Royal London Hospital,
London, UK

Regina Keenan BSc
Senior Dietitian in Hepatobiliary Surgery
St Vincent's University Hospital
Dublin, Ireland

Richard Keld MD MRCP
Consultant Gastroenterologist
Wrightington, Wigan and Leigh NHS
Foundation Trust
Wigan, UK

Tanya Klopper M Nutr RD
Head of Dietetics, Macmillan Oncology Dietitian
Royal Surrey County Hospital
Guildford, UK

Vikas Kumar PhD
Postdoctoral Researcher
Ohio State University
Ohio, USA

Simon Lal PhD FRCP
Consultant Gastroenterologist
Salford Royal NHS Foundation Trust
Salford, UK

Rachel Lewis BSc RD
Clinical Lead Dietitian Critical Care
Glangwili Hospital
Carmarthen, UK

Anke Liebert PhD
Research Fellow
University College London
London, UK

Miranda C. E. Lomer PhD RD
Senior Consultant Dietitian in Gastroenterology
Guy's and St Thomas' NHS Foundation Trust and
King's College London
London, UK

Angela M. Madden PhD RD
Principal Lecturer in Nutrition and Dietetics
University of Hertfordshire
Hatfield, UK

Luca Marciani PhD
Lecturer in Gastrointestinal MRI
Nottingham University Hospitals and University
of Nottingham
Nottingham, UK

Catherine McAnenny BSc RD
Clinical Specialist Dietitian Liver Transplantation
Royal Infirmary of Edinburgh
Edinburgh, UK

Laura M. McGeeney MSc RD
Specialist Hepatology and Liver Transplant Dietitian
Cambridge University Hospitals NHS Trust
Cambridge, UK

Alison Morton BSc RD
Clinical Specialist Dietitian
Leeds Teaching Hospital NHS Trust
Leeds, UK

Maria O'Sullivan PhD MINDI
Associate Professor in Human Nutrition
Trinity College Dublin
Dublin, Ireland

Niamh O'Sullivan BSc MINDI
Clinical Specialist Dietitian in Liver Disease
St Vincent's University Hospital
Dublin, Ireland

Gareth Parkes PhD MRCP
Consultant Gastroenterologist
Barts Health NHS Trust
London, UK

Anu Paul MS FRCS
Clinical Fellow in Paediatric Surgery
King's College Hospital NHS Foundation Trust
London, UK

Mary Phillips BSc RD
Hepato-pancreaticobiliary Specialist Dietitian
Royal Surrey County Hospital
Guildford, UK

Nina C. Powell MSc RD
Specialist Hepatology and Liver Transplant Dietitian
Cambridge University Hospitals NHS
Foundation Trust
Cambridge, UK

Tara Raftery BSc MINDI
Research Fellow
Trinity College Dublin
Dublin, Ireland

David S. Sanders MD FRCP
Consultant Gastroenterologist
Royal Hallamshire Hospital
Sheffield, UK

Jeremy D. Sanderson MD FRCP
Consultant Gastroenterologist
Guy's and St Thomas' NHS Foundation Trust and
King's College London
London, UK

S. Mark Scott PhD
Co-Director, Gastrointestinal Physiology Unit
Wingate Institute of Neurogastroenterology,
Queen Mary University of London
London, UK

Clare Shaw PhD RD
Consultant Dietitian
Royal Marsden NHS Foundation Trust
London, UK

Sue Shepherd PhD AdvAPD
Senior Lecturer in Nutrition and Dietetics
La Trobe University
Melbourne, Australia

Amit Kumar Sinha PhD
Postdoctoral Fellow
University of Antwerp
Antwerp, Belgium

Chris Speed BSc
Senior Trial Manager
Newcastle University
Newcastle upon Tyne, UK

Heidi Staudacher M Nutr Diet RD
NIHR Doctoral Research Fellow
King's College London and Guy's and
St Thomas' NHS Foundation Trust
London, UK

Katherine Stephens BSc
Research Fellow
University of Reading
Reading, UK

Dallas M. Swallow PhD
Professor of Human Genetics
University College London
London, UK

Rami Sweis PhD MRCP
Consultant Gastroenterologist
University College London Hospital
London, UK

Mark G. Thomas PhD
Professor of Evolutionary Genetics
University College London
London, UK

Natasha A. Vidas BSc RD
Specialist Hepatology Dietitian
King's College Hospital NHS Foundation Trust
London, UK

Gemma E. Walton PhD
Postdoctoral Research Fellow
University of Reading
Reading, UK

Han-ping Wang PhD
Principal Scientist
Ohio State University
Ohio, USA

David Westaby MA FRCP
Lead Clinician for Pancreatobiliary Services
Imperial College Healthcare NHS Foundation Trust
London, UK

Kevin Whelan PhD RD
Professor of Dietetics
King's College London
London, UK

Physiology and function of the gastrointestinal and hepatobiliary tract

Chapter 1.1

Physiology and function of the mouth

Michael P. Escudier
King's College London and Guy's and St Thomas' NHS Foundation Trust London, UK

1.1.1 Physiology

The mouth is an important organ as it is the entry point into the gastrointestinal (GI) tract and damage and disease can compromise dietary intake. Even very minor disorders can have a profound impact on nutritional status.

Anatomy

The oral cavity consists of a number of structures.

The lips surround the mouth and comprise skin externally and a mucous membrane (which has many minor salivary glands) internally, which together with saliva ensure adequate lubrication for the purposes of speech and mastication.

The cheeks make up the sides of the mouth and are similar in structure to the lips with which they are continuous but differ in containing a fat pad in the subcutaneous tissue. On the inner surface of each cheek, opposite the upper second molar tooth, is an elevation that denotes the opening of the parotid duct which leads back to the parotid gland located in front of the ear.

The palate (roof of the mouth) is concave and formed by the hard and soft palate. The hard palate is formed by the horizontal portions of the two palatine bones and the palatine portions of the maxillae (upper jaws). The hard palate is covered by thick mucous membrane that is continuous with that of the gingivae. The soft palate is continuous with the hard palate anteriorly and with the mucous membrane covering the floor of the nasal cavity posteriorly. The soft palate is made up of a fibrous sheet together with the glossopalatine and pharyngopalatine muscles and the uvula hangs freely from its posterior border.

The floor of the mouth can only be seen when the tongue is raised and is formed by the mucosa overlying the mylohyoid muscle. In the midline is the lingual frenum (a fold of mucous membrane), on either side of which is the opening of the submandibular duct from the associated submandibular gland.

The gingivae form a collar around the neck of the teeth and consist of mucous membranes connected by thick fibrous tissue to the periosteum surrounding the bones of the jaw. The gingivae are highly vascular and well innervated.

The teeth are important in mastication and in humans, who are omnivores, they enable both plant and animal tissue to be chewed effectively. Each tooth consists of a crown, which varies in shape dependent on the position in the mouth, and one or more roots. There are eight permanent teeth in each quadrant, consisting of two incisors, a canine, two premolars and three molars, resulting in a total of 32 permanent teeth.

The tongue is a highly mobile, muscular organ in the floor of the mouth which is important in speech, chewing and swallowing. In conjunction with the cheeks, it guides food between the upper and lower teeth until mastication is complete. The taste buds situated on the tongue are responsible for the sensation of taste (salt, bitter, sweet and sour).

Advanced Nutrition and Dietetics in Gastroenterology, First Edition. Edited by Miranda Lomer.
© 2014 John Wiley & Sons, Ltd. Published 2014 by John Wiley & Sons, Ltd.

Table 1.1.1 Contribution of groups of salivary glands to overall saliva production at rest and during eating

	Resting %	Stimulated %
Parotid	20	50
Submandibular	65	49
Sublingual	8	
Minor	7	1

Function

The main role of the mouth is to prepare food for swallowing via the oesophagus and its subsequent passage to the stomach. The first phase of this process is mastication (chewing) which requires activity in the muscles of mastication (masseter, temporalis, medial and lateral pterygoids and buccinator). Chewing helps digestion by reducing food to small particles and mixing it with the saliva secreted by the salivary glands. The saliva lubricates and moistens dry food whilst the movement of the tongue against the hard palate produces a rounded mass (bolus) of food which can be swallowed.

The saliva required for this process is produced by the three paired major salivary glands (parotid, submandibular and sublingual), together with the many minor salivary glands throughout the oropharynx. The total daily production of saliva is around 500 mL, with the rate of production around 0.35 mL/min at rest which increases to 2.0 mL/min during eating and falls to 0.1 mL/min during sleep. The contribution of the various glands varies at rest and during eating (Table 1.1.1).

In addition to its role in digestion and taste, saliva produces a film which coats the teeth and mucosa and helps to cleanse and lubricate the oral cavity. It also prevents dessication of the oral mucosa and acts as a barrier to oral microbiota [1], both physically and through its antimicrobial activity. The buffers within it also help to maintain optimal pH for the action of the salivary amylase and maintain the structure of the teeth.

Role in digestion

Very little digestion of food occurs in the oral cavity. However, saliva does contain the enzyme amylase which begins the chemical process of digestion by catalysing the breakdown of starch into sugars.

Box 1.1.1 Challacombe dry mouth scale

One point for each feature to a maximum of 10

- Mirror sticks to one buccal mucosa
- Mirror sticks to both buccal mucosa
- Mirror sticks to tongue
- Saliva frothy
- No saliva pooling in floor of mouth
- Tongue shows loss of papillae
- Altered (smooth) gingival architecture
- Glassy appearance to oral mucosa
- Cervical caries (more than two teeth)
- Tongue highly fissured
- Tongue lobulated
- Debris on palate

1.1.2 Measurement and assessment of function

Salivary function is the most commonly assessed measure of oral function and can be achieved clinically by using the Challacombe dry mouth scale (Box 1.1.1).

A reasonable indication of salivary function may be obtained by measuring the resting (unstimulated) salivary flow over a period of 10 min. In health, the rate will normally be around 0.35 mL/min with a range of 0.2–0.5 mL/min. However, this will be reduced in the presence of xerostomic medications or underlying conditions such as Sjögren's syndrome and a value below 0.2 mL/min requires further investigation and below 0.1 mL/min is indicative of an underlying condition or disease process. Whilst the stimulated parotid flow rate may also be determined, neither is particularly reliable and hence both should only be viewed as indicative rather than diagnostic.

1.1.3 Dental disease

The oral cavity is home to around 500 different microbial species. These bacteria together with saliva and other particles constantly form a sticky, colourless 'plaque' on the surface of teeth. Brushing and flossing help to remove this layer which is intimately involved in the development of dental caries and gingivitis. Plaque that is not removed can harden and form calculus which requires professional cleaning by a dentist or dental hygienist to prevent the development of periodontal disease which can lead to the destruction of the dental support structures and eventually loss of the affected tooth or teeth.

Whilst both dental caries and periodontal disease have been common for many years, non-carious tooth surface loss, particularly in the form of erosion, is a more recent development and is associated with modern lifestyle and dietary intake.

Dental caries

Dental caries can occur at any stage throughout life and is one of the most common preventable diseases in childhood [2]. In developed countries there has been a fall in the lifetime experience of dental caries by at least 75% since the 1960s but it still remains a concern in children from low socioeconomic groups and immigrants from outside Western Europe.

The occurrence of decay requires the presence of teeth, oral micobiota, carbohydrate and time. Following a meal, oral microbiota in plaque on the tooth surface ferment carbohydrate to organic acids. This rapid acid production lowers the pH at the enamel surface below the level (the critical pH) at which enamel will dissolve. When the carbohydrate supply is exhausted, the pH within plaque rises, due to the outward diffusion of the acids and their metabolism and neutralisation, and remineralisation of enamel can occur. Dental caries only progresses when demineralisation is greater than remineralisation.

As a result, the risk of dental decay is greatly increased by the intake of fermentable carbohydrate, e.g. sugars, at a frequency which results in the pH remaining below the critical level (the highest pH at which there is a net loss of enamel from the teeth, which is generally accepted to be about 5.5 for enamel). This risk can be negated by the total avoidance of sugar or at least minimised by limiting the frequency of intake, e.g. no between-meals consumption.

Periodontal disease

The presence of bacteria on the gingiva causes inflammation (gingivitis), resulting in the gums becoming red and swollen and often bleeding easily. Gingivitis is a mild form of gum disease that can usually be reversed with regular tooth brushing and flossing. This form of gum disease does not include any loss of bone or support tissue.

If gingivitis is not treated, the inflammation can spread and result in the loss of attachment of the gum to the tooth and the development of 'pockets' that are colonised by bacteria. The body's immune system fights these bacteria and as a by-product the body's natural response and bacterial toxins break down the bone and connective tissue that support the teeth. If this condition remains untreated, the teeth may eventually become mobile and require removal.

While some people are more susceptible than others to periodontal disease, smoking is one of the most significant risk factors and also reduces the chances of successful treatment. Periodontal disease has been reported as a potential risk factor for cardiovascular disease, poorly controlled diabetes and preterm low birth weight [3].

Non-carious tooth surface loss

Regular consumption of acidic foods and drinks can reduce the pH below the critical level and the surface layer of enamel is then lost through a combination of erosion, attrition (action of teeth on teeth) and abrasion (by foodstuffs). Over time, the full thickness of the enamel may be lost in this way, leaving exposed dentine which is often associated with sensitivity to temperature changes. This situation may be avoided by limiting the intake of acidic food and drink, e.g. carbonated drinks.

1.1.4 Oral manifestations of gastrointestinal disease

Oral manifestations can arise either as a direct presentation of the condition itself or secondary to the effects of the condition or its treatment.

Malabsorption may lead to iron, vitamin B12 or folate deficiency whilst blood loss is most commonly associated with iron deficiency. In all cases, a deficiency state may occur, resulting in anaemia. This can present with depapillation of the tongue (glossitis), a burning sensation affecting the oral mucosa, angular cheilitis or oral ulceration. Correction of the underlying deficiency state will therefore be associated with their improvement and resolution.

Medical therapy commonly involves the use of corticosteroids or other immunosuppressive medications. Both of these increase the risk of opportunistic infections and hence oral candidosis [4] is frequently seen in the form of angular cheilitis (redness, crusting and splitting of the corners of the mouth), denture stomatitis (erythema of the mucosa in contact with the fit surface of a denture), acute pseudomembranous candidosis or oral soreness/burning affecting the tongue or oral mucosa. Some medications, e.g. methotrexate, may also cause oral ulceration which will only resolve on cessation of the treatment.

In contrast, disease-specific presentations vary and are discussed below.

Gastro-oesophageal reflux disease

Due to the high acidity of the gastric contents (pH 1), chronic gastro-oesophageal reflux disease may result in erosion of the teeth [5]. This classically affects the palatal aspect of the upper anterior teeth but may extend further to affect the upper premolar and molar teeth.

Coeliac disease

Coeliac disease may present with oral ulceration or dental enamel defects and, less commonly, atrophic glossitis. In addition, whilst the caries indexes are often lower than in unaffected individuals, they may experience delay in tooth eruption [6].

Crohn's disease and orofacial granulomatosis

The precise relationship between Crohn's disease and orofacial granulomatosis remains unclear [7]. They share many orofacial manifestations including cervical lymphadenopathy, lip swelling, angular cheilitis, mucosal tags, full-thickness gingivitis, submandibular duct 'staghorning', fibrous banding and oral ulceration [8].

The oral ulceration seen may arise in relation to an associated deficiency state or medical therapy when it is usually aphthoid in appearance. However,

when it takes a linear form and occurs in the sulci, it is suggestive of underlying GI involvement requiring further investigation [8].

Crohn's disease may also rarely present with pyostomatitis gangrenosum (chronic ulceration) affecting the tongue or oral mucosa [9].

Ulcerative colitis

Oral features of ulcerative colitis are generally secondary to the underlying condition or its treatment. Rarely, pyostomatitis vegetans (a generalised ulceration of the oral mucosa) may be the initial presentation of previously occult ulcerative colitis [10].

Irritable bowel syndrome (IBS)

A significant number of patients with IBS also have orofacial pain such as facial arthromyalgia (16%, [11]) or persistent orofacial pain (atypical facial pain, atypical odontalgia) [12]. Conversely, IBS has been shown to be present in many (64%) patients diagnosed with facial arthromyalgia [11].

References

1. Altarawneh S, Bencharit S, Mendoza L, et al. Clinical and histological findings of denture stomatitis as related to intraoral colonization patterns of Candida albicans, salivary flow, and dry mouth. *International Journal of Prosthodontics* 2013; **22**(1): 13–22.
2. Selwitz RH, Ismail AI, Pitts NB. Dental caries. *Lancet* 2007; **369**: 51–59.
3. Ameet MM, Avneesh HT, Babita RP, Pramod PM. The relationship between periodontitis and systemic diseases – hype or hope? *Journal of Clinical and Diagnostic Research* 2013; **7**(4): 758–762.
4. Weerasuriya N, Snape J. Oesophageal candidiasis in elderly patients: risk factors, prevention and management. *Drugs and Aging* 2008; **25**(2): 119–130.
5. Ranjitkar S, Kaidonis JA, Smales RJ. Gastroesophageal reflux disease and tooth erosion. *International Journal of Dentistry* 2012; Article ID 479850.
6. Pastore L, Carroccio A, Compilato D, Panzarella V, Serpico R, Lo Muzio L. Oral manifestations of celiac disease. *Journal of Clinical Gastroenterology* 2008; **42**(3): 224–232.
7. Campbell HE, Escudier MP, Patel P, Challacombe SJ, Sanderson JD, Lomer MC. Review article: cinnamon- and benzoate-free diet as a primary treatment for orofacial granulomatosis. *Alimentary Pharmacology and Therapeutics* 2011a; **34**(7): 687–701.

8. Campbell H, Escudier M, Patel P, et al. Distinguishing orofacial granulomatosis from Crohn's disease: two separate disease entities? *Inflammatory Bowel Disease* 2011b; **17**(10): 2109–2115.

9. Thrash B, Patel M, Shah KR, Boland CR, Menter A. Cutaneous manifestations of gastrointestinal disease: part II. *Journal of the American Academy of Dermatology* 2013; **68**(2): 211.

10. Nico MM, Hussein TP, Aoki V, Lourenço SV. Pyostomatitis vegetans and its relation to inflammatory bowel disease, pyoderma gangrenosum, pyodermatitis vegetans, and pemphigus. *Journal of Oral Pathology and Medicine* 2012; **41**(8): 584–588.

11. Whitehead W, Palsson O, Jones K. Systematic review of the comorbidity of irritable bowel syndrome with other disorders: what are the causes and implications? *Gastroenterology* 2002; **122**: 1140–1156.

12. Stabell N, Stubhaug A, Flægstad T, Nielsen CS. Increased pain sensitivity among adults reporting irritable bowel syndrome symptoms in a large population-based study. *Pain* 2013; **154**(3): 385–392.

Chapter 1.2

Physiology and function of the oesophagus

Rami Sweis

University College London Hospital, London, UK

The oesophagus co-ordinates the transport of food and fluid from the mouth to the stomach. The oesophagogastric junction (OGJ) is a physiological barrier which reduces reflux of gastric contents. In harmony, these processes limit contact of the swallowed bolus, refluxed acid and other chemicals with oesophageal mucosa. Disruption of function can interrupt bolus delivery or induce gastro-oesophageal reflux. Symptoms produced may range in severity from heartburn and regurgitation to dysphagia and pain.

1.2.1 Anatomy

Oesophagus

The oesophagus is a muscular tube connecting the pharynx to the stomach. The cervical oesophagus extends distally from the cricopharyngeus and the thoracic oesophagus terminates at the hiatal canal before it flares into the gastric fundus. The muscularis propria consists of the outer longitudinal and inner circular muscle layers. The musculature is divided into the proximal striated and mid-distal smooth muscle. This proximal 'transition zone' is located one-third of the distance from the pharynx and is the site with the weakest force of peristaltic contractions [1].

Histologically, the oesophageal wall is composed of the mucosa, submucosa and muscularis mucosa. The oesophageal body is lined by non-keratinised stratified squamous epithelium which abruptly joins with the glandular gastric columnar epithelium at the squamocolumnar junction. This can be the site of mucosal change associated oesophagitis and Barrett's oesophagus.

The antireflux barrier

The OGJ is not a clearly identifiable sphincter but its sphincter-like properties can be defined functionally as a high-pressure zone between the stomach and oesophagus. Sphincter competence is dependent on the integrity and overlap of the intrinsic lower oesophageal sphincter (LOS) and diaphragmatic crura. A separation, hiatus hernia, is associated with disruption of LOS integrity, loss of the intra-abdominal LOS segment and an increased susceptibility to gastro-oesophageal reflux.

1.2.2 Physiology and function

Voluntary swallowing initiates with 'deglutitive inhibition' of the smooth muscle oesophagus and LOS. This reflex relaxation is nitric oxide mediated and permits passage of the bolus with minimal resistance. The subsequent excitatory, predominantly cholinergic, activity produces a progressive wave of smooth muscle excitation. A co-ordinated peristalsis clears the bolus from the oesophagus.

The LOS exhibits a continuous resting (basal) tone which relaxes on stimulation of the intramural nerves such as during deglutitive inhibition (swallowing). Disruption of this physiological process may impact on bolus transport and induce symptoms

Advanced Nutrition and Dietetics in Gastroenterology, First Edition. Edited by Miranda Lomer.
© 2014 John Wiley & Sons, Ltd. Published 2014 by John Wiley & Sons, Ltd.

Box 1.2.1 Co-ordinated peristaltic activity

Co-ordinated peristaltic activity is a multistep process which usually requires:

- a pharyngeal 'pump' – to push food and fluid through the oesophagus
- gravity – whereby bolus weight contributes to its aboral progress
- appropriate relaxation *and* opening of the oesophagogastric junction
- effective oesophageal motor function – deglutitive inhibition followed by co-ordinated peristaltic contraction
- a positive oesophagogastric pressure drop.

(Box 1.2.1). A representative normal swallow using high-resolution manometry is presented in Figure 1.2.1.

Spontaneous LOS relaxations normally occur as a response to gastric postprandial distension and bloating: 'transient lower oesophageal sphincter relaxation' (TLOSR). LOS relaxation can also follow peristaltic activity: 'swallow-induced lower oesophageal sphincter relaxation' (SLOSR). Gastro-oesophageal reflux and belch occur when there is equalisation of pressure between the stomach and oesophagus (common cavity) (Figure 1.2.2). Patients with gastro-oesophageal reflux disease (GORD) do not have an increased frequency of TLOSRs; rather, the tendency of reflux to occur during these events is greater [2]. The effectiveness of oesophageal clearance of refluxed material is an important contributor to the severity of GORD [3–5]. Other determinants of GORD include the presence and size of a hiatus hernia, increasing age and obesity as well as the calorie and fat content of the diet [6,7].

Measurement and assessment of function

In the absence of disease on endoscopy and failure to respond to empirical therapy, guidelines recommend manometry and ambulatory reflux testing [8,9]. Recent advances in technology provide better insight into the assessment of oesophageal function and disease.

Manometry

Peristalsis and OGJ activity can be measured with manometry. Conventional manometry (4–8 sensors) measures the circumferential contraction, pressure wave duration and peristaltic velocity of single water swallows. High-resolution manometry (HRM; 21–36 sensors) is an advance on conventional systems as it provides a compact, spatiotemporal representation of oesophageal pressure activity. In addition, it can measure the forces that drive movement of food and fluid through the oesophagus and OGJ [10]. An uninterrupted well-co-ordinated peristalsis defines oesophageal motility while the presence of a positive pressure gradient in the absence of obstruction describes whether this motility is effective and likely to clear the bolus [11] (see Figure 1.2.1). Thus HRM improves diagnostic sensitivity to peristaltic dysfunction as symptoms and mucosal damage are more likely to occur as a result of disturbed bolus transport and poor clearance [5]. Furthermore, recent advances in methodology have shown how HRM can also facilitate the assessment of swallowing behaviour (eating and drinking) when symptoms are more likely to be triggered [5,12,13] (Box 1.2.2).

Ambulatory reflux studies

Gastro-oesophageal reflux disease (GORD) occurs when gastric contents pass into the oesophagus at an increased frequency, are not effectively cleared or are perceived in an exaggerated manner. This can lead to mucosal damage and/or symptoms with varying degrees of severity. Presenting symptoms alone are an unreliable guide to identifying oesophageal dysfunction [14,15]. Objective testing is required to avoid inappropriate medical and surgical therapy. Ambulatory pH monitoring provides an assessment of oesophageal acid exposure and symptoms. Standard testing is performed using a 24-hour nasopharyngeal pH catheter (with or without impedance, see next section). Diagnosis is made based on measurements of oesophageal acid exposure (e.g. total number of reflux events and percent time reflux events cause a pH drop below a threshold of 4) as well as the association of reflux events with symptoms. Measurements can

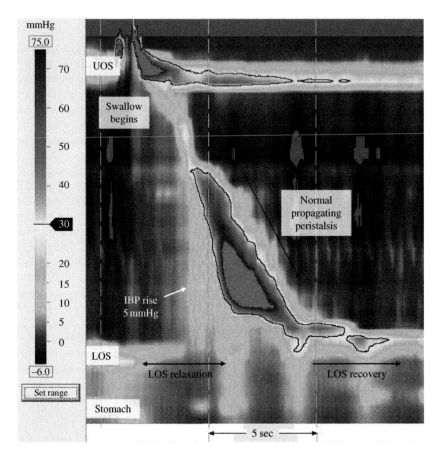

Figure 1.2.1 High-resolution manometry of a normal swallow, with pressure data presented as a spatiotemporal plot. Sensors are spaced at <2 cm intervals which provide a vivid depiction of oesophageal pressure activity from the pharynx to the stomach with changes in pressure represented as changes in colour (in clinical practice). Deglutitive inhibition is seen as the synchronous relaxation of the upper oesophageal sphincter (UOS) and lower oesophageal sphincter (LOS) followed by a co-ordinated peristalsis with increasing pressure duration as it progresses distally. Important landmarks are highlighted. Images acquired by 36-channel SSI Manoscan 360. IBP, intrabolus pressure.

be further subdivided into upright and supine. However, intolerance to the nasal catheter can influence the result.

Multiple intraluminal impedance with pH monitoring (MII-pH)

Oesophageal symptoms are often related to disturbed bolus transport rather than acid reflux [16]. Also symptoms may persist despite effective acid suppression as acid-reducing medications do not influence the frequency or volume of *non-acid* reflux episodes [17,18]. Multiple intraluminal impedance (MII) can determine the direction of bolus movement, the success or failure of bolus transit and the proximal extent of the refluxate. Furthermore, it can discriminate between liquid and gas reflux. When combined with a pH sensor (MII-pH), it can differentiate between acid (pH <4), weakly acid (pH 4–7) or weakly alkaline (pH >7) reflux [19]. Therefore, MII-pH is considered to be more sensitive than standard pH testing, with up

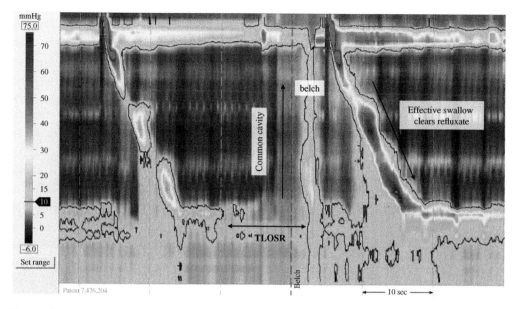

Figure 1.2.2 Transient lower oesophageal sphincter relaxation followed shortly afterwards by a common cavity during which there is equalisation of pressure between the stomach and oesophagus when reflux is most likely to occur. The event is terminated and the oesophagus is cleared of refluxed contents with the arrival of a well-co-ordinated primary peristalsis. Oesophageal and lower oesophageal sphincter pressures return to baseline levels following completion of peristalsis. TLOSR, transient lower oesophageal sphincter relaxation.

Box 1.2.2   Hierarchical analysis of high-resolution manometry

Hierarchical analysis of high-resolution manometry studies according to the Chicago Classification whereby pathology in the OGJ is considered first. Major motility disorders (achalasia, absent peristalsis, diffuse oesophageal spasm and extreme hypertensive disorders) are never found in healthy individuals, are commonly associated with impaired bolus transport and, in turn, often lead to symptoms. The significance of peristalsis abnormalities described in 'Other motility disorders' is not clear as these can also be found in asymptomatic individuals [20].

I. OGJ obstruction
Achalasia
Classic (non-relaxing LOS + aperistalsis + dilated oesophagus)
Compression (non-relaxing LOS + aperistalsis + oesophageal pressurisation)
Vigorous (non-relaxing LOS + oesophageal spasm)

Other obstruction
Eosinophilic oesophagitis
Benign or malignant stricture
Post surgery (e.g. antireflux procedure)

II. Major motility disorder
Absent peristalsis
Diffuse spasm
Jackhammer oesophagus (nutcracker with extreme pressures)

III. Other motility disorders
Weak peristalsis
Frequent failed peristalsis
Hypertensive peristalsis
Rapid contractility

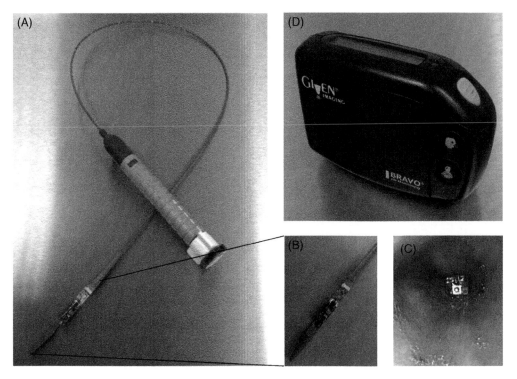

Figure 1.2.3 Bravo delivery system. The delivery device (A, B) is normally inserted orally through the pharynx. Markings on the delivery device depict the distance from the incisors. The capsule is deployed at the proximal LOS high-pressure zone (C). The receiver remains with the patient (via belt clip or shoulder pouch) for the duration of the study (D). The capsule falls off spontaneously at a median of 5 days. Complications requiring its early removal are rare.

to 20% improvement in diagnostic yield [21]. Indications for its use are the same as for standard ambulatory pH studies. In those with established GORD but ongoing symptoms despite optimal medical therapy, MII-pH can be performed while *on* acid reducing medication in order to identify if (non-acid) reflux is the culprit or to exclude breakthrough acid reflux. In addition, in the assessment of atypical disease (e.g. laryngopharyngeal reflux, aerophagia, supragastric belching, cough).

Wireless pH monitoring (Bravo®)

Wireless pH monitoring (Bravo®, Given Imaging) is an endoscopically placed, catheter-free, ambulatory pH monitoring system (Figure 1.2.3). Bravo® is a viable option for those who are intolerant to the nasal catheter [6]. It can measure for

prolonged periods (at least 48 h) [22,23] and is especially suitable for patients with intermittent symptoms [22,24] or those with persistent typical symptoms whose catheter-based study was inconclusive [25]. However, Bravo® cannot discriminate between liquid and gas reflux nor can it differentiate between acid and nonacid reflux.

1.2.3 Pathology

Motility

An important advance of the modern HRM-based classification (the Chicago Classification) [26–28] is that it is hierarchical; the OGJ is considered first because pathology within the OGJ will influence oesophageal function above [20] (see Box 1.2.2). In addition, the Chicago Classification makes a clear distinction between dysmotility that is 'never seen in normal individuals' (Major motility disorders) and that which may be merely 'outside the normal range'. In the former, treatment is usually directed at correcting the underlying pathology whereas in the latter, therapy often targets symptoms [29,30].

Achalasia, a 'Major motility disorder', is characterised by a non-relaxing LOS and the absence of oesophageal peristalsis. The Chicago Classification further categorises achalasia into three subtypes, each with its own response to medical (pneumatic dilation and botulinum toxin) and surgical (Heller myotomy) therapy [31,32] (see Box 1.2.2). Left untreated, the compression subtype (an HRM diagnosis) is thought to 'decompensate' and lead to classic achalasia. Furthermore, this compression subtype has the best response to all forms of therapy (botulinum toxin, dilatation, myotomy) classic achalasia [33,34]. On the other hand, many hypertensive oesophageal disorders can also be found in asymptomatic individuals and have shown varying degrees of success with therapy. Nitrates, calcium channel blockers and sildenafil can influence function in some but often tricyclic antidepressants and selective serotonin receptor inhibitors are required to target symptoms [35,36].

Gastro-oesophageal reflux disease

Gastro-oesophageal reflux disease is subclassified into erosive oesophagitis, endoscopy-negative reflux disease (positive oesophageal acid exposure and/or reflux-symptom association with normal endoscopy) and functional heartburn (negative oesophageal acid exposure, negative reflux-symptom association, poor response to acid-reducing medication with normal endoscopy but ongoing symptoms) [37,38]. Differentiating between erosive oesophagitis, endoscopy-negative reflux disease and functional heartburn is essential to target appropriate therapy and oesophageal physiology studies are required to secure a diagnosis. In addition, an assessment of GORD should also be sought in patients presenting with dysphagia as oesophageal dysfunction can be exacerbated by or be a consequence of reflux disease.

1.2.4 Conclusion

In conclusion, GORD and dysphagia are common in the community and can be associated with significant morbidity and reduced quality of life. Furthermore, chronic reflux is related to the rising incidence of oesophageal adenocarcinoma, especially in those with Barrett's oesophagus [39]. Such concerns emphasize the importance of appropriate and early investigation and management. In the absence of disease on endoscopy and failure to respond to empirical therapy, guidelines recommend manometry and ambulatory reflux testing. Advances in technology and methodology have revolutionised the way the oesophagus is investigated and provide a more 'realistic' assessment of function which can help guide therapy.

References

1. Meyer GW, Austin RM, Brady CE 3rd, Castell DO. Muscle anatomy of the human esophagus. *Journal of Clinical Gastroenterology* 1986; **8**(2): 131–134.
2. Sifrim D, Holloway R. Transient lower esophageal sphincter relaxations: how many or how harmful? *American Journal of Gastroenterology* 2001; **96**(9): 2529–2532.
3. Anggiansah A, Taylor G, Marshall RE, Bright NF, Owen WA, Owen WJ. Oesophageal motor responses to gastro-oesophageal reflux in healthy controls and reflux patients. *Gut* 1997; **41**(5): 600–605.
4. Bredenoord AJ, Hemmink GJ, Smout AJ. Relationship between gastro-oesophageal reflux pattern and severity of mucosal damage. *Neurogastroenterology and Motility* 2009; **21**(8): 807–812.
5. Fox MR, Bredenoord AJ. Oesophageal high-resolution manometry: moving from research into clinical practice. *Gut* 2008; **57**(3): 405–423.
6. Lee J, Anggiansah A, Anggiansah R, Young A, Wong T, Fox M. Effects of age on the gastroesophageal junction, esophageal motility, and reflux disease. *Clinical Gastroenterology and Hepatology* 2007; **5**(12): 1392–1398.
7. Fox M, Barr C, Nolan S, Lomer M, Anggiansah A, Wong T. The effects of dietary fat and calorie density on esophageal acid exposure and reflux symptoms. *Clinical Gastroenterology and Hepatology* 2007; **5**(4): 439–444.
8. Bodger K, Trudgill N. *Guidelines for Oesophageal Manometry and pH Monitoring*. London: British Society of Gastroenterology, 2006.
9. National Institute for Health and Clinical Excellence. *Catheterless Oesophageal pH Monitoring*. London: National Institute for Health and Clinical Excellence, 2006.
10. Pandolfino JE, Bulsiewicz WJ. Evaluation of esophageal motor disorders in the era of high-resolution manometry and intraluminal impedance. *Current Gastroenterology Report* 2009; **11**(3): 182–189.

11. Fox M, Bredenoord AJ. High resolution manometry: moving from research into clinical practice. *Gut* 2008; **57**: 405–423.

12. Sweis R, Anggiansah A, Wong T, Kaufman E, Obrecht S, Fox M. Normative values and inter-observer agreement for liquid and solid bolus swallows in upright and supine positions as assessed by esophageal high-resolution manometry. *Neurogastroenterology and Motility* 2011; **23**: 509.

13. Sweis R, Anggiansah A, Wong T, Brady G, Fox M. Assessment of esophageal dysfunction and symptoms during and after a standardized test meal: development and clinical validation of a new methodology utilizing high-resolution manometry. *Neurogastroenterol Motil* 2014; **26**: 215–228.

14. Costantini M, Crookes PF, Bremner RM, et al. Value of physiologic assessment of foregut symptoms in a surgical practice. *Surgery* 1993; **114**(4): 780–786; discussion 786–787.

15. Klauser AG, Schindlbeck NE, Muller-Lissner SA. Symptoms in gastro-oesophageal reflux disease. *Lancet* 1990; **335**(8683): 205–208.

16. Bernhard A, Pohl D, Fried M, Castell DO, Tutuian R. Influence of bolus consistency and position on esophageal high-resolution manometry findings. *Digestive Diseases and Sciences* 2008; **53**: 1198–1205.

17. Mainie I, Tutuian R, Agrawal A, Adams D, Castell DO. Combined multichannel intraluminal impedance-pH monitoring to select patients with persistent gastro-oesophageal reflux for laparoscopic Nissen fundoplication. *British Journal of Surgery* 2006; **93**(12): 1483–1487.

18. Emerenziani S, Zhang X, Blondeau K, et al. Gastric fullness, physical activity, and proximal extent of gastroesophageal reflux. *American Journal of Gastroenterology* 2005; **100**(6): 1251–1256.

19. Sifrim D, Castell D, Dent J, Kahrilas PJ. Gastro-oesophageal reflux monitoring: review and consensus report on detection and definitions of acid, non-acid, and gas reflux. *Gut* 2004; **53**(7): 1024–31.

20. Bredenoord AJ, Fox M, Kahrilas PJ, Pandolfino JE, Schwizer W, Smout AJ. Chicago classification criteria of esophageal motility disorders defined in high resolution esophageal pressure topography. *Neurogastroenterology and Motility* 2012; **24** Suppl 1: 57–65.

21. Bredenoord AJ, Weusten BL, Timmer R, Conchillo JM, Smout AJ. Addition of esophageal impedance monitoring to pH monitoring increases the yield of symptom association analysis in patients off PPI therapy. *American Journal of Gastroenterology* 2006; **101**(3): 453–459.

22. Scarpulla G, Camilleri S, Galante P, Manganaro M, Fox M. The impact of prolonged pH measurements on the diagnosis of gastroesophageal reflux disease: 4-day wireless pH studies. *American Journal of Gastroenterology* 2007; **102**(12): 2642–2647.

23. Pandolfino JE, Richter JE, Ours T, Guardino JM, Chapman J, Kahrilas PJ. Ambulatory esophageal pH monitoring using a wireless system. *American Journal of Gastroenterology* 2003; **98**(4): 740–749.

24. Hirano I, Zhang Q, Pandolfino JE, Kahrilas PJ. Four-day Bravo® pH capsule monitoring with and without proton pump

25. Sweis R, Fox M, Anggiansah A, Wong T. Prolonged, wireless pH-studies have a high diagnostic yield in patients with reflux symptoms and negative 24-h catheter-based pH-studies. *Neurogastroenterology and Motility* 2011; **23**: 419–426.

26. Kahrilas PJ, Ghosh SK, Pandolfino JE. Esophageal motility disorders in terms of pressure topography: the Chicago Classification. *Journal of Clinical Gastroenterology* 2008; **42**(5): 627–635.

27. Pandolfino JE, Ghosh SK, Rice J, Clarke JO, Kwiatek MA, Kahrilas PJ. Classifying esophageal motility by pressure topography characteristics: a study of 400 patients and 75 controls. *American Journal of Gastroenterology* 2008; **103**(1): 27–37.

28. Pandolfino JE, Fox MR, Bredenoord AJ, Kahrilas PJ. High-resolution manometry in clinical practice: utilizing pressure topography to classify oesophageal motility abnormalities. *Neurogastroenterology and Motility* 2009; **21**(8): 796–806.

29. Hobson AR, Furlong PL, Sarkar S, et al. Neurophysiologic assessment of esophageal sensory processing in noncardiac chest pain. *Gastroenterology* 2006; **130**(1): 80–88.

30. Fox M, Schwizer W. Making sense of oesophageal contents. *Gut* 2008; **57**(4): 435–438.

31. Pandolfino JE, Kwiatek MA, Nealis T, Bulsiewicz W, Post J, Kahrilas PJ. Achalasia: a new clinically relevant classification by high-resolution manometry. *Gastroenterology* 2008; **135**(5): 1526–1533.

32. Boeckxstaens G, Zaninotto G. Achalasia and esophago-gastric junction outflow obstruction: focus on the subtypes. *Neurogastroenterology and Motility* 2012; **24** Suppl 1: 27–31.

33. Pandolfino JE, Kwiatek MA, Nealis T, Bulsiewicz W, Post J, Kahrilas PJ. Achalasia: a new clinically relevant classification by high-resolution manometry. *Gastroenterology* 2008; **135**(5): 1526–33.

34. Boeckxstaens G, Zaninotto G. Achalasia and esophago-gastric junction outflow obstruction: focus on the subtypes. *Neurogastroenterol Motil* 2012; **24** Suppl 1: 27–31.

35. Fox M, Sweis R, Wong T, Anggiansah A. Sildenafil relieves symptoms and normalizes motility in patients with oesophageal spasm: a report of two cases. *Neurogastroenterology and Motility* 2007; **19**(10): 798–803.

36. Pandolfino JE, Roman S, Carlson D, et al. Distal esophageal spasm in high-resolution esophageal pressure topography: defining clinical phenotypes. *Gastroenterology* 2011; **141**(2): 469–475.

37. Fass R, Sifrim D. Management of heartburn not responding to proton pump inhibitors. *Gut* 2009; **58**(2): 295–309.

38. Galmiche JP, Clouse RE, Balint A, et al. Functional esophageal disorders. *Gastroenterology* 2006; **130**(5): 1459–1465.

39. Lagergren J, Bergstrom R, Lindgren A, Nyren O. Symptomatic gastroesophageal reflux as a risk factor for esophageal adenocarcinoma. *New England Journal of Medicine* 1999; **340**(11): 825–831.

inhibitor therapy. *Clinical Gastroenterology and Hepatology* 2005; **3**(11): 1083–1088.

Chapter 1.3

Physiology and function of the stomach

Luca Marciani and Mark Fox
University of Nottingham, Nottingham, UK

1.3.1 Physiology, anatomy and function

The human stomach is a J-shaped organ of the gastrointestinal (GI) tract, located between the oesophagus and the duodenum, and it has a key role in digestion and absorption. The main anatomical regions are shown in Figure 1.3.1. The stomach's main functions are to store and break down food and deliver digesta to the small intestine.

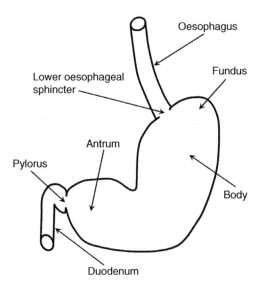

Figure 1.3.1 Schematic diagram of the human stomach.

The stomach receives boluses of food via the lower oesophageal sphincter. It is able to reduce gastric wall tone via a vagally mediated reflex ('accommodation') which allows the reservoir to expand and accommodate increasing amounts of food without important increases in intragastric pressure [1]. In addition to 'receptive' accommodation mediated by mechanoreceptors in the gastric wall, once nutrients pass into the small intestine the gastric response is modulated by chemoreceptors and osmoreceptors to ensure that gastric emptying through the pylorus is controlled and optimized for efficient digestion [1,2].

During intragastric food processing, the stomach secretes hydrochloric acid, lipase and pepsin. This process is regulated by the central and enteric nervous system and neuroendocrine cell networks [3]. These secretions together with salivary enzymes active within the bolus start the chemical breakdown of food. At the same time, highly co-ordinated antropyloroduodenal contractions effect mechanical breakdown (trituration) of solid food. Gastric emptying is ultimately the result of these co-ordinated actions, controlled opening of the pylorus and antroduodenal differences in pressure which drive gastric emptying [4,5]. Liquids empty faster than solids, which are first triturated to small particles, usually less than 3 mm in size, to promote chemical digestion and absorption after delivery to the duodenum and small intestine [6]. Other physical factors such as meal viscosity, the density and breaking strength of food particles also affect the rate of gastric emptying [6–8].

Advanced Nutrition and Dietetics in Gastroenterology, First Edition. Edited by Miranda Lomer.
© 2014 John Wiley & Sons, Ltd. Published 2014 by John Wiley & Sons, Ltd.

1.3.2 Measurement and assessment of gastric function

Measurement of gastric function has improved understanding of the physiological response to food in health and disease and in response to dietary or pharmacological intervention. A number of tests are available and are briefly described in the following sections [9].

Gastric accommodation and sensation

Gastric accommodation can be evaluated using the barostat test. This involves intubating the subjects orally using a double-lumen catheter with a plastic bag on the tip. The balloon is commonly placed in the proximal stomach. An electronic barostat device is then used to control expansions of the bag to assess, for example, volume expansion during pressure-guided distension or after delivery of a test meal [10]. This is the 'standard test' of gastric accommodation though availability is limited, the method is invasive and the presence of a balloon in the stomach affects gastric relaxation. Gastric sensation elicited by barostat distension paradigms leads to brain cortical activations that can be assessed using functional brain magnetic resonance imaging (MRI) and positron emission tomography (PET) methods [11,12].

A simple and inexpensive alternative to the barostat is the drink test [13]. This involves ingesting water or a nutrient drink at a given rate until the maximum tolerated volume is reached. Subjective scores of sensation are collected during and after the test. The results are not easy to interpret due to variation in gastric capacity and the merits of this test are debated.

Conventional ultrasound has been used to measure the area of the proximal stomach after a meal in a sagittal section and the maximal diameter in an oblique frontal section [14]. Three-dimensional reconstruction of ultrasound images integrates this information and gives volume measurements; however, the technique is user dependent and can be used only with liquid meals.

The distribution of gastric contents within the stomach on scintigraphy provides some impression of gastric accommodation [15]. Another nuclear medicine test that can measure change in gastric volumes is single photon emission computed tomography (SPECT). This method involves injecting intravenously a ^{99m}Tc-labelled compound which is taken up in the mucosa. A dual-headed gamma camera is used to measure the radiation emitted and reconstruct axial images of the stomach. A three-dimensional image can be reconstructed later; however, the temporal and spatial resolution are limited compared to MRI.

Magnetic resonance imaging is an emerging technique used to assess fasting and postprandial gastric volumes [16] due to the lack of ionising radiation, multiplanar imaging, speed and excellent contrast between different organs and intragastric meal components. It has been used to evaluate the effects of the barostat balloon in the stomach [17], finding that the bag increased postprandial gastric volumes. Cross-sections of the fundus [18] and maximum antral diameters following model meals [7] have also been measured using MRI and changes in these variables correlate closely with sensation of fullness and other symptoms in health and disease [8,19].

Gastric contractility

Antroduodenal motility can be measured using intraluminal manometry by passing a catheter nasogastrically through the pylorus and into the proximal duodenum. The catheter has a varying number of water-perfused or solid-state sensors. These detect the periodical stomach wall contractions and the pressure amplitude profiles with time can be displayed and analysed [20].

The high-resolution and high-speed capabilities of MRI allow imaging of the stomach serially at intervals of a few seconds. These images can be played as motility 'movies' and subsequently postprocessed to measure motility in terms of antral contractions, frequency, speed and percentage occlusion [21–24]. An interesting finding from MRI studies is the lack of correlation between meal volumes and antral contractility that suggests these contractions are highly stereotyped after a meal and do not determine the rate of gastric emptying through the pylorus [5,25]. Dynamic gamma scintigraphy can measure antral motility but this requires higher radiation doses and the resolution is poor.

Gastric emptying

Gastric emptying can be measured by labelling test meals with ^{13}C stable isotopes such as octanoic acid. The label is absorbed in the small intestine during digestion, metabolised to $^{13}CO_2$ and then expelled with the breath. As such, serial breath samples are taken at baseline and postprandially to calculate the increase of $^{13}CO_2$ with time, which is then assumed to be proportional to gastric emptying [26]. This is an advance on the oral paracetamol absorption under the assumption that the appearance in the blood is directly related to gastric emptying [27].

Using imaging, the simple radiopaque marker test involves the subject ingesting a number (about 20) of small radiopaque pellets with a test meal and following their emptying with fluoroscopy [28]. Results depend on the size and density of the pellets and test meal composition.

Gastric scintigraphy involves the patient eating a radiolabelled meal and measuring the gamma radiation emitted from the 'region' of the stomach using a gamma camera. This is carried out at various time points to measure the postprandial gastric emptying curve. The normal range of results depends on the test meal, though simplified protocols have been reported [29] and standardised scrambled egg substitute test meals have been validated in multicentre studies [30]. It is a widely used test and so far considered the 'gold standard' although it involves a radiation dose to the subject and results correlate only poorly with patient symptoms [31].

Wireless capsule pills that can measure pH, pressure and temperature have recently appeared on the market. Subjects swallow the pills with a test meal and a receiver worn on the belt records data continuously. The time at which the pill detects a step change up in pH is taken as the time at which the pill is emptied from the stomach [32]. However, given their large size and indigestibility, the emptying of a pill from the stomach is due to strong phase III contractions and not the fed pattern of meal emptying, making interpretation of the data difficult.

A different approach that uses pills to measure gastric emptying is based on magnetically marked solid pills that are ingested by the subjects with a meal and their spatial location monitored over time using non-invasive magnetic source imaging methods [33]. This method is elegant, but requires the use of superconducting quantum interference device (SQUID) magnetometers and has limited applications, mostly to monitor the dissolution of dosage forms for pharmaceutical use.

As described, ultrasound, SPECT and MRI can all measure cross-sections or entire volumes of the stomach. As such, they have all been employed to measure gastric emptying. MRI in particular can measure serially intragastric gas and meal volumes from which one can assess the gastric emptying curves [34,35]. Of particular interest is MRI's ability to observe the intragastric fate of many food materials and their mixing and dilution [8,36–39].

1.3.3 Pathology

Reflux

Gastro-oesophageal reflux disease (GORD) is a very common disorder caused by the return of gastric contents ('reflux') back to the oesophagus, causing inflammation (e.g. oesophagitis) or symptoms (e.g. heartburn, acid regurgitation). Changes in gastric structure have been reported in patients with GORD that compromise the putative 'flap-valve' mechanism of the gastro-oesophageal reflux barrier. Additionally, delayed gastric emptying is common in patients with severe disease, prolonging the period after the meal during which reflux can occur.

Disorders of gastric emptying (gastroparesis)

Gastroparesis is a condition in which gastric emptying is delayed. It is classically found in diabetic patients but can be linked to connective tissue diseases, related to previous gastric surgery or have no clear cause (idiopathic). In diabetes, abnormal gastric emptying impairs glucose control and intake and digestion of nutrients and medications. Symptoms include prolonged fullness, nausea and vomiting after meals; however, a clear link between delayed emptying and symptoms is observed only in very severe cases. Rather, typical symptoms are associated more closely with impaired gastric accommodation and psychosocial factors as seen in functional dyspepsia.

Rapid gastric emptying can cause symptoms due to 'dumping' of nutrients into the small intestine which leads to a powerful neurohormonal response that can cause nausea but also faintness and other symptoms related to insulin-induced hypoglycaemia. In addition, rapid emptying can impair digestion and tolerance of certain nutrients (e.g. fat).

Functional dyspepsia

Functional dyspepsia is thought to be a heterogeneous condition characterised by specific gastric motor and sensory abnormalities. Symptoms include fullness, nausea, bloating and epigastric pain. Impaired gastric accommodation is linked to early satiety and weight loss, delayed gastric emptying to prolonged fullness and nausea, and visceral hypersensitivity to epigastric pain. It may be that breakdown of the dynamic, neurohormonal and functional response to food underlies all these abnormalities.

Rumination

Rumination is a behavioural disorder in which, responding to dyspeptic or reflux symptoms, patients subconsciously contract their abdominal muscles, forcing gastric contents back to the mouth repeatedly after meals. At this point, the patient often swallows the food again (hence 'rumination') or spits out the food, which can lead to undernutrition. This condition is often mistaken for vomiting or reflux disease; however, it does not respond to antiemetics or antacid medication and requires behavioural therapy.

Cyclic vomiting

Cyclic vomiting syndrome is a rare condition characterised by paroxysmal bouts of severe nausea and vomiting lasting several days separated by periods of normal health. It may be triggered by cannabis use; however, most cases are idiopathic and are thought to be linked to autonomic nerve dysfunction.

Acute gastroenteritis

Gastric infection is unusual except for *Helicobacter pylori* (see next section). However, ingestion of contaminated food can cause nausea and vomiting either directly due to toxins or indirectly due to infection and dysfunction of the small or large intestine.

Helicobacter pylori

Helicobacter pylori, a spiral-shaped bacterium located in the mucous layer of the stomach, may inhibit or promote acid secretion and causes different diseases depending on how the infection affects the stomach. Distal (antral) gastritis increases the production of gastric acid and increases the risk of duodenal ulceration. Conversely, generalised atrophic gastritis decreases the production of gastric acid with an increased risk of gastric cancer.

Gastric cancer

Gastric cancer usually arises in the glandular epithelium ('adenocarcinoma') although rare cancers of the smooth muscle ('leiomyosarcoma') and immune cells ('lymphoma') can also occur. The risk of adenocarcinoma is increased by smoking, alcohol abuse, certain factors in the diet (e.g. nitrites derived from preservatives) and, most importantly, atrophic gastritis induced by *Helicobacter pylori* infection. These cancers usually present in an advanced stage due to obstruction of food passage through the stomach with pain and vomiting or progressive anaemia. Treatment options are often limited and less than one in five patients survives more than 5 years.

References

1. Camilleri M. Integrated upper gastrointestinal response to food intake. *Gastroenterology* 2006; **131**(2): 640–658.
2. Kwiatek MA, Menne D, Steingoetter A, et al. Effect of meal volume and calorie load on postprandial gastric function and emptying: studies under physiological conditions by combined fiber-optic pressure measurement and MRI. *American Journal of Physiology* 2009; **297**(5): G894–G901.

3. Schubert ML, Gastric secretion. *Current Opinion in Gastroenterology* 2010; **26**(6): 598–603.

4. Indireshkumar K, Brasseur JG, Faas H, et al. Relative contributions of 'pressure pump' and 'peristaltic pump' to gastric emptying. *American Journal of Physiology-Gastrointestinal and Liver Physiology* 2000; **278**(4): G604–G616.

5. Kwiatek MA, Fox MR, Steingoetter A, et al. Effects of clonidine and sumatriptan on postprandial gastric volume response, antral contraction waves and emptying: an MRI study. *Neurogastroenterology and Motility* 2009; **21**(9): 928–e71.

6. Meyer JH, Dressman J, Fink AS, Amidon G. Effect of size and density on gastric emptying of indigestible solids. *Gastroenterology* 1985; **88**(5): 1502.

7. Marciani L, Gowland PA, Fillery-Travis A, et al. Assessment of antral grinding of a model solid meal with echo-planar imaging. *American Journal of Physiology* 2001; **280**(5): G844–G849.

8. Marciani L, Gowland PA, Spiller RC, et al. Effect of meal viscosity and nutrients on satiety, intragastric dilution, and emptying assessed by MRI. *American Journal of Physiology* 2001; **280**(6): G1227–G1233.

9. Parkman HP, Jones MP. Tests of gastric neuromuscular function. *Gastroenterology* 2009; **136**(5): 1526–1543.

10. Ang D. Measurement of gastric accommodation: a reappraisal of conventional and emerging modalities. *Neurogastroenterology and Motility* 2011; **23**(4): 287–291.

11. Ladabaum U, Roberts TP, McGonigle DJ. Gastric fundic distension activates fronto-limbic structures but not primary somatosensory cortex: a functional magnetic resonance imaging study. *Neuroimage* 2007; **34**(2): 724–732.

12. Vandenberghe J, Dupont P, van Oudenhove L, et al. Regional cerebral blood flow during gastric balloon distention in functional dyspepsia. *Gastroenterology* 2007; **132**(5): 1684–1693.

13. Hjelland IE, Ofstad AP, Narvestad JK, Berstad A, Hausken T. Drink tests in functional dyspepsia: which drink is best? *Scandinavian Journal of Gastroenterology* 2004; **39**(10): 933–937.

14. Gilja OH, Hausken T, Odegaard S, Berstad A. Monitoring postprandial size of the proximal stomach by ultrasonography. *Journal of Ultrasound in Medicine* 1995; **14**(2): 81–89.

15. Troncon LE, Bennett RJ, Ahluwalia NK, Thompson DG. Abnormal intragastric distribution of food during gastric emptying in functional dyspepsia patients. *Gut* 1994; **35**(3): 327–332.

16. Marciani L. Assessment of gastrointestinal motor functions by MRI: a comprehensive review. *Neurogastroenterology and Motility* 2011; **23**(5): 399–407.

17. De Zwart IM, Haans JJ, Verbeek P, Eilers PH, de Roos A, Masclee AA. Gastric accommodation and motility are influenced by the barostat device: assessment with magnetic resonance imaging. *American Journal of Physiology-Gastrointestinal and Liver Physiology* 2007; **292**(1): G208–G214.

18. Coleman NS, Marciani L, Blackshaw E, et al. Effect of a novel 5-HT3 receptor agonist MKC-733 on upper gastrointestinal motility in humans. *Alimentary Pharmacology and Therapeutics* 2003; **18**(10): 1039–1048.

19. Fruehauf H, Goetze O, Steingoetter A, et al. Intersubject and intrasubject variability of gastric volumes in response to isocaloric liquid meals in functional dyspepsia and health. *Neurogastroenterology and Motility* 2007; **19**(7): 553–561.

20. Camilleri M, Hasler WL, Parkman HP, Quigley EM, Soffer E. Measurement of gastrointestinal motility in the GI laboratory. *Gastroenterology* 1998; **115**(3): 747–762.

21. Wright J, Evans D, Gowland P, Mansfield P. Validation of antroduodenal motility measurements made by echo-planar magnetic resonance imaging. *Neurogastroenterology and Motility* 1999; **11**(1): 19–25.

22. Marciani L, Young P, Wright J, et al. Antral motility measurements by magnetic resonance imaging. *Neurogastroenterology and Motility* 2001; **13**(5): 511–518.

23. Schwizer W, Fraser R, Borovicka J, Crelier G, Boesiger P, Fried M. Measurement of gastric emptying and gastric motility by magnetic resonance imaging (MRI). *Digestive Diseases and Sciences* 1994; **39**(12): S101–S103.

24. Kunz P, Crelier GR, Schwizer W, et al. Gastric emptying and motility: assessment with MR imaging: preliminary observations. *Radiology* 1998; **207**(1): 33–40.

25. Kwiatek MA, Steingoetter A, Pal A, et al. Quantification of distal antral contractile motility in healthy human stomach with magnetic resonance imaging. *Journal of Magnetic Resonance Imaging* 2006; **24**(5): 1101–1109.

26. Szarka LA, Camilleri M, Vella A, et al. A stable isotope breath test with a standard meal for abnormal gastric emptying of solids in the clinic and in research. *Clinical Gastroenterology and Hepatology* 2008; **6**(6): 635–643.

27. Willems M, Quartero AO, Numans ME. How useful is paracetamol absorption as a marker of gastric emptying? A systematic literature study. *Digestive Diseases and Sciences* 2001; **46**(10): 2256–2262.

28. Stotzer PO, Fjalling M, Gretarsdottir J, Abrahamsson H. Assessment of gastric emptying – comparison of solid scintigraphic emptying and emptying of radiopaque markers in patients and healthy subjects. *Digestive Diseases and Sciences* 1999; **44**(4): 729–734.

29. Camilleri M, Zinsmeister AR, Greydanus MP, Brown ML, Proano M. Towards a less costly but accurate test of gastric emptying and small bowel transit. *Digestive Diseases and Sciences* 1991; **36**(5): 609–615.

30. Tougas G, Eaker EY, Abell TL, et al. Assessment of gastric emptying using a low fat meal: establishment of international control values. *American Journal of Gastroenterology* 2000; **95**(6): 1456–1462.

31. Karamanolis G, Caenepeel P, Arts J, Tack J. Association of the predominant symptom with clinical characteristics and pathophysiological mechanisms in functional dyspepsia. *Gastroenterology* 2006; **130**(2): 296–303.

32. Kuo B, McCallum RW, Koch KL, et al. Comparison of gastric emptying of a nondigestible capsule to a radiolabelled meal in healthy and gastroparetic subjects. *Alimentary Pharmacology and Therapeutics* 2008; **27**(2): 186–196.

33. Weitschies W, Kotitz R, Cordini D, Trahms L. High-resolution monitoring of the gastrointestinal transit of a magnetically marked capsule. *Journal of Pharmaceutical Sciences* 1997; **86**(11): 1218–1222.

34. Schwizer W, Maecke H, Fried M. Measurement of gastric emptying by magnetic resonance imaging in humans. *Gastroenterology* 1992; **103**: 369–376.

35. Goetze O, Steingoetter A, Menne D, et al. The effect of macro-nutrients on gastric volume responses and gastric emptying in humans: a magnetic resonance imaging study. *American Journal of Physiology* 2007; **292**(1): G11–G17.

36. Boulby P, Gowland P, Adams V, Spiller RC. Use of echo planar imaging to demonstrate the effect of posture on the intragastric distribution and emptying of an oil/water meal. *Neurogastroenterology and Motility* 1997; **9**(1): 41–47.

37. Boulby P, Moore R, Gowland P, Spiller RC. Fat delays empty-ing but increases forward and backward antral flow as assessed by flow-sensitive magnetic resonance imaging. *Neurogastroenterology and Motility* 1999; **11**(1): 27–36.

38. Kunz P, Feinle-Bisset C, Faas H, et al. Effect of ingestion order of the fat component of a solid meal on intragastric fat distribution and gastric emptying assessed by MRI. *Journal of Magnetic Resonance Imaging* 2005; **21**(4): 383–390.

39. Treier R, Steingoetter A, Goetze O, et al. Fast and optimized T1 mapping technique for the noninvasive quantification of gastric secretion. *Journal of Magnetic Resonance Imaging* 2008; **28**(1): 96–102.

Chapter 1.4

Physiology and function of the small intestine

Paul A. Blaker and Peter Irving
Guy's and St Thomas' NHS Foundation Trust, London, UK

The main functions of the small intestine are to complete the digestion of food through co-ordinated motility and secretion and to facilitate the absorption of water, electrolytes and nutrients. Approximately 9 L of fluid derived from oral intake (1.5 L) and exocrine secretions (7.5 L) enter the small intestine each day. Ninety per cent of this is reabsorbed in the small intestine with a further 8% absorbed in the colon. As such, only 100–150 mL of fluid is lost in faeces each day. The average length of the small intestine is 6.9 m but structural adaptations including mucosal folds, villi and microvilli mean that its surface area is 200–500 m². The first 100 cm of the small intestine are highly adapted to the absorption of nutrients, whereas the more distal portions are involved in reclaiming fluid and electrolytes. The small intestine is able to absorb far in excess of the body's requirements and as such, large portions of this organ can be removed without deleterious effects. However, changes in absorption and secretion homeostasis can rapidly lead to diarrhoea, dehydration, electrolyte disturbance and malnutrition.

1.4.1 Anatomy and histology

The small intestine includes three substructures termed the duodenum, jejunum and ileum, which extend sequentially from the gastric pylorus to the ileocaecal valve. The wall comprises an outer serous coat (tunica serosa), a layer of smooth muscle fibres (muscularis externa), submucosa consisting of dense connective tissue, a thin layer of smooth muscle (mucularis mucosa) and a mucosal layer (tunica mucosa) covered by epithelial cells (Figure 1.4.1). The tunica mucosa is thrown into numerous subfolds, creating the intestinal villi, which contain a dense blood capillary and lymphatic network that supplies the epithelial cells. Enterocytes are the most abundant epithelial cells (80%) and are characterised by the presence of enterocytic microvilli (brush border) that further increases the small intestinal surface area. Goblet cells are interspersed between enterocytes and secrete mucus that acts as a protective coat and lubricant. Tubular intestinal glands are found at the base of the villi (crypts of Lieberkuhn), which contain cells that differentiate into enterocytes, goblet cells, endocrine, paracrine and immune cells (Paneth cells). Changes in the cellular structure between sections of the small intestine allow for functional subspecialisation (Table 1.4.1).

Duodenum

The duodenum is approximately 25–35 cm in length and is split into four parts. It starts as the duodenal bulb, which arises from the gastric pylorus, and ends at the ligament of Treitz, where it joins the jejunum at the duodenojejunal flexure. The common bile duct enters the small intestine in the second part of the duodenum via the ampulla of Vater.

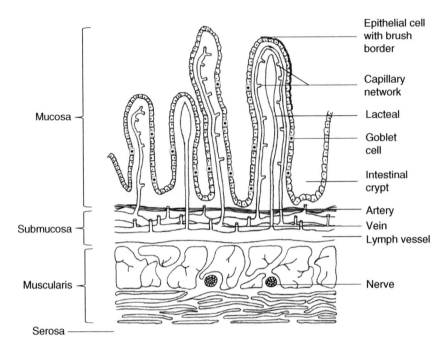

Figure 1.4.1   Structure of the small intestine.

Table 1.4.1   Differences in the ultrastructure and function of the small intestine

Layer	Duodenum	Jejunum	Ileum
Serosa	No change	No change	No change
Muscularis externa	Longitudinal and circular smooth muscle supplied by Auerbach's plexus	Similar to duodenum	Similar to duodenum
Submucosa	Brunner's glands +++ Meissner's plexus	Brunner's glands +	Brunner's glands +
Muscularis mucosae	No change	No change	No change
Lamina propria	No Peyer's patches	No Peyer's patches	Peyer's patches +++
Intestinal epithelium	Simple columnar Goblet cells Endocrine cells Paracrine cells Paneth cells	Villi longer than duodenum	Villi shorter than duodenum
Sodium content	145 mmol/L		125 mmol/L
Specialised functions	Iron and folate absorption	Iron and folate absorption in proximal jejunum Absorption of vitamin B1 and B2	Vitamin B12 and bile salt absorption in terminal ileum Absorption of vitamin C

The duodenum is distinguished from other parts of the small intestine by the presence of numerous Brunner's glands which secrete urogastrone (human epidermal growth factor), which is required for epithelial cell proliferation [1]. Consequently, the tips of the villi are continuously shed into the lumen and replaced by new cells from the crypts of Lieberkuhn. As such, the entire small intestine epithelium is renewed every 2–6 days.

Jejunum and ileum

The jejunum is approximately 2.5 m in length, whereas the length of the ileum is more variable (average 2–4 m). Both are contained within the peritoneum and are suspended by a mesentery. Most of the jejunum lies in the left upper quadrant of the abdomen, whereas the ileum mainly occupies the right lower quadrant. The jejunal folds are larger than those found in the duodenum or ileum.

1.4.2 Physiology and function

The gastric antrum sieves liquid chyme through the remaining solid matter in the stomach and delivers a continuous slow rate of gastric contents into the duodenum. The presence of chyme in the small intestine leads to the release of the hormones cholecystokinin (CCK) and secretin, which stimulate secretion of bicarbonate and pancreatic enzymes, and cause contraction of the gallbladder, which releases bile [2–4]. Proteins and peptides are degraded into amino acids through the action of pancreatic trypsin, chymotrypsin and elastase and subsequently by enzymes on the brush border. Lipids are degraded into fatty acids and glycerol and following emulsification by bile salts, triglycerides are split into free fatty acids and monoglycerides by pancreatic lipase. Carbohydrates may be broken down by pancreatic amylase into oligosaccharides or may pass into the colon where they are metabolised by GI microbiota. Brush border enzymes including dextrinase, glycoamylase, maltase, sucrase and lactase further break down oligosaccharides into monosaccharides prior to absorption. It is estimated that up to 65% of the adult population demonstrate a deficiency in lactase activity.

Reflex peristaltic waves mediated by musculo-motor neurones propel the small intestinal contents at a rate of 1–2 cm/min, meaning that it takes an average of 2–6 h to reach the colon [5]. The intensity of the muscular contractions is influenced by the nature of the ingested food. Solid foods induce greater activity than liquid meals, and those that are high in glucose cause greater stimulation than ones high in fat.

Several mechanisms are involved in the absorption of nutrients by enterocytes, including passive diffusion, cytosis, active transfer and carrier-mediated transport [6]. Uptake of water is driven by the absorption of sodium (Na^+), potassium (K^+) and organic compounds and occurs through the formation of osmotic gradients. The absorption of Na^+ is mediated by several different mechanisms including specific transmembrane carrier proteins.

1.4.3 Investigation of the small intestine

Correct diagnosis and management of small intestinal pathology are dependent on accurate history taking, clinical examination and specialist investigations. Non-bloody liquid stools greater than 1.5 L a day strongly suggest disease of the small intestine and weight loss may signify malabsorption. Here we summarise the key small intestinal investigations and describe their relevance to pathology.

Blood tests

Anaemia is detected on a full blood count (FBC). Iron deficiency anaemia is characterised by red cell microcytosis (low mean corpuscular volume, MCV), low serum ferritin and iron, low transferrin saturation and a high total iron-binding capacity. The most common causes of iron deficiency anaemia are a lack of dietary iron, gastrointestinal bleeding or proximal small intestinal pathology. Low serum folate may suggest disease in the duodenum or proximal jejunum, and is associated with a macrocytic anaemia (high MCV). Vitamin B12 deficiency also causes macrocytic anaemia and may be due to inadequate intake, autoimmune destruction of gastric parietal cells or antibodies to intrinsic factor (pernicious anaemia), pancreatic exocrine deficiency or disease in the terminal ileum.

Albumin is a protein synthesized in the liver that can be measured in blood tests. Hypoalbuminaemia may be due to a number of different causes but when associated with a history consistent with small intestinal disease, it may suggest protein-losing enteropathy or small intestinal inflammation [7].

Coeliac serology forms part of a screen for small intestinal pathology given the high prevalence of coeliac disease in northern Europeans (1 in 300–500). Antitissue transglutaminase (anti-tTG) is the best test, and is also useful to monitor response to gluten withdrawal.

Endoscopy

Upper gastrointestinal endoscopy (OGD) detects mucosal abnormalities in the oesophagus, stomach and duodenum. It also allows biopsies to be taken and is therefore the gold standard test in coeliac disease. Furthermore, OGD offers potential for therapeutic intervention in the management of upper gastrointestinal bleeding. Enteroscopes are longer than standard gastroscopes and allow deeper intubation of the small intestine.

Wireless capsule endoscopy involves swallowing a pill containing a small camera which transmits images to a receiver as it passes through the small intestine, allowing them to be viewed at a later date. This technique is particularly useful in the diagnosis of small intestinal vascular lesions and sites of inflammation that cannot be reached with conventional endoscopy [8] but is contraindicated in patients with small intestinal strictures and does not permit biopsies to be taken.

Radiology

A plain abdominal X-ray is useful in the diagnosis of intestinal obstruction. However, to provide intraluminal or mucosal detail, either enterography or enteroclysis is needed. Enterography, or small intestine follow-through, involves the ingestion of barium with X-rays being taken as it moves through the small intestine, thus potentially demonstrating small intestinal dilation, mucosal thickening, strictures, fistulae and tumours. Enhanced mucosal detail may be obtained through enteroclysis in which barium is rapidly infused through a nasoduodenal

or nasojejunal tube. Computed tomography (CT) allows for better examination of intra- and extraluminal structures than barium X-rays but also involves ionising radiation exposure. Small intestinal magnetic resonance imaging (MRI) is an alternative to CT and, because it does not involve radiation exposure, has an increasingly important role to play in patients who require repeated imaging such as those with small intestinal Crohn's disease.

Hydrogen breath tests

Breath tests are used to identify incomplete absorption of sugars such as lactose and fructose by the small intestine. If incompletely absorbed, the sugars will be fermented by colonic microbiota, resulting in the production of hydrogen which can be detected in exhaled breath. The test results may aid dietary advice on carbohydrate restriction.

Bacterial overgrowth in the proximal small intestine can be detected by using lactulose or glucose as the test sugar. The concept of distal small intestinal bacterial overgrowth is somewhat more controversial and is probably overdiagnosed by lactulose breath tests, the majority of positive results probably being explained by rapid transit of lactulose through the small intestine to the caecum [9].

Tests for malabsorption

Several other tests are sometimes used for the investigation of malabsorption, including xylose absorption (through detection of urinary xylose concentrations 5 h after oral ingestion), measurement of faecal alpha-1 antitrypsin (as a marker of protein-losing enteropathy) and measurement of faecal fat over 3 days following an orally administered fat load of 70 g to detect fat malabsorption. The latter is sometimes combined with measurement of faecal elastase as a marker of exocrine pancreatic function, with low enzyme concentrations denoting pancreatic insufficiency.

Bile malabsorption study (SeHCAT scan)

Normally bile acids are produced in the liver, stored in the gallbladder and released into the duodenum in response to a meal; 90% of bile acids are reabsorbed in the terminal ileum and circulated via the portal vein back to the liver. The presence of excess bile acids in the colon can result in diarrhoea. Malabsorption of bile salts may occur in patients with terminal ileal disease or following its resection. In such cases, diarrhoea may respond to treatment with bile salt sequestrants such as cholestyramine which chelates bile salts/acids [10,11]. In patients with short ileal resections (<1 m), the liver is able to synthesize sufficient replacement bile acids to maintain normal fat absorption. However, in long ileal resections (>1 m), it is unable to do so, resulting in fat malabsorption and, consequently, steatorrhoea [12]. Such patients will usually respond to dietary fat restriction. To maintain energy requirements, dietary fats may need to be substituted with medium-chain triglyceride (MCT) oil, since MCTs are absorbed directly into the portal vein without the need for bile acids/salts. Bile acid malabsorption can be detected using a radiolabelled synthetic bile acid scan (SeHCAT).

1.4.4 Pathology

Villous atrophy

Malabsorption occurs when there is a failure to absorb nutrients from the GI tract. It is either generalised or specific to a particular molecule (e.g. lactose), which may have associated clinical consequences. For example, fat malabsorption leads not only to steatorrhoea but also to malabsorption of the fat-soluble vitamins A, D, E and K. The causes of malabsorption are myriad; the major ones are listed in Table 1.4.2. The symptoms of malabsorption are variable but diarrhoea, undernutrition and fatigue are common (Table 1.4.3).

In Western countries, the most common cause of villous atrophy is coeliac disease, in which small intestinal inflammation occurs in response to the ingestion of gluten. The disease usually affects the duodenum and jejunum and is characterised by loss of the normal finger-like villi (villous atrophy), which decreases the surface area available for absorption. Coeliac serology and duodenal biopsy are diagnostic and the majority of patients respond to a gluten-free diet. Infections such as *Tropheryma whippelii* (Whipple's disease), tropical sprue and giardia may also lead to villous atrophy.

Inflammation

Inflammation affecting the small intestine may be either acute or chronic. Acute inflammation is often related to infection or medications (for example, non-steroidal inflammatory drugs).

Small intestinal Crohn's is a cause of chronic inflammation. Crohn's disease most commonly affects the terminal ileum and right colon whereas isolated duodenal or jejunal disease is rare [13]. Crohn's disease affecting the proximal small intestine can present with weight loss, iron deficiency anaemia and protein-losing enteropathy, whereas distal small intestinal inflammation presents with the more typical symptoms associated with Crohn's disease, including abdominal pain and diarrhoea [14]. Over time, complications such as strictures, penetration of inflammation through the intestinal wall or perforation may occur and 50–60% of patients will require surgery for Crohn's disease within 5 years of diagnosis [13,15].

Infection

There are several different mechanisms by which bacterial and viral infections may interfere with the normal absorptive and secretory functions of the small intestine to cause diarrhoea and malabsorption. For example, the enterotoxin of *Vibrio cholerae* stimulates chloride secretion, leading to secretory diarrhoea and copious fluid losses [16]. Enteropathogenic *Escherichia coli* (EPEC), which is a common cause of traveller's diarrhoea, impairs intestinal permeability [17] while rotavirus, the major cause of infantile gastroenteritis, limits fluid absorption [18].

Hypertonic oral rehydration solution (ORS) is able to reduce fluid losses from the small intestine by stimulating Na^+ and glucose transport, which concomitantly facilitates the absorption of water. This simple intervention is responsible for saving many millions of lives, particularly in developing countries.

Table 1.4.2 Causes of malabsorption

Changes in small intestinal contents	Changes in the small intestinal mucosa	Changes outside the small intestine	Inadequate small intestinal length
Inadequate mixing of contents (motility disorders, post gastrectomy)	Loss of intestinal villi (coeliac disease, Whipple's disease, tropical sprue)	Lymphatic obstruction (primary and secondary lymphangiectasia)	Congenital short bowel Short bowel syndrome after intestinal resection
Bacterial overgrowth	Inflammation of small intestinal mucosa (Crohn's disease, diffuse small intestinal vasculitis, NSAID-induced enteropathy, infection)		Malabsorption following gastric bypass surgery
Lack of bile salts (obstruction to the flow of bile, disruption of the enterohepatic circulation)			Enterocolic and enteroenteric fistulation
Exocrine pancreatic dysfunction			

NSAID, non-steroidal anti-inflammatory drug.

Table 1.4.3 Clinical consequences of specific micronutrient deficiencies

Deficient micronutrient	Clinical consequence
Vitamin A	Night blindness
Vitamin B1	Wernicke's encephalopathy
	Wernicke–Korsakoff syndrome
Vitamin B6	Dermatitis, peripheral neuropathy, angular cheilitis
Vitamin B12	Anaemia, altered mood, subacute combined degeneration of the spinal cord
Vitamin C	Scurvy
Vitamin D	Osteomalacia
Vitamin E	Neuropathy, myopathy, immunosuppression
Vitamin K	Impaired clotting (extrinsic clotting pathway – factors 2, 7, 9, 10)
Iron	Anaemia, glossitis, angular stomatitis
Calcium	Osteopenia/osteoporosis, muscle spasm, cardiac arrhythmias
Copper	Myelopathy, peripheral neuropathy, optic neuropathy
Magnesium	End-organ resistance to parathyroid hormone leading to hypocalcaemia. Cardiac arrhythmias, myopathy, fatigue
Selenium	Cardiomyopathy
Zinc	Acrodermatitis enteropathica, reduced fertility

Tumours of the small intestine

Benign tumours of the small intestine are rare and are usually derived from either the smooth muscle layers (leiomyoma), fat within the submucosa (lipoma) or from the enteric nervous system (neuroma). Occasionally large lesions may present with small intestinal obstruction or occult gastrointestinal bleeding but most are asymptomatic. Primary malignant lesions of the small intestine are very rare. In up to 1% of the population, tumours derived from enterochromaffin cells (carcinoid tumours) may be found.

In general, these are small, benign lesions found in the appendix but are more likely to become malignant if located in the small intestine. Such tumours may cause symptoms such as flushing, diarrhoea, sweating and shortness of breath (carcinoid syndrome).

Short bowel syndrome

Short bowel syndrome describes problems arising from a reduced small intestinal length, usually following surgical resection. If less than 1 m of small intestine remains, enteral nutrition alone may be inadequate. Patients with short bowel syndrome may present with dehydration, malabsorption, weight loss and micronutrient deficiencies. Occasionally, parenteral nutrition is required to supplement feeding but oral feeding should still be encouraged where possible to prevent GI atrophy.

1.4.5 Conclusion

The small intestine is a highly adapted organ with the capacity to absorb water and nutrients far in excess of the body's requirements. Whilst large portions of the small intestine can be resected without deleterious effects, changes in absorption and secretion homeostasis, for example in gastroenteritis, can cause copious diarrhoea, malabsorption and undernutrition. There are myriad diagnostic tests for the detection of small intestinal pathology and their application should be directed by accurate clinical history taking and examination. Furthermore, disease of the small intestine should be considered in any patient presenting with systemic symptoms occurring as a result of micronutrient deficiency.

References

1. Goodlad RA, Wilson TJ, Lenton W, Gregory H, Mccullagh KG, Wright NA. Effects of urogastrone (epidermal growth factor) on the intestinal epithelium. *Zeitschrift fur Gastroenterologie Verhandlungsband* 1988; **23**: 171–177.
2. Poitras P, Modigliani R, Bernier JJ. Effect of a combination of gastrin, secretin, cholecystokinin, glucagon, and gastric inhibitory polypeptide on jejunal absorption in man. *Gut* 1980; **21**(4), 299–304.
3. Dockray GJ. Cholecystokinin. *Current Opinion in Endocrinology, Diabetes and Obesity* 2012; **19**(1): 8–12.
4. Villanger O, Veel T, Raeder MG. Secretin causes H+/HCO3- secretion from pig pancreatic ductules by vacuolar-type H(+)-adenosine triphosphatase. *Gastroenterology* 1995; **108**(3): 850–859.
5. Worsoe J, Fynne L, Gregersen T, et al. Gastric transit and small intestinal transit time and motility assessed by a magnet tracking system. *BMC Gastroenterology* 2011; **11**: 145.
6. Sanderson J, Mallinson C. Basic functions of the gut. In: Brostoff J, Challacombe S (eds) *Food Allergy and Intolerance.* London: Saunders, 2002, pp. 17–35.
7. Braamskamp MJ, Dolman KM, Tabbers MM. Clinical practice. Protein-losing enteropathy in children. *European Journal of Pediatrics* 2010; **169**(10): 1179–1185.
8. Fisher LR, Hasler WL. New vision in video capsule endoscopy: current status and future directions. *Nature Reviews. Gastroenterology and Hepatology* 2012; **9**(7): 392–405.
9. Gibson PR, Barrett JS. The concept of small intestinal bacterial overgrowth in relation to functional gastrointestinal disorders. *Nutrition* 2010; **26**(11–12): 1038–1043.
10. Johnston I, Nolan J, Pattni SS, Walters JR. New insights into bile acid malabsorption. *Current Gastroenterology Reports* 2011; **13**(5): 418–425.
11. Money ME, Camilleri M. Review: Management of postprandial diarrhea syndrome. *American Journal of Medicine* 2012; **125**(6): 538–544.
12. Stevens T, Conwell D. Pancreatic enzyme replacement and bile acid therapy. In: Matarese L, Steiger E, Seidner D (eds) *Intestinal Failure and Rehabilitation: A Clinical Guide.* Boca Raton, FL: CRC Press, 2005, pp. 167–175.
13. Louis E, Collard A, Oger AF, Degroote E, Aboul Nasr El Yafi FA, Belaiche J. Behaviour of Crohn's disease according to the Vienna classification: changing pattern over the course of the disease. *Gut* 2001; **49**(6): 777–782.
14. Sands B, Siegel C. Crohn's disease. In: Feldman M, Friedman L, Brandt L (eds) *Sleisenger & Fordtran's Gastrointestinal and Liver Disease*, 9th edn. Philadelphia: Saunders Elsevier, 2010.
15. Tonelli F, Paroli GM. [Colorectal Crohn's disease: indications to surgical treatment]. *Annali Italiani di Chirurgia* 2003; **74**(6): 665–672.
16. Camilleri M, Nullens S, Nelsen T. Enteroendocrine and neuronal mechanisms in pathophysiology of acute infectious diarrhea. *Digestive Diseases and Sciences* 2012; **57**(1): 19–27.
17. Navaneethan U, Giannella RA. Mechanisms of infectious diarrhea. *Nature Clinical Practice. Gastroenterology and Hepatology* 2008; **5**(11): 637–647.
18. Lundgren O, Peregrin AT, Persson K, Kordasti S, Uhnoo I, Svensson L. Role of the enteric nervous system in the fluid and electrolyte secretion of rotavirus diarrhea. *Science* 2000; **287**(5452): 491–495.

Chapter 1.5

Physiology and function of the colon

Emma V. Carrington and S. Mark Scott

Queen Mary University of London, London, UK

The colon is the principal organ of the distal gastrointestinal tract. It plays a vital role in fluid and electrolyte homeostasis, digestion of food, absorption of nutrients, propulsion of intestinal contents and ultimately expulsion of waste products. Disorders of colonic function such as irritable bowel syndrome, inflammatory bowel disease, chronic constipation and diarrhoea are highly prevalent and cause significant morbidity with a negative impact on quality of life and consequently high socioeconomic costs. A keen understanding of colonic function is therefore required for the successful management of gastrointestinal disease.

1.5.1 Anatomy

Embryology

The primitive intestine begins to form in the third week of gestation. It arises secondary to ventral folding of the embryonic yolk sac and results in a tubular structure, lined with endoderm (ultimately forming the colonic mucosa) and covered with mesoderm (from which arises the surrounding muscle and serosa) [1]. This subsequently develops into foregut, midgut and hindgut regions, an understanding of which allows an appreciation of each section's resultant blood supply, lymphatic drainage and neuronal innervation. The colon is derived from the midgut and hindgut regions (the midgut spanning from the second part of the duodenum to the

middle third of the transverse colon and the hindgut extending from the middle third of the transverse colon to the rectum) [2].

Structure

The colon begins at the caecum and terminates with the rectum. It comprises six sections: caecum, ascending colon, transverse colon, descending colon, sigmoid colon and rectum. The junction of the ascending and transverse colon is commonly referred to as the hepatic flexure and the junction of the transverse and descending colon as the splenic flexure.

The caecum lies in the right iliac fossa, is completely covered by peritoneum and is therefore intraperitoneal. It is approximately 6 cm in length, without mesentery and is relatively mobile. Longitudinal muscle bands called teniae coli (which continue throughout the colon) converge at the base of the appendix, a vestigial organ that originates from its posterior surface.

The ascending colon is a continuation of the caecum. This extends upwards along the lateral side of the abdominal wall towards the right upper quadrant of the abdomen. It is approximately 15 cm in length and is covered on its anterior and lateral surfaces by peritoneum (therefore considered retroperitoneal). Once it has reached the inferior surface of the right lobe of the liver, it turns to form the transverse colon, which passes in front of the second part of the duodenum and the head of the pancreas. Following a further turn beneath the spleen, it

Advanced Nutrition and Dietetics in Gastroenterology, First Edition. Edited by Miranda Lomer.
© 2014 John Wiley & Sons, Ltd. Published 2014 by John Wiley & Sons, Ltd.

carries on to become the descending colon, which lies retroperitoneally on the left lateral side of the abdominal wall and is approximately 30 cm long. As the colon continues into the pelvis, it becomes known as the sigmoid colon, which finally terminates as the rectum [3].

Aside from its location at the periphery of the abdominal cavity, the colon may be characterised by the presence of teniae coli and appendices epiploicae (small fatty tags attached to the serosa surface). It is thrown into concertina-like saccular folds referred to as haustra, which are thought to be important for mixing of intestinal contents.

Vascular supply

The vascular supply of the colon is determined by its embryological origin. Structures derived from the midgut receive arterial supply from branches of the superior mesenteric artery and are drained by tributaries of the superior mesenteric vein and thence into the portal system. Distal to the middle third of the transverse colon (hindgut in origin), tissue receives arterial supply derived from the inferior mesenteric artery. Similarly, venous drainage is via tributaries of the inferior mesenteric vein (which also subsequently drains into the portal system).

Neuronal innervation

Colonic innervation is derived from four sources: the enteric, extrinsic afferent, sympathetic and parasympathetic nervous systems.

The enteric nervous system is composed of a number of nerve plexi within the GI wall and is principally responsibly for regulation of colonic motility. The two major plexi are the myenteric plexus and the submucosal plexus. The interstitial cells of Cajal provide the functional link between the nerve processes of the plexi and the muscle cells.

The extrinsic afferent nerves provide sensory innervation of the colon and rectum. The proximal colon receives this supply from the vagus nerve and the distal colon and rectum receive this supply from S1 and S2. It is thought that this innervation is primarily responsible for the conscious perception of rectal filling as well as the initiation of propulsion required for defaecation [4].

Sympathetic and parasympathetic supplies also act to modulate sensory and motor activity. Midgut structures derive this innervation from the superior mesenteric plexus and hindgut structures from the pelvic splanchnic nerves via the inferior mesenteric plexus. Generally speaking, parasympathetic activity exhibits an excitatory effect on colonic function, increasing colonic motility and secretory activity. By contrast, sympathetic activity inhibits colonic tone and motility [5].

1.5.2 Function

The colon has evolved to perform four major functions:

(1) propulsion of colonic contents towards the rectum and anus for eventual expulsion
(2) absorption of water and electrolytes from intraluminal contents
(3) absorption of short-chain fatty acids produced by resident microbiota
(4) defaecation.

Propulsion of intestinal contents

The term 'colonic motility' is used to describe the mixing and propulsive movements of the colon that allow for digestion, absorption and transit of intraluminal contents.

The mechanisms responsible for absorption in the colon are slow and the colonic microbiota are facilitated by the speed and orientation of mixing movements. Distal propulsion of contents is therefore gradual to allow for mixing and uniform contact with the colonic mucosa. Contents take roughly 12–30 h to traverse the length of the colon, compared to 2–4 h in the small intestine (which is four or five times greater in length).

Colonic motility patterns are complex. Co-ordinated activity between the terminal ileum, caecum and proximal colon is required to deliver chyme from the terminal ileum to the colon. Contents become increasingly solid as water is absorbed and they are transported aborally toward the rectum for eventual evacuation.

Two forms of colonic contractile activity have been described: propagating pressure sequences

(PSs) (sometimes referred to as high- and low-amplitude propagating pressure sequences) and segmental contractions. Antegrade movement of colonic contents is generally as a result of proximally originating PSs. Frequency significantly increases after waking and/or meal ingestion and may be of high (with a >100 mmHg rise in colonic pressure over a significant length) or lower amplitude (2–5 mmHg increase in pressure). Both high- and low-amplitude PSs are equally likely to produce colonic movement [6].

Localised mixing of colonic contents is achieved through segmental contractions, accounting for the majority of colonic activity. These can be considered as more limited areas of activity facilitating contact with the colonic mucosa principally for absorption of water and other contents.

Disorders of colonic motility can result in impaired stool propulsion and abdominal pain, distension, constipation and diarrhoea.

Water and electrolyte homeostasis

Absorption of water and electrolytes is one of the principal functions of the colon. Roughly 1500 mL of effluent reaches the ileocaecal valve each day and the healthy colon will generally resorb 90% of the fluid from this, resulting in the formation of 200 g of solid stool.

Water absorption is intimately associated with sodium reabsorption and occurs primarily in the ascending and transverse colon [5]. Intraluminal Na^+ passively diffuses into colonocytes via apical channels in response to a negative electrochemical gradient (maintained through the presence of electrogenic Na^+/K^+ pumps present on their basolateral membrane). Absorption of water then follows the resultant osmotic gradient via a paracellular pathway and is controlled by both aldosterone and antidiuretic hormone (ADH). Aldosterone acts to increase K^+ secretion/Na^+ conservation and ADH increases apical membrane water permeability.

Chloride is also actively absorbed from the colonic lumen. It is transported through the apical membrane via $Cl^-HCO_3^-$ channels. Secretion of HCO_3^- acts to neutralise acidic compounds produced through bacterial fermentation.

Digestion and absorption

Although the majority of digestion and absorption occurs in the stomach and small intestine, the colon also plays a role in nutrient salvage through the process of fermentation [5]. The colon contains approximately 10^{11}–10^{12} bacteria per gram of contents [7] and these bacteria have the ability to break down carbohydrates and proteins into short-chain fatty acids (SCFAs). If required, this can supply to up to 15% of an individual's total energy requirements [8].

The production of SCFAs depends on a number of factors including the constituents of luminal contents, gut transit time and microbial variety. As colonic microbiota will preferentially ferment carbohydrates over proteins, saccharolytic fermentation is predominant in the proximal ascending colon whereas proteolysis is more common in the distal colon.

The three end-products of fermentation are acetate, butyrate and propionate. Although butyrate only accounts for approximately 20% of total SCFA production, it is of particular importance as it is the primary energy source for the colonic mucosa and plays a major role in cellular differentiation and proliferation [9]. Additionally, there is a degree of evidence suggesting that butyrate has anti-inflammatory and anticarcinogenic properties.

Absorption of SFCAs is both passive and active in nature and results in sodium absorption and bicarbonate excretion. The colon is particularly proficient at SFCA absorption (as only 10% of those produced are excreted) [9].

Recognition of the benefits of saccharolytic fermentation has led to the development of prebiotics, probiotics and synbiotics.

In addition to the production of SFCAs, colonic microbiota also play a role in the production of vitamin synthesis, notably vitamin K, biotin (vitamin B7) and niacin (vitamin B3).

Defaecation

Effective defaecation is a result of the successful co-ordinated function of the colon, rectum and anus and is under central, spinal and enteric neural control [10]. A number of factors influence defaecatory frequency including diet, intraluminal contents, colonic transit, behaviour and posture. There is variability in defaecatory frequency between individuals but studies suggest that 99% of the healthy population open their bowels between three times per day and three times per week [11].

Consumption of food produces a near immediate increase in colonic motor activity. Food content affects the degree of colonic response as it has been shown that a fat-rich meal induces colonic motor activity to a greater extent than a protein- or carbohydrate-rich meal [12].

The process of defaecation constitutes four distinct phases: the basal phase (characterised by a change in colonic motor activity, usually precipitated by waking or meal ingestion), the predefaecatory phase (during which gradual rectal distension produces an awareness of rectal filling), expulsion (following a conscious desire to evacuate) and termination (characterised by contraction of the external anal sphincter and closure of the anal canal) [10].

1.5.3 Measurement and assessment of function

Assessment of colonic motility and transit is usually indicated in patients with symptoms of infrequent evacuation. At the present time, two radiological methods for the assessment of transit are routinely employed to look indirectly at colonic motor function: radiopaque marker studies and colonic scintigraphy. Colonic manometry can be employed to look directly at colonic contractile activity.

Radiopaque marker studies

This technique is the simplest method for study of colonic transit times (either total or segmental) [13]. This study is often used for the evaluation of patients with symptoms of persistent constipation. Radiopaque markers contained in a degradable capsule are ingested and plain abdominal X-rays are subsequently taken to determine marker distribution. Segmental colonic transit times can be estimated by administration of different-shaped markers on consecutive days.

Conventionally, this study involves the ingestion of 24 markers on day 1 and the performance of a single plain radiograph on day 6, but in reality there are significant differences in practice between centres, making interinstitution comparisons difficult. The upper limit of normal colonic transit time is around 72 h and delayed transit may be secondary to a primary colonic dysmotility or disorders of evacuation. Further testing with either colonic scintigraphy and/or evacuation proctography is often required to establish a definitive diagnosis.

Colonic scintigraphy

Colonic scintigraphy is a radioscintigraphic method for studying colonic motility. A radioisotope, usually ^{111}In (indium), is bound to a non-absorbable substance, e.g. diethylenetriamine penta-acetic acid (DTPA), and is either ingested orally with water, or delivered direct to the colonic lumen via an ingestible enteric-coated capsule (i.e. that degrades in the caecum). For data analysis, the colon is generally divided into regions of interest. Time-distribution analysis enables information about activity in a given region of interest to be determined at any one time or for the overall study [14,15].

Colonic manometry

Direct evaluation of changes in intracolonic pressure is termed 'colonic manometry'. This technique utilises an intraluminal device with the ability to detect pressure changes that occur as a result of phasic contractions of circular colonic muscle. As opposed to radiopaque marker studies and colonic scintigraphy, which provide an indirect assessment of intraluminal movement, colonic manometry is able to characterise specific patterns and phases of colonic motor activity, giving the clinician a greater appreciation of differences in regional function. Regrettably, colonic manometry is an invasive procedure (requiring colonoscopy for placement of the catheter) and for this reason a paucity of data are available in both health and disease, limiting its use in clinical practice [16].

1.5.4 Conclusion

The colon is a complex and responsive structure with function dependent not only on external events and influence of other organs, but also the maintenance of a stable microbiota. The impact of diet should not be underestimated. Diseases characterised by disorders of colonic function are common; for example, chronic constipation affects 3% of individuals and diverticular disease may affect up to 60% of the population over 60 years of age [17,18]. Maintenance of colonic health is therefore fundamental to ensure a satisfactory quality of life.

References

1. Pokorny WJ, Rothenberg SS, Brandt ML. Growth and development. In: O'Lery JP, Capote LR (eds) *The Physiologic Basis of Surgery*, 5th edn. Philadelphia: Lippincott Williams and Wilkins, 1996.
2. Wexner SD, Jorge JM. Anatomy and embryology of the anus, rectum and colon. In: Corman ML (ed) *Colon and Rectum Surgery*. Philadelphia: Lippincott Williams and Wilkins, 2005.
3. Whitaker RH, Borley NR. *Instant Anatomy*. Oxford: Wiley-Blackwell, 2010.
4. Brookes SJ, Dinning PG, Gladman MA. Neuroanatomy and physiology of colorectal function and defaecation: from basic science to human clinical studies. *Neurogastroenterology and Motility* 2009; 21(Suppl 2): 9–19.
5. Szmulowicz UM, Hull TL. Colonic physiology. In: Beck DE, Roberts PL, Saclarides TJ, Senagore AJ, Stamos MJ, Wexner S (eds) *The ASCRS Textbook of Colon and Rectal Surgery*. New York: Springer, 2011.
6. Dinning PG, Szczesniak MM, Cook IJ. Proximal colonic propagating pressure waves sequences and their relationship with movements of content in the proximal human colon. *Neurogastroenterology and Motility* 2008; 20: 512–520.
7. Cummings JH, Macfarlane GT. The control and consequences of bacterial fermentation in the human colon. *Journal of Applied Bacteriology* 1991; 70: 443–459.
8. Hamer HM, Jonkers D, Venema K, Vanhoutvin S, Troost FJ, Brummer RJ. Review article: the role of butyrate on colonic function. *Alimentary Pharmacology and Therapeutics*, 2008; 27: 104–119.
9. Wong JM, de Souza R, Kendall CW, Emam A, Jenkins DJ. Colonic health: fermentation and short chain fatty acids. *Journal of Clinical Gastroenterology* 2006; 40: 235–243.
10. Palit S, Lunniss PJ, Scott SM. The physiology of human defecation. *Digestive Diseases and Sciences* 2012; 57: 1445–1464.
11. Connell AM, Hilton C, Irvine G, Lennard-Jones JE, Misiewicz JJ. Variation of bowel habit in two population samples. *British Medical Journal* 1965; 2: 1095–1099.
12. Rao SS, Kavelock R, Beaty J, Ackerson K, Stumbo P. Effects of fat and carbohydrate meals on colonic motor response. *Gut* 2000; 46: 205–211.
13. Hinton JM, Lennard-Jones JE, Young AC. A new method for studying gut transit times using radioopaque markers. *Gut* 1969; 10: 842–847.
14. Notghi A, Hutchinson R, Kumar D, Smith NB, Harding LK. Simplified method for the measurement of segmental colonic transit time. *Gut* 1994; 35: 976–981.
15. Notghi A, Kumar D, Panagamuwa B, Tulley NJ, Hesslewood SR, Harding LK. Measurement of colonic transit time using radionuclide imaging: analysis by condensed images. *Nuclear Medicine Communications* 1993; 14: 204–211.
16. Scott SM. Manometric techniques for the evaluation of colonic motor activity: current status. *Neurogastroenterology and Motility* 2003; 15: 483–513.
17. Parks TG. Natural history of diverticular disease of the colon. *Clinics in Gastroenterology* 1975; 4: 53–69.
18. Sonnenberg A, Koch TR. Epidemiology of constipation in the United States. *Diseases of the Colon and Rectum* 1989; 32: 1–8.

Chapter 1.6

Physiology and function of the pancreas

Yiannis N. Kallis[1] and David Westaby[2]
[1]Barts Health NHS Trust, London, UK
[2]Imperial College Healthcare NHS Trust, London, UK

1.6.1 Anatomy, physiology and function

The pancreas is a retroperitoneal organ located in the upper abdomen. It extends transversely between the concavity of the duodenum and the spleen, and lies posteroinferior to the stomach. The medial aspect of the pancreas receives a blood supply from branches of the gastroduodenal and superior mesenteric arteries, whilst branches of the splenic artery supply the bulk of the pancreatic body and tail. Blood drains into the portal venous system via the superior mesenteric and splenic veins. Lymph drainage of the pancreas is via splenic, coeliac and superior mesenteric lymph nodes, which are common sites of metastatic cancer spread.

The pancreas performs both exocrine and endocrine functions and plays a central role in digestion and glucose metabolism. Pancreatic exocrine secretions drain into the medial aspect of the second part of the duodenum via tributaries that form the main pancreatic duct. The duct enters the duodenum at the ampulla of Vater, into which the common bile duct also drains. Outflow is controlled by a smooth muscle sphincter termed the sphincter of Oddi. Endocrine cells of the pancreas release hormones directly into the bloodstream.

The exocrine pancreas consists of units called acini, which are arranged into lobules and drain into the main pancreatic duct. They make up 98% of the pancreatic mass and are responsible for the production of digestive enzymes and pancreatic fluid.

Enzymes, such as trypsin, chymotrypsin, lipase, phospholipase A2 and amylase, are stored as inactive precursors within secretory granules and are released under neurohormonal control. These proenzymes are activated by intestinal enteropeptidases only upon reaching the duodenum, thereby preventing pancreatic autodigestion due to premature activation. Dysregulation of these mechanisms is thought to underpin the pathogenesis of pancreatitis. Enzymes are released in large quantities for the early digestion of proteins, fats and carbohydrates. Pancreatic ductal cells secrete approximately 2 L of bicarbonate-rich fluid daily to neutralise duodenal chyme and optimise conditions for digestion.

Exocrine function is governed by multiple neurohormonal pathways triggered by the process of eating. The autonomic nervous system directly induces pancreatic enzyme release via vagal parasympathetic efferents in response to cephalic stimuli (e.g. the sight and smell of food), and also after gastric distension. Duodenal exposure to food and acidity induces the release of gut hormones from specialised intestinal enteroendocrine cells. Cholecystokinin governs acinar cell degranulation and secretin is primarily responsible for alkaline pancreatic secretion.

Endocrine cells are distributed throughout the pancreas in spherical clusters called islets of Langerhans, which are criss-crossed by a dense network of capillaries. Beta-cells, the predominant cell type, are responsible for insulin production and alpha-cells synthesise glucagon, both key hormones

Advanced Nutrition and Dietetics in Gastroenterology, First Edition. Edited by Miranda Lomer.
© 2014 John Wiley & Sons, Ltd. Published 2014 by John Wiley & Sons, Ltd.

in glucose homeostasis. Other cell types secrete inhibitors of pancreatic exocrine secretion, such as somatostatin, which also have inhibitory effects on islet cell function.

1.6.2 Measurement and assessment of function

Structural assessment

Cross-sectional imaging with arterial phase contrast-enhanced computed tomography (CT) scanning is the gold standard for detection of pancreatic lesions and for assessment of complications of acute and chronic pancreatitis [1]. Magnetic resonance imaging (MRI) is a suitable alternative and can provide more detailed information about pancreatic ductal anatomy, via magnetic resonance cholangio-pancreatography (MRCP). Ultrasound scanning is of limited utility because overlying intestinal gas frequently obscures views.

The role of endoscopic ultrasound in the investigation of pancreatic disease is rapidly expanding. It is particularly helpful in the staging of pancreatic cancer and the diagnosis of pancreatic cystic lesions [2]. Fine needle aspiration facilitates histological diagnosis and large pancreatic cysts can be managed by transgastric stent insertion.

Assessment of function

Acute pancreatic inflammation is typified by release of enzymes into the bloodstream, and simple assays are widely available to quantify serum amylase and lipase in the diagnosis of acute pancreatitis.

Pancreatic exocrine insufficiency is common in chronic pancreatic disease, though clinically evident malabsorption only usually occurs after 85–90% reduction in enzyme production. Endocrine insufficiency is typically a late feature and is manifest by the development of diabetes.

A variety of assays of exocrine function are available though many are expensive and time consuming, and most are rarely performed. Measurement of faecal elastase is a useful screening tool for moderate or severe pancreatic insufficiency and is commercially available [3]. Elastase is exclusively

produced by the pancreas, is not enterally absorbed, and has largely replaced quantification of faecal fat or chymotrypsin as the assay of choice. Faecal fat excretion of more than 7 g per day (100 g daily fat intake) is considered indicative of fat malabsorption, though may represent intestinal disorders as well as pancreatic disease. Direct analysis of endoscopically obtained duodenal aspirates following pancreatic stimulation is laborious and costly and largely obsolete.

Quantification of exocrine function can also be performed by indirect assessment of enzymatic activity. The pancreolauryl and PABA (N-benzoyl-L-tyrosyl-p-aminobenzoic acid) tests are two such assays, whereby orally administered, labelled compounds are digested by luminal pancreatic enzymes, releasing substrates quantifiable in urine. They are only reliable for detecting severe insufficiency and are not widely available.

1.6.3 Pathology

Acute pancreatitis is a condition of sudden onset usually precipitated by acute pancreatic injury. Common causes include gallstones and alcohol, though drugs, trauma and other rare triggers are also recognised. Its severity can range from mild to life threatening, and a number of prognostic scoring systems have been developed [4]. Its pathophysiology involves the premature activation of pancreatic enzymes leading to tissue autodigestion and necrosis, which can also trigger a systemic inflammatory response syndrome. Early treatment is largely supportive, and later management is often focused on local complications such as fluid collections or abscesses [5]. The role and timing of enteral feeding during an acute episode are under ongoing review [6]. Identification and removal of precipitating factors are important to prevent future episodes. Occasionally patients may experience recurrent discrete episodes classified as acute relapsing pancreatitis.

Chronic pancreatitis is defined by abdominal pain, which is often intractable, and involves irreversible fibrosis, atrophy and calcification of the gland. It may involve features of exocrine or endocrine insufficiency. The most common cause is excess alcohol consumption, though many cases are classified as idiopathic. Other aetiologies include inherited genetic abnormalities, autoimmune disorders and conditions associated with impaired pancreatic drainage (e.g. pancreas divisum). The pathogenesis of chronic pancreatitis is increasingly recognised as multifactorial [7]. Treatment incorporates avoidance of precipitating factors and adequate analgesia, though supplementation of exocrine/endocrine function and maintenance of nutrition are also important aspects. Endoscopic or surgical procedures to improve pancreatic duct drainage may be required.

Ductal adenocarcinoma is the most common pancreatic malignancy and is often locally advanced or metastatic upon presentation. Surgical resection offers the only prospect of a cure, but a majority of cancers are inoperable at the time of diagnosis [8]. Palliative chemotherapy and relief of biliary or gastric outlet obstruction with endoscopic stenting or surgery are the mainstays of treatment.

Neuroendocrine tumours are commonly located in the pancreas. They are a heterogenous group of tumours of variable metastatic potential, with a more favourable prognosis [9]. They may cause symptoms by dysregulated release of hormones such as insulin, glucagon or gut hormones (e.g. gastrin). Surgical resection and somatostatin analogues are mainstays of treatment.

Cystic lesions of the pancreas are often found incidentally on abdominal imaging. They can be divided into simple cysts, pseudocysts or true cystic neoplasms. Management of these lesions is focused on defining their malignant potential [10]. Size and characterisation of the cyst are key, and endoscopic ultrasound has advanced this field significantly. Surgical resection is considered where lesions are symptomatic or have high malignant potential.

References

1. Bharwani N, Patel S, Prabhudesai S, Fotheringham T, Power, N. Acute pancreatitis: the role of imaging in diagnosis and management. *Clinical Radiology* 2011; **66**: 164–175.
2. Thornton GD, Mcphail MJ, Nayagam S, Hewitt MJ, Vlavianos P, Monahan KJ. Endoscopic ultrasound guided fine needle aspiration for the diagnosis of pancreatic cystic neoplasms: a meta-analysis. *Pancreatology* 2013; **13**: 48–57.
3. Loser C, Mollgaard A, Folsch UR. Faecal elastase 1: a novel, highly sensitive, and specific tubeless pancreatic function test. *Gut* 1996; **39**: 580–586.
4. Gravante G, Garcea G, Ong SL, et al. Prediction of mortality in acute pancreatitis: a systematic review of the published evidence. *Pancreatology* 2009; **9**: 601–614.
5. UK Working Party on Acute Pancreatitis. UK guidelines for the management of acute pancreatitis. *Gut* 2005; **54**(Suppl 3): iii1–9.
6. Petrov MS, Pylypchuk RD, Emelyanov NV. Systematic review: nutritional support in acute pancreatitis. *Alimentary Pharmacology and Therapeutics* 2008; **28**: 704–712.
7. Conwell DL, Banks PA. Chronic pancreatitis. *Current Opinion in Gastroenterology* 2008; **24**: 586–590.
8. Ghaneh P, Costello E, Neoptolemos JP. Biology and management of pancreatic cancer. *Postgraduate Medical Journal* 2008; **84**: 478–497.
9. Ramage JK, Ahmed A, Ardill J, et al. Guidelines for the management of gastroenteropancreatic neuroendocrine (including carcinoid) tumours (NETs). *Gut* 2012; **61**: 6–32.
10. Tanaka M, Fernandez-del Castillo C, Adsay V, et al. International consensus guidelines 2012 for the management of IPMN and MCN of the pancreas. *Pancreatology* 2012; **12**: 183–197.

Chapter 1.7

Physiology and function of the hepatobiliary tract

Yiannis N. Kallis[1] and David Westaby[2]
[1]Barts Health NHS Trust, London, UK
[2]Imperial College Healthcare NHS Trust, London, UK

1.7.1 Anatomy, physiology and function

The liver is situated in the right hypochondrium and is split into right and left lobes. It can be further divided into eight functional segments according to vascular supply and biliary drainage [1]. Inflow of blood is via a dual supply, with approximately 25% derived from the hepatic artery and 75% from the portal vein, which drains the gastrointestinal tract, pancreas and spleen. Both vessels enter the liver at the hilum and subdivide into smaller branches, running in structures called portal tracts, also composed of bile ducts and lymphatics. Blood perfuses the liver within sinusoids before draining via tributaries to form the hepatic vein, which enters the inferior vena cava just beneath the diaphragm.

Histologically, liver parenchyma is arranged into units called lobules, defined by a central hepatic venule and multiple peripheral portal tracts [2]. Hepatocytes are organised into three-dimensional plates separated by sinusoids, which are lined by fenestrated endothelium through which blood can readily permeate. Kupffer cells (liver macrophages) and hepatic stellate cells (fibroblast-like collagen-producing cells) lie in close approximation [3]. Spatially, hepatocytes are classified into three zones, with those around portal tracts in zone 1 receiving the most oxygenated blood and those in zone 3 around hepatic venules the least [4].

Bile caniliculi form a dense meshwork around hepatocytes and fuse to form bile ducts within portal tracts. The right and left hepatic ducts join at the hilum to form the common hepatic duct. The cystic duct drains the gallbladder and fuses with the common hepatic duct to form the common bile duct. The latter enters the duodenum at the ampulla of Vater (see Chapter 1.5).

The gallbladder is located in the abdomen under the right lobe of the liver. It is a pear-shaped sac, with average volume of 50 mL and length of 9 cm in healthy adults (range 4–14 cm), and is connected to the gastrointestinal tract via the cystic duct and common bile duct [5]. Its function is to concentrate and store bile produced in the liver and to release this into the duodenum when required for digestion. Release of bile is achieved by muscular contraction of the gallbladder in response primarily, but not exclusively, to gut hormones, especially cholecystokinin (CCK), that are stimulated by the products of digestion in the gastrointestinal tract. In the small intestine, bile is essential for the emulsification of dietary fat.

Carbohydrate metabolism

The liver plays a major role in glucose homeostasis and is the main store of glycogen. It assimilates excess glucose into glycogen within hepatocytes under insulin control. Conversely, hepatic glycogenolysis makes

---

Advanced Nutrition and Dietetics in Gastroenterology, First Edition. Edited by Miranda Lomer.
© 2014 John Wiley & Sons, Ltd. Published 2014 by John Wiley & Sons, Ltd.

glucose readily available to other organs as the first response to starvation. Thereafter, the liver can also release glucose via gluconeogenesis from non-carbohydrate substrates such as lactate, amino acids (alanine and glutamine) and glycerol. During prolonged starvation, hepatic fatty acids are metabolised by beta-oxidation to ketone bodies, an important energy source for organs such as the brain.

Protein metabolism

The liver regulates plasma amino acid levels by controlling amino acid transamination and gluconeogenesis. All circulating plasma proteins except gamma-globulins are synthesised by the liver. Approximately 10–12 g of albumin is produced daily, helping to maintain oncotic pressure and transport water-insoluble compounds. Coagulation cascade factors, including fibrinogen, are produced in the liver, as are acute phase and complement proteins. The liver is the primary site of nitrogen excretion via amino acid transamination and oxidative deamination, leading to the formation of ammonia, which is subsequently converted to urea and excreted renally.

Lipid metabolism

Following dietary fat absorption, the liver synthesises triglycerides from free fatty acids for redistribution around the body within very low-density lipoproteins (VLDL). Likewise, hepatic fatty acid oxidation can be utilised for energy release. The liver controls production of circulating lipoproteins which transport insoluble fats through the bloodstream. Cholesterol formation, excretion and redistribution are also under hepatic regulation. Circulating cholesterol is taken up via hepatic low-density lipoprotein (LDL) receptors, and cholesterol can be formed *de novo* from hepatic acetyl-CoA. Cholesterol esterification to fatty acids also takes place in the liver.

The liver is a store for several vitamins and minerals, including vitamins A, D, B12, iron and copper, and is the site of 25-hydroxylation of cholecalciferol.

Bile acid and bilirubin metabolism

Bile is composed of water, electrolytes, bile acids, bilirubin, phospholipids, cholesterol and conjugated waste products, with approximately 600 mL

produced each day [6]. In fasted states, approximately half is syphoned off to the gallbladder where it is concentrated. It is actively secreted at the hepatocyte canalicular membrane via bile transporter proteins, with biliary ductular epithelium also contributing. It facilitates the emulsification and digestion of fats and provides an alkaline pH for optimal pancreatic enzyme function. It is also the main vehicle for the elimination of hydrophobic waste products such as bilirubin. Bile formation is stimulated by secretin and inhibited by somatostatin. After ingestion of a meal, cholecystokinin stimulates gallbladder contraction and sphincter of Oddi relaxation.

Primary bile acids are synthesised from cholesterol in the liver and these are converted into secondary bile acids by GI microbiota. Ninety-five per cent of these are reabsorbed in the terminal ileum, returned to the liver in the portal venous circulation and resecreted into bile, termed the enterohepatic circulation [7]. Bilirubin is formed from erythrocyte breakdown, conjugated with glucuronic acid in the liver to render it water soluble and excreted within bile. Some is reabsorbed via the enterohepatic circulation after bacterial hydrolysis to urobilinogen.

Drug and hormone metabolism

Most xenobiotics, including alcohol, are inactivated in the liver by cytochrome P450-mediated processes such as methylation or hydroxylation, and excreted in bile or urine after conjugation by hepatic transferases [8]. The liver is a key site of the catabolism of hormones such as oestrogens, insulin, growth hormone, glucocorticoids and parathyroid hormone. Angiotensinogen is produced in the liver and helps regulate blood pressure.

Immunological function

As part of the reticuloendothelial system, the liver is a crucial site of gut-derived antigen presentation to Kupffer cells, NK cells and sinusoidal endothelium transported in the portal venous circulation [9]. It is also involved in adaptive immunity via lymphocyte trafficking from the GI tract. Impaired immunity and recurrent sepsis are common consequences of hepatic dysfunction.

1.7.2 Measurement and assessment of function

Blood tests

Liver function tests (LFTs) can be subdivided into true tests of liver synthetic and excretory function, and markers of liver injury measured by cellular enzyme release. Alanine aminotransferase (ALT) and aspartate aminotransferase (AST) are enzymes predominantly located in hepatocytes and their release into serum reflects hepatocellular damage. Alkaline phosphatase (ALP) and gamma-glutamyl transpeptidase (gamma-GT) are chiefly found in biliary canaliculae and serum rises indicate intrahepatic cholestasis as well as extrahepatic bile duct damage or obstruction. ALP is also located in other tissues such as bone and placenta, and gamma-GT is an enzyme inducible by certain drugs and alcohol. Commonly measured indices of liver function are bilirubin, albumin and prothrombin time. Advanced liver impairment can be associated with renal failure, hence serum sodium and creatinine concentrations are included in scoring systems of liver dysfunction such as MELD and UKELD [10,11].

Blood tests can help determine the cause of liver injury, and include viral hepatitis serology, immunoglobulins, autoantibody profiles, serum iron and copper indices and a metabolic screen. Alphafetoprotein (AFP) and Ca19.9 are tumour markers associated with hepatocellular carcinoma (HCC) and cholangiocarcinoma, respectively, though their clinical utility is limited.

Imaging

Ultrasound scanning is usually the first modality employed to define anatomy in hepatobiliary investigation. The presence of liver lesions, gallbladder stones, biliary obstruction, portal hypertension or ascites can be readily detectable. Fatty liver infiltration gives an echo 'bright' signal. Doppler is used to interrogate blood flow and detect portal or hepatic venous occlusion.

Cross-sectional imaging with contrast-enhanced triple phase computed tomography (CT) or magnetic resonance imaging (MRI) can better define hepatic or biliary mass lesions and gives a clearer indication of liver size and architecture. HCC can be diagnosed on radiological characteristics alone, obviating the need for biopsy. CT or MRI scanning is also invaluable in the management of cholangiocarcinoma to define anatomical relationships to blood vessels and bile ducts and thus determine surgical resectability. MR cholangiopancreatography is the 'gold standard' modality to delineate the biliary tree and can detect calculi, strictures or diffuse cholangiopathy.

Hepatobiliary iminodiacetic acid (HIDA) scanning is a dynamic radionucleotide test of bile flow and is still sometimes used in the investigation of the jaundiced patient to determine if cholestasis is of hepatic or biliary origin.

Endoscopy

Upper gastrointestinal (GI) endoscopy is used for the diagnosis and treatment of complications of portal hypertension such as oesophageal or gastric variceal bleeding. Endoscopic retrograde cholangiopancreatography (ERCP) is the therapeutic modality of choice in the management of bile duct stones or strictures.

Interventional radiology

Percutaneous transhepatic cholangiography (PTC) is sometimes performed when ERCP is unsuccessful. The biliary tree is accessed under fluoroscopic guidance and obstruction can be relieved by internal or external stenting. It is particularly useful in the context of complex hilar strictures.

Fluoroscopically guided cannulation of the hepatic vein via a transjugular approach can allow the measurement of hepatic and portal venous pressure in the management of portal hypertension, and can offer an alternative approach to obtaining a liver biopsy. The transjugular placement of an intrahepatic portosystemic shunt (TIPSS) can control variceal bleeding when endoscopy has failed [12]. Hepatic arterial angiography is employed to embolise liver tumours such as HCC, which have a dense hepatic arterial supply.

Liver biopsy

Histological examination of liver tissue is frequently invaluable in the diagnosis of parenchymal liver disease and in the characterisation of liver or biliary mass lesions [13]. Estimation of liver fibrosis permits the staging of chronic liver disease and establishes a diagnosis of cirrhosis. Most liver biopsies are performed percutaneously under ultrasound guidance, though transjugular and laparoscopic approaches are alternatives.

1.7.3 Pathology

Liver disease is often asymptomatic and can be present for many years before diagnosis. Symptoms occur late and are characterised by jaundice or features of hepatic decompensation such as ascites, peripheral oedema, encephalopathy or portal hypertensive GI bleeding.

Severe acute liver injury is rare though may rapidly lead to liver failure. Paracetamol overdose is the most common cause, though other aetiologies such as idiosyncratic drug reactions, viral hepatitis and autoimmune liver disease are recognised.

Chronic liver disease is characterised by a balance between progressive fibrosis and attempts at liver regeneration. Cirrhosis is the hallmark of advanced liver disease and can herald the development of liver dysfunction and HCC. Undernutrition and loss of muscle mass are common features. Excess alcohol consumption, non-alcoholic fatty liver disease (NAFLD) and chronic hepatitis C are the most common causes in the developed world. Other important aetiologies include hepatitis B, haemochromatosis and immune disorders such as primary biliary cirrhosis (PBC), primary sclerosing cholangitis (PSC) and autoimmune hepatitis. Management includes the withdrawal or treatment of the causative agent where possible, and the treatment of complications of liver decompensation. Liver transplantation can offer good medium-term survival in end-stage disease [14].

Biliary disorders are characterised by upper abdominal pain, jaundice, fever or weight loss. Gallstone disease can present with biliary colic,

obstructive jaundice or cholangitis. Isolated strictures of the biliary tree may be benign or malignant and usually present with LFT derangement and jaundice. Diffuse stricturing of the biliary tree is distinctive of a cholangiopathy, e.g. PSC or autoimmune cholangiopathy. Biliary obstruction can also occur from extrinsic compression, such as from intrahepatic or lymph node metastases.

Worldwide, common disorders affecting the gallbladder are the formation of stones, functional dyskinesia, cancer of the gallbladder and steatocholecystitis [15–18].

Hepatocellular carconoma typically arises in the context of cirrhosis, though it can occur in the precirrhotic liver in conditions such as hepatitis B and NAFLD. Benign liver lesions such as haemangioma, adenoma and focal nodular hyperplasia (FNH) are also common. Primary biliary tract cancer (gallbladder carcinoma and cholangiocarcinoma) is a relatively common malignancy and carries a poor overall prognosis [19].

References

1. Couinaud, C. *Le Foie: Études anatomiques et chirurgicales [The Liver: Anatomical and Surgical Studies]* (in French). Paris: Masson, 1957.
2. Dooley J, Lok A, Burroughs A, Heathcote J. *Sherlock's Diseases of the Liver and Biliary System.* Oxford: Wiley-Blackwell, 2011.
3. Friedman SL. The virtuosity of hepatic stellate cells. *Gastroenterology* 1999; **117**: 1244–1246.
4. Bacon B, O'Grady J, di Bisceglie A, Lake J. *Comprehensive Clinical Hepatology.* Oxford: Elsevier Health Sciences, 2006.
5. Gropper SS, Smith JL, Groff JL. *Advance Nutrition and Human Metabolism,* 5th edn. Belmont, CA: Wadworth Publishing Company, 2008.
6. Redinger RN, Small DM. Bile composition, bile salt metabolism and gallstones. *Archives of Internal Medicine* 1972; **130**: 618–630.
7. Dowling RH. The enterohepatic circulation. *Gastroenterology* 1972; **62**: 122–140.
8. Danielson PB. The cytochrome P450 superfamily: biochemistry, evolution and drug metabolism in humans. *Current Drug Metabolism* 2002; **3**: 561–597.
9. Racanelli V, Rehermann B. The liver as an immunological organ. *Hepatology* 2006; **43**: S54–S62.
10. Kamath PS, Wiesner RH, Malinchoc M, et al. A model to predict survival in patients with end-stage liver disease. *Hepatology* 2001; **33**: 464–470.
11. Neuberger J, Gimson A, Davies M, et al. Selection of patients for liver transplantation and allocation of donated livers in the UK. *Gut* 2008; **57**: 252–257.

12. Boyer TD, Haskal ZJ. American Association for the Study of Liver Diseases Practice Guidelines: the role of transjugular intrahepatic portosystemic shunt creation in the management of portal hypertension. *Journal of Vascular and Interventional Radiology* 2005; **16**: 615–629.

13. Rockey DC, Caldwell SH, Goodman ZD, Nelson RC, Smith AD, for the American Association for the Study of Liver. Liver biopsy. *Hepatology* 2009; **49**: 1017–1044.

14. Lucey MR, Terrault N, Ojo L, et al. Long-term management of the successful adult liver transplant: 2012 practice guideline by the American Association for the Study of Liver Diseases and the American Society of Transplantation. *Liver Transplantation* 2013; **19**: 3–26.

15. Tsai CJ, Leitzmann MF, Willett WC, Giovannucci EL. Macronutrients and insulin resistance in cholesterol gallstone disease. *American Journal of Gastroenterology* 2008; **103**: 2932–2939.

16. Eslick GD. Epidemiology of gallbladder cancer. *Gastroenterology Clinics of North America* 2010; **39**: 307–330.

17. Hansel SL, di Baise JK. Functional gallbladder disorder: gallbladder dyskinesia. *Gastroenterology Clinics of North America* 2010; **39**: 369–379.

18. Stinton LM, Myers RP, Shaffer EA. Epidemiology of gallstones. *Gastroenterology Clinics of North America* 2010; **39**: 157–169.

19. Khan SA, Davidson BR, Goldin RD, et al. Guidelines for the diagnosis and treatment of cholangiocarcinoma: an update. *Gut* 2012; **61**: 1657–1669.

Gastrointestinal microbiota

Katherine Stephens, Gemma E. Walton and Glenn R. Gibson
University of Reading, Reading, UK

Bacteria are associated with all areas of the human body from the skin to the genitourinary, respiratory and gastrointestinal (GI) tracts [1]. The GI tract is the most heavily populated, with the majority of the total bacterial population of humans residing therein. A highly diverse ecosystem exists, with the collective bacterial species within the human GI tract totalling in the thousands [2,3]. The results of the MetaHIT Consortium (Metagenomics of the Human Intestinal Tract, www.metahit.eu/) indicate that any one of 1000–1150 different species could populate the human GI tract, with at least 160 species residing in an individual [4]. Given these large numbers, although there is great potential for diversity in the GI microbiota between different humans, there is considerable stability in some species, with a core of 18 species being found in all those in the MetaHIT Consortium, and a core of 57 species found in 90% of subjects [4].

1.8.1 Composition

The GI tract has evolved to become a functional organ comprising anatomically distinct areas. The digestive process starts in the oral cavity, then moves through the stomach, small and large intestine and finally the rectum. This passage allows the presence of several microbial niches due to different environmental conditions, such as acidity in the stomach, varying retention times and different nutrient availabilities (Table 1.8.1). Physicochemical variables are contributing factors to the diverse community of micro-organisms residing in the GI tract (see Table 1.8.1). Within the intestinal tract, genomic analysis has shown the number of micro-organisms to be approximately 10^{13} to 10^{14} in total [5], with the overall microbiome (the combined genome of all the micro-organisms) approximately 100 times greater than the human genome [4]. Within the large intestine, there is also variation in diversity of species within specific compartments, such as the mucosa, lumen and epithelium [6]. The small intestinal sites, duodenum, jejunum and ileum, also comprise differing numbers and species.

Micro organisms residing within the GI tract carry out many necessary roles, for example in metabolism, immune defence and GI physiology [7]. Some are associated with health benefits whereas others are known to be potentially pathogenic. Lactobacilli and bifidobacteria are associated with many positive effects and have been used in various health food products as probiotics. A possible reason for this could be their ability to prevent commensal and potentially pathogenic microbial population levels from increasing through various inhibitory mechanisms [8–11]. Potential pathogens include *Clostridium difficile*, *Escherichia coli* and *Helicobacter pylori* which have been connected with antibiotic-associated diarrhoea, vomiting and stomach ulcers respectively [12,13].

Although each individual has a distinctive microbiome, the majority of key players remain the same but in varying quantities.

Advanced Nutrition and Dietetics in Gastroenterology, First Edition. Edited by Miranda Lomer.
© 2014 John Wiley & Sons, Ltd. Published 2014 by John Wiley & Sons, Ltd.

Table 1.8.1   Summary of microbiota associated with the GI tract in humans

Site	Approximate numbers per mL	Examples of microbial types	Environmental factors	References
Oral cavity	$10^{8/9}$	*Streptococcus* spp. *Viellonella* spp. *Prevotella* spp. *Actinomyces* spp *Klebsiella* spp.	Anaerobic and aerobic	57, 58
Stomach	10^3	*H. pylori* *Lactobacillus* spp. *Veillonella* spp. *Staphylococcus* spp. *Streptococcus* spp.	Microaerophilic Low pH due to gastric acidity from hydrochloric acid Presence of pepsin Rapid transit	14, 58, 59
Small intestine (ileum, jejunum, duodenum)	10^3–10^8	*Lactobacillus* spp. *Veillonella* spp. Yeasts *Staphylococcus* spp. *Streptococcus* spp.	Anaerobic Presence of bile salts and pancreatic secretions	60
Large intestine	10^{12}	*Bifidobacterium* spp. *Lactobacillus* spp. *Clostridium* spp. *Bacteroides* spp. *Enterobacteriaceae* spp. *Staphylococcus* spp. Acetogens Methanogens Sulphate-reducing bacteria *Proteus* spp. *Fusobacterium* spp. *Eubacterium* spp. *Roseburia* spp.	Anaerobic Dietary residues available for fermentation, as well as indigenous sources Favourable pH for microbial growth Slow transit (ca. 24–72 h)	60

1.8.2 Functions of the human gastrointestinal tract

A main function of the GI microbiota is modulation of the immune system. Germ-free mice have been extensively used in studies investigating the involvement of the microbiota in immune response development [14]. The microbiota can form a protective barrier which decreases the chance of pathogen invasion by possibly occupying receptor sites in the GI tract [14]. The micro organisms compete by several different mechanisms, such as nutrient scavenging, receptor occupation and the production of antimicrobial substances, which can elicit a specific or non-specific effect such as the modulation of pH. Antimicrobial substances produced in the GI tract include acids, antimicrobial peptides (AMPs), defensins, cathelicidins and C type lectins, all of which are capable of targeting bacterial cell walls, thus controlling population levels of commensal organisms or aiding protection against pathogens [15,16].

Competition plays a vital role in immune defence, helping to prevent potential pathogen invasion.

Specialised GI tract lymphoid tissues produce secretory immunoglobin A (IgA) [17] which neutralises receptors on target bacteria, allowing some control over the GI microbiota [18]. Activation of IgA is due to localised GI dendritic cells, which sample the luminal micro organisms; therefore antibodies against GI microbiota have already been developed.

A number of features aid in the control of GI population levels, for example IgA and AMPs. Dendritic cells (DCs) are specialised white blood cells which act as antigen-presenting cells (APCs); they sample the intestinal lumen, and therefore GI microbiota, and are able to secrete antibodies to neutralise any potential growing threat [18]. Distinguishing between threats involves Toll-like receptors which are expressed on eukaryotic cells; these have a unique function of recognising conserved regions within bacterial membranes [19]. Due to this ability, signalling molecules such as cytokines can elicit an inflammatory response [20]. Antimicrobial peptides have the ability to work across the GI tract; they are localised towards the intestinal mucosa, preventing the expansion of microbes throughout the lumen and minimising contact with host GI tract epithelium [21]. Lactic acid bacteria produce lactate and acetate, which can be detrimental to other microbes, through their ability to disrupt bacterial outer membranes [22].

The GI tract must also be able to tolerate microbes and not always elicit an immune response. This can be achieved in three different ways: a physical barrier between host cells and bacterial cells, antigen modification on bacterial cells or modifying immune responsive cells in the GI tract [14]. DC's are specialised in the GI tract to induce and stimulate T-cell differentiation into T-helper cells and T-regulatory cells, an alternative to cytotoxic T-cells which can damage the GI tract epithethial lining [23]. Another potential problem is lipopolysaccharide (LPS) on the gram-negative bacterium's outer membrane; host recognition of LPS can lead to septic shock or low-grade chronic inflammation [24]. To overcome this, LPS toxicity can be reduced by phosphorylation [25]. In mice, it has been shown that GI epithelial cells inherit a tolerance to LPS endotoxin [26].

Bacterial metabolism is a key part of the microbiota. They are able to breakdown non-digestible food products into short-chain fatty acids (SCFA). Such substrates include non-starch polysaccharides (NSP), starch, oligosaccharides, proteins and amino acids [27]. These organic acids can be used for growth and energy, not only for themselves but as a secondary source for the host [28]. Acetate, propionate and butyrate are the main SCFAs produced and have various impacts on human metabolism and the immune system [28,29]. Butyrate is involved in cytokine development as an essential signalling molecule and provides structural aid in the intestinal epithelium; it also stimulates apoptosis and therefore is an important growth regulator for colonocytes [30,31]. Acetate can aid intestinal inflammation during an immune response, allowing for more immune cells to translocate to the infected site via G-protein-coupled receptors. Acetate is also metabolised in muscle and other systemic tissues [32]. Propionate has been shown to lower cholesterol concentration [33]. SCFAs also have abilities in AMP generation, aiding in immune system defence [5].

Studies have shown that microbial GI composition plays a role in human brain development and behaviour, with germ-free mice displaying higher anxiety issues and less motor control than conventionally raised animals [34]. *Bifidobacterium infantis* has been shown to regulate the metabolism of tryptophan, an amino acid involved in the production of serotonin showing a potential link between GI micro-organisms and neurotransmitter concentrations [35]. As such, the GI microbiota may have an additional impact on host psychology. The microbiota have also been shown to interfere with the hypothalamic-pituitary-adrenal axis – interactions between the hypothalamus, pituitary and adrenal glands [36]. The GI microbiota have been associated with the control of different signalling molecules such as neurotransmitters. These connections suggest that the GI microbiota have an impact on host response to stress as well as mood/psychological disorders [37,38].

1.8.3 Factors influencing composition of the microbiota

The establishment of the native microbiota can be observed from birth and continues to develop throughout life. During pregnancy, the infant's intestinal tract is thought to be devoid of micro-organisms. The delivery method of the infant can result in distinctive colonisation patterns. Natural birth delivery, where the infant passes through the birthing canal, results in the infant ingesting the mother's commensal vaginal and faecal microbiota [39]. A caesarean birth results in the first colonisers being those from the hospital environment; species such as *Staphylococcus epidermis* and other *Staphylococcus* spp and *Propionibacterium* have been noted in caesarean births [40,41]. Facultative anaerobes are the first GI tract colonisers due to the infant GI tract having positive oxidation/reduction potential [8]. Examples include *E. coli, Enterococcus faecium, Enterococcus faecalis, Pseudomonas* spp, *Aeromonas* spp, *Klebsiella* spp and *Enterobacter* spp [36,38]. Oxygen is rapidly utilised by initial invaders, thus creating anaerobic conditions which allow the colonisation of strict anaerobes [37]. Examples of such strict anaerobic bacterial genera include *Bifidobacterium* spp, *Bacteroides* spp and *Clostridium* spp [42].

From birth, diet will also affect the initial colonisers, particularly in the case of breast as opposed to formula feeding, with the former having a preponderance of bifidobacteria. Much research has shown that the initial microbiota composition can have an impact on subsequent colonisation which may later influence the health of the individual [14]. For example, early colonisers of lactobacilli have been associated with a lower number of allergies [43]. After 3 years of age, post breastfeeding and weaning, the GI tract starts to stabilise and over time a more established microbiota is developed [44]. In general, breastfed infants have reduced risks of infections and more chronic issues in later life [39].

In the elderly population the microbiota is more changeable [45]. Composition varies and the diversity of micro-organisms has been observed to decrease [46]. Factors which can affect this altered organisation over time include loss of appetite and therefore less nutrient availability, decrease in saliva secretion, decrease in vitamin synthesis, tooth decay, potential mutations in cancer suppression genes, immunological changes, decreases in nutrient absorption and intestinal transit time and sensitivity [47,48]. *Lactobacillus* spp and *Bifidobacterium* spp have been observed to be lower in elderly volunteers whereas *Bacteroides*, enterococci, enterobacteria and *Clostridia* levels were fairly similar or even higher than in younger adults [49].

Diet can affect bacterial diversity in the GI tract. Non-digestible nutrients will become available to the microbiota; certain species may thrive depending on substrate availability and type [42]. The energy can be harboured for their own metabolic processes or can be available to the host. Diet cannot always provide the vital nutrients the body needs to function, and in this context, the microbiota is important for the synthesis of certain vitamins [28].

Microbial infection can occur at any stage of life. The usual treatment consists of a recommended antibiotic to which the proposed bacterial infection shows sensitivity. However, antibiotic use may also have an impact on the normal indigenous microbiota which can lead to complex issues such as diarrhoea or pseudomembranous colitis [50]. Commensal micro-organisms such as lactobacilli and bifidobacteria may decrease [20]. As a result, opportunistic micro-organisms such as *C. difficile* and yeasts such as *Candida albicans* may be better able to multiply due to less competition; these then may have the ability to cause further illnesses, such as antibiotic-associated diarrhoea (AAD) [13,20]. Other issues include vitamin deficiencies, as members of the microbiota contribute to the vitamin requirements of the host [51]. The severity of deficiencies is dictated by a series of factors including dosage and duration of antibiotic treatment, range of potential microbial targets, route of transmission of the treatment, pharmacokinetics of the drug and how easily it can be metabolised [52]. Clindamycin is an antibiotic commonly used for individuals suffering with a health issue caused by an anaerobe, its wide range of targets making it a useful drug on its own and in combination with others. Although this drug is effective, it has a negative impact on commensal GI micro-organisms, allowing for an increase in *C. difficile* and therefore the risk of colitis, diarrhoea and bloating [51,53].

A growing predicament with the use of antibiotics is increasing bacterial resistance – commensal to commensal or commensal to pathogen [52]. With growing resistance to antibiotic treatments, it is more likely that micro organisms can transfer resistant genes

Box 1.8.1 Examples of factors that may affect the composition of the GI microbiota, adapted from Fooks and Gibson [61]

Other microbiota
Type of feeding
Amount, chemical composition and availability of growth substrates
Availability of colonisation sites
Immunological interactions
Individual fermentation
Strategies by the bacteria
Intestinal transit time
Gut pH
Redox potential
Availability of inorganic electron acceptors
Production of bacterial metabolites
Presence of antimicrobial compounds
Xenobiotic compounds
Age of the host
Peristalsis
Host genetics
Physical activity levels
Antibiotics
Disease state
Stress

studies contradicting one another. However, what is clear is that the microbiota can markedly affect host health.

The microbiota are a crucial component of the human body, required not only in manufacturing necessities such as vitamins and SCFAs but also for the digestive process to occur optimally. Their role in immune defence is of great magnitude and the human body would be at much higher risk of infection without the protection of the commensal microbiota. However, there are also negative effects, which can be mostly controlled through a healthy lifestyle. Our knowledge of the relationship between the host and their microbiota is developing further, with new studies providing more insight into the complex network of our GI system.

References

1. Van de Guchte M, Serror P, Chervaux C, Smokvina T, Ehrlich SD, Maguin E. Stress responses in lactic acid bacteria. *Antonie Van Leeuwenhoek International Journal of General and Molecular Microbiology* 2002; **82**(1–4): 187–216.

2. Ley RE, Peterson DA, Gordon JI. Ecological and evolutionary forces shaping microbial diversity in the human intestine. *Cell* 2006; **124**(4): 837–848.

3. Frank DN, Amand ALS, Feldman RA, Boedeker EC, Harpaz N, Pace NR. Molecular-phylogenetic characterization of microbial community imbalances in human inflammatory bowel diseases. *Proceedings of the National Academy of Sciences of the United States of America* 2007; **104**(34): 13780–13785. Available at www.pnas.org.

4. Qin J, Li R, Raes J, et al. A human gut microbial gene catalogue established by metagenomic sequencing. *Nature* 2010; **464**(7285): U59–U70.

5. Gill SR, Pop M, DeBoy RT, et al. Metagenomic analysis of the human distal gut microbiome. *Science* 2006; **312**(5778): 1355–1359.

6. Zoetendal EG, von Wright A, Vilpponen-Salmela T, Ben-Amor K, Akkermans AD, de Vos WM. Mucosa-associated bacteria in the human gastrointestinal tract are uniformly distributed along the colon and differ from the community recovered from feces. *Applied and Environmental Microbiology* 2002; **68**(7): 3401–3407.

7. Clemente JC, Ursell LK, Parfrey LW, Knight R. The impact of the gut microbiota on human health: an integrative view. *Cell* 2012; **148**(6): 1258–1270.

8. Penders J, Thijs C, Vink C, et al. Factors influencing the composition of the intestinal microbiota in early infancy. *Pediatrics* 2006; **118**(2): 511–521.

9. Gibson GR. Dietary modulation of the human gut microflora using the prebiotics oligofructose and inulin. *Journal of Nutrition* 1999; **129**(7): 1438S–1441S.

to one another via horizontal transfer, e.g. bacterial conjugation. An example of this was the transfer of beta-lactamase on a plasmid from a resistant *E. coli* strain to an initially susceptible strain in a child taking amoxicillin [54]. It is now thought that over a short antibiotic treatment period, resistant strains can remain for several years which may lead to less successful treatment and higher costs due to failure to eradicate pathogenic infection and the evolution of superbugs [55].

Dysbiosis of the GI microbiota can occur, influencing microbiota composition and leading to potential health problems (Box 1.8.1). A common cause of dysbiosis is inflammation, which is associated with many GI-related diseases [56]. Current research has shown a connection between the microbiota and health issues such as obesity, diabetes, cancer, autism, allergies, inflammatory bowel disease and irritable bowel syndrome. There is much debate about the exact species involved in these disorders, with some

10. Shah NP. Functional cultures and health benefits. *International Dairy Journal* 2007; **17**(11): 1262–1277.

11. De Vrese M, Schrezenmeir J. Probiotics, prebiotics, and synbiotics. In: Stahl U, Donalies UE, Nevoigt E (eds) *Food Biotechnology*. Belgium: Springer Reference, 2008, pp. 1–66.

12. Blaser MJ, Chyou PH, Nomura A. Age at establishment of Helicobacter-pylori infection and gastric-carcinoma, gastric-ulcer, and duodenal-ulcer risk. *Cancer Research* 1995; **55**(3): 562–565.

13. McFarland LV. Meta-analysis of probiotics for the prevention of antibiotic associated diarrhea and the treatment of *Clostridium difficile* disease. *American Journal of Gastroenterology* 2006; **101**(4): 812–822.

14. Sekirov I, Russell SL, Antunes LC, Finlay BB. Gut microbiota in health and disease. *Physiological Reviews* 2010; **90**(3): 859–904.

15. Salzman NH, Underwood MA, Bevins CL. Paneth cells, defensins, and the commensal microbiota: a hypothesis on intimate interplay at the intestinal mucosa. *Seminars in Immunology* 2007; **19**(2): 70–83.

16. Hooper LV. Opinion: Do symbiotic bacteria subvert host immunity? *Nature Reviews Microbiology* 2009; **7**(5): 367–374.

17. Cerutti A, Rescigno M. The biology of intestinal immuno-globulin A responses. *Immunity* 2008; **28**(6): 740–750.

18. Begley M, Gahan CG, Hill C. The interaction between bacteria and bile. *FEMS Microbiology Reviews* 2005; **29**(4): 625–651.

19. Aderem A, Ulevitch RJ. Toll-like receptors in the induction of the innate immune response. *Nature* 2000; **406**(6797): 782–787.

20. Noverr MC, Huffnagel GB. Does the microbiota regulate immune responses outside the gut? *Trends in Microbiology* 2004; **12**(12): 562–568.

21. Sugimoto S, Abdullah Al M, Sonomoto K. Molecular chaperones in lactic acid bacteria: physiological consequences and biochemical properties. *Journal of Bioscience and Bioengineering* 2008; **106**(4): 324–336.

22. Alakomi HL, Skytta E, Saarela M, Mattila-Sandholm T, Latva-Kala K, Helander IM. Lactic acid permeabilizes gram-negative bacteria by disrupting the outer membrane. *Applied and Environmental Microbiology* 2000; **66**(5): 2001–2005.

23. Jernberg C, Lofmark S, Edlund C, Jansson JK. Long-term ecological impacts of antibiotic administration on the human intestinal microbiota. *ISME Journal* 2007; **1**(1): 56–66.

24. Beutler B, Rietschel ET. Innate immune sensing and its roots: the story of endotoxin. *Nature Reviews Immunology* 2003; **3**(2): 169–176.

25. Bates JM, Akerlund J, Mittge E, Guillemin K. Intestinal alka-line phosphatase detoxifies lipopolysaccharide and prevents inflammation in zebrafish in response to the gut microbiota. *Cell Host and Microbe* 2007; **2**(6): 371–382.

26. Lotz M, Gutle D, Walther S, Menard S, Bogdan C, Hornef MW. Postnatal acquisition of endotoxin tolerance in intestinal epithelial cells. *Journal of Experimental Medicine* 2006; **203**(4): 973–984.

27. Guarner F, Malagelada JR. Gut flora in health and disease. *Lancet* 2003; **361**(9356): 512–519.

28. Kau AL, Ahern PP, Griffin NW, Goodman AL, Gordon JI. Human nutrition, the gut microbiome and the immune system. *Nature* 2011; **474**(7351): 327–336.

29. Cummings JH, Macfarlane GT. Role of intestinal bacteria in nutrient metabolism (Reprinted from *Clinical Nutrition* 1997; **16**: 3). *Journal of Parenteral and Enteral Nutrition* 1997; **21**(6): 357–365.

30. Bird JJ, Brown DR, Mullen AC, et al. Helper T cell differentiation is controlled by the cell cycle. *Immunity* 1998; **9**(2): 229–237.

31. Peng L, He Z, Chen W, Holzman IR, Lin J. Effects of butyrate on intestinal barrier function in a Caco-2 cell monolayer model of intestinal barrier. *Pediatric Research* 2007; **61**(1): 37–41.

32. Maslowski KM, Vieira AT, Ng A, et al. Regulation of inflammatory responses by gut microbiota and chemoattractant receptor GPR43. *Nature* 2009; **461**(7268): 1282–1286.

33. Pereira DI, Gibson GR. Effects of consumption of probiotics and prebiotics on serum lipid levels in humans. *Critical Reviews in Biochemistry and Molecular Biology* 2002; **37**(4): 259–281.

34. Heijtza RD, Wang S, Anuar F, et al. Normal gut microbiota modulates brain development and behavior. *Proceedings of the National Academy of Sciences of the United States of America* 2011; **108**(7): 3047–3052.

35. Desbonnet L, Garrett L, Clarke G, Bienenstock J, Dinan TG. The probiotic *Bifidobacteria infantis*: an assessment of potential antidepressant properties in the rat. *Journal of Psychiatric Research* 2008; **43**(2): 164–174.

36. Adlerberth I, Wold AE. Establishment of the gut microbiota in Western infants. *Acta Paediatrica* 2009; **98**(2): 229–238.

37. Fanaro S, Chierici R, Guerrini P, Vigi V. Intestinal microflora in early infancy: composition and development. *Acta Paediatrica* 2003; **91**(Suppl 441): 48–55.

38. Adlerberth I, Carlsson B, Deman P, et al. Intestinal colonization with Enterobacteriaceae in Pakistani and Swedish hospital-delivered infants. *Acta Paediatrica Scandinavica* 1991; **80**(6–7): 602–610.

39. O'Toole PW, Claesson MJ. Gut microbiota: changes throughout the lifespan from infancy to elderly. *International Dairy Journal* 2010; **20**(4): 281–291.

40. Heavey PM, Rowland IR. The gut microflora of the developing infant: microbiology and metabolism. *Microbial Ecology in Health and Disease* 1999; **11**(2): 75–83.

41. Dominguez-Bello MG, Costello EK, Contreras M, et al. Delivery mode shapes the acquisition and structure of the initial microbiota across multiple body habitats in newborns. *Proceedings of the National Academy of Sciences of the United States of America* 2010; **107**(26): 11971–11975.

42. Rotimi VO, Duerden BI. The development of the bacterial-flora in normal neonates. *Journal of Medical Microbiology* 1981; **14**(1): 51–62.

43. Round JL, Mazmanian SK. The gut microbiota shapes intestinal immune responses during health and disease. *Nature Reviews Immunology* 2009; **9**(5): 313–323.

44. Mackie RI, Sghir A, Gaskins HR. Developmental microbial ecology of the neonatal gastrointestinal tract. *American Journal of Clinical Nutrition* 1999; **69**(5): 1035S–1045S.

45. Claesson MJ, Cusack S, O'Sullivan O, et al. Composition, variability, and temporal stability of the intestinal microbiota of the elderly. *Proceedings of the National Academy of Sciences of the United States of America* 2011; **108**: 4586–4591.

46. Maukonen J, Matto J, Kajander K, Mattila-Sandholm T, Saarela M. Diversity and temporal stability of fecal bacterial populations in elderly subjects consuming galacto-oligosaccharide containing probiotic yoghurt. *International Dairy Journal* 2008; **18**(4): 386–395.

47. Lovat LB. Age related changes in gut physiology and nutritional status. *Gut* 1996; **38**(3): 306–309.

48. Majumdar AP. Regulation of gastrointestinal mucosal growth during aging. *Journal of Physiology and Pharmacology* 2003; **54**(Suppl 4): 143–154.

49. He T, Harmsen HJ, Raangs GC, Welling GW. Composition of faecal microbiota of elderly people. *Microbial Ecology in Health and Disease* 2003; **15**(4): 153–159.

50. Dethlefsen L, Huse S, Sogin ML, Relman DA. The pervasive effects of an antibiotic on the human gut microbiota, as revealed by deep 16S rRNA sequencing. *PLOS Biology* 2008; **6**(11): 2383–2400.

51. Levy J. The effects of antibiotic use on gastrointestinal function. *American Journal of Gastroenterology* 2000; **95**(1): S8–S10.

52. Jernberg C, Lofmark S, Edlund C, Jansson JK. Long-term impacts of antibiotic exposure on the human intestinal microbiota. *Microbiology* 2010; **156**: 3216–3223.

53. Bartlett JG. Antibiotic-associated diarrhea. *New England Journal of Medicine* 2002; **346**(5): 334–339.

54. Karami N, Martner A, Enne VI, Swerkersson S, Adlerberth I, Wold AE. Transfer of an ampicillin resistance gene between two *Escherichia coli* strains in the bowel microbiota of an infant treated with antibiotics. *Journal of Antimicrobial Chemotherapy* 2007; **60**(5): 1142–1145.

55. Lofmark S, Jernberg C, Jansson JK, Edlund C. Clindamycin-induced enrichment and long-term persistence of resistant Bacteroides spp. and resistance genes. *Journal of Antimicrobial Chemotherapy* 2006; **58**(6): 1160–1167.

56. Shanahan F. Inflammatory bowel disease: immunodiagnostics, immunotherapeutics, and ecotherapeutics. *Gastroenterology* 2001; **120**(3): 622–635.

57. Kolenbrander PE, Andersen RN, Blehert DS, Egland PG, Foster JS, Palmer RJ. Communication among oral bacteria. *Microbiology and Molecular Biology Reviews* 2002; **66**(3): 486–505.

58. Tlaskalova-Hogenova H, Stepankova R, Kozakova H, et al. The role of gut microbiota (commensal bacteria) and the mucosal barrier in the pathogenesis of inflammatory and autoimmune diseases and cancer: contribution of germ-free and gnotobiotic animal models of human diseases. *Cellular and Molecular Immunology* 2011; **8**(6): 110–120.

59. Dethlefsen L, Eckburg PB, Bik EM, Relman DA. Assembly of the human intestinal microbiota. *Trends in Ecology and Evolution* 2006; **21**(9): 517–523.

60. Tiihonen K, Ouwehand AC, Rautonen N. Human intestinal microbiota and healthy ageing. *Ageing Research Reviews* 2010; **9**(2): 107–116.

61. Fooks LJ, Gibson GR. Probiotics as modulators of the gut flora. *British Journal of Nutrition* 2002; **88**: S39–S49.

Gastrointestinal tract and appetite control

Jaimini Cegla and Stephen R. Bloom
Imperial College London, London, UK

Despite fluctuations in food intake and physical activity, healthy adults maintain a relatively constant weight over decades. However, as stated by the laws of thermodynamics, if less energy is expended than consumed then the excess energy will be stored. It is calculated that an average North American man will increase his weight by 9.1 kg between 25 and 35 years of age, as a consequence of a mere 0.3% imbalance between energy consumed and energy expended over this period [1]. It is therefore of no surprise that, as a result of readily available high-energy food and our sedentary lifestyles, obesity has become a growing global epidemic. The converse is true in disorders that culminate in reduced energy intake such as anorexia nervosa. An understanding of the mechanisms that control body weight, by co-ordinating food intake and energy expenditure, is key in unravelling the pathogenesis of disordered energy homeostasis in gastrointestinal disease.

1.9.1 Role of the gut neuroendocrine system in appetite regulation

Several neural, hormonal and psychological factors control the complex process known as appetite. The hypothalamus and brainstem receive these peripheral neural and hormonal signals and co-ordinate a response in order to achieve energy homeostasis. Two discrete populations of neurones present in the arcuate nucleus (ARC) of the hypothalamus with opposing effects on food intake are crucial in this process: medially located orexigenic neurones (i.e. those stimulating appetite) express neuropeptide Y (NPY) and agouti-related peptide (AgRP), and anorexigenic neurones (i.e. those inhibiting appetite) in the lateral ARC express pro-opiomelanocortin (POMC) and cocaine and amphetamine-regulated transcript (CART) [2]. Additionally, ARC neurones also project onto the paraventricular nucleus (PVN) of the hypothalamus where important efferent pathways regulating energy expenditure arise.

The important inputs to this intricate neural network are twofold. Firstly, the short-term signals that govern meal ingestion are primarily regulated by the 'gut–brain axis' and secondly, information regarding long-term energy stores is signalled via leptin, an adipose-derived hormone [3]. This 'gut–brain axis' exists to contribute to the short-term feelings of satiety and hunger, by transmitting information from the gastrointestinal tract to the hypothalamus and brainstem, via gut hormones and the vagus nerve (see Figure 1.9.1). The majority of these gut hormones are anorexigenic and include peptide tyrosine- tyrosine (PYY), pancreatic polypeptide (PP), glucagon-like peptide-1(GLP-1), oxyntomodulin (OXM) and cholecystokinin (CCK). The only truly orexigenic hormone to be discovered thus far is ghrelin. These hormones act in concert as meal initiators and terminators [4].

These endogenous gut hormones act on the central nervous system either via the circulation

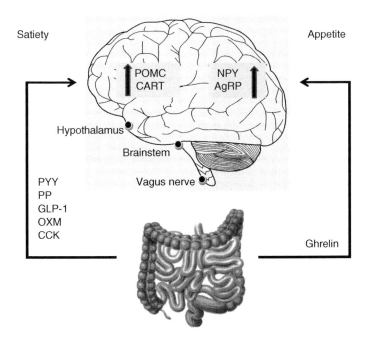

Figure 1.9.1 Mechanism of gut hormone action. Hormones released from the gastrointestinal tract into the circulation act on the brain to modulate appetite. Three sites are known to be of key importance: the hypothalamus, brainstem and vagus nerve. AgRP, agouti-related peptide; CART, cocaine- and amphetamine-regulated transcript; CCK, cholecystokinin; GLP-1, glucagon-like peptide 1; NPY, neuropeptide Y; POMC, pro-opiomelanocortin; OXM, oxyntomodulin; PP, pancreatic polypeptide; PYY, peptide tyrosine-tyrosine.

through areas deficient in the blood–brain barrier, such as the median eminence of the hypothalamus and the area postrema [5] or via receptors of vagal afferents, together with stretch receptors and nutrient chemoreceptors [6]. These signals converge in the nucleus of the tractus solitarius (NTS) of the brainstem and are integrated with information from higher brain centres relaying reward drive and mood to regulate appetite and control energy expenditure. In this chapter, a review of the key gut hormones implicated in appetite regulation is undertaken.

1.9.2 Peptide tyrosine-tyrosine

Peptide tyrosine-tyrosine is a member of the PP-fold family of peptides, which also includes the anorexigenic PP and the orexigenic neurotransmitter NPY, all sharing a common tertiary structure. PYY exists endogenously in two forms: peptide tyrosine-tyrosine$_{1-36}$ and PYY$_{3-36}$ [7]. Enzymatic cleavage of

secreted PYY$_{1-36}$ at the amino terminal by the enzyme dipeptidyl peptidase IV (DPP-IV) gives rise to PYY$_{3-36}$ [8], the predominant form of circulating PYY.

Peptide tyrosine-tyrosine is released postprandially by the L-cells of the distal gut in proportion to the energy content consumed. Plasma PYY$_{3-36}$ concentrations rise within 15 min of food ingestion, well before nutrients reach the colon or rectum where it is released, implicating a neural or hormonal mechanism for its release [9]. PYY$_{3-36}$ concentrations peak 1–2 h postprandially and remain elevated for up to 6 h [10]. Protein-rich meals cause the greatest increase in PYY concentrations compared to other macronutrients [11]. The effects of PYY are thought to be mediated centrally via the G-protein-coupled Y receptors, in particular the Y2 receptor [12], which is densely expressed in the ARC. Peptide tyrosine-tyrosine may also exert its actions via the vagus nerve which also expresses the Y2 receptor [13]. Interestingly, obese individuals have lower fasting PYY$_{3-36}$ concentrations than their lean counterparts, suggesting that obesity is a 'PYY-deficient' state [10].

Peptide tyrosine-tyrosine changes occur in several gastrointestinal disorders. PYY concentration in tissue extracts from the ileum and colon of patients with Crohn's colitis and ulcerative colitis has been found to be lower than in controls [14]. Furthermore, rectal and fasting plasma PYY concentrations have been reported to be reduced in patients with ulcerative colitis. This decrease in PYY could contribute to the development of the symptoms seen in inflammatory bowel disease; for example, diarrhoea may be brought about by hindering the ileal brake and loss of inhibition of intestinal transit. Conversely, total PYY concentrations have recently been found to be increased, both pre- and postprandially, in patients with Crohn's disease affecting the small intestine. It appears that enhanced enteroendocrine cell responses may play a role in feeding disturbance and weight loss [15]. In patients with coeliac disease, basal and postprandial plasma concentrations of PYY are elevated. These elevated concentrations of PYY normalise within 8 months on a gluten-free diet [16]. PYY concentrations in cerebrospinal fluid (CSF) have been found to be elevated in normal-weight bulimic patients abstinent for a month from pathological eating behaviour. However, CSF PYY concentrations were not affected in women who had recovered from anorexia [17]. Plasma concentrations of PYY have not yet been investigated in this group of patients.

1.9.3 Pancreatic polypeptide

Pancreatic polypeptide is an amidated 36-amino acid peptide, structurally similar to PYY. It is released postprandially under vagal control from pancreatic islet PP cells, in proportion to caloric intake. A biphasic response is observed postprandially and concentrations remain elevated for up to 6 h after a meal [18]. Pancreatic polypeptide is thought to mediate its effects via the Y4 receptor, which is highly expressed in the brainstem and ARC [19].

Fasting plasma concentrations of PP are lower in obese individuals, as is the second phase of release after food consumption [20]. Children with Prader–Willi syndrome, a condition characterised by hyperphagia and obesity, have reduced fasting and postprandial concentrations of PP [21]. In contrast, increased concentrations of PP are observed in patients with anorexia nervosa [22]. Pancreatic polypeptide release is reduced in patients with slow transit constipation, but increased in those with functional diarrhoea [23]. Levels are unchanged in patients with coeliac disease [24] but patients with ulcerative colitis have significantly elevated fasting PP concentrations [25].

1.9.4 Glucagon-like peptide 1

Glucagon-like peptide 1 is a product of proglucagon, secreted by enteroendocrine L-cells in the intestine. After a meal, it is released in response to direct L-cell stimulation by nutrients within the GI lumen, and indirectly via neuronal pathways within the enteric nervous system. Glucagon-like peptide 1_{1-37} is processed intracellularly to generate the 7–37 and 7–36 amide peptides. Glucagon-like peptide 1 is inactivated by dipeptidyl peptidase-4 (DPP-4) which processes GLP-1_{7-37} and GLP-1_{7-36} amide to GLP-1_{9-36} amide.

Glucagon-like peptide 1 binds the G-protein-coupled GLP-1 receptor expressed by pancreatic islet cells as well as brain, heart and lung tissue [26]. The actions of GLP-1 are best characterised in the beta cell where GLP-1 exerts an incretin effect, the stimulation of glucose-dependent insulin release from pancreatic beta cells [27]. Therefore, until recently, the focus on GLP-1 has been largely as an antidiabetic agent and two long-acting analogues of GLP-1, exenatide and liraglutide, are licensed for the treatment of diabetes.

In contrast to insulin, however, GLP-1 causes a decrease in body weight [28]. Acute intravenous injection of GLP-1 reduces appetite and energy intake [29]. This effect has been observed in lean, obese and diabetic volunteers. The actions of GLP-1 on appetite are likely to be related to a direct effect on the central nervous system (CNS) via activation of POMC-expressing neurones in the ARC, as well as through delayed gastric emptying [30].

In gastrointestinal disease, circulating concentrations of GLP-1 can be affected. In both ulcerative colitis and Crohn's disease, postprandial GLP-1 responses are augmented [31]. In coeliac disease, concentrations are unaffected [32]. Research into GLP-1 physiology in these inflammatory gastrointestinal conditions is limited and thus far, the emphasis of investigation has been in the field of diabetes and obesity. It is well established that obese subjects have diminished postprandial GLP-1 responses compared to lean controls, but improved secretion is observed after weight loss [33]. The mechanism by which obesity affects GLP-1 secretion is not known but may be related to the insulin resistance that accompanies weight gain, and which also impairs GLP-1 release. The prospect of using long-acting analogues of GLP-1 as a treatment for obesity is eagerly anticipated.

1.9.5 Oxyntomodulin

Also formed by the cleavage of proglucagon, OXM is secreted by the L-cells postprandially, in proportion to energy intake [34]. In addition to reducing appetite, OXM delays gastric emptying and reduces gastric acid secretion [35]. Furthermore, chronic administration of OXM causes rats to lose more weight than pair-fed controls, suggesting that its weight loss effect may be mediated by an increase in energy expenditure [36].

Although OXM is a dual agonist at both the glucagon and GLP-1 receptors, the anorectic effects of OXM are abolished in GLP-1 receptor knockout mice, suggesting that its action on appetite control is primarily via the GLP-1 receptor [37]. OXM concentrations in gastrointestinal disease have not been well studied.

1.9.6 Cholecystokinin

Cholecystokinin is released postprandially from the I-cells of small intestine, and also co-localises with PYY in L-cells. After a meal, CCK is secreted in response to saturated fat, long-chain fatty acids, amino acids and small peptides that would normally result from protein digestion [38]. After lipid ingestion, CCK is released and binds CCK1 receptors, thereby stimulating release of PYY and inhibition of ghrelin [39]. Both of these hormones act to further inhibit food intake. Postprandial secretion of

CCK also stimulates pancreatic enzyme secretion and gallbladder contraction, leading to release of bile salts into the duodenum, promoting protein and fat digestion [38]. In addition, CCK is implicated in other gastrointestinal functions, including gastric emptying [40].

Cholecystokinin appears to have a role in the pathogenesis of gallstone disease. Recent studies have shown that postprandial concentrations of CCK are higher in patients with reduced gallbladder contractility, predisposing them to gallstone disease, compared to their healthy counterparts. Interestingly, CCK1 receptor expression in the gallbladders of these patients was lower [41]. This finding is supported by the phenotype of CCK1 receptor knockout mice, in which the prevalence of gallstones is markedly increased [42].

In patients with Crohn's disease, postprandial CCK concentrations were markedly increased compared to a control group, and patients with ulcerative colitis and diverticulitis. This excessive postprandial release of CCK may be responsible for the delayed gastric emptying observed in these patients [31]. Similarly in *Giardia* enteritis, elevated postprandial CCK concentrations were correlated with anorectic symptoms upon feeding and treatment led to normalisation of CCK concentrations and symptoms [43].

1.9.7 Ghrelin

Ghrelin is a 28-amino acid peptide that is acylated by the enzyme ghrelin O-acyltransferase (GOAT) and secreted from the gastric fundus. It binds to the growth hormone secretagogue receptor type 1 (GHSR) and stimulates release of growth hormone from the pituitary gland [44]. It is the only true orexigenic gut hormone to have been discovered thus far.

Plasma ghrelin concentrations are highest preprandially, both when meals are provided at scheduled times and when individuals are allowed to eat at will [45]. Fasting ghrelin concentrations are low in obese subjects and chronically high in patients with weight loss due to anorexia nervosa or dietary restriction [46]. In lean people, concentrations decrease after a test meal but do not change in patients with obesity [47]. There is recent evidence that diet-induced obesity may blunt the orexigenic effects of ghrelin. High-fat feeding renders NPY/AgRP neurones relatively ghrelin resistant [48], and diets high in fat directly inhibit the hyperphagic effect of ghrelin [49]. Furthermore, ghrelin interacts with neurones in the ventral tegmental area of the brain and may provide a link between the GI tract and central control of stress-induced eating of 'comfort foods' [50].

Ghrelin seems to be affected in several gastrointestinal diseases. Serum ghrelin concentrations are significantly higher in patients with active ulcerative colitis and Crohn's disease compared to those in remission or controls. Levels were positively correlated with erythrocyte sedimentation rate and C-reactive protein and negatively correlated with nutritional status parameters [51]. In children with coeliac disease, serum ghrelin was higher than those of controls and negatively correlated with Body Mass Index (BMI). Ghrelin concentrations decreased after 6 months of gluten-free diet compared with the concentrations detected on admission [52]. *Helicobacter pylori* infection is associated with reduced circulating ghrelin concentrations independent of sex and BMI. Ghrelin concentrations increased, however, 12 weeks after successful *H. pylori* eradication [53]. In patients with gastric cancer, ghrelin in the gastric mucosa is affected. Gastrectomy decreased the plasma concentration, regardless of the extent of gastric resection [54]. Ghrelin serum concentrations were significantly lower in colon cancer patients compared with controls [55].

1.9.8 Conclusion

In conclusion, the GI tract is now recognised as an endocrine organ that secretes a variety of hormones. These gut hormones play a crucial role in the control of appetite and hence energy homeostasis. Changes in gut hormones concentrations have been identified in several gastrointestinal disorders but the molecular mechanisms by which individual diseases are affected still need to be resolved. Furthermore, the clinical implications of these changes are yet to be elucidated.

Acknowledgements

JC has no financial interests to declare. SRB is an inventor of United Kingdom patent application nos. PCT/GB02/04082 and PCT/GB/04/00017 and was a consultant for Thiakis, now a subsidiary of Pfizer.

References

1. Rosenbaum M, Leibel RL, Hirsch J. Obesity. *New England Journal of Medicine* 1997; **337**: 396–407.
2. Schwartz MW, Woods SC, Porte Jr D, Seeley RJ, Baskin DG. Central nervous system control of food intake. *Nature* 2000; **404**: 661–671.
3. Morris DL, Rui LY. Recent advances in understanding leptin signaling and leptin resistance. *American Journal of Physiology - Endocrinology and Metabolism* 2009; **297**: E1247–E1259.
4. Chaudhri OB, Field BC, Bloom SR. Gastrointestinal satiety signals. *International Journal of Obesity* 2008; **32**(Suppl 7): S28–S31.
5. Peruzzo B, Pastor FE, Blazquez JL, et al. A second look at the barriers of the medial basal hypothalamus. *Experimental Brain Research* 2000; **132**: 10–26.
6. Jobst EE, Enriori PJ, Cowley MA. The electrophysiology of feeding circuits. *Trends in Endocrinology and Metabolism* 2004; **15**: 488–499.
7. Grandt D, Schimiczek M, Struk K, et al. Characterization of two forms of peptide YY, PYY(1–36) and PYY(3–36), in the rabbit. *Peptides* 1994; **15**: 815–820.
8. Medeiros MD, Turner AJ. Processing and metabolism of peptide-YY: pivotal roles of dipeptidylpeptidase-IV, aminopeptidase-P, and endopeptidase-24.11. *Endocrinology* 1994; **134**: 2088–2094.
9. Adrian TE, Ferri G, Bacarese-Hamilton AJ, Fuessl HS, Polak JM, Bloom SR. Human distribution and release of a putative new gut hormone, peptide YY. *Gastroenterology* 1985; **89**: 1070–1077.
10. Batterham RL, Cohen MA, Ellis SM. Inhibition of food intake in obese subjects by peptide YY3-36. *New England Journal of Medicine* 2003; **349**: 941–948.
11. Batterham RL, Heffron H, Kapoor S, et al. Critical role for peptide YY in protein-mediated satiation and body-weight regulation. *Cell Metabolism* 2006; **4**: 223–233.
12. Grandt D, Teyssen S, Schimiczek M, et al. Novel generation of hormone receptor specificity by amino terminal processing of peptide YY. *Biochemical and Biophysical Research Communications* 1992; **186**: 1299–1306.
13. Koda S, Date Y, Murakami N, et al. The role of the vagal nerve in peripheral PYY3-36-induced feeding reduction in rats. *Endocrinology* 2005; **146**: 2369–2375.
14. Koch TR, Roddy DR, Go VL. Abnormalities of fasting serum concentrations of peptide YY in the idiopathic inflammatory bowel disease. *American Journal of Gastroenterology* 1987; **82**: 321–326.

15. Moran G, Leslie FC, McLaughlin JT. Crohn's disease affecting the small bowel is associated with reduced appetite and elevated levels of circulating gut peptides. *Clinical Nutrition* 2013; **32**(3): 404–411.

16. Sjölund K, Ekman R. Inceased plasma level of peptide YY in coeliac disease. *Scandinavian Journal of Gastroenterology* 1988; **23**: 297–300.

17. Gendall KA, Kaye WH, Altemus M, McConaha CW, La Via MC. Leptin, neuropeptide Y, and peptide YY in long-term recovered eating disorder patients. *Biological Psychiatry* 1999; **46**: 292–299.

18. Adrian TE, Bloom SR, Bryant MG, Polak JM, Heitz PH, Barnes AJ. Distribution and release of human pancreatic polypeptide. *Gut* 1976; **17**: 940–944.

19. Bard JA, Walker MW, Branchek TA, Weinshank RL. Cloning and functional expression of a human y4 subtype receptor for pancreatic-polypeptide, neuropeptide-y, and peptide yy. *Journal of Biological Chemistry* 1995; **270**: 26762–26765.

20. Lassmann V, Vague P, Vialettes B, Simon MC. Low plasma-levels of pancreatic-polypeptide in obesity. *Diabetes* 1980; **29**: 428–430.

21. Zipf WB, Odorisio TM, Cataland S, Dixon K. Pancreatic-polypeptide responses to protein meal challenges in obese but otherwise normal children and obese children with Prader–Willi syndrome. *Journal of Clinical Endocrinology and Metabolism* 1983; **57**: 1074–1080.

22. Fujimoto S, Inui A, Kiyota N. Increased cholecystokinin and pancreatic polypeptide responses to a fat-rich meal in patients with restrictive but not bulimic anorexia nervosa. *Biological Psychiatry* 1997; **41**(10): 1068–1070.

23. Preston DM, Adrian TE, Christofides ND, Lennard-Jones JE, Bloom SR. Positive correlation between symptoms and circulating motilin, pancreatic polypeptide and gastrin concentrations in functional bowel disorders. *Gut* 1985; **26**(10): 1059–1064.

24. Besterman HS, Bloom SR, Sarson DL, et al. Gut-hormone profile in coeliac disease. *Lancet* 1978; **1**(8068): 785–788.

25. Besterman HS, Mallinson CN, Modigliani R, et al. Gut hormones in inflammatory bowel disease. *Scandinavian Journal of Gastroenterology* 1983; **7**: 845–852.

26. Thorens B. Expression cloning of the pancreatic beta-cell receptor for the gluco-incretin hormone glucagon-like peptide-1. *Proceedings of the National Academy of Sciences of the United States of America* 1992; **89**(18): 8641–8645.

27. Kreymann B, Williams G, Ghatei MA, Bloom SR. Glucagonlike peptide-1 7–36 – a physiological incretin in man. *Lancet* 1987; **2**(8571): 1300–1304.

28. Zander M, Madsbad S, Madsen JL, Holst JJ. Effect of 6-week course of glucagon-like peptide 1 on glycaemic control, insulin sensitivity, and beta-cell function in type 2 diabetes: a parallel-group study. *Lancet* 2002; **359**(9309): 824–830.

29. Verdich C, Flint A, Gutzwiller JP, Naslund E, Beglinger C, Hellstrom PM. A meta-analysis of the effect of glucagon-like peptide-1 (7–36) amide on ad libitum energy intake in humans. *Journal of Clinical Endocrinology and Metabolism* 2001; **86**(9): 4382–4389(a).

30. Willms B, Werner J, Holst JJ, Orskov C, Creutzfeldt W, Nauck MA. Gastric emptying glucose responses, and insulin secretion after a liquid test meal: effects of exogenous glucagon-like peptide-1 (GLP-1)-(7–36) amide in type 2 (noninsulin-dependent) diabetic patients. *Journal of Clinical Endocrinology and Metabolism* 1996; **81**(1): 327–332.

31. Keller J, Beglinger C, Holst JJ, Andresen V, Layer P. Mechanisms of gastric emptying disturbances in chronic and acute inflammation of the distal gastrointestinal tract. *American Journal of Physiology, Gastrointestinal and Liver Physiology* 2009; **297**(5): G861–G868.

32. Caddy GR, Ardill JE, Fillmore D, et al. Plasma concentrations of glucagon-like peptide-2 in adult patients with treated and untreated coeliac disease. *European Journal of Gastroenterology and Hepatology* 2006; **18**: 195–202.

33. Verdich C, Toubro S, Buemann B, Lysgard MJ, Juul HJ, Astrup A. The role of postprandial releases of insulin and incretin hormones in meal-induced satiety-effect of obesity and weight reduction. *International Journal of Obesity and Related Metabolic Disorders* 2001; **25**: 1206–1214(b).

34. Le Quellec A, Kervran A, Blache P, Ciurana AJ, Bataille D. Oxyntomodulin-like immunoreactivity: diurnal profile of a new potential enterogastrone. *Journal of Clinical Endocrinology and Metabolism* 1992; **74**: 1405–1409.

35. Schjoldager B, Mortensen PE, Myhre J, Christiansen J, Holst J. Oxyntomodulin from distal gut. Role in regulation of gastric and pancreatic functions. *Digestive Diseases and Sciences* 1989; **34**: 1411–1419.

36. Dakin CL, Small CJ, Park AJ, Seth A, Ghatei MA, Bloom SR. Repeated ICV administration of oxyntomodulin causes a greater reduction in body weight gain than in pair-fed rats. *American Journal of Physiology – Endocrinology and Metabolism* 2002; **283**: E1173–E1177.

37. Baggio LL, Huang Q, Brown TJ, Drucker DJ. Oxyntomodulin and glucagon-like peptide-1 differentially regulate murine food intake and energy expenditure. *Gastroenterology* 2004; **127**: 546–558.

38. Rehfeld JF, Bungaard JR, Friis-Hansen L, Goetze JP. On the tissue-specific processing of procholecystokinin in the brain and gut – a short review. *Journal of Physiology and Pharmacology* 2003; **54**(4): 73–79.

39. Degen L, Drewe J, Piccoli F, et al. Effect of CCK-1 receptor blockade on ghrelin and PYY secretion in men. *American Journal of Physiology – Regulatory, Integrative and Comparative Physiology* 2007; **292**: R1391–R1399.

40. Fried M, Erlacher U, Schwizer W, et al. Role of cholecystokinin in the regulation of gastric emptying and pancreatic enzyme secretion in humans. Studies with the cholecystokinin-receptor antagonist loxiglumide. *Gastroenterology* 1991; **101**: 503–511.

41. Zhu J, Han T-Q, Chen S. Gallbladder motor function, plasma cholecystokinin and cholecystokinin receptor of gallbladder in cholesterol stone patients. *World Journal of Gastroenterology* 2005; **11**: 1685–1689.

42. Wang DQ-H, Schmitz F, Kopin AS. Targeted disruption of the murine cholecystokinin-1 receptor promotes intestinal cholesterol absorption and susceptibility to cholesterol cholelithiasis. *Journal of Clinical Investigation* 2004; **114**: 521–528.

43. Dizdar V, Spiller R, Singh G, et al. Relative importance of abnormalities of CCK and 5-HT (serotonin) in Giardia-induced

post-infectious irritable bowel syndrome and functional dyspepsia. *Alimentary Pharmacology and Therapeutics* 2010; **31**(8): 883–891.

44. Kojima M, Hosoda H, Date Y, Nakazato M, Matsuo H, Kangawa K. Ghrelin is a growth-hormone-releasing acylated peptide from stomach. *Nature* 1999; **402**(6762): 656–660.

45. Cummings DE, Frayo RS, Marmonier C, Aubert R, Chapelot D. Plasma ghrelin levels and hunger scores in humans initiating meals voluntarily without time- and food-related cues. *American Journal of Physiology – Endocrinology and Metabolism* 2004; **287**(2): E297–E304.

46. Ariyasu H, Takaya K, Tagami T, et al. Stomach is a major source of circulating ghrelin, and feeding state determines plasma ghrelin-like immunoreactivity levels in humans. *Journal of Clinical Endocrinology and Metabolism* 2001; **86**: 4753–4758.

47. English PJ, Ghatei MA, Malik IA, Bloom SR, Wilding JP. Food fails to suppress ghrelin levels in obese humans. *Journal of Clinical Endocrinology and Metabolism* 2002; **87**(6): 2984.

48. Briggs DI, Enriori PJ, Lemus MB, Cowley MA, Andrews ZB. Diet-induced obesity causes ghrelin resistance in arcuate NPY/AgRP neurons. *Endocrinology* 2010; **151**: 4745–4755.

49. Gardiner JV, Campbell D, Patterson M, et al. The hyperphagic effect of ghrelin is inhibited in mice by a diet high in fat. *Gastroenterology* 2010; **138**: 2468–2476.

50. Chuang JC, Perello M, Sakata I, et al. Ghrelin mediates stress-induced food-reward behavior in mice. *Journal of Clinical Investigation* 2011; **121**: 2684–2692.

51. Ates Y, Degertekin B, Edril A, Yaman H, Dagalp K. Serum ghrelin levels in inflammatory bowel disease with relation to disease activity and nutrition status. *Digestive Diseases and Sciences* 2008; **53**: 2215–2221.

52. Selimoglu MA, Altinkaynak S, Ertekin V, Akcay F. Serum ghrelin levels in children with celiac disease. *Journal of Clinical Gastroenterology* 2006; **40**(3): 191–194.

53. Osawa H, Kita H, Ohnishi H, et al. Changes in plasma ghrelin levels, gastric ghrelin production, and body weight after Helicobacter pylori cure. *Journal of Gastroenterology* 2006; **41**: 954–961.

54. An JY, Choi MG, Noh JH, Sohn TS, Jin DK, Kim S. Clinical significance of ghrelin concentration of plasma and tumor tissue in patients with gastric cancer. *Journal of Surgical Research* 2007; **143**: 344–349.

55. D'Onghia V, Leoncini R, Carli R, et al. Circulating gastrin and ghrelin levels in patients with colorectal cancer: correlation with tumour stage. Helicobacter pylori infection and BMI. *Biomedicine and Pharmacotherapy* 2007; **61**: 137–141.

Dietary components relevant to gastrointestinal health

Chapter 2.1

Fibre and gastrointestinal health

Vikas Kumar,[1] Amit Kumar Sinha,[2] Han-ping Wang[1] and Gudrun De Boeck[2]
[1]Ohio State University, Ohio, USA
[2]University of Antwerp, Antwerp, Belgium

The term 'fibre' was first used by Eben Hipsley in 1953. During his observations he found that populations with fibre-rich diets tended to have lower rates of pregnancy toxaemia [1]. In 1976, Trowell defined fibre as the component of plant foods that resisted digestion by enzymes produced by humans [2].

Dietary fibre is a group of non-digestible plant polysaccharides which escapes digestion and absorption in the upper gastrointestinal (GI) tract and is termed non-starch polysaccharides (NSPs). Plant ingredients generally contain a mixture of both water-soluble and insoluble fibre. Soluble fibre disperses when mixed with water and has the ability to increase the viscosity of digesta which slows down the diffusion of digestive enzymes and the absorption of nutrients. This reduction in absorption lowers postprandial glucose, cholesterol and insulin responses, which has significant implications for the prevention and management of insulin-resistant and type 2 diabetes.

Soluble fibre is mainly found inside the cells of fruits, vegetables, beans and oat bran, and consists of pectins, gums and mucilages. Insoluble fibre possesses high water-binding capacity, renders faecal content softer and bulkier, and allows easy luminal passage [3], thereby playing a crucial role in the correct functioning of the GI tract. Cellulose, lignin and hemicellulose contain insoluble fibre and are widely found in wheat, whole grains, fruits and vegetables.

A major proportion of NSPs escapes the small intestine nearly intact, and is fermented by commensal microbiota residing in the caecum and colon into short-chain fatty acids (SCFAs), promoting normal laxation. Short-chain fatty acids have a number of health-promoting effects such as maintaining normal GI structure and function, preventing or alleviating colon-based diarrhoea, lowering colonic pH, inhibiting growth of pathogenic organisms [4], improving mineral utilisation, stimulating proliferation of colonic epithelial cells, thereby increasing the absorptive capacity of the epithelium, and stimulating colonic blood flow and fluid and electrolyte uptake. Non-starch polysaccharides may benefit human health by reducing and/or limiting the risk of both acute and chronic diseases, such as infectious diarrhoea, obesity, diabetes, colorectal cancer, neonatal necrotising enterocolitis and inflammatory bowel disease through various mechanisms including a physiological effect on the GI tract, colonic fermentation, immunomodulation and a prebiotic effect [4,5]. Subsequently, NSP intake can be viewed as a marker of a healthy diet and higher dependency on fibre-supplemented food reflects a healthier lifestyle [5].

2.1.1 Classification of non-starch polysaccharides

According to Phillips [6], the 2009 meeting of the Codex Committee on Nutrition and Foods for Special Dietary Uses finally agreed upon the following definition – that NSPs are carbohydrate polymers with ≥10 monomeric units which are not hydrolysed by the endogenous enzymes in the small intestine of humans and belong to the following categories.

(1) Edible carbohydrate polymers naturally occurring in food as consumed.
(2) Carbohydrate polymers, which have been obtained from raw food material by physical, enzymatic or chemical means and which have been shown to have a physiological effect or benefit to health as established by mostly accepted scientific proof from competent authorities.
(3) Synthetic carbohydrate polymers which have been shown to have a physiological benefit to health as demonstrated by generally accepted scientific evidence from competent authorities [7].

Fibre from different sources may vary in a number of physical and chemical characteristics. Even though fibre was conventionally classified according to solubility, additional properties, such as viscosity and fermentability, are now being recognized as more important in terms of specific physiological benefits [8] (Table 2.1.1). Generally, soluble fibres are fermented and have a higher viscosity than insoluble fibres. Nevertheless, most soluble fibres are not viscous (e.g. acacia gum, partially hydrolysed guar gum), whereas a few of the insoluble fibres may be well fermented (e.g. finely ground soy polysaccharides) [8].

2.1.2 Clinical effect of non-starch polysaccharides

Dietary supplementation of fibre has a wide array of beneficial health effects as already described. It is well known that the human GI tract is less suited to the modern high-fat, energy-rich and low-volume diets of urbanised countries but better suited to cope with a diet rich in NSP with a large volume. Consequently, low NSP intake is associated with many Western diseases such as obesity, type 2 diabetes and gastrointestinal disorders. Based on various scientific reports, it is apparent that the majority of the clinical effect of NSP intake is promoted by the fibre-mediated alterations in the functional processes of the GI tract. As such, this chapter will highlight the health-promoting effects of NSPs on the GI tract and the key mechanisms associated with modulating the clinical benefits of fibre intake.

Physiological effects of fibre on the GI tract

Dietary intake of fibre influences the entire GI tract from mouth to anus. Foods rich in fibre have lower energy density and take longer to empty from the stomach. Water-soluble fibre usually delays gastric emptying and slows the transit of food materials through the small intestine, consequently increasing nutrient absorption time [9]. In the GI tract (particularly the small intestine), fibre can elicit responses of a wide variety of gut hormones that serve as incretins to stimulate insulin release and affect appetite [10]. Fibre can also bind with bile acids and impede micelle formation, thus increasing faecal excretion of bile acids and cholesterol [11]. Consumption of a diet low in NSP could lead to watery stools and the addition of pectin significantly reduces the occurrence of watery stools and promotes normalisation of colonic fluid composition [12]. Reports suggest that consumption of pectin and soy polysaccharides increases colonic water absorption, probably mediated via SCFA production, suggesting that reduction in luminal SCFA levels in antibiotic-associated colitis may be responsible for diarrhoea [13]. Ramakrishna and Mathan (1993) further confirmed that acute watery diarrhoea is associated with a reduction in luminal SCFAs and a decrease of net water and sodium absorption in the colon [14].

Short-chain fatty acids also stimulate colonic blood flow and smooth muscular activity [15]. The greater blood flow enhances tissue oxygenation and transport of absorbed nutrients. The mechanism of action of SCFAs on blood flow may involve local neural networks as well as chemoreceptors together

Table 2.1.1 Classification of non-starch polysaccharides based on three physicochemical characteristics [5,8,55]

Types	Properties	Solubility	Fermentability*	Viscosity*
Acacia gum	A non-viscous, soluble fibre obtained as an exudate from the branches and stems of *Acacia senegal* and *Acacia seyal*. A highly branched, high molecular weight molecule consisting of galactose, arabinose, rhamnose and glucuronic acid units.	Soluble	Fermentable	
Guar gum	Guar gum is produced by milling the endosperm of the guar seed. The major polysaccharide is galactomannan. Galactomannans are highly viscous and are therefore used as food ingredients for their thickening, gelling and stabilising properties.	Soluble		Non-viscous
Partially hydrolysed guar gum (PHGG)	The structure consists of a mannose backbone with galactose side units. PHGG is a soluble fibre with only marginal effects on viscosity, yet it seems to retain the ability of native guar gum to lower glucose and insulin levels.	Soluble	Fermentable	Viscous
Inulin, oligofructose and fructo-oligosaccharides	Inulin, oligofructose (OF) and fructo-oligosaccharides (FOS) belong to a larger class called inulin-type fructans, which refers to all linear fructans that contain beta-2,1 fructosyl-fructose glycosidic bonds. These molecules differ in chain length and method of extraction or synthesis, yet nomenclature is inconsistent in the literature. In general, inulin refers to molecules with an average degree of polymerisation ≥10, whereas FOS and OF refer to shorter chain molecules. FOS, OF and inulin are non-viscous, soluble fibres obtained from a number of foods (primarily chicory root) or produced synthetically by adding fructose units to a sucrose molecule via beta-1,2 linkages (FOS only).	Soluble	Fermentable	Non-viscous
Pectin	Pectins are mainly present in the cell wall and intracellular tissues of many fruits and berries, and consist of galacturonic acid units with rhamnose interspersed in a linear chain. Pectins frequently have side chains of neutral sugars, and the galactose units may be esterified with a methyl group, a feature that allows for its viscosity.	Soluble	Fermentable	Non-viscous

(*Continued*)

Table 2.1.1 Continued

Types	Properties	Solubility	Fermentability*	Viscosity*
Hemicellulose A	Its structure is that of an acidic xylan, a linear chain of beta-D-xylopyranosyl units, bonded together by (1->4) glycosidic links, containing single alpha-D-xylopyranosyl and 4-O-methyl-alpha-D-glucopyranuronosyl residues.	Soluble		
Oat fibre	Oat beta-glucans are non-starch polysaccharides. Like starch, oat beta-glucans are composed of glucose molecules in long chains but the binding between glucose mononers differs from starch. It has both $(1 \rightarrow 4)$- and $(1 \rightarrow 3)$ linkages. About 70% of the links are beta$(1 \rightarrow 4)$- and the rest are beta$(1 \rightarrow 3)$. The distribution is not random. The mixed linkages that form oat beta-glucans are important for their physical properties, such as viscosity and solubility. The GI tract does not contain enzymes that can digest oat beta-glucans.	Soluble		Viscous
Mixed-linked beta-glucans	Mixed-linked beta-glucans occur exclusively in members of the monocotyledon family Poaceae, to which the cereals and grasses belong, and in related families of the order Poales. Mixed-linked beta-glucans are also referred as $(1 \rightarrow 3,1 \rightarrow 4)$- beta-D-glucans or cereal beta-glucans. They are linear, unbranched polysaccharides in which beta-D-glucopyranosyl monomers are polymerised through both beta$(1 \rightarrow 4)$- and beta$(1 \rightarrow 3)$ linkages.	Soluble		
Polydextrose polyol	Polydextrose polyol is a water-soluble specialty carbohydrate which is manufactured from glucose. It is a complex carbohydrate and traditionally used as a bulking agent in foods. It is like other polyols and can be used as a sugar and fat replacer. It is particularly valuable in the production of low-calorie foods.	Soluble		
Psyllium	Psyllium refers to the husk of psyllium seeds and is a very viscous mucilage in aqueous solution. The psyllium seed, also known as plantago or flea seed, is small, dark, reddish-brown, odourless and nearly tasteless. *P. ovata*, known as blond or Indian plantago seed, is the species from which husk is usually derived.	Soluble		

Wheat dextrin	Wheat dextrins are a group of low molecular weight carbohydrates produced by the hydrolysis of starch or glycogen. Dextrins are mixtures of polymers of D-glucose units linked by alpha$(1 \rightarrow 4)$ or alpha$(1 \rightarrow 6)$ glycosidic bonds. Dextrins can be produced from starch from malting and mashing and during digestion by the enzyme amylase.	Soluble		
Cellulose	Cellulose is the main structural component of all cell walls in cereal grains and is a linear homopolymer of beta$(1 \rightarrow 4)$ linked glucose units. Cellulose chains are long flat linear ribbons of glucose units with molecular weights of over 1,000,000. The beta$(1 \rightarrow 4)$ linkage between the glucose units holds the chain in a flat conformation so cellulose chains can align next to each other and form numerous hydrogen bonds between the sugar hydroxyl groups. Cellulose quantity in whole grains can vary from species to species and is largely a consequence of the thickness of the husk and seed coat.	Insoluble	Non-fermentable	Viscous
Soy polysaccharide	Soy polysaccharides are obtained from soy cotyledon and consist of a number of fibre components, including cellulose, hemicelluloses, lignin and pectin-like molecules. Although soy polysaccharides are typically 75–85% insoluble, they have been shown to be highly fermentable in humans, probably because of their small particle size.	Insoluble	Fermentable	Viscous
Resistant starch	Resistant starch refers to starch and products of starch digestion that are not absorbed in the small intestine and pass to the colon. It can be classified according to the characteristics that make it resistant to digestion (physically inaccessible, granular form, retrograded or chemically modified).	Insoluble	Fermentable	Viscous
Hemicellulose B	This hemicellulose seems to be a homogeneous polysaccharide with an apparent molecular weight of 35,000. Its structure is that of an acidic arabinoxylan, a linear chain of beta-D-xylopyranosyl units, bonded together by $(1 \rightarrow 4)$ glycosidic links, containing a single L-arabinofuranosyl, alpha-D-xylopyranosyl and 4-O-methyl-alpha-D-glucopyranuronosyl residues joined by glycosidic links.	Insoluble		

(*Continued*)

Table 2.1.1 Continued

Types	Properties	Solubility	Fermentability*	Viscosity*
Lignin	Lignin is a highly branched polymer composed of phenylpropanoid units and is found within 'woody' plant cell walls, covalently bound to fibrous polysaccharides.	Insoluble		
Outer pea fibre	Outer pea fibre is an insoluble fibre obtained from the hulls of the field pea and is composed of hemicelluloses, cellulose and pectic substances. It is primarily used to enhance the fibre content of products, without modifying functional or technical properties, and increases stool weight in healthy individuals.	Insoluble	Non-fermentable	Viscous
Resistant dextrins	Indigestible components of starch hydrolysates, as a result of heat and enzymatic treatment, yield indigestible dextrins that are also called resistant maltodextrins. The average molecular weight of resistant maltodextrins is 2000 daltons and they consist of polymers of glucose containing alpha$(1 \rightarrow 4)$ and alpha$(1 \rightarrow 6)$ glucosidic bonds, as well as $1 \rightarrow 2$ and $1 \rightarrow 3$ linkages.	Other		
Chitin and chitosan	Chitin is an amino-polysaccharide containing beta$(1 \rightarrow 4)$ linkages as are present in cellulose. Chitosan is the deacetylated product of chitin. Both chitin and chitosan are found in the exoskeletons of shrimp, crabs and lobsters and in the cell walls of most fungi.	Other		
Polydextrose	Polydextrose is a polysaccharide that is synthesised by random polymerisation of glucose and sorbitol. Polydextrose serves as a bulking agent in foods and sometimes as a sugar substitute. It is not digested or absorbed in the small intestine and is partially fermented in the large intestine, with the remnants excreted in the faeces.	Other		

*Fermentability and viscosity will vary depending on degree of water solubility and additionally for viscosity, physical form, molecular weight and concentration.

with direct effects on smooth muscle cells. Production of SCFAs in the colon also tends to activate the upper GI tract musculature and the ileocolonic brake directly in a dose-dependent manner [16]. Consumption of fermentable carbohydrate, inulin and beet fibre can also increase the bioavailability of various minerals such as calcium, magnesium and zinc in the colon [17].

Clinical effect of NSP intake on the GI tract

Dietary intake of NSPs can affect gastrointestinal health, in particular in relation to structural and physiological functions of the colonic wall, the mucus layer, immune function and its microbial ecosystem.

Gastrointestinal structure and health

A healthy GI tract is vital as it is the main site of digestion, absorption and substrate redistribution, and acts as a barrier to prevent foreign materials of dietary or microbial origin crossing into the internal body cavity. The effect of NSPs on the GI tract seems to be dependent on the ability of different fibre types to increase digesta viscosities. In the GI lumen, NSPs may have a major effect on the dynamic process of small intestinal cell turnover, crypt cell proliferation rates, migration along the crypt-villus axis, and cell extrusion from the villous apex via apoptosis and cell sloughing or invagination [18]. The production of SCFAs from bacterial fermentation of NSP is important both for protecting the health of the large intestinal wall and for stimulating repair in a damaged colon. The SCFAs, particularly butyrate and to a certain extent propionate, stimulate the proliferation of caecal crypt cells in normal human mucosa *in vitro* [19]. Increased epithelial cell proliferation in colonic crypts was also demonstrated in humans fed oat bran and oat gum [20].

The complete mechanisms by which SCFAs stimulate cell proliferation and growth of the small intestine are still poorly understood but it is likely that this effect is mediated by a systemic mediatory mechanism [21]. SCFAs also act as a potent stimulus

for colonic sodium and water absorption, as observed in humans [14,16]. Besides, SCFAs have a number of other favourable properties and relevance for GI structure and function as summarised below [22].

- Type of fibre (monosaccharide composition and chemical structure)
- Physical nature of the fibre (e.g. particle size and method of fibre preparation)
- Rate of hydrolysis of fibre
- Mix of different fibre types consumed
- Amount of fibre consumed
- Duration of fibre intake
- Colonic retention time (in turn stimulated by distension, bile acids, stimulation of mucosa by particulate matter and possibly distal fermentation and SCFA production)
- Other dietary components
- Colonic microbiota profiles

These properties may be of importance in maintaining the normal structure and function of the GI tract and preventing colonic-based abnormalities [23]. Ulcerative colitis has been linked with reduced faecal concentrations of SCFAs, impairment in butyrate oxidation and increased lactic acid levels during acute exacerbations [24].

Gastrointestinal mucus layer

The mucus layer of the GI tract is an important barrier lining. It provides lubrication and protects GI epithelium from the luminal stress of damaging agents, shear forces, toxins, enzymatic and acid degradation [25]. It also acts as a substrate for the gastrointestinal microbiota, serves as an antioxidant and facilitates the removal of micro-organisms [26]. It may also serve as a barrier to mucosal transport by reducing absorption of cholesterol [26] and have direct antioxidative effects in the GI tract [27]. The factors inducing intestinal mucus production and the associated dynamics are illustrated in Figure 2.1.1. The effects of different types of NSP on the intestinal mucus barrier have been assessed in a range of animal models, suggesting that alginates, wheat bran, ispaghula husk and ulvan benefit the protective potential of the

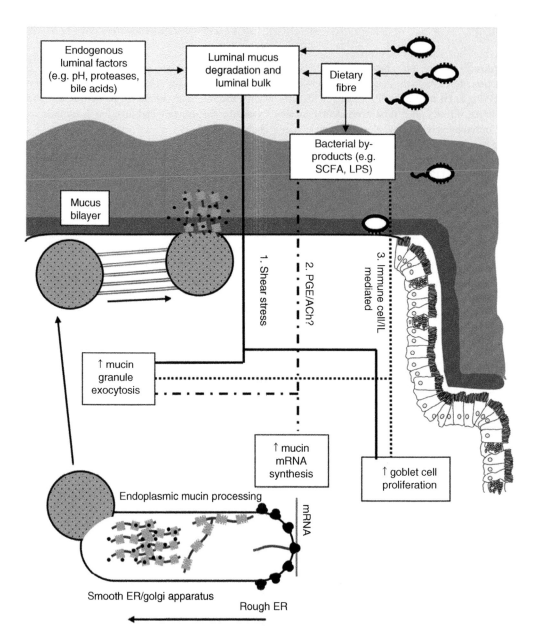

Figure 2.1.1 Modulation of mucus barrier dynamics by luminal factors in the intestine. A complex interplay of luminal factors of bacterial, endogenous and dietary origin results in luminal bulk and mucus degradation. The epithelium may respond to increased or decreased luminal stress by altering rates of mucin granule exocytosis, mucin mRNA synthesis or goblet cell proliferation. Luminal stress triggers three putative pathways that result in an epithelial response. 1. Shear stress or colonic distension results in triggering of the mucosal mechanoreceptors. 2. Prostaglandins or acetylcholine are released as a result of either increased luminal bulk or enteroendocrine cell response to changes in the luminal milieu. 3. Direct (e.g. bacterial adherence to epithelium) or indirect (e.g. chains to bacterial by-products) sensing of changes to the luminal bacterial populations by the GALT results in an immune-type response, driven by interleukins or other local mediators. These three pathways appear to drive different epithelial responses that drive mucin secretion. Within mucin production, proteins are synthesised with the rough endoplasmic reticulum, then glycosylated and polymerised. Prior to encapsulation in secretory vesicles, mucins are tightly packed into granules, in high calcium ion (*black dots*) concentration. As the vesicles join to the apical membrane, mucins rapidly swell upon hydration and separate from Ca++. ER, endoplasmic reticulum; LPS, lipopolysaccharide; PGE, prostaglandins; SCFA, short-chain fatty acids. Source: Allen and Flemstrom [25]; Brownlee et al. [28]; Brownlee [35]. Reproduced with permission from Elsevier.

colonic mucus layer and prevent bacterial translocation [28]. These effects are likely to occur through direct mechanical mechanisms or indirectly by regulating mucosal metabolism via SCFAs derived from fibre fermentation [29]. These effects may also be of great importance for protecting and repairing the GI tract, such as in patients with ulcerative colitis, ileal pouchitis, colonic anastomoses and short bowel syndrome [30]. The potential effects of fibre on components of the GI barrier and possible mechanisms involved are summarised in Table 2.1.2.

Gastrointestinal immunity

The GI tract is involved in a range of immune functions. Gut-associated lymphoid tissue (GALT) is dependent on dietary constituents, particularly those that stimulate the growth of health-promoting colonic microbiota [31,32]. In this respect, it has been reported that the constituents of dietary fibres such as inulin and other oligofructoses stimulate growth of bifidobacteria and lactobacilli in the colon. These bacterial colonies generate SCFAs and stimulate the GI immune system [32]. Other potential beneficial health effects include protection from infection, inducing vitamin and antioxidant production, reducing the number of potentially harmful bacteria, supporting digestion and absorption, bulking activity to prevent constipation and a reduction in the risk of colorectal cancer [31,32]. Despite all these potential implications, there are a limited number of studies favouring a role for NSPs in GI immune function [33]. Further studies are required to elucidate how NSPs intakes affect the GI microbiota and GI immune function.

Colonic microbiota

The colonic microbiota contains a large and diverse population of predominantly anaerobic bacteria. Non-starch polysaccharides are an important fuel for different groups of colonic microbiota and play a profound role in regulating their number and diversity. In the absence of NSPs or other luminal energy sources, colonic bacteria will utilise intestinal mucus as an energy substrate. As bacteria require the necessary enzymes to break down saccharide bonds of the diverse range of NSPs, fibre will clearly affect the dynamics of the microbiota.

The GI microbiota, besides being a component of the GI barrier, plays an important role in fermenting NSPs to produce SCFAs and acidify the colon environment. Therefore, the presence of any fermentable NSPs is likely to cause a reduction in colonic pH which is beneficial for the development of bacteria such as bifidobacteria and lactobacilli, and detrimental to the growth of potential pathogenic species by inducing colonisation resistance, blocking epithelial attachment and promoting secretion of bactericidal substances [34]. Studies suggest that NSPs like chitosan, inulin and alginate can limit the production of potentially harmful metabolites of the microbiota [35]. There is now a growing consensus that certain NSPs may be able to stimulate the growth of specific types of colonic bacteria which deliver a prebiotic effect. Also, high-fibre diet supplements have the potential to improve microbial balance in the colon by reducing coliform population [36].

Effects on stool frequency and consistency

Constipation is a common disorder affecting many people in Western countries [37]. Inadequate NSP intake has been suggested as the major cause for the prevalence of constipation [23]. The main symptoms are low stool frequency, long transit time, difficult stool expulsion, dry stools and incomplete rectal emptying. Treatment in the first instance is usually by dietary supplementation of fibre; the lack of enzymatic degradation of NSPs in the small intestine helps to increase faecal bulk [37]. Increased bulk in the colon is the best documented mechanism for the laxative effect of fibre [37]. It has been confirmed that the laxative effect of fibre occurs substantially through greater faecal mass (and not any other effect) as consumption of indigestible

Table 2.1.2 Potential effects of fibre on components of the gastrointestinal barrier and on bacterial translocation, and possible mechanisms [22]

Component of GI barrier	Types of fibre	Potential effects	Possible mechanisms
GI mucus	Very well fermented	Qualitative and quantitative alteration in mucus composition	Direct mechanical effects Indirect effects by modulation of mucosal metabolism by end-productsof fermentation
	Well fermented	Possible influence on intestinal microbiota Increased potential resistance to bacterial enzymes Protection from oxidative damage	Increased thickness of unstirred water layer
GI mucosa and muscle wall	Well fermented and less well fermented	Stimulation of proliferation (proximal/mid colon by well-fermented fibres and distal colon by less well-fermented fibres)	Direct (energy source) or systemic effects of SCFA Indirect effects of SCFA (decrease caecal pH, increase GI blood flow, autonomic nervous system effects) Influence of faecal bulk and particle size of fibres Influence of luminal viscosity
	Less well fermented	Maintenance of intestinal muscle bulk	Stimulation of gut hormones and peptides Abrasive action
	Well fermented	Protection from oxidative damage	Abrasive action Direct scavenging of radicals Chelating agent
GI microbiota	Very well fermented	Stimulation of microbiota	Substrate for proliferation
		Maintenance of healthy balance of end-products	Carbohydrate metabolism
		Detrimental effects on growth of pathogens	Production of SCFA
		Colonisation resistance	Displacement of pathogens
	Well fermented (inulin, OF and FOS)	Stimulation of specific microbiota, e.g. bifidobacteria	Preferred substrate for selective proliferation
GI immune function	Well fermented and less well fermented	Immunoregulatory effects on colonic epithelium	Regulation of gene transcription, protein synthesis of genes and gene products via butyrate
Systemic immune function	Not yet well established	Possible effects on non-specific and cell-mediated immunity	Via SCFA
Bacterial translocation	Less well fermented	Decreased bacterial translocation	Effects related to improving components of the GI barrier Binding of bacteria, toxins, bile acids Blocking bacterial adherence to the mucosa Altering microbial cell wall structures

FOS, fructo-oligosaccharide; SCFA, short-chain fatty acid.

plastic 'bran' flakes promoted laxation and increased stool output [38]. Increased bulk stimulates passage through the colon, resulting in faster transit time and thus a reduced time available for water reabsorption. All these factors together result in an increased stool weight with a softer composition [39].

The bulking effects of NSPs are reported to be greatest with cereal fibre [5]. However, soluble fibre is generally less effective in increasing stool mass. Diverticular disease is a herniation of the colon and is associated with chronic constipation in elderly people; increased consumption of NSPs from mainly cereal foods could relieve such disorders [40].

These studies clearly signify that dietary supplementation of NSPs has great potential for improving the GI health of people in many developed countries where NSP intake is relatively low [5]. The actual NSP dose required for prevention of constipation is not certain but would seem to be around 20–25 g/person/day [37].

Non-starch polysaccharides and GI tract-related cancers

Globally, 13% of annual mortality is due to cancer. Around 35% of cancer deaths are probably related to unhealthy dietary habits which are directly linked to GI tract-related abnormalities such as colorectal cancer, oesophageal cancer and gastric cancer [41]. Growing scientific investigation and epidemiological data suggest that sufficient NSP intakes may reduce the risk of these cancers.

Colorectal cancer

Colorectal cancers cause more than 655,000 deaths annually across the world and are the third most commonly diagnosed cancers. They are also ranked third among cancer deaths in the USA [42]. Cumulative data from various countries suggested that increased consumption of NSPs may reduce the risk of colorectal cancer [43, 44].

The possible mechanisms by which NSPs may protect against colon cancer include direct absorption of the carcinogen and excretion into faeces, anti-initiation effects such as prevention of carcinogen activation or prevention of mutations, the production of SCFAs (predominantly acetic, propionic and butyrate) that can result in alterations in microbial community and also changes to their metabolic activities in terms of the formation of genotoxins, carcinogens and tumour promoters [45]. Short-chain fatty acids also lower colonic pH, resulting in lower production of secondary bile acids which are involved in colonic carcinogenesis [46], synergistic interaction between dietary substrates (prebiotics) and beneficial bacteria (probiotics) in the colon [47] which mitigates colon cancer by the suppression of DNA damage in colonic mucosal cells, manifested by modification in the activity and expression of mutated *ras* genes by *Bifidobacterium longum* [47]. Increased stool bulk and reduction in intestine transit time [48], antiprogression effects such as scavenging or apoptotic effects [49] and soluble fibre (e.g. short-chain fructo-oligosaccharides, polydextrose and beta-glucan) can concomitantly develop GALT, possibly via stimulation of anti-tumoural immunity by modulation of colonic physiology and/or production of immunoglobulin A [41]. The detailed mechanism is illustrated in Figure 2.1.2.

Gastric cancer

After colorectal cancer, stomach cancer is the next most frequent and the second leading cause of cancer death globally. Data from epidemiological and experimental studies suggested that diet plays an important role in the incidence of gastric cancer. A 10-year study in Italy (between 1997 and 2007) with 230 subjects showed an inverse relationship between risk of gastric cancer and consumption of soluble fibre, insoluble fibre, lignin and fibre derived from vegetables or fruit [50]. Although the associated mechanism is unclear, it is postulated that a reduced transit time from a high NSP intake might reduce the prolonged exposure of stomach tissue to carcinogens [50].

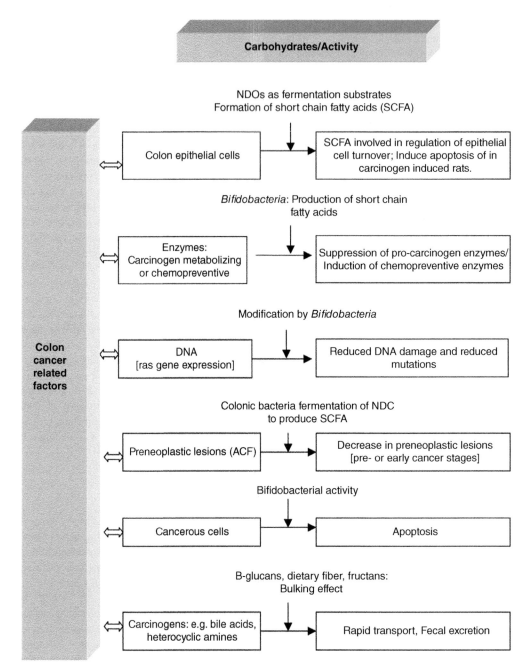

Figure 2.1.2 Roles of fibre in colon cancer protection. Source: Niba & Niba [54]. Reproduced with permission from Emerald Group Publishing Ltd. NDOs Non-digestible oligosaccharides.

Oesophageal cancer

Compared to colorectal and stomach cancer, the occurrence of oesophageal cancer is very minor and accounts for about 1% of total diagnosed cancers in the USA. However, the number of cases of oesophageal cancer is increasing rapidly worldwide. A 5-year case study from Soler et al. recommended that consumption of a diet which included soluble and insoluble fibre, and fibre from agricultural products (grains, vegetables and fruits), had a significant protective role against oesophageal cancer [51]. Likewise, Mulholland et al. confirmed that dependence on a diet high in NSPs reduces the incidence of Barrett's oesophagus and oesophageal adenocarcinoma by 56% [52].

Three mechanisms by which NSP intake can reduce the risk of oesophageal cancer have been hypothesised. First, by a reduction in the glycaemic response, as NSP is known to slow down digestion and absorption of carbohydrates, consequently reducing hyperinsulinaemia and the formation of insulin-like growth factor (IGF) [51]. Second, by lowering plasma levels of systemic inflammatory markers such as interleukin-6, which is likely to play a vital role in the incidence of carcinogenesis [53]. Third, by the mechanical removal or binding of damaged cells and/or carcinogens from the epithelial surface of the oesophagus which also reduces the risk of gastro-oesophageal reflux symptoms.

In summary, high NSP intakes or fibre supplements have health-promoting and disease-protective effects. These clinical implications include reducing the risk of diabetes, obesity, gastrointestinal cancer and certain gut-associated abnormalities. Consequently, there is a growing consensus that in the future, fibre supplements are likely to become a standard component of almost all types of food products. However, it is important that only ideal amounts of fibre should be considered on a routine basis; overconsumption might cause undesirable side-effects such as bloating, diarrhoea and excessive gas production.

References

1. Hipsley EH. Dietary "fibre" and pregnancy toxaemia. *British Medical Journal* 1953; **2**(4833): 420–422.

2. Trowell H. Definition of dietary fiber and hypotheses that it is a protective factor in certain diseases. *American Journal of Clinical Nutrition* 1976; **29**(4): 417–427.

3. Davidson MH McDonald A. Fiber: forms and functions. *Nutrition Research* 1998; **18**: 617–624.

4. Scott KP, Duncan SH, Flint HJ. Dietary fiber and the gut microbiota. *Nutrition Bulletin* 2008; **33**: 201–211.

5. Kumar V, Sinha AK, Makkar HP, De Boeck G, Becker K. Dietary role of nonstarch polysaccharides in human nutrition: a review. *Critical Reviews in Food Science and Nutrition* 2012; **52**(10): 899–935.

6. Phillips GO. Dietary fibre: a chemical category or a health ingredient? *Bioactive Carbohydrate and Dietary Fibre* 2013; **1**: 3–9.

7. Cummings JH, Mann JI, Nishida C, Vorster HH. Dietary fibre: an agreed definition. *Lancet* 2009; **373**(9661): 365–366.

8. Klosterbuer A, Roughead ZF, Slavin J. Benefits of dietary fiber in clinical nutrition. *Nutrition in Clinical Practice* 2011; **26**(5): 625–635.

9. Cummings JH. The effect of dietary fiber on fecalweight and composition. In: Spiller G (ed) *Dietary Fiber in Human Nutrition*. Boca Raton, FL: CRC Press, 2001, pp. 183–252.

10. Anderson JW. Dietary fiber and associated phytochemicals in prevention and reversal of diabetes. In: Pasupuleti VK, Anderson JW (eds) *Nutraceuticals, Glycemic Health and Type 2 Diabetes*. Ames, IA: Blackwell Publishing Professional, 2008, pp. 111–142.

11. Kirby RW, Anderson JW, Sieling B, et al. Oat-bran intake selectively lowers serum low-density lipoprotein cholesterol concentrations of hypercholesterolemic men. *American Journal of Clinical Nutrition* 1981; **34**: 824–829.

12. Fleming SE, Choi YS, Fitch DM. Absorption of short-chain fatty acids from the rat cecum in vivo. *Journal of Nutrition* 1991; **121**: 1787–1797.

13. Clausen MR, Bonnen H, Tvede M, Mortensen PB. Colonic fermentation to short-chain fatty acids is decreased in antibiotic associated diarrhea. *Gastroenterology* 1991; **101**: 1497–1504.

14. Ramakrishna BS, Mathan VI. Colonic dysfunction in acute diarrhoea – the role of luminal short chain fatty acids. *Gut* 1993; **34**: 1215–1218.

15. Mortensen FV, Hessov I, Birke H, Korsgaad N, Nielsen H. Microcirculatory and trophic effects of short chain fatty acids in the human rectum after Hartmann's procedure. *British Journal of Surgery* 1991; **78**: 1208–1211.

16. Topping DL, Clifton PM. Short-chain fatty acids and human colonic function: role of resistant starch and non starch polysaccharides. *Physiological Reviews* 2001; **81**: 1031–1064.

17. Coudray C, Bellanger J, Castiglia-Delavaud C, Remesy C, Vermorel M, Rayssiguier Y. Effects of soluble or partly soluble dietary fibers supplementation on absorption and balance of calcium, magnesium, iron and zinc in healthy young men. *European Journal of Clinical Nutrition* 1997; **51**: 375–380.

18. Lynn ME, Mathers JC, Parker DS. Increasing luminal viscosity stimulates crypt cell proliferation throughout the gut. *Proceedings of the Nutrition Society* 1994; **53**: 226.

19. Wasan HS, Goodlad RA. Fiber-supplemented foods may damage your health. *Lancet* 1996; **348**: 319–320.

20. Malkki Y, Virtanen E. Gastrointestinal effects of oat bran and oat gum – a review. *Journal of Food Science and Technology* 2001; **34**: 337–347.

21. Sakata T, Inagaki A. Organic acid production in the large intestine: implication for epithelial cell proliferation and cell death. In: Piva A, Bach Knudsen KE, Lindberg JE (eds) *The Gut Environment of Pigs*. Nottingham: Nottingham University Press, 2001, pp. 85–94.

22. Green CJ. Fiber in enteral nutrition. *South African Journal of Clinical Nutrition* 2000; **13**(4): 150–160.

23. Green CJ. Fibre in enteral nutrition. *Clinical Nutrition* 2001; **20**(1): 23–39.

24. Vernia P, Caprilli R, Latella G, Barbetti F, Magliocca M, Cittadini M. Fecal lactate and ulcerative colitis. *Gastroenterology* 1988; **95**: 1564–1568.

25. Allen A, Flemstrom G. Gastroduodenal mucus bicarbonate barrier: protection against acid and pepsin. *American Journal of Physiology - Cell Physiology* 2005; **288**(1 57-1): C1–C19.

26. Satchithanandam S, Klurfeld DM, Calvert RJ, Cassidy MM. Effects of dietary fibers on gastrointestinal mucin in rats. *Nutrition Research* 1996; **16**: 1163–1177.

27. Kohen R, Shadmi V, Kakunda A, Rubinstein A. Prevention of oxidative damage in the rat jejunal mucosa by pectin. *British Journal of Nutrition* 1993; **69**: 789–800.

28. Brownlee IA, Dettmar PW, Strugala V, Pearson JP. The interaction of dietary fibres with the colon. *Current Nutrition and Food Science* 2006; **2**(3): 243–264.

29. Barcelo A, Claustre J, Moro F, Chayvialle JA, Cuber JC, Plaisancie P. Mucin secretion is modulated by luminal factors in the isolated vascularly perfused rat colon. *Gut* 2000; **46**: 218–224.

30. Welters CF, Deutz NE, Dejong CH, Soeters PB, Heineman E. Supplementation of enteral nutrition with butyrate leads to increased portal efflux of amino acids in growing pigs with short bowel syndrome. *Journal of Pediatric Surgery* 1996; **3**: 526–529.

31. Anderson JW, Baird P, Davis RH, et al. Health benefits of dietary fiber. *Nutrition Reviews* 2009 **67**: 188–205.

32. Vos AP, M'Rabet L, Stahl B, Boehm G, Garssen J. Immunemodulatory effects and potential working mechanisms of orally applied nondigestible carbohydrates. *Critical Reviews in Immunology* 2007; **27**: 97–140.

33. Watzl B, Girrbach S, Roller M. Inulin, oligofructose and immunomodulation. *British Journal of Nutrition* 2005; **93**(Suppl): S49–S55.

34. Tungland BC. Fructooligosaccharides and other fructans: structures and occurrence, production, regulatory aspects, food applications and nutritional health significance. In: Eggleston G, Côté GL (eds) *Oligosaccharides in Food and Agriculture*. Washington, DC: ACS Press, 2003, pp. 135–152.

35. Brownlee IA. The physiological roles of dietary fibre. *Food Hydrocolloids* 2011; **25**: 238–250.

36. Bird AR. Prebiotics: a role for dietary fiber and resistant starch? *Asia Pacific Journal of Clinical Nutrition* 1999; **8**: 32–36.

37. Topping D. Cereal complex carbohydrates and their contribution to human health. *Journal of Cereal Science* 2007; **46**: 220–229.

38. Lewis SJ, Heaton KW. The intestinal effects of bran-like plastic particles: is the concept of 'roughage' valid after all? *European Journal of Gastroenterology and Hepatology* 1997; **9**: 553–557.

39. Brandt LA. Prebiotics enhance gut health. *Prepared Foods* 2001; **170**(9): 7–10.

40. Baghurst PA, Rohan TE. High-fiber diets and reduced risk of breast cancer. *International Journal of Cancer* 2006; **56**(2): 173–176.

41. Gao Y, Yue J. Dietary fiber and human health. In: Yu L, Tsao R, Shahidi F (eds) *Cereals and Pulses: Nutraceutical Properties and Health Benefits*. Hoboken, NJ: John Wiley & Sons, 2012.

42. American Cancer Society. *Cancer Facts and Figures 2008*. Atlanta, GA: American Cancer Society, 2008.

43. Coudray C, Demigné C, Rayssiguier Y. Effects of dietary fibers on magnesium absorption in animals and humans. *Journal of Nutrition* 2003; **133**: 1–4.

44. McIntyre A, Gibson PR, Young GP. Butyrate production from dietary fiber and protection against large bowel cancer in a rat model. *Gut* 1993; **34**: 386–391.

45. Kaur N, Gupta A. Applications of inulin and oligofructose in health and nutrition. *Journal of Biosciences* 2002; **27**(7): 703–714.

46. Marteau P, Boutron-Ruault MC. Nutritional advantages of probiotics and prebiotics. *British Journal of Nutrition* 2002; **87**(2): 153–157.

47. Reddy BS. Possible mechanisms by which pro- and prebiotics influence colon carcinogenesis and tumor growth. *Journal of Nutrition* 1999; **129**: 1478–1482.

48. Harris PJ, Triggs CM, Roberton AM, Watson ME, Ferguson LR. The adsorption of heterocyclic aromatic amines by model dietary fibres with contrasting compositions. *Chemico-Biological Interactions* 1996; **100**: 13–25.

49. Ferguson LR, Chavan RR, Harris PJ. Changing concepts of dietary fiber: implications for carcinogenesis. *Nutrition and Cancer* 2001; **39**(2): 155–169.

50. Francesca B, Lorenza S, Cristina B, Paola B, Eva N, La Carlo V. Dietary fiber and stomach cancer risk: a case-control study from Italy. *Cancer Causes and Control* 2009; **20**: 847–853.

51. Soler M, Bosetti C, Franceschi S, et al. Fiber intake and the risk of oral, pharyngeal and esophageal cancer. *International Journal of Cancer* 2001; **91**: 283–287.

52. Mulholland HG, Cantwell MM, Anderson LA, et al. Glycemic index, carbohydrate and fiber intakes and risk of reflux esophagitis, Barrett's esophagus, and esophageal adenocarcinoma. *Cancer Causes and Control* 2009; **20**: 279–288.

53. Ma Y, Griffith JA, Chasan-Taber L, et al. Association between dietary fiber and markers of systemic inflammation in the women's health initiative observational study. *Nutrition* 2008; **24**: 941–949.

54. Niba LL, Niba SH. Role of non-digestible carbohydrates in colon cancer protection. *Nutrition and Food Science* 2003; **33**(1): 28–33.

55. Tsai AC, Mott EL, Owen GM, Bennick MR, Lo GS, Steinke FH. Effects of soy polysaccharide on gastrointestinal functions, nutrient balance, steroid excretions, glucose tolerance, serum lipids, and other parameters in humans. *American Journal of Clinical Nutrition* 1983; **38**: 504–511.

Chapter 2.2

Short-chain fermentable carbohydrates

Sue Shepherd

La Trobe University, Melbourne, Australia

Carbohydrates are classified chemically according to the number of component molecules (degree of polymerisation, DP). The type of bond that exists between the monomers (alpha or beta) is also important as it affects the structure and/or digestibility of the carbohydrate [1]. Carbohydrate terminology has changed over the years, and the current classifications are described in Table 2.2.1 [2]. Sucrose, lactose, maltose, maltodextrin and starches are hydrolysed by gastrointestinal enzymic action to their constituent monosaccharides glucose, galactose and fructose prior to absorption. Classification of carbohydrates according to their digestibility in a normally functioning small intestine is described in Table 2.2.2.

2.2.1 Gastrointestinal effects of short-chain fermentable carbohydrates

Short-chain fermentable carbohydrates include fructose, lactose, polyols, fructo-oligosaccharides (FOS)/fructans and galacto-oligosaccharides (GOS). These are small molecules that may be poorly absorbed in the small intestine. These then arrive into the large intestine, which is populated by the gastrointestinal microbiota. Luminal bacteria rapidly ferment these to hydrogen, carbon dioxide and short-chain fatty acids [3]. The major source of gas production in the lumen is via bacterial fermentation, the principal substrate being carbohydrates.

How rapidly these are fermented is dictated by the chain length of the carbohydrate; oligosaccharides and sugars are more rapidly fermented compared with polysaccharides such as soluble dietary fibre [4]. Gas, bloating and distension may occur due to rapid fermentation.

Small sugars are highly osmotic. When these are not absorbed in the small intestine, they are delivered into the colonic lumen, together with water due to their osmotic effect. Thus, if sufficient short-chain carbohydrates reach the colon, GI function may be disturbed via effects on motility and/or via the effect of the osmotic load (similar to that utilised by the disaccharide laxative lactulose). Thus, short-chain carbohydrates that are poorly absorbed are reasonable candidates for dietary triggers of luminal distension and irritable bowel syndrome (IBS) symptoms (see Chapter 3.19 Irritable bowel syndrome dietary management).

There have been numerous studies in support of the concept that exceeding the tolerated dose of fructose and lactose causes malabsorption. These unabsorbed sugars and osmotically entrapped water together with electrolytes increase the liquidity of luminal contents and affect GI motility, including speeding up GI transit. This effect is utilised by lactulose, sorbitol and polyethylene glycol in their role as laxatives. Provocation tests with lactose, fructose, FOS or sorbitol cause abdominal symptoms such as bloating, pain, excess wind, nausea and disturbed stool output (diarrhoea and/or constipation) in many people, especially those with IBS [5–7].

Advanced Nutrition and Dietetics in Gastroenterology, First Edition. Edited by Miranda Lomer.
© 2014 John Wiley & Sons, Ltd. Published 2014 by John Wiley & Sons, Ltd.

Table 2.2.1 Classification of dietary carbohydrates

Class	Degree of polymerisation	Subgroup	Examples
Sugars	1–2	Monosaccharides	Glucose, fructose, galactose
		Disaccharides	Sucrose, lactose, maltose, trehalose
		Polyols	Sorbitol, mannitol, lactitol, xylitol, erythritol, isomalt, maltitol
Oligosaccharides	3–9	Malto-oligosaccharides (alpha-glucans)	Maltodextrins
		Non-alpha-glucan oligosaccharides	Raffinose, stachyose, fructo-oligosaccharides, galacto-oligosaccharides, polydextrose
Polysaccharides	>10	Starch (alpha-glucan)	Amylose, amylopectin, modified starches
		Non-starch polysaccharides	Cellulose, hemicellulose, pectin, arabinoxylans, beta-glucan, fructans, plant gums and mucilages, hydrocolloids

Table 2.2.2 Dietary carbohydrates classified according to digestibility

Classification	Name	Constituent monosaccharides
Digestible		
Monosaccharide	Glucose	n/a
	Fructose	n/a
	Galactose	n/a
Disaccharide	Sucrose	Glucose + fructose
	Lactose	Glucose + galactose
	Maltose	Glucose + glucose
Oligosaccharide	Maltodextrin	Glucose polymer
Polysaccharide	Starch	Glucose polymer
Non-digestible		
Polyols*		
Oligosaccharide	Inulin-type fructans (short chain, e.g. fructo-oligosaccharides, oligofructose)	Fructose polymer (glucose terminal end)
	Galacto-oligosaccharides (e.g. raffinose, stachyose)	Galactose polymer (glucose terminal end)
Polysaccharide	Inulin-type fructans (long chain, e.g. inulin)	Fructose polymer (glucose terminal end)
	Arabinoxylans	Xylose with side chains of arabinose
	Resistant starch	Glucose polymer
	Non-starch polysaccharides	

*Considered here as a non-digestible carbohydrate.

2.2.2 Short-chain fermentable carbohydrates (FODMAPs)

Fructose, lactose, polyols, fructans and GOS are widely distributed in foods and have collectively been termed FODMAPs [8,9] (Table 2.2.3). FODMAP is an acronym referring to fermentable oligosaccharides (fructans, galacto-oligosaccharides), disaccharides (lactose), monosaccharides (free fructose) and polyols.

Subclassification of FODMAPs

FODMAPs can be subclassified into two categories.

(1) *FODMAPs that are poorly absorbed in some people: fructose, lactose, polyols* – as the capacity to absorb these varies between individuals, the symptoms will also vary. Breath testing may be useful to determine if there is successful absorption.
(2) *FODMAPs that are not absorbed in anyone: fructans and GOS* – these are always fermented in the colon, and a certain amount will result in symptoms in susceptible individuals.

Fructose

Fructose is a monosaccharide found in three main forms in the diet: as free fructose (present, for instance, in fruits and honey); as a constituent of the disaccharide sucrose; or as fructans, a polymer of fructose usually in oligosaccharide form (discussed later in this section) [10].

Intestinal absorption of free fructose The majority of fructose absorption occurs via two transporters in the brush border epithelium of the small intestine [11].

- *GLUT5* – a facultative transporter (i.e. it depends upon a concentration gradient for movement of fructose across the membrane), which is specific for fructose. This is a glucose-*independent* pathway of fructose absorption.
- *GLUT2* – a low-affinity, facultative transporter that will carry glucose, fructose and galactose. In this pathway, glucose facilitates the uptake of fructose. This is a glucose-*dependent* pathway for fructose absorption.

Fructose malabsorption People with fructose malabsorption (which differs from hereditary fructose intolerance) have impairment in the glucose-independent pathway (GLUT5), whilst the glucose-dependent (GLUT2) pathway remains functioning. The proportion of people who can completely absorb a load of fructose depends upon the load given; approximately 60% of people can completely absorb 35 g of fructose but this is reduced to 20% when 50 g is given [12,13].

Provocation studies where fructose loads are given to people with fructose malabsorption induce symptoms of wind, bloating, abdominal discomfort, nausea and disturbed stool output in many more subjects with IBS than in those without IBS [14–17]. These observations led to the research proving that the malabsorption of dietary fructose is a trigger for symptoms in patients with IBS and that removal of fructose from the diet leads to symptomatic improvement.

Lactose

Lactose is a disaccharide that occurs naturally in the milk from any mammal, including cow, sheep and goat. Lactose must be hydrolysed to its two constituent monosaccharides, glucose and galactose, in order to be absorbed. The enzyme lactase hydrolyses lactose and is secreted by cells in the brush border lining the small intestine. If insufficient lactase is produced, then lactose can be malabsorbed. Lactase insufficiency is present in a proportion of adults and children, varying with ethnicity [18]. Malabsorption of lactose (which can be detected by breath hydrogen testing, a lactose tolerance test or lactase activity determined from small intestinal biopsy) indicates that lactose should be considered a fermentable sugar (FODMAP) in that person. For further information about lactose malabsorption see Chapter 3.15 Lactose malabsorption and nutrition.

Polyols

Polyols, also called sugar alcohols, include sorbitol and mannitol as the most commonly occurring in foods, and also include xylitol and maltitol. Polyols occur naturally in foods and may also be used as a low-energy sweetener, where the laxative effect must be indicated on the food label.

Table 2.2.3 Details of FODMAPs

FODMAP	Structure / composition	Alternative names	Gastrointestinal absorption	Significant sources
Fructans	Oligo- and polysaccharides of fructose with a glucose terminal end. Most have beta(1 → 2) bond but may have beta(2 → 6) bond	Fructo-oligosaccharides (FOS) or oligofructose (OF) Degree of polymerisation (DP) <10 Inulins: DP >10	Human small intestine does not produce a hydrolase, therefore is incapable of breaking the beta(1 → 2) bond	Major dietary sources of fructans are wheat and onions Inulin is also increasingly being used as a food additive, being promoted as a prebiotic
Galacto-oligosaccharides (GOS)	Oligosaccharides with a beta-fructosidic bond and an alpha-galactosidic bond	Raffinose consists of one fructose, one glucose and one galactose molecule Stachyose contains one glucose, one fructose and two galactose molecules	Humans do not produce galactosidases, therefore are incapable of hydrolysing the galactosidic linkages of stachyose and raffinose to their monosaccharide constituents	Legumes (e.g. baked beans, red kidney beans, borlotti beans, soy beans), lentils, chickpeas
Polyols and polydextrose		Sugar alcohols including sorbitol, mannitol, xylitol, erythritol, isomalt, maltitol	Polyols are poorly absorbed in the small intestine via 'pores' Polydextrose behaves in a similar way to polyols	Naturally occurring, e.g. sorbitol and mannitol Food additives: sorbitol, xylitol, mannitol, maltitol
Fructose	Six-carbon monosaccharide (hexose)		Absorbed via two mechanisms, glucose-independent facilitated transport and glucose-dependent fructose co-transport Well absorbed when ingested in equimolar combination with glucose (e.g. as sucrose)	Present in three forms in food: • as free fructose (fruits, honey) • as a constituent of the disaccharide sucrose, or • as an oligosaccharide form of fructans
Lactose	Disaccharide: constituent monosaccharides are glucose and galactose		Absorption is dependent upon the brush border enzyme lactase, which hydrolyses lactose Lactase deficiency is common, affecting approximately 10% of Caucasians and >90% of Chinese	Present in cow, goat and sheep milk Tolerance of dietary sources of lactose will vary according to production of lactase Sources are milk, ice cream, yoghurt, low-fat soft cheeses

Polyol absorption across the small intestine is slow. Polyols do not have specific active transport systems in the epithelium of the small intestine and are most probably absorbed by passive diffusion. There are three main variables that affect the rate of absorption of polyols.

- The size of the polyol. Diffusion of polyols occurs through 'pores' in the epithelium and therefore ability to absorb relates to molecular size. For example, the 4-carbon polyol erythritol is well absorbed in the jejunum but the 6-carbon mannitol is not [19]. The size of the pore for uptake of polyols is also important, as there is variation of pore size along the small intestine with larger pores found proximally and smaller pores found distally.
- How quickly matter transits through the jejunum. Polyols will be inefficiently absorbed in fast transit.
- Presence of disease in the mucosa of the gastrointestinal tract may reduce pore size, reducing polyol absorption, for example in active coeliac disease [20].

This therefore explains why the (limited) studies performed on the absorption of sorbitol and mannitol have produced substantial individual variation and that the amount available for fermentation varies according to dose [21].

Fructans

Fructans are linear or branched fructose polymers that contain a beta1–2 linkage between fructose molecules. They are present as the naturally occurring storage carbohydrates of a variety of vegetables, including onions, garlic, leeks and artichokes, fruits such as watermelon, and in cereals [22–24]. Wheat is a major source of fructans in the diet, and contains 1–4% fructans on solid matter [25]. Additional sources of fructans are inulin (mostly as a long-chain fructan) and FOS, which are increasingly being added to foods for their putative prebiotic effects. The terminology used for fructose polymers (fructans) is varied, but it is generally accepted that <10 units DP are termed oligofructose or fructo-oligosaccharide and >10 units DP are termed inulin. Short-chain fructans have a slightly sweet taste; the sweetness decreases with increasing DP (26), such that inulins with a DP >20 do not have a sweet taste at all [26].

The fate of fructans differs significantly from that of free fructose. Fructans cannot be transported across the epithelium and are malabsorbed because the small intestine lacks hydrolases capable of breaking fructose-fructose bonds. This has been confirmed in studies which have shown that 34–90% of ingested fructans can be recovered from small intestinal output in subjects with an ileostomy [27–29]. The loss of inulin during transit through the small intestine is seemingly due to hydrolysis by either enzymes or acids, and also probably via microbial degradation from the microbiota that permanently colonise the distal small intestine [26]. The majority have resisted digestion in the small intestine, and arrive into the large intestine where they are fermented by the colonic bacteria.

Research interest in fructans has increased in recent years as they may have wide-ranging beneficial effects on health [30,31]. Proposed health benefits include suppressing the growth of potential pathogens in the colon, increasing stool bulking capacity and minimising risk of constipation, increasing calcium absorption, maintaining the integrity of the GI mucosal barrier and increasing colonic mucus production, stimulating the gastrointestinal immune system and reducing the risk of colorectal cancer.

The reported physiological effects of fructans are not all positive. Fructans can trigger gastrointestinal symptoms including gastro-oesophageal reflux [32], bloating, flatulence and abdominal pain [33–35]. There is some evidence in experimental animals that fructans may have negative effects on health by causing an injury response in the colonic epithelium (increased colonic epithelial turnover and mucus production), decreasing epithelial barrier function and increasing susceptibility to salmonella infection [36]. Only some of these animal observations have been shown in human studies [37,38] but baseline dietary intake of fructose and fructans was not well controlled, raising some question about the validity of the results.

Galacto-oligosaccharides (GOS)

Galacto-oligosaccharides are polymers of galactose with fructose and glucose at the terminal ends. The most common are raffinose (comprising one

Table 2.2.4 Examples of high FODMAP foods

Fruit and fruit products	Vegetables and vegetable products	Milk products	Grain and starch foods	Legumes, nuts and Seeds	Others
Apple	Artichoke –globe	Cow's milk (full fat, low fat, skimmed)	Barley-, rye- and wheat-based: bread, crackers, pasta, couscous, gnocchi, noodles, croissants, muffins, crumpets	Cashews	Agave
Apricot	Artichoke –Jerusalem	Custard		Chickpeas	Chicory-based drinks
Blackberry	Asparagus	Dairy desserts		Legumes (e.g. red kidney beans, soy beans, borlotti beans)	Fructo-oligosaccharides
Boysenberry	Cauliflower	Evaporated milk			High-fructosecorn syrup
Custard apple	Garlic	Goat's milk (full fat, low fat, skimmed)		Lentils	Honey
Fruit juice (apple, pear, mango, tropical)	Leek	Ice cream		Pistachios	Inulin
	Mushroom	Milk powder			Salts – onion, garlic, vegetable
Fruit leather (strap bars)	Onion	Sheep's milk (full fat, low fat, skimmed)			Sweeteners: sorbitol (420), mannitol (421), xylitol (967), maltitol (965), isomalt (953)
Fruit-based muesli bar	Shallot	Sweetened condensed milk			
Mango	Snow peas				
Nashi fruit	Spring onion (white part)				
Nectarine	Sugar snap peas				
Peach					
Pear					
Persimmon					
Plum					
Tamarillo					
Watermelon					

Table 2.2.5   Examples of low FODMAP foods (*indicates foods that contain a lesser amount of FODMAPs – these can be eaten, but not in large amounts)

Fruit and fruit products	Vegetables and vegetable products	Milk products	Grain and starch foods	Legumes, nuts and Seeds	Others
Avocado*	Alfalfa	Hard cheeses,	Cracker*	Almonds*	Garlic-infused
Banana	Bamboo shoots	e.g. Blue vein,	Buckwheat	Chia seeds	olive oil
Blueberry	Bean sprouts	Brie, Cheddar,	Corn	Hazelnuts*	Herbs
Canteloupe	Beans (green)	Colby, Edam,	Gluten-free	Linseed	Spices
Carambola	Beetroot*	Feta, Gouda,	bread & cereal	(flaxseed)	Ginger
Cherries*	Bok choy	Mozzarella,	products	Poppy seeds	Small amounts
Dragon fruit	Broccoli*	Parmesan, Swiss	Millet	Pumpkin seeds	of regular milk
Dried fruit*	Brussels	Butter	Oats	(pepita)	as an ingredient
Durian	sprouts*	Cream	Oat bran	Sesame seeds	Maple syrup
Grapefruit	Butternut	Margarine	Polenta	Sunflower seeds	Golden syrup
Grapes	pumpkin*	Oat milk	Quinoa	Tahini*	Sugar (sucrose),
Honeydew	Cabbage	Rice milk	Rice		glucose, any
melon	(savoy)*	Lactose-free ice	Sweet biscuit*		other artificial
Kiwifruit	Capsicum	cream			sweeteners not
Lemon	Carrot	Lactose-free			ending in 'ol'
Lime	Cauliflower	yoghurt			(e.g. aspartame)
Longon*	Celery*	Fromage frais*			
Lychee*	Chives	Yoghurt – cow,			
Mandarin	Choy sum	sheep, goat*			
Orange	Cucumber	Soft cheeses,*			
Passionfruit	Eggplant	e.g. cottage,			
Pawpaw	Endive	ricotta, quark,			
Pineapple	Fennel bulb*	cream cheese,			
Pomegranate*	Green peas*	mascarpone,			
Prickly pear	Lettuce	crème fraiche			
Rambutan*	Olives				
Raspberry	Parsnip				
Rhubarb	Potato				
Strawberry	Pumpkin (Jap)				
Tangelo	Radish				
	Rocket				
	Silverbeet				
	Spinach				
	Spring onion				
	(green part only)				
	Squash				
	Swede				
	Sweet corn*				
	Sweet potato*				
	Tomato				
	Turnip				
	Zucchini				

galactose, one glucose and one fructose unit) and stachyose (comprising two galactose, one glucose and one fructose unit). The most significant dietary sources of GOS are legumes, including baked beans, red kidney beans, borlotti beans, soy beans, lentils and chickpeas. Humans do not produce alpha-galactosidase, so there is no hydrolysis of the galactosidic linkages of GOS to their monosaccharides. Hence they are delivered into the colon and are fermented by colonic bacteria.

Sugar malabsorption and breath tests

Malabsorption of fructose, lactose and sorbitol can be diagnosed with breath testing for hydrogen or methane production after ingestion of the sugar in test volumes. Symptoms do not correlate with the degree of hydrogen or methane production [14] but this is not surprising since symptoms are not the direct result of the malabsorption, but rather a result of the response of the gut-brain axis to the malabsorbed carbohydrate. In breath test studies comparing patients with IBS-like symptoms and healthy subjects, symptoms generated during the test are of increased frequency and severity in patients with IBS-like symptoms compared to healthy subjects [14–17].

FODMAP content of foods

The FODMAP content of food varies and so cut-off values have been established to classify foods as suitable and problematic. Cut-off values were based on careful clinical observation, which included obtaining feedback from patients regarding foods that they identified as triggers for symptoms. The foods reported by patients as being problematic have been examined for trends in the pooled food composition table. Foods and beverages containing:

- >0.2 g fructose in excess of glucose per serving size
- >0.3 g of oligosaccharides per serving size
- >0.5 g total polyols (sorbitol and mannitol) per serving size
- >4 g lactose per serving size

were reported by patients to consistently induce symptoms [39]. Therefore cut-off figures at these

levels have been established. Foods and beverages containing FODMAPs below these levels are not considered problematic as clinical experience suggests these are not regularly reported to induce symptoms. This approach aims to avoid unnecessary overrestriction of the diet [9].

Examples of problematic and favourable foods related to FODMAP content are shown in Tables 2.2.4 and 2.2.5. Problematic foods are foods exceeding the cut-off figures.

References

1. FAO. *Carbohydrates in Human Nutrition*. Report of a Joint FAO/WHO Expert Consultation, Rome, 14–18 April 1997. FAO Food and Nutrition Paper 66. Rome: Food and Agriculture Organisation, 1998.

2. Cummings JH, Stephen AM. Carbohydrate terminology and classification. *European Journal of Clinical Nutrition* 2007; 61 **Suppl 1**: S5–18.

3. Oku T, Nakamura S. Comparison of digestibility and breath hydrogen gas excretion of fructo-oligosaccharide, galactosyl-sucrose, and isomalto-oligosaccharide in healthy human subjects. *European Journal of Clinical Nutrition* 2003; **57**: 1150–1156.

4. Wong J, Jenkins D. Carbohydrate digestibility and metabolic effects. *Journal of Nutrition* 2007; **137**: 2539S–2546S.

5. Truswell AS, Seach JM, Thorburn AW. Incomplete absorption of pure fructose in healthy subjects and the facilitating effect of glucose. *American Journal of Clinical Nutrition* 1988; **48**: 1424–1430.

6. Hyams JS. Sorbitol intolerance: an unappreciated cause of functional gastrointestinal complaints. *Gastroenterology* 1983; **84**: 30–33.

7. Goldstein R, Braverman D, Stankiewicz H. Carbohydrate malabsorption and the effect of dietary restriction on symptoms of irritable bowel syndrome and functional bowel complaints. *Israel Medical Association Journal* 2000; **2**: 583–587.

8. Shepherd, SJ Parker FJ, Muir JG, Gibson PR Dietary triggers of abdominal symptoms in patients with irritable bowel syndrome- randomised placebo-controlled evidence. *Clinical Gastroenterology and Hepatology* 2008; **6**(7): 765–771.

9. Gibson PR, Shepherd SJ. Evidence-based dietary management of functional gastrointestinal symptoms: The FODMAP approach. *Journal of Gastroenterology and Hepatology* 2010; **25**: 252–258.

10. Rumessen JJ. Fructose and related food carbohydrates. Sources, intake, absorption, and clinical implications. *Scandinavian Journal of Gastroenterology* 1992; **27**: 819–828.

11. Gibson PR, Newnham E, Barrett JS, Shepherd SJ, Muir JG. Review article: fructose malabsorption and the bigger picture. *Alimentary Pharmacology and Therapeutics* 2007; **25**(4): 349–363.

12. Barrett JS, Irving PM, Shepherd SJ, et al. Comparison of the prevalence of fructose and lactose malabsorption across

chronic intestinal disorders. *Alimentary Pharmacology and Therapeutics* 2009; **30**: 165–174.

13. Rumessen JJ, Gudmand-Hoyer E. Absorption capacity of fructose in healthy adults. Comparison with sucrose and its constituent monosaccharides. *Gut* 1986; **27**: 1161–1168.

14. Kneepkens CM, Vonk RJ, Fernandes J. Incomplete intestinal absorption of fructose. *Archives of Disease in Childhood* 1984; **59**: 735–738.

15. Nelis GF, Vermeeren MA, Jansen W. Role of fructose-sorbitol malabsorption in the irritable bowel syndrome. *Gastroenterology* 1990; **99**: 1016–1020.

16. Fernandez-Banares F, Esteve-Pardo M, de Leon R, et al. Sugar malabsorption in functional bowel disease: clinical implications. *American Journal of Gastroenterology* 1993; **88**: 2044–2050.

17. Symons P, Jones MP, Kellow JE. Symptom provocation in irritable bowel syndrome. Effects of differing doses of fructose-sorbitol. *Scandinavian Journal of Gastroenterology* 1992; **27**: 940–944.

18. Lomer MC, Parkes GC, Sanderson JD. Review article: lactose intolerance in clinical practice – myths and realities. *Alimentary Pharmacology and Therapeutics* 2008; **27**: 93–103.

19. Fordtran JS, Rector FC Jr, Ewton MF, Soter N, Kinney J. Permeability characteristics of the human small intestine. *Journal of Clinical Investigation* 1965; **44**: 1935–1944.

20. Fordtran JS, Rector FC, Locklear TW, Ewton MF. Water and solute movement in the small intestine of patients with sprue. *Journal of Clinical Investigation* 1967; **46**: 287–298.

21. Langkilde AM, Andersson H, Schweizer TF, Würsch P. Digestion and absorption of sorbitol, maltitol and isomalt from the small bowel. A study in ileostomy subjects. *European Journal of Clinical Nutrition* 1994; **48**: 768–775.

22. Muir J, Shepherd SJ, Rosella O, Rose R, Barrett J, Gibson P. Fructan and free fructose content of common Australian vegetables and fruit. *Journal of Agricultural and Food Chemistry* 2007; **55**: 6619–6627.

23. Muir JG, Rose R, Rosella O, et al. Measurement of short-chain carbohydrates (FODMAPs) in common Australian vegetables and fruit by high performance liquid chromatography (HPLC) with evaporative light-scattering detection (ELSD). *Journal of Agricultural and Food Chemistry* 2009; **57**: 554–565.

24. Biesiekierski JR, Rosella O, Rose R, et al. Quantification of fructans, galacto-oligosaccharides and other short-chain carbohydrates in processed grains and cereals *Journal of Human Nutrition and Dietetics* 2011; **24**(2): 154–176.

25. Nilsson U, Dahlqvist A. Cereal fructosans: Part 2 – characterisation and structure of wheat fructosans. *Food Chemistry* 1986; **22**: 95–106.

26. Bach Knudsen KE, Hessov I. Recovery of inulin from Jerusalem artichoke (Helianthus tuberosus L.) in the small intestine of man. *British Journal of Nutrition* 1995; **74**: 101–113.

27. Tack J, Fried M, Houghton LA, Spicak J, Fisher G. Systematic review: the efficacy of treatments for irritable bowel syndrome – a European perspective. *Alimentary Pharmacology and Therapeutics* 2006; **24**: 183–205.

28. Drossman D, Whitehead W, Camilleri M. Irritable bowel syndrome: a technical review for practice guideline development. *Gastroenterology* 1997; **112**: 2120–2137.

29. Hungin APS, Whorwell PJ, Tack J, Mearin F. The prevalence, patterns and impact of irritable bowel syndrome: an international survey of 40,000 subjects. *Alimentary Pharmacology and Therapeutics* 2003; **17**: 643–650.

30. Van Loo J, Coussement P, de Leenheer L, Hoebregs H, Smits G. On the presence of inulin and oligofructose as natural ingredients in the western diet. *Critical Reviews in Food Science and Nutrition* 1995; **35**: 525–552.

31. Nyman M. Fermentation and bulking capacity of indigestible carbohydrates: the case of inulin and oligofructose. *British Journal of Nutrition* 2002; **87 Suppl 2**: S163–168.

32. Piche T, des Varannes SB, Sacher-Huvelin S, Holst JJ, Cuber JC, Galmiche JP. Colonic fermentation influences lower esophageal sphincter function in gastroesophageal reflux disease. *Gastroenterology* 2003; **124**: 894–902.

33. Stone-Dorshow T, Levitt MD. Gaseous response to ingestion of poorly absorbed fructo-oligosaccharide sweetener. *American Journal of Clinical Nutrition* 1987; **46**: 61–65.

34. Rumessen JJ, Gudmand-Hoyer E. Functional bowel disease: malabsorption and abdominal distress after ingestion of fructose, sorbitol, and fructose-sorbitol mixtures. *Gastroenterology.*1988; **95**: 694–700.

35. Briet F, Achour L, Flourie B, et al. Symptomatic response to varying levels of fructo-oligosaccharides consumed occasionally or regularly. *European Journal of Clinical Nutrition* 1995; **49**: 501–507.

36. Bovee-Oudenhoven IMJ, ten Bruggencate SJM, Lettink-Wissink MLG, van der Meer R. Dietary fructo-oligosaccharides and lactulose inhibit intestinal colonisation but stimulate translocation of salmonella in rats. *Gut* 2003; **52**: 1572–1578.

37. Ten Bruggencate SJM, Bovee-Oudenhoven IMJ, Lettink-Wissink MLG, Katan MB, van der Meer R. Dietary fructooligosaccharides affect intestinal barrier function in healthy men. *Journal of Nutrition* 2006; **136**: 70–74.

38. Scholtens PAMJ, Alles MS, Willemsen LEM, et al. Dietary fructo-oligosaccharides in healthy adults do not negatively affect faecal cytotoxicity: a randomised, double-blind, placebo-controlled crossover trial. *British Journal of Nutrition* 2006; **95**: 1143–1149.

39. Vitasoy 2012: www.soy.com.au/hcp/wp-content/uploads/2012/07/Vitasoy-Nutrition-News-June-2012-Edition.pdf, accessed 23 December 2013.

Chapter 2.3

Probiotics and the gastrointestinal microbiota

Mary Hickson

Imperial College Healthcare NHS Foundation Trust and Imperial College London, London, UK

2.3.1 Criteria for classification as a probiotic

Probiotics are defined as 'live micro-organisms, which, when administered in adequate amounts, confer a health benefit on the host' [1]. There are three key points to note in this definition. First, the micro-organisms must be alive. Although *in vitro* and animal studies have shown that dead or fragments of bacteria may have positive physiological effects, there are no human studies yet to support this [2]. Second, the micro-organism must be administered in adequate amounts. It is important to ensure that doses used are supported by evidence of efficacy. Finally, to be called 'probiotic' the micro-organism must have been shown to confer a health benefit on the host. Regulations will soon ensure that probiotics will have rigorous evidence to support the use of this term. This problem has been addressed in guidance on the evaluation of probiotics in food (Box 2.3.1). In future, this approach should help reduce misuse of the term 'probiotic' and improve the quality of products and information available to the consumer.

It is also critical to understand that the effects of probiotic bacteria and yeasts are strain specific and specific to the disease or diagnosis in question (the nomenclature of bacteria is described in Box 2.3.2). For example, *Lactobacillus rhamnosus* GG demonstrates a probiotic effect in the prevention of antibiotic-associated diarrhoea [3]. Other strains of *L .rhamnosus* may not have this effect, and likewise other species in the genus *Lactobacillus* may not act as probiotics. This is because individual strains exhibit different specific characteristics, such as resistance to gastric acid and bile, ability to colonise the mucosa, and antimicrobial activity [4].

Given that each strain has specific attributes, different strains will offer varying benefits in different disease states. Thus, there is no one universal 'probiotic'; each bacterium may help resolve symptoms in specific circumstances. It is also worth noting that generic health claims (such as improving well-being or health) made by probiotic manufacturers are unlikely to be substantiated by evidence. It is highly debatable whether good health can be further improved simply by modulating the gastrointestinal microbiota. The European Food Standards Agency (EFSA) is currently reviewing health claims made by food manufacturers so in future claims will not be allowed unless supported by sound evidence. As of 2013, no probiotic product has had a health claim approved by this body.

2.3.2 Safety

Probiotics in food products are generally regarded as safe in healthy populations, as demonstrated by their extensive use over centuries, with few reported adverse consequences. However, there are specific at-risk groups.

Probiotic bacteria can cause infective episodes if they translocate from the gastrointestinal tract to

---

Advanced Nutrition and Dietetics in Gastroenterology, First Edition. Edited by Miranda Lomer.
© 2014 John Wiley & Sons, Ltd. Published 2014 by John Wiley & Sons, Ltd.

Box 2.3.1   Summary of the FAO/WHO guidelines for the evaluation of probiotics in food

1. The probiotic must be identified at the genus, species and strain level
   - The gold standard for species identification is DNA–DNA hybridization; 16S rRNA sequence determination is a suitable substitute, particularly if phenotypic tests are used for confirmation
   - Strain typing should be performed by pulsed-field gel electrophoresis
   - Strain should be deposited in an international culture collection so scientists are able to replicate published research on the strain
2. The probiotic's functional characteristics should be defined
   - Using both *in vitro* and animal assessments (e.g. resistance to bile acids and gastric acidity, adherence to mucosa, activity against pathogenic bacteria, etc.)
   - Choice of assessments should be based on relevance to the probiotic function in the target host
   - *In vitro* testing should correlate with *in vivo* performance, e.g. *in vitro* resistance to bile salts should correlate with gastric survival *in vivo*
3. The probiotic should be fully assessed for safety
   - Non-pathogenic
   - Not carrying transferable antibiotic resistance genes
   - No detrimental metabolic activities, e.g. bile salt deconjugation, toxin production, haemolytic activity
   - Assessment of side-effects during human studies
   - Surveillance of adverse incidents in consumers
   - Susceptible to antibiotics
4. The probiotic should possess clinically documented and validated health effects
   - At least one phase 2 human study (testing efficacy, i.e. randomised double-blind placebo-controlled trial)
   - Preferably with independent confirmation of results by another centre
   - Adverse events should be monitored and incidents reported
   - Where appropriate phase 3 effectiveness trial to compare probiotic with standard treatment of a specific condition
5. The probiotic should be appropriately labelled
   - Contents – genus, species, strain designation
   - Minimum numbers of viable bacteria at end of shelf-life
   - Proper storage conditions
   - Corporate contact details for consumer information.

Adapted from FAO/WHO [1].

---

extraintestinal sites, such as regional lymph nodes, spleen, liver, bloodstream, heart valves or other tissues. Bacterial translocation is caused by a defective intestinal barrier, immunosuppression or gastrointestinal prematurity, and may result in bacteraemia, sepsis and multiple organ failure [5]. However, cases of probiotic administration leading to bacteraemia or fungaemia are rare. In 2003 an expert panel concluded that 'Current evidence suggests that the risk of infection with probiotic *Lactobacilli* or *Bifidobacteria* is similar to that of infection with commensal strains, and that consumption of such products presents a negligible risk to consumers, including immuno-compromised hosts' [6]. More recently, a systematic review of

probiotics and nutritional support identified reports of 32 patients with infections of *L. rhamnosus GG* or *Saccharomyces boulardii* but this is most probably due to their extensive use rather than particular virulence [7]. The review identified the risks for probiotic-related infections as central venous catheter *in situ* and critical illness or impaired immune function leading to increased likelihood of bacterial translocation. Delivery of large doses of bacteria via postpyloric feeding tubes was also identified as a possible risk factor due to an increase in non-infectious complications [8] and mortality [9] in severely ill patients. Nevertheless, other trials have delivered probiotic bacteria via jejunal feeding tubes with no reported adverse events [7].

Box 2.3.2 Micro-organism nomenclature

All organisms are organised into taxonomic trees to describe their classification, with ever increasing specificity moving down the tree structure. This is an example for one particular bacterial strain.

1. Division, e.g. Firmicutes
2. Class, e.g. Bacilli
3. Order, e.g. Lactobacillales
4. Family, e.g. Lactobacillaceae
5. Genus, e.g. Lactobacillus
6. Species, e.g. rhamnosus
7. Strain, e.g. GG

The last three taxa make up the given name for the organism: *Lactobacillus rhamnosus GG*, which by convention is written in italics.

Three other recent reviews have explored the safety of probiotics in all patient groups [5,10,11]. *L. rhamnosus* GG, *L. casei* and *Bacillus subtilis* are species and strains that have caused bacteraemia and *S. boulardii* has caused fungaemia. Immunocompromised adults and neonates are identified as at risk, but there is no clear description of how to precisely define immunocompromise. The presence of a central venous catheter, impaired intestinal barrier, postpyloric delivery of the probiotic and cardiac valve disease are also highlighted as increasing the risk of infection. However, the reviews also note that infections are very rare and are not reported in most trials of probiotics, even those studying immunocompromised groups, such as those with HIV and neonates.

It should be noted that there are difficulties in linking infections to the specific probiotic strain, particularly if only phenotypic identification techniques are used. Ideally, genotypic methods should be used in order to identify the precise strain causing the infection and matching it to the probiotic strain. Lactobacilli are ubiquitous in the human diet and commonly occur in the GI tract and therefore many strains are indistinguishable from probiotic lactobacilli using phenotypic techniques alone. The data in the literature do not always refer to certain probiotic infection since the infective bacteria may not have been conclusively identified. Strain specificity is critical when evaluating the benefits of bacteria and it is equally important in considering safety profiles, and so the safety of each proposed probiotic bacterium should be individually assessed. Equally, the risk of using a probiotic should be carefully weighed against the benefits it may confer.

2.3.3 Review of different probiotics

A variety of micro-organisms have been studied to explore their probiotic effect, including various strains of *Escherichia, Enterococcus, Bacillus* and the yeast *S. boulardii*, but the most commonly proposed organisms are *Lactobacillus* and *Bifidobacterium* strains.

For commercial production, these organisms are purified, grown and multiplied, concentrated and preserved. They can then be incorporated into products in one of three basic ways.

(1) Added as a culture to a food with little or no opportunity for culture growth (e.g. juice).
(2) Included in the production of a fermented food and allowed to grow (e.g. yoghurt).
(3) Concentrated, dried and then packaged as powders, capsules or tablets, which can contain a range of bacterial numbers.

There is little research about the impact of formulation on probiotic efficacy, so no particular delivery vehicle can currently be viewed as superior. However, the product should be produced with adequate quality control to ensure viability of the bacteria and a good shelf-life.

There are various probiotic products available and these contain single strains, mixtures of bacteria or one or more active strains mixed with standard yoghurt cultures (not shown to have probiotic properties). Mixtures have invariably been tested as such, and so it is impossible to identify which bacterium within the mixture has the beneficial effect. Claims have been made for their benefit in a wide variety of conditions from allergy, dental caries and vaginosis to a range of gastrointestinal disorders and diarrhoea of several causes.

One of the issues associated with recommending the use of probiotics is their variable availability in different countries. For example, there is a large body of evidence for *L. rhamnosus* GG in preventing antibiotic-associated diarrhoea, but it may be difficult to find a reliable source if there is limited availability in a particular country. The internet does make purchasing of probiotics easier but the quality of the product is not always guaranteed. Care is needed in ensuring the products contain only the claimed probiotic bacteria, in the claimed numbers, and will deliver viable bacteria to their site of action.

It is worth noting that while probiotic bacteria are commonly added to yoghurt, there is little research on the standard yoghurt starter cultures. Yoghurt is made by the fermentation of milk by *Lactobacillus delbrueckii* subsp *bulgaricus* and *Streptococcus thermophilus*, plus *L. acidophilus* and *Bifidobacterium animalis lactis* in bio-yoghurt. There is little evidence that any of these strains offer beneficial effects. Where research has examined live yoghurt and bio-yoghurt specifically, the results are equivocal. For example, in the prevention of antibiotic-associated diarrhoea (AAD), Conway et al. [12] showed no benefit for either standard or bio-yoghurt, whereas Beniwal et al. [13] showed a reduction in AAD incidence from 24% to 12%. Both studies had a variety of limitations.

2.3.4 Effects in the gastrointestinal tract

The healthy human GI tract contains around 10 times as many bacteria as there are cells in the human body. Most of these bacteria (termed the microbiota) co-exist with the human host, either providing a functional benefit or doing no harm. Experiments using germ-free animals have shown that the microbiota plays an important role in growth, synthesis of vitamins, development of the immune system and even behaviour [14]. The microbiota is extremely varied with up to 1000 different bacterial species, together containing 100 times as many genes as the human genome. This genetic pool is referred to as the microbiome [15]. Relatively little is known about the human microbiota or the microbiome, although there are now major projects ongoing to define them and establish how the bacteria and their genes interact with the human host [14].

Since little is known about the human GI microbiota, it is not surprising that the mechanisms of action of probiotic bacteria are poorly understood. Primarily *in vitro* and animal experiments have started to elucidate these mechanisms. Three broad areas of possible action have been proposed: modulation of the host's immune system; antimicrobial activity; and other mechanisms relating to indirect action on pathogens, the host or food components. It is certain that the mechanism of action will vary between strains, yet again reflecting strain specificity.

There is evidence that probiotics can act on a range of immune cells involved in both innate and adaptive immunity, including intestinal epithelial cells, dendritic cells, monocytes, macrophages, B-lymphocytes, natural killer cells and T-cells. Intestinal epithelial cells form a critical barrier function in the GI tract and there is evidence that some probiotics can enhance this and prevent the destructive effects of pathogenic bacteria through the suppression of TNF-alpha and NF-kappaB pathways and by enhancing mucin secretion [16]. Actions can also influence these cells to alter cytokine secretion, favouring anti-inflammatory pathways [17]. Dendritic cells are antigen-presenting cells acting as messengers that shape the subsequent T-cell responses. They may interact with probiotics either directly via their dendrites, which can extend into the GI lumen, or indirectly via M-cells. Certain probiotics have been shown to downregulate the proinflammatory pathways, although the particular cytokine profile depends on the stimulus (e.g. strain of pathogenic bacteria) and the strain of probiotic [17]. This enhanced anti-inflammatory cytokine profile may also be influenced via monocytes and macrophages. The key cytokines that appear to be modulated are interleukin (IL)-12 and IL-10, the former enhancing cellular immunity and the latter inhibiting the inflammatory response [17].

Vaccination trials have offered insights into immunoglobulin release from B-lymphocytes, suggesting that certain probiotics can enhance the production of specific antibodies in response to vaccinations [18,19]. Other human studies have used the activity of natural killer cells as an outcome and shown that activity can increase in probiotic-supplemented groups, suggesting improved immune function [20,21]. Evidence also points to induction of regulatory T-cells (T_{reg}), which have a key role in immunological tolerance. Data are accumulating to suggest that T_{reg} cells are involved in the immunopathology related to a range of inflammatory conditions, such as inflammatory bowel disease. Research is now being targeted towards understanding the abilities of bacteria to induce the development of these T_{reg} cells, since this may offer a mechanism by which to control inflammatory diseases of the GI tract [16].

Probiotic bacteria have also been shown to have antimicrobial activities which limit the proliferation and actions of pathogenic bacteria in the GI tract. There is mainly *in vitro* evidence to suggest that this is achieved by reducing the pH of the GI lumen, inhibiting bacterial adherence and translocation or by producing antibacterial substances and stimulating defensin release. Defensins are cysteine-rich cationic peptides produced by the intestinal epithelial cells active against bacteria, fungi and viruses, and some probiotics stimulate their release to increase antimicrobial activity [22]. Probiotics have also been shown to produce their own antimicrobial substances, termed bacteriocins, further contributing to their beneficial actions [17]. Evidence suggests that some of these actions require the probiotics to be present in the GI tract before colonisation by the pathogen, explaining the efficacy of many probiotics in prevention rather than treatment of GI disease [23].

Lastly, evidence from animal models indicates that some probiotics can directly inhibit pathogenic bacterial toxins. For example, the action of *Clostridium difficile* toxin was limited in rats pretreated with *S. boulardii*, resulting in reduction in the binding of toxin A to the intestinal brush border and consequently a reduction in intestinal fluid secretion and intestinal permeability [24].

This uncertainty about how probiotic bacteria confer their benefits makes it difficult to ascertain what effects different bacterial strains may have. Much more research is required to establish these mechanisms of action, firstly so that currently available probiotics can be better understood but also so that it will be easier to identify the most promising strains of bacteria to confer benefit in a particular disease state.

2.3.5 Assessing potential probiotics for efficacy

It is important to understand the critical design and reporting issues when appraising published research to make an accurate assessment of the study's

---

Box 2.3.3 Criteria for the critical appraisal of studies of probiotic efficacy

The authors reporting the study should provide:

1. the name of the precise strain/s used
2. details of the product in which the probiotic is delivered, with manufacturer's details (if it is successful you may wish to obtain the product)
3. the content of probiotic in the delivery product (colony forming units (cfu) per gram or mL)
4. information about how the product reaches the patient, particularly if the product is delivered to inpatients (so this can be replicated)
5. the frequency of dose
6. the total daily dose of bacteria delivered (cfu/day)
7. evidence of the viability of the bacteria in the product up to the stated shelf-life
8. evidence of safety assessment, i.e. reported adverse events
9. evidence that the bacteria reach the site of action in the GI tract
10. evidence for the mode of action (theoretically if not specifically studied)
11. length of time the patient received the daily dose (bacteria may take some time to achieve an effect) and length of follow-up (how long did the beneficial effect last?)

Plus the usual criteria for randomised controlled trials, e.g. double-blind, placebo-controlled, intention to treat analysis, low drop-out, representative sample, etc.

---

quality. Box 2.3.3 summarises these key criteria. Once efficacy is established, it is also important to show that the products can be easily acquired and successfully delivered to patients, that they are consumed in sufficient amounts, and that any costs are outweighed by the savings.

References

1. FAO/WHO. *Evaluation of Health and Nutritional Properties of Probiotics in Food including Powder Milk with Live Lactic Acid Bacteria.* Joint FAO/WHO Expert Consultation Group. Cordoba, Argentina: Food and Agriculture Organization of the United Nations and World Health Organization, 2001.
2. Taverniti V, Guglielmetti S. The immunomodulatory properties of probiotic microorganisms beyond their viability (ghost

probiotics: proposal of paraprobiotic concept). *Genes and Nutrition* 2011; **6**(3): 263–274.

3. McFarland LV. Meta-analysis of probiotics for the prevention of antibiotic associated diarrhea and the treatment of Clostridium difficile disease. *American Journal of Gastroenterology* 2006: **101**(4): 812–822.

4. Jacobsen CN, Rosenfeldt Nielsen V, Hayford AE, et al. Screening of probiotic activities of forty-seven strains of Lactobacillus spp. by in vitro techniques and evaluation of the colonization ability of five selected strains in humans. *Applied and Environmental Microbiology* 1999; **65**(11): 4949–4956.

5. Liong MT. Safety of probiotics: translocation and infection. *Nutrition Reviews* 2008; **66**(4): 192–202.

6. Borriello SP, Hammes WP, Holzapfel W, et al. Safety of probiotics that contain lactobacilli or bifidobacteria. *Clinical Infectious Diseases* 2003; **36**(6): 775–780.

7. Whelan K, Myers CE. Safety of probiotics in patients receiving nutritional support: a systematic review of case reports, randomized controlled trials, and nonrandomized trials. *American Journal of Clinical Nutrition* 2010; **91**(3): 687–703.

8. Rayes N, Seehofer D, Theruvath T, et al. Supply of pre- and probiotics reduces bacterial infection rates after liver transplantation – a randomized, double-blind trial. *American Journal of Transplantation* 2005; **5**(1): 125–130.

9. Besselink MG, van Santvoort HC, Buskens E, et al. Probiotic prophylaxis in predicted severe acute pancreatitis: a randomised, double-blind, placebo-controlled trial. *Lancet* 2008; **371**(9613): 651–659.

10. Boyle RJ, Robins-Browne RM, Tang ML. Probiotic use in clinical practice: what are the risks? *American Journal of Clinical Nutrition* 2006; **83**(6): 1256–1264.

11. Hammerman C, Bin-Nun A, Kaplan M. Safety of probiotics: comparison of two popular strains. *British Medical Journal* 2006; **333**(7576): 1006–1008.

12. Conway S, Hart A, Clark A, Harvey I. Does eating yogurt prevent antibiotic-associated diarrhoea? A placebo-controlled randomised controlled trial in general practice. *British Journal of General Practice* 2007; **57**(545): 953–959.

13. Beniwal RS, Arena VC, Thomas L, et al. A randomized trial of yogurt for prevention of antibiotic-associated diarrhea. *Digestive Diseases and Sciences* 2003; **48**(10): 2077–2082.

14. Turnbaugh PJ, Ley RE, Hamady M, Fraser-Liggett CM, Knight R, Gordon JI. The human microbiome project. *Nature* 2007; **449**(7164): 804–810.

15. Hooper LV, Gordon JI. Commensal host-bacterial relationships in the gut. *Science* 2001; **292**(5519): 1115–1118.

16. Shida K, Nanno M. Probiotics and immunology: separating the wheat from the chaff. *Trends in Immunology* 2008; **29**(11): 565–573.

17. Ng SC, Hart AL, Kamm MA, Stagg AJ, Knight SC. Mechanisms of action of probiotics: recent advances. *Inflammatory Bowel Diseases* 2008; **15**(2): 300–310.

18. Isolauri E, Joensuu J, Suomalainen H, Luomala M, Vesikari T. Improved immunogenicity of oral D x RRV reassortant rotavirus vaccine by Lactobacillus casei GG. *Vaccine* 1995; **13**(3): 310–312.

19. Fang H, Elina T, Heikki A, Seppo S. Modulation of humoral immune response through probiotic intake. *FEMS Immunology and Medical Microbiology* 2000; **29**(1): 47–52.

20. Gill HS, Cross ML, Rutherfurd KJ, Gopal PK. Dietary probiotic supplementation to enhance cellular immunity in the elderly. *British Journal of Biomedical Science* 2001; **58**(2): 94–96.

21. Takeda K, Suzuki T, Shimada SI, Shida K, Nanno M, Okumura K. Interleukin-12 is involved in the enhancement of human natural killer cell activity by Lactobacillus casei Shirota. *Clinical and Experimental Immunology* 2006; **146**(1): 109–115.

22. Preidis GA, Hill C, Guerrant RL, Ramakrishna BS, Tannock GW, Versalovic J. Probiotics, enteric and diarrheal diseases, and global health. *Gastroenterology* 2011; **140**(1): 8–14.

23. Parkes GC, Sanderson JD, Whelan K. The mechanisms and efficacy of probiotics in the prevention of Clostridium difficile-associated diarrhoea. *Lancet Infectious Diseases* 2009; **9**(4): 237–244.

24. Pothoulakis C, Kelly CP, Joshi MA, et al. Saccharomyces boulardii inhibits Clostridium difficile toxin A binding and enterotoxicity in rat ileum. *Gastroenterology* 1993; **104**(4): 1108–1115.

Chapter 2.4

Prebiotics and gastrointestinal health

Kevin Whelan
King's College London, London, UK

The composition of the gastrointestinal (GI) micro-biota is dramatically influenced by diet, with the first description of differences in the numbers of luminal bifidobacteria between breastfed and for-mula-fed infants occurring in the late 1800s [1]. However, the ability of certain dietary constituents to impact specifically on the GI microbiota, the mechanisms through which they do so, and the potential clinical application for the management of disease have only recently been explored in depth.

Habitual long-term diet has been shown to strongly associate with different clusters of bacteria in the colon, termed 'enterotypes'. For example, high intakes of protein and animal fat are associ-ated with the *Bacteroides* enterotype and high intakes of carbohydrate are associated with the *Prevotella* enterotype [2]. In terms of short-term dietary changes, acute feeding studies show that altering fat and non-starch polysaccharide intakes alters the microbiota but does not change these enterotypes [3].

Many exogenous dietary components, as well as endogenous material (e.g. sloughed enterocytes, red blood cells), are metabolised by the GI microbiota through fermentation and produce short-chain fatty acids (SCFA). The main dietary substrates that undergo bacterial metabolism are non-digestible carbohydrates that escape digestion and absorption in the upper GI tract (commonly termed dietary fibre), including non-starch polysaccharides (e.g. pectins, guar gum, hemicellulose), non-digestible oligosaccharides (e.g. fructans, galactans) and resist-ant starch, in addition to some disaccharides and monosaccharides that are conditionally non-digestible (e.g. in lactose maldigestion, fructose maldigestion). Many of these non-digestible carbohydrates are substrates for bacterial fermentation and therefore support the growth of a wide range of bacteria in the GI tract. However, since 1995, extensive research has demonstrated that some non-digestible carbo-hydrates stimulate specific microbiota (e.g. bifido-bacteria) and these are termed prebiotics [4].

2.4.1 Prebiotic definitions, characteristics and classes

Prebiotics are non-digestible, fermentable food components that result in 'the selective stimulation of growth and/or activity of one or a limited number of microbial genera/species in the GI microbiota that confer health benefits to the host' [5]. This is the most recent definition and updates earlier versions to account for the fact that prebiotics can influence the activity, as well as the numbers, of specific bacteria.

There are three essential characteristics of a prebiotic: (i) its resistance to digestion in the upper GI tract; (ii) its ability to be fermented by the host microbiota; and (iii) for this to impact on the growth or activity of specific bacteria only [5]. Resistance to small intestinal digestion is the result of humans lacking enzymes that hydrolyse the various poly-mer bonds. This allows the prebiotic to reach the colon intact and undergo fermentation, but only by a limited number of genera/species.

Advanced Nutrition and Dietetics in Gastroenterology, First Edition. Edited by Miranda Lomer.
© 2014 John Wiley & Sons, Ltd. Published 2014 by John Wiley & Sons, Ltd.

Table 2.4.1 Selection of compounds with proven prebiotic properties

Generic name	Class	Common source and manufacture	Degree of polymerisation (DP) Range	Degree of polymerisation (DP) Average
Inulin (mixed length)	Inulin-type fructan (ITF)	Extracted from chicory or other sources	2–60	12
Inulin (high molecular weight)	Inulin-type fructan	Physical purification of inulin from chicory	10–60	25
Fructo-oligosaccharides (FOS)	Inulin-type fructan	Generally from enzymatic synthesis from sucrose	2–9	3.6
Oligofructose (OF)	Inulin-type fructan	Generally from partial enzymatic hydrolysis of inulin	2–9	4
Galacto-oligosaccharides (GOS) or trans-GOS	Galactans	Enzymatic transgalactosylation of lactose	2–9	—

The most common classes of prebiotics are inulin-type fructans (e.g. inulin, oligofructose, fructo-oligosaccharides) and galactans (galacto-oligosaccharides, e.g. stachyose, raffinose) (Table 2.4.1). Lactulose, the synthetic non-digestible carbohydrate used as an osmotic laxative for constipation, is also a prebiotic but is rarely used in functional food preparations and therefore is not reviewed here. The potential prebiotic properties of other novel oligosaccharides (e.g. isomalto-oligosaccharides, soybean oligosaccharides) are also under investigation.

Inulin-type fructans (ITF) consist of linear polymers of fructose monomers joined by beta($2 \rightarrow 1$) linkages, some of which also have a terminal glucose monomer. The major ITFs are inulin, oligofructose (OF) and fructo-oligosaccharides (FOS), which are defined based upon their source and the number of monomers in the polymer chain (degree of polymerisation, DP) (see Table 2.4.1). In general, inulin has a wide-ranging polymer length (DP 2–60), whereas OF and FOS have a shorter length (DP 2–10) [5]. Inulin-type fructans are found in very large amounts in chicory root (35.7–47.6 g/100 g), which is the most common source for commercial preparations of inulin, but is also present in Jerusalem artichoke (16–20 g/100 g) and garlic

(9–16 g/100 g) [6]. ITFs are found in small amounts in cereals such as wheat (1–4 g/100 g), which is actually the most common dietary source in the United Kingdom [7] and the United States [8] due to its widespread consumption.

Galactans include the prebiotics galacto-oligosaccharides (GOS), which are short polymers (DP usually <10) of galactose monomers joined by beta($1 \rightarrow 6$), beta($1 \rightarrow 3$) and/or beta($1 \rightarrow 4$) linkages to a terminal glucose monomer [9]. Galacto-oligosaccharides are widely contained and consumed within pulses, where the type of linkages may differ.

2.4.2 Evidence of selective stimulation of gastrointestinal microbiota

The first key human study to demonstrate the prebiotic effect compared the impact of 15 g/day of oligofructose or inulin, in a randomized, cross-over trial of eight healthy people consuming a controlled diet. Both compounds resulted in almost a 1 $\log_{10}$ increase in luminal bifidobacteria [10].

Many *in vitro*, animal, human and even some clinical studies have now demonstrated the ability of ITFs and GOS to stimulate the growth of bifidobacteria (the prebiotic effect), and these have been extensively reviewed and tabulated elsewhere [5]. Indeed, some studies in healthy humans have also shown increases in other bacteria including lactobacilli [10] and *Faecalibacterium prausnitzii* [11]. Although not frequently investigated *in vivo*, the increase in bifidobacteria following prebiotic supplementation (sometimes referred to as bifidogenesis) has been shown to be at the expense of a range of other bacteria including reductions in clostridia [10]and bacteroides [12]. Interestingly, the majority of prebiotic studies use supplements and the effect of prebiotics naturally occurring in foods has received little attention in the literature. Therefore, the effects of a diet high in ITFs (e.g. chicory, onion, wheat) and GOS (e.g. beans, pulses) are as yet unclear.

The mechanism of how prebiotics are able to selectively stimulate the growth of specific bacteria has until recently received little attention in the literature. In one study it was shown that some bacteria have 'fructan utilisation locus' genes that enable them to acquire and ferment ITFs [13]. Studies in mice have shown that the functional expression of the 'fructan utilisation locus' in different bacteria was highly predictive of the ability of that strain to be selectively stimulated when the mice were fed inulin [13]. Therefore it is thought that during prebiotic supplementation, bacteria with the ability to express genes coding for fructan utilisation are better able to access the carbon source in the ITF, use it for bacterial metabolism and therefore are better able to proliferate, a process of competitive selection.

The capacity of a prebiotic to stimulate the growth of specific bacteria can depend on a number of factors including the physiochemical characteristics and dose of the prebiotic used and the host microbiota.

First, the physiochemical characteristics of the prebiotic can have functionally important effects. In general, ITFs with shorter DP (OF, FOS) are more rapidly fermented which potentially allows fermentation to start earlier in the colon, whereas those with a longer DP (long-chain inulin) have a more prolonged fermentation, that might enable fermentation to continue to the latter regions of the colon. With regard to GOS, some researchers consider that variations in the proportions of the beta$(1 \rightarrow 6)$,

beta$(1 \rightarrow 3)$ and beta$(1 \rightarrow 4)$ linkages result in varying degrees of fermentability [9], and therefore commercial preparations that vary in the proportions of these linkages are available.

Second, in general, higher doses result in a greater impact of prebiotics on the GI microbiota [14,15]. However, bloating and flatulence can occur at high doses due to excessive gas production during fermentation. Therefore, careful dose–response studies have been undertaken that investigate the dose that elicits the greatest impact on the microbiota without a significant increase in GI symptoms. For example, in a study of short-chain FOS given at a range of doses, the greatest impact on bifidobacteria occurred at 10 g/day and 20 g/day, but the higher dose also resulted in increased frequency and severity of flatulence, resulting in 10 g/day being recommended as the optimal dose of short-chain FOS to be used in healthy people [15].

Third, the composition of the host GI microbiota can affect the responsiveness to prebiotics. Numerous studies have shown that the baseline concentration of bifidobacteria negatively correlates with the magnitude of the increase in bifidobacteria following consumption of ITFs [16]. This relationship may have important consequences, as those people with the lowest concentrations of bifidobacteria (and therefore with the most to benefit from supplementation) are likely to respond the most. However, this observation has not been consistently shown and there is even evidence of people who do (responders) and do not (non-responders) experience an increase in bifidobacteria following GOS supplementation [14].

The factors resulting in the interindividual differences in response to prebiotic supplementation require further investigation.

2.4.3 Clinical applications of prebiotics

An in-depth review has recently been published regarding the physiological effects of prebiotics on GI function, immune function and mineral absorption [5]. Some prebiotics suppress the growth of enteropathogens, such as clostridia, and although this was thought to be due to a process of colonisation resistance by increased numbers of bifidobacteria, this has not been conclusively demonstrated [17]. There is evidence from many animal studies that some prebiotics stimulate innate and adaptive immunity of the GI tract as well as the systemic immune system, but human studies are only recently emerging [18]. Furthermore, as with other non-digestible carbohydrates, prebiotics are fermentable and produce a range of products, such as SCFAs, that themselves have health-promoting activities, including water absorption and acidification of the GI tract.

In view of these potential mechanisms, a small number of disparate studies has been undertaken on the effects of prebiotics in managing GI disorders. Here, their role in the management of GI infection, Crohn's disease and irritable bowel syndrome (IBS) is addressed.

In GI infectious diarrhoea, one research group undertook randomised controlled trials (RCTs) and found that OF (12 g/day) had no impact on the duration of antibiotic-associated diarrhoea [19] but that in a separate study it did reduce the relapse rate in the secondary prevention of *Clostridium difficile* infection [20] (Table 2.4.2). Meanwhile, an RCT of 5.5 g/day of GOS showed a reduction in the incidence of travellers' diarrhoea when healthy people travelled to areas of low to high risk for gastroenteritis [21]. However, in the latter study no formal testing for enteropathogenic colonisation or microbiota analysis was undertaken.

Crohn's disease is a chronic relapsing and remitting inflammatory bowel disease characterised by discontinuous transmural inflammation, ulceration and stricturing anywhere in the GI tract. There is considerable evidence that the GI microbiota is directly involved in the pathogenesis of Crohn's disease, including animal models that do not develop disease until their GI tract becomes colonised with bacteria, the discovery of Crohn's disease susceptibility loci/genes whose function is bacterial recognition (CARD15/NOD2) and bacterial processing and extensive evidence of altered GI microbiota (termed dysbiosis), including lower bifidobacteria and *Faecalibacterium prausnitzii* in patients with Crohn's disease [22]. Two large RCTs have investigated the mixtures of OF/inulin at doses of 15 g/day [23] or 20 g/day [24] but neither found a significant impact on Crohn's disease activity, nor

on concentrations of bifidobacteria or *F. prausnitzii* when comparing the prebiotic with the placebo (see Table 2.4.2).

Irritable bowel syndrome is a functional GI disorder characterised by abdominal pain and altered stool output in the absence of an organic cause. There is also evidence that the GI microbiota may be involved in the pathogenesis of IBS, including a greater risk following gastroenteritis, evidence of dysbiosis such as lower bifidobacteria in patients with diarrhoea-predominant IBS and elevated luminal gas production in IBS [25]. Few RCTs have investigated the role of prebiotics in the management of IBS, and only two have shown benefit (see Table 2.4.2) [25]. Fructo-oligosaccharides (5 g/day) were shown to lower composite symptom scores in an RCT of people with functional bowel disorders [26] and trans-GOS (3.5 g/day) has been shown to lower bloating and improve global symptom relief in patients with IBS [27]. However, both studies experienced large attrition rates and were not analysed as intention to treat. Other studies have shown worsening symptoms during supplementation of some prebiotics in IBS, and this is actually the basis for the effectiveness of a diet low in fermentable oligosaccharides, disaccharides, monosaccharides and polyols (FODMAP)s in IBS (see Chapter 3.9). Clearly, the role of modifying the microbiota and fermentation in IBS is important, and whilst prebiotic supplementation and the low FODMAP diet may at first seem to be conflicting approaches, clearly the physiochemical structure and the dose of prebiotic are likely to be important in determining its efficacy.

Evidence of the interaction between prebiotics, the GI microbiota and the management of disease is now emerging. Currently, there is limited but expanding evidence for specific prebiotics in specific clinical settings, alongside interindividual differences in response to supplementation. Therefore, where studies show increases in bifidobacteria (and any associated physiological or clinical response) following prebiotic supplementation, this can only be assumed to occur for that prebiotic, at that dose and in that population. In clinical practice, advice should therefore be specific to the product, dose and disorder investigated in clinical trials.

Table 2.4.2 Clinical trials of prebiotic supplementation in a range of gastrointestinal disorders

Reference	Study details	Intervention	Differences between intervention and placebo
Lewis et al. [20]	**C. difficile-associated diarrhoea** Secondary prevention in inpatients with *C. difficile* infection Randomised, double-blind trial 142 patients, 30-day intervention period	(1) OF (12 g/day) (2) Placebo (12 g/day)	**Microbiota**: Higher bifidobacteria in prebiotic group **Clinical**: Lower relapse of *C. difficile* in the prebiotic group (8% vs 34%)
Drakoularakou et al. [21]	**Travellers' diarrhoea** Primary prevention in people travelling to low/high-risk area Randomised, double-blind trial 159 people, intervention period was for 7 days prior to, and for duration of, holiday	(1) GOS (5.5 g/day) (2) Placebo (5.5 g/day)	**Clinical**: Lower incidence of travellers' diarrhoea in the prebiotic group (23% vs 38%)
Benjamin et al. [23]	**Crohn's disease** Primary treatment of active Crohn's Randomised, double-blind trial 103 patients, 4-week intervention period	(1) OF/inulin (15 g/day) (2) Placebo (15 g/day)	**Microbiota**: No difference in bifidobacteria or *F. prausnitzii* **Clinical**: No difference in remission rates between groups (11% vs 20%). Greater severity of flatulence and pain in the prebiotic group
Joossens et al. [24]	**Crohn's disease** Primary management of active/inactive Crohn's Randomised, double-blind trial 40 patients, 4-week intervention period	(1) OF/inulin (20 g/day) (2) Placebo (20 g/day)	**Microbiota**: No differences in any microbiota measured **Clinical**: No difference in disease activity, even in subgroup with active disease
Paineau et al. [26]	**Functional bowel disorder** Primary management of functional symptoms Randomised, double-blind trial 50 patients, 6-week intervention period	(1) FOS (5 g/day) (2) Placebo (5 g/day)	**Clinical**: Lower composite symptom score and greater reduction in abdominal pain in the prebiotic group
Silk et al. [27]	**Irritable bowel syndrome** Primary management of IBS symptoms Randomised, double-blind, cross-over trial 44 patients, 4-week intervention period	(1) Placebo, then 3.5 g/day GOS (2) Placebo, then 7.0 g/day GOS (3) Placebo, then placebo	**Microbiota**: Higher bifidobacteria in both the prebiotic groups **Clinical**: Lower scores for flatulence, bloating and global relief in the low-dose group. Higher composite score in the high-dose group compared with placebo

FOS, fructo-oligosaccharides; **GOS**, galacto-oligosaccharide; **OF**, oligofructose.

References

1. Tissier H. *Recherches sur la flore intestinale de nourissons (Research on the intestinal flora of infants).* PhD thesis. France: University of Paris, 1898.
2. Arumugam M, Raes J, Pelletier E, et al. Enterotypes of the human gut microbiome. *Nature* 2011; **473**: 174–180.
3. Wu GD, Chen J, Hoffmann C, et al. Linking long-term dietary patterns with gut microbial enterotypes. *Science* 2011; **334**: 105–108.
4. Gibson GR, Roberfroid MB. Dietary modulation of the human colonic microbiota: introducing the concept of prebiotics. *Journal of Nutrition* 1995; **125**: 1401–1412.
5. Roberfroid M, Gibson GR, Hoyles L, et al. Prebiotic effects: metabolic and health benefits. *British Journal of Nutrition* 2010; **104**(S2): S1–S63.
6. Van Loo J, Coussement P, de Leenheer L, Hoebregs H, Smits G. On the presence of inulin and oligofructose as natural ingredients in the western diet. *Critical Reviews in Food Science and Nutrition* 1995; **35**: 525–552.
7. Dunn S, Datta A, Kallis S, Law E, Myers CE, Whelan K. Validation of a food frequency questionnaire to measure intakes of inulin and oligofructose. *European Journal of Clinical Nutrition* 2011; **65**: 402–408.
8. Moshfegh AJ, Friday JE, Goldman JP, Chug Ahuja JK. Presence of inulin and oligofructose in the diets of Americans. *Journal of Nutrition* 1999; **129**(Suppl 7): S1407–S1411.
9. Lamsal BP. Production, health aspects and potential food uses of dairy prebiotic galactooligosaccharides. *Journal of Food Science and Agriculture* 2012; **92**(10): 2020–2028.
10. Gibson GR, Beatty ER, Wang X, Cummings JH. Selective stimulation of bifidobacteria in the human colon by oligofructose and inulin. *Gastroenterology* 1995; **108**: 975–982.
11. Ramirez-Farias C, Slezak K, Fuller Z, Duncan A, Holtrop G, Louis P. Effect of inulin on the human gut microbiota: stimulation of *Bifidobacterium adolescentis* and *Faecalibacterium prausnitzii*. *British Journal of Nutrition* 2009; **101**: 541–550.
12. Davis LM, Martínez I, Walter J, Goin C, Hutkins RW. Barcoded pyrosequencing reveals that consumption of galacto-oligosaccharides results in a highly specific bifidogenic response in humans. *PLOS One* 2011; **6**(9): e25200.
13. Sonnenburg ED, Zheng H, Joglekar P, et al. Specificity of polysaccharide use in intestinal bacteroides species determines diet-induced microbiota alterations. *Cell* 2010; **141**: 1241–1252.
14. Davis LM, Martínez I, Walter J, Hutkins R. A dose dependent impact of prebiotic galactooligosaccharides on the intestinal microbiota of healthy adults. *International Journal of Food Microbiology* 2010; **144**: 285–292.
15. Bouhnik Y, Vahedi K, Achour L, et al. Short-chain fructo-oligosaccharide administration dose-dependently increases fecal bifidobacteria in healthy humans. *Journal of Nutrition* 1999; **129**: 113–116.
16. De Preter V, Vanhoutte T, Huys G, Swings J, Rutgeerts P, Verbeke K. Baseline microbiota activity and initial bifidobacteria counts influence responses to prebiotic dosing in healthy subjects. *Alimentary Pharmacology and Therapeutics* 2008; **27**: 504–513.
17. Hopkins MJ, Macfarlane GT. Nondigestible oligosaccharides enhance bacterial colonization resistance against Clostridium difficile in vitro. *Applied and Environmental Microbiology* 2003; **69**: 1920–1927.
18. Lomax AR, Calder PC. Prebiotics, immune function, infection and inflammation: a review of the evidence. *British Journal of Nutrition* 2009; **101**: 633–658.
19. Lewis S, Burmeister S, Cohen S, Brazier J, Awasthi A. Failure of dietary oligofructose to prevent antibiotic-associated diarrhoea. *Alimentary Pharmacology and Therapeutics* 2005; **21**: 469–477.
20. Lewis S, Burmeister S, Brazier J. Effect of the prebiotic oligofructose on relapse of *Clostridium difficile*-associated diarrhea: a randomized, controlled study. *Clinical Gastroenterology and Hepatology* 2005; **3**: 442–448.
21. Drakoularakou A, Tzortzis G, Rastall RA, Gibson GR. A double-blind, placebo-controlled, randomized human study assessing the capacity of a novel galacto-oligosaccharide mixture in reducing travellers' diarrhoea. *European Journal of Clinical Nutrition* 2010; **64**: 146–152.
22. Manichanh C, Borruel N, Casellas F, Guarner F. The gut microbiota in IBD. *Nature Reviews Gastroenterology and Hepatology* 2012; **9**: 599–608.
23. Benjamin JL, Hedin CRH, Koutsoumpas A, et al. A randomised, double blind placebo controlled trial of fructo-oligosaccharides in active Crohn's disease. *Gut* 2011; **60**: 923–929.
24. Joossens M, de Preter V, Ballet V, et al. Effect of oligofructose-enriched inulin (OF-IN) on bacterial composition and disease activity of patients with Crohn's disease: results from a double-blinded randomised controlled trial. *Gut* 2012; **61**: 958.
25. Whelan K. Probiotics and prebiotics in the management of irritable bowel syndrome: a review of recent clinical trials and systematic reviews. *Current Opinion in Clinical Nutrition and Metabolic Care* 2011; **14**: 581–587.
26. Paineau D, Payen F, Panserieu S, et al. The effects of regular consumption of short-chain fructo-oligosaccharides on digestive comfort of subjects with minor functional bowel disorders. *British Journal of Nutrition* 2008; **99**: 311–318.
27. Silk DB, Davis A, Vulevic J, Tzortzis G, Gibson GR. Clinical trial: the effects of a trans-galactooligosaccharide prebiotic on faecal microbiota and symptoms in irritable bowel syndrome. *Alimentary Pharmacology and Therapeutics* 2009; **29**: 508–518.

SECTION 3

Gastrointestinal disorders

Chapter 3.1

Orofacial granulomatosis and nutrition

Helen Campbell, Jeremy D. Sanderson and Miranda C. E. Lomer
Guy's and St Thomas' NHS Foundation Trust and King's College London, London, UK

The term 'orofacial granulomatosis' (OFG) is a descriptor for the presentation of granulomatous inflammation which affects, most noticeably, the lips and face but invariably intraoral features are also present and can include swelling, erythema, nodules, tags and ulcers [1]. Orofacial granulomatosis is rare and the incidence is unknown although the highest reported published patient numbers are from Scotland. Approximately one quarter of patients present with a concurrent diagnosis of Crohn's disease and more rarely a diagnosis of Melkersson Rosenthal syndrome is appropriate when facial palsy and fissured tongue are additional clinical findings [2]. Both children and adults can be affected. The diagnosis is made through oral examination and the gold standard histological diagnostic criteria require the presence of non-casaeating granulomas observed in the biopsies taken from the disease sites.

3.1.1 Aetiology

The aetiology is unknown. Hypotheses have included allergic, infective and genetic causes [3]. However, the majority of studies have been limited by the rarity of the disease. Allergic causes have received most coverage, with oral exposure to foods, dental hygiene products and dental materials being implicated in the disease process for some patients.

3.1.2 Treatments

Treatments have involved exclusion of suspected allergens but where this fails, topical immunosuppression such as topical steroids or tacrolimus is used, often prior to systemic immunosuppression [4,5]. It is not uncommon for patients to also present with accompanying candidiasis or bacterial infections, particularly in fissures, which can exacerbate disease and may require treatment with topical antifungals or antibiotic therapies [6]. Intralesional steroids can offer benefit but are unpleasant and recurrence is common although more recently, a succession of injections with accompanying use of anaesthetic nerve block has been described as inducing long-term remission [7]. Oral steroids often have some initial benefit but recurrence is common [8,9]. Azathioprine has been used but does not tend to have an immediate response. However, it shows some promise, particularly in those with a concurrent diagnosis of Crohn's disease [10]. Anti-tumour necrosis factor (TNF)-alpha has been used in refractory OFG but reports are rare and again long-term response is not always satisfactory [11].

Dietary treatments have involved exclusion diets and have demonstrated some resolution when the offending food can be readily identified [12]. The most frequently used dietary treatment avoids cinnamon and benzoate [13]. Elemental diets have shown some promise, particularly in children, but this has its limitations in terms of palatability and acceptability [14].

Advanced Nutrition and Dietetics in Gastroenterology, First Edition. Edited by Miranda Lomer.
© 2014 John Wiley & Sons, Ltd. Published 2014 by John Wiley & Sons, Ltd.

3.1.3 History of the cinnamon- and benzoate-free diet

Sensitivity to cinnamon and benzoates was first observed in patients with OFG in 1997 when patch testing in a small group of patients indicated a higher rate of benzoic acid sensitivity [15]. In 2000, Wray et al. undertook a retrospective review of patch test data in 1252 patients with oral disease, of whom 261 had OFG [16]. A high rate of sensitivity to perfumes and flavourings, and in particular benzoic acid and cinnamaldehyde sensitivity, was illustrated and the authors reported improvement through avoidance of these compounds. They also reported chocolate sensitivity in OFG. In 2006, White et al. demonstrated improvement in 72% of patients who could comply with this diet and subsequently a cinnamon- and benzoate-free diet became the primary therapy employed in the management of OFG [17].

3.1.4 Mechanisms involved in dietary avoidance of cinnamon and benzoates in orofacial granulomatosis

The immunopathological mechanisms for the observed response to dietary avoidance of cinnamon and benzoates are not clear. However, other rare reports of allergic reactions have implicated benzoates, mainly in asthma and allergic contact dermatitis [18]. One postulated but unproven theory includes the potential for a type 4 reaction involving a T-cell response. Another suggests a possible late-phase IgE-dependent response. A further hypothesis suggests that benzoates are too small to act as allergens but they may act as haptens that potentially bind to proteins in the mouth that then trigger a reaction [19,20]. Additionally, sodium benzoate has been shown to suppress a Th1 pathway [21]. The implication is that sodium benzoate is not an allergen itself but aggravates an allergic response by suppressing the Th1 pathway and in doing so, allows a Th2 response to flourish in the presence of an allergen. This too could apply in OFG. However, contradicting

this theory is a study in which 10 patients with OFG were predominantly found to have a Th1 profile in keeping with Crohn's disease. However, more recently, discovery of a novel subepithelial dendritic B-cell which expresses IgE in the lips of patients with OFG has contributed to a hypothesis of a possible contribution of a Th2 pathway and an IgE-mediated response [22].

The mechanisms involving the role of cinnamon and benzoates in OFG are not understood and much work is still required to appreciate the immunological impact this diet might have.

3.1.5 Sources of cinnamon and benzoates

Benzoates

Benzoates are naturally present in plant foods and are also added to foods as preserving agents (Table 3.1.1) [23–27]. Sources of added benzoates can include drinks, chewing gums, biscuits, cakes, yoghurts, pickles, sauces, preserved fish and meat. A maximum dose of 150 mg/kg can be added and the highest likely exposures would be from soft drinks [28,29]. Natural sources of benzoic acid are found in plant foods, most commonly in berry fruits but also in other sources such as spinach, pumpkin and spices (Table 3.1.2) [23–27].

Cinnamon

Cinnamon (*Cinnamomum zeylanium* N.) originates from Sri Lanka and is a spice used in a variety of medicinal and culinary industries [30]. The compound that patients appear most sensitive to is cinnamaldehyde [16], which is the component that gives cinnamon its rich aroma and flavour. Cinnamaldehyde is also present naturally in blueberries [25]. Cinnamon is also a natural source of benzoic acid and is used as an ingredient for both sweet and savoury foods, chewing gums, sweets, chocolates, cakes and other baked goods. It is also used in toothpastes, mouthwashes and other cosmetics and hygiene products as both a perfume and antimicrobial preserving agent. It is perhaps

Table 3.1.1 Preservatives to be avoided on the cinnamon- and benzoate-free diet

*Preservative	E number
Benzoic acid	E210
Sodium benzoate	E211
Potassium benzoate	E212
Calcium benzoate	E213
Ethyl 4-hydroxybenzoate or ethyl para-hydroxybenzoate	E214
Ethyl 4-hydroxybenzoate, sodium salt or sodium ethyl para-hydroxybenzoate	E215
#Propyl 4-hydroxybenzoate or propyl para-hydroxybenzoate	*E216*
#Propyl 4-hydroxybenzoate, sodium salt or sodium para-hydroxybenzoate	*E217*
Methyl 4-hydroxybenzoate or methyl para-hydroxybenzoate	E218
Methyl 4-hydroxybenzoate, sodium salt or sodium methyl-hydroxybenzoate	E219

*All food labels need to be checked for these preservatives which are most commonly found in soft drinks but can potentially be added to jams, sauces, pickles, yoghurts, salad dressings, ketchups, cakes, biscuits, preserved delicatessen foods and other preserved foods.
#Banned in the European Union but might be available in imported goods.

most recognised for its use in Asian-style cooking and curries.

In terms of food labelling, any spice is only required to be fully labelled if it exceeds 2% of the food product [31,32]. Consequently, any food with 'spice' or 'spice mix' on the food ingredients label requires avoidance on a cinnamon- and benzoate-free diet in case the spices used include cinnamon. Garam masala is a mix of spices used in Indian curries and usually contains cinnamon. A similar spice known as cassia (*Cinnamomum cassia Presi*) is often used as a cheaper alternative to cinnamon [33]. Often thought to be inferior in flavour, it is primarily sourced from China, Vietnam and Indonesia and requires avoidance on the cinnamon- and benzoate-free diet. In contrast to cinnamon, cassia has received

some negative publicity associated with its high level of coumarin which is thought to be carcinogenic.

3.1.6 Treating with a cinnamon- and benzoate-free diet

Orofacial granulomatosis is a complex and distressing condition that requires a high level of input, and a multidisciplinary approach is most often useful. Disease-specific expertise is rare but access to oral medicine specialists, gastroenterology and dietetics provides the optimal healthcare approach.

Following a diagnosis of OFG, dietary management is often used first. Patch testing was originally employed to help determine sensitivity to cinnamaldehyde and benzoates and this initiated the dietary avoidance of cinnamon and benzoates. However, a recent review of response to the cinnamon- and benzoate-free diet, irrespective of patch test results, indicated that patients were no more likely to respond to the diet if they had positive patch test results to either cinnamaldehyde or benzoates [3]. The recommendation is therefore to trial exclusion of cinnamon and benzoates first line both as a treatment and as a means to identify possible sensitivities to these compounds.

The cinnamon- and benzoate-free diet should be tried for an initial period of 12 weeks. The diet is considered nutritionally adequate and so no routine micronutrient supplementation is necessary unless a diet history reveals other food aversions or intolerances that might otherwise impact on micronutrient status. If no improvement is observed then other treatments should be considered. If there is symptom improvement, it may be appropriate to consider reintroducing foods to try and identify any specific food intolerances and improve the variety of the patient's diet. One food should be introduced at a time and can be gradually increased to a normal portion size over a 4-day period. During this time, the patient should remain on an otherwise cinnamon- and benzoate-free diet but providing no reactions are observed with the foods tested, then these can also be included.

Table 3.1.2 Main sources of cinnamon and benzoates

Foods to avoid	Alternatives
Herbs and spices Cinnamon, cloves, nutmeg, sage, curry powder, all spice, mixed spice, garum masala. Check food products (e.g. curries, puddings, sweet and savoury baked goods, cereals with added cinnamon)	Salt, pepper, single herbs and spices (e.g. cumin, coriander, turmeric, chilli, paprika, basil, marjoram, oregano, mint, etc.)
Drinks Any drinks with added flavourings (e.g. most soft drinks, squash, flavoured waters, flavoured spirits and alco-pops), tea including black, rooibos and green tea or any herbal teas with tea leaves, chai tea, chicory drinks, camp coffee or liquid coffees, non-alcoholic grape drinks, mulled wine and fruit juices from 'not allowed' fruits (e.g. berry juices, prune juice, peach or papaya juice, tropical juices with these additions)	Coffee, fruit, herbal infusions, fruit juices from 'allowed' fruits (e.g. orange, apple, grapefruit juice). Red or white wines, unflavoured spirits with more than 15% alcohol, whisky, cider, beer, lager
Fruit and vegetables Avocado, pumpkin, kidney beans, soya beans, spinach, berries (e.g. blackberries, cranberries, blueberries, strawberries, raspberries), prunes, peaches, papaya, nectarines, dried fruits, jams made from these fruits or jams with added flavourings and benzoates. Fruit sauces or compotes. Tomato puree , sundried tomatoes, passata	All other fresh and frozen fruits (e.g. apples, oranges, pears, bananas, satsumas, tangerines, melon, pineapple, grapefruit, lemon, lime, grapes, mangoes) or vegetables (e.g. broccoli, cauliflower, cabbage, carrots, green beans, runner beans, broad beans, spring greens, lettuce, cucumber, onion, peppers, bean sprouts, rhubarb, fresh tomatoes
Sweet and savoury snacks Sweets with cinnamon, chocolate and chocolate-containing sweets, sweets with added flavourings, spiced mix, Bombay mix, flavoured crisps	Plain or salted nuts, crisps and seeds, sugar, honey, molasses, syrups, icing sugar, sweets without added flavourings (e.g. toffee, honeycomb, fudge, mints)
Meat, fish dairy Delicatessen-bought meat and fish, preserved meats and fish with added benzoates, meat and fish with added spices, sweet or savoury yoghurts and cheeses with added 'not allowed' fruits and spices. Blue and Gorgonzola cheese	Any other meat or fish without added benzoates or sauces with added flavourings. Eggs, milk, all other cheeses, and yoghurts without 'not allowed' ingredients, cream cheese, sour cream

Unlike allergic reactions, OFG recurrence can often be delayed and so patients should appreciate that reactions can occur sometimes up to 24 h after exposure to the food.

Practical considerations on a cinnamon and benzoate free diet

Tables 3.1.1 and 3.1.2 provide dietary guidance for a cinnamon- and benzoate-free diet. Tools to help with the dietary management of OFG can be sourced from www.kcl.ac.uk/ofg.

There are other dietary factors to consider.

Flavourings

Flavourings are added to many foods and are labelled as 'flavourings' or 'natural flavourings' [32]. Consequently, the flavour compound added is not known to the consumer. Over 2000 flavourings exist for use in the European Union [28] and some of these compounds contain cinnamon and benzoate derivatives. For example, balsam of Peru is used in a wide range of products including cosmetics and perfumes, pharmaceuticals, food flavourings, sweets, chocolates, drinks, pastries and cigarettes [34]. The main chemical components include benzoic acid, cinnamic acid, benzyl benzoate, benzyl cinnamate, cinnamyl cinnamate, vanillin and nerolidol. It is recommended that where possible, products with added flavourings are avoided on the cinnamon- and benzoate-free diet.

Chocolate

Patients with OFG can have sensitivity to chocolate and positive results on patch testing have been reported [16]. Cinnamon and certain flavourings with cinnamon and benzoate derivatives can be added to chocolate. It is not known if patients react to the cocoa or the other food additives in chocolate. Chocolate is therefore avoided as part of the cinnamon- and benzoate-free diet.

Tomato

Raw tomatoes contain trace amounts of benzoates [35] and anecdotally patients report that concentrated tomato sources induce symptoms. Recently, cinnamic acid (a phenolic acid structurally similar to benzoic acid and component of cinnamon) has been found in tomatoes [36]. Quantification of these compounds in tomato concentrates is not available. However, it is likely that the concentration will be considerably higher than for raw tomatoes which have a very high water content. Tomato puree and concentrated sources of tomato are avoided on the cinnamon- and benzoate-free diet but fresh tomato (cooked or uncooked) can be used as an alternative.

Soya

Soya is a natural source of benzoates. Soya is used increasingly in food manufacturing, as soya flour added to breads and baked goods, while soya lecithin, sourced from soya oil, is added to a whole range of foods as a lubricant and emulsifier. It is

added to margarines, baked goods, cereals, yoghurts, puddings and many more products. The amount of soya and therefore the amount of benzoic acid from these sources is very low so soya avoidance is not required on the cinnamon- and benzoate-free diet [37].

Cosmetics and toiletries

Benzoates are also used as preservatives in oral medicines and medicinal topical creams, cosmetics, hygiene products and oral hygiene products [38]. Dermal absorption of benzoates and related compounds can occur but no studies exist specifically in OFG in terms of the contributions this might make to the disease. It is suggested that where possible, benzoates are avoided through these sources, particularly with creams, sunscreens, lip balms, soaps and toothpastes that are used directly on affected areas. With respect to oral hygiene products, tartar control toothpastes and mouthwashes are often key sources and labels on all other toothpastes and mouthwashes need to be observed. Avoidance of benzoates is often harder for creams, sunscreen and balsams but these can sometimes be found in health food shops, and products designed for babies are occasionally suitable. Specialist stockists on the internet can be helpful, particularly for sunscreens.

References

1. Wiesenfeld D, Ferguson MM, Mitchell DN, et al. Oro-facial granulomatosis – a clinical and pathological analysis. *Quarterly Journal of Medicine* 1985; **54**(213): 101–113.
2. Campbell H, Escudier M, Patel P, et al. Distinguishing orofacial granulomatosis from Crohn's disease: two separate disease entities? *Inflammatory Bowel Diseases* 2011; **17**(10): 2109–2115.
3. Campbell HE, Escudier MP, Patel P, Challacombe SJ, Sanderson JD, Lomer MC. Review article: cinnamon- and benzoate-free diet as a primary treatment for orofacial granulomatosis. *Alimentary Pharmacology and Therapeutics* 2011; **34**(70): 687–701.
4. Casson DH, Eltumi M, Tomlin S, Walker-Smith JA, Murch SH. Topical tacrolimus may be effective in the treatment of oral and perineal Crohn's disease. *Gut* 2000; **47**(3): 436–440.
5. Leao JC, Hodgson T, Scully C, Porter S. Review article: orofacial granulomatosis. *Alimentary Pharmacology and Therapeutics* 2004 15; **20**(10): 1019–1027.

6. Gibson J, Wray D, Bagg J. Oral staphylococcal mucositis: a new clinical entity in orofacial granulomatosis and Crohn's disease. *Oral Surgery, Oral Medicine, Oral Pathology, Oral Radiology and Endodontics* 2000; **89**(2): 171–176.

7. Sakuntabhai A, Macleod RI, Lawrence CM. Intralesional steroid injection after nerve block anesthesia in the treatment of orofacial granulomatosis. *Archives of Dermatology* 1993; **129**(4): 477–480.

8. Williams AJ, Wray D, Ferguson A. The clinical entity of orofacial Crohn's disease. *Quarterly Journal of Medicine* 1991; **79**(289): 451–458.

9. Van der Waal RI, Schulten EA, van der Meij EH, van de Scheur MR, Starink TM, van der Waal I. Cheilitis granulomatosa: overview of 13 patients with long-term follow-up – results of management. *International Journal of Dermatology* 2002; **41**(4): 225–229.

10. Plauth M, Jenss H, Meyle J. Oral manifestations of Crohn's disease. An analysis of 79 cases. *Journal of Clinical Gastroenterology* 1991; **13**(1): 29–37.

11. Elliott T, Campbell H, Escudier M, et al. Experience with anti-TNF-alpha therapy for orofacial granulomatosis. *Journal of Oral Pathology and Medicine* 2011; **40**(1): 14–19.

12. Ferguson MM, MacFadyen EE. Orofacial granulomatosis – a 10 year review. *Annals of the Academy of Medicine, Singapore* 1986; **15**(3): 370–377.

13. Campbell H, Escudier M, Patel P, et al. Distinguishing orofacial granulomatosis from crohn's disease: two separate disease entities? *Inflammatory Bowel Diseases* 2011; **17**(10): 2109–2115.

14. Kiparissi F, Lindley K, Hill S, Milla P, Shah N, Elawad M. Orofacial granulomatosis is a separate entity of Crohn's disease comprising and allergic component. *Journal of Pediatric Gastroenterology and Nutriton* 2006; **42**(5): E3.

15. Armstrong DK, Biagioni P, Lamey PJ, Burrows D. Contact hypersensitivity in patients with orofacial granulomatosis. *American Journal of Contact Dermatology* 1997; **8**(1): 35–38.

16. Wray D, Rees SR, Gibson J, Forsyth A. The role of allergy in oral mucosal diseases. *Quarterly Journal of Medicine* 2000; **93**(8): 507–511.

17. White A, Nunes C, Escudier M, et al. Improvement in orofacial granulomatosis on a cinnamon- and benzoate-free diet. *Inflammatory Bowel Diseases* 2006; **12**(6): 508–514.

18. Wuthrich B. Food-induced cutaneous adverse reactions. *Allergy* 1998; **53**(46 Suppl): 131–135.

19. Hannuksela M, Haahtela T. Hypersensitivity reactions to food additives. *Allergy* 1987; **42**(8): 561–575.

20. Taylor SL, Dormedy ES. Flavorings and colorings. *Allergy* 1998; **53**(46 Suppl): 80–82.

21. Brahmachari S, Pahan K. Sodium benzoate, a food additive and a metabolite of cinnamon, modifies T cells at multiple steps and inhibits adoptive transfer of experimental allergic encephalomyelitis. *Journal of Immunology* 2007; **179**(1): 275–283.

22. Patel P, Barone F, Nunes C, et al. Subepithelial dendritic B cells in orofacial granulomatosis. *Inflammatory Bowel Diseases* 2010; **16**(6): 1051–1060.

23. Cressey P, Jones S. Levels of preservatives (sulfite, sorbate and benzoate) in New Zealand foods and estimated dietary exposure. *Food Additives and Contaminants. Part A Chemistry, Analysis, Control, Exposure and Risk Assessment* 2009; **265**: 604–613.

24. Heimhuber B, Herrmann K. Benzoe-, Phylessig-, 3-Phenylpropan- und Zimtsaure sowie benzoglucosen in einigen Obst-und Fruchtgemusearten. *Deutsche Lebensmittel-Rundschau* 1990; **86**: 205–209.

25. Herrmann K. Occurrence and content of hydroxycinnamic and hydroxybenzoic acid compounds in foods. *Critical Reviews in Food Science and Nutrition* 1989; **28**(4): 315–347.

26. Toyoda M, Ito Y, Isshiki K, et al. Estimation of daily intake of many kinds of food additives according to the market basket studies in Japan. *Journal of the Japanese Society of Nutrition and Food Science* 1983; **36**(6): 489–497.

27. Toyoda M, Ito Y, Isshiki K, et al. Daily intake of preservatives, benzoic acid, dhydroacetic acid, propionic acid and their salts, and esters of *p*-hydroxybenzoic acid in Japan. *Journal of Japanese Society of Nutrition and Food Science* 1983; **36**(6): 467–480.

28. European Council and Commission Directives. Statutory Instrument No. 1971, *The Flavourings in Food Regulations*, 1992.

29. European Parliament and Council Directive No 95/2/EC of 20 February 1995 on food additives other than colours and sweeteners. *Official Journal of the European Union* 1995; **L61**: 18.3, 1.

30. Singletary K. Cinnamon: overview of health benefits 160. *Nutrition Today* 2008; **43**(6): 263–266.

31. Food Standards Agency. *Food Labelling: Clear Food Labelling Guidance*. London: Food Standards Agency, 2008.

32. Food Standards Agency. The Food Labelling Regulations 1996: *Guidance Notes on Quantitative Ingredients Declarations ('QUID')*. London: Food Standards Agency, 2008.

33. Abraham K, Wohrlin F, Lindtner O, Heinemeyer G, Lampen A. Toxicology and risk assessment of coumarin: focus on human data. *Molecular Nutrition and Food Research* 2010; **54**(2): 228–239.

34. Hausen B, Simatupang T, Bruhn G, Evers P, Koenig W. Identification of new allergenic constituents and proof of evidence for coniferyl benzoate in balsam of peru. *American Journal of Contact Dermatitis* 1995; **6**(4): 199–208.

35. Sieber R, Butikofer U, Bosset JO, Ruegg M. Benzoic acid as a natural component of foods – a review. *Mitteilungen aus dem Gebiete der Lebensmitteluntersuchung und Hygiene* 1989; **80**(3): 345–362.

36. Amado A, Jacob SE. [Contact dermatitis caused by foods]. *Actas Dermosifiliograficas* 2007; **98**(7): 452–458.

37. Nagarajah R, Campbell H, Sanderson JD, Lomer MC. Dietary management of orofacial granulomatosis: quantification of benzoates in foods and cosmetics 83. *Journal of Human Nutrition and Dietetics* 2008; **21**(4): 397–398.

38. Nair B (Food and Drug Administration). Final Report on the Safety Assessment of Benzyl Alcohol, Benzoic Acid, and Sodium Benzoate. *International Journal of Toxicology* 2001; **20**(Suppl 3): 23–50.

Chapter 3.2

Eosinophilic oesophagitis and nutrition

Stephen E. Attwood and Stuart Allan
North Tyneside General Hospital, North Shields, UK

Eosinophilic oesophagitis (EoE) is an underrecognised chronic relapsing-remitting disease that is characterised by damage to the oesophageal mucosa by eosinophils. It can affect adults and children alike. In a large percentage of patients it presents as intermittent dysphagia but can cause severe social embarrassment, emergency admission to hospital, undernutrition and weight loss. It seems to have a strong link with atopy and many of the target therapies are similar to those used in asthma. Dietary omissions seem to play a strong role in the management of paediatric EoE and have a place in adult EoE but have limitations due to compliance. EoE is a very problematic condition but with careful input from a multidisciplinary team, good outcomes may be achieved.

3.2.1 Definition

Eosinophilic oesophagitis is a disease characterised by the presence of a large number of a special type of white blood cell, the eosinophil, that can cause inflammation in the oesophagus. It has recently been defined as 'a chronic, immune/antigen-mediated disease characterized clinically by symptoms related to esophageal dysfunction and histologically by eosinophil-predominant inflammation' [1]. Prior to 1990 it was very rarely recognised, and since then an increasing number of patients have been presenting throughout the Western world [2]. In the past many patients were assumed to have a variant of acid gastro-oesophageal reflux disease, but resistant to acid suppression therapy. Now it is recognised that

EoE is not usually related to acid reflux and it does not usually respond to acid suppression therapy. The true prevalence of EoE remains unclear but it has been postulated that it may affect 400 per 100,000 people in the UK [3]. In children, it has been predicted that as many as 8.9 per 100,000 are affected [4], roughly the same number as in Crohn's disease.

3.2.2 Typical symptoms

Eosinophilic oesophagitis manifestation is quite variable and begins at any age but is usually more common in younger males (M:F 3:1) [5]. The symptoms range in nature and severity. Dysphagia is the most common presentation and is largely intermittent but can be a continuous problem. In some, this intermittent dysphagia can present as an oesophageal food bolus obstruction requiring emergency attendance to hospital. For most, however, there is often severe social embarrassment as the patient attempts to relieve the obstruction. In children aged less than 9, regurgitation and failure to thrive are a common presentation. Unusual symptoms often prove a chronic element to the disease and are usually related to change in oesophageal structure. Dysphagia during every meal would suggest narrowing of the oesophagus either as a stricture to one part or a continuous narrowing of the oesophageal lumen. Weight loss and undernutrition may occur but only affect the most severe minority.

Advanced Nutrition and Dietetics in Gastroenterology, First Edition. Edited by Miranda Lomer.
© 2014 John Wiley & Sons, Ltd. Published 2014 by John Wiley & Sons, Ltd.

3.2.3 Diagnosis

A flexible endoscopy of the oesophagus with biopsy to look for the eosinophils in the mucosal lining is the essential test and should be done on everyone with unexplained swallow difficulties. Patients with assumed gastro-oesophageal reflux who do not respond to the usual acid suppression medications should also be examined by endoscopy and biopsy. A guideline of finding >15 eosinophils per high power field under the microscope is useful, although many patients have much higher densities of eosinophil infiltration. The endoscopy also identifies whether strictures, rings or other endoscopic abnormalities are present.

3.2.4 Natural history

Eosinophilic oesophagitis is a relapsing-remitting condition which is sometimes progressive over many years but in others remission can occur without relapse later. In adults, it is uncommon for symptoms to disappear without recurrence [6]. In children, the condition differs as some studies have shown that relapse can be prevented with successful dietary therapy [7,8].

3.2.5 Causation – dietary or aeroallergens?

It is thought that EoE is a condition driven by exposure to allergens (either swallowed or inhaled), with a focal allergic reaction in the oesophageal mucosa. Some studies have also proven a strong association with other forms of atopy [9]. It is characterised by the presence of eosinophils within oesophageal stroma that are sensitised to eotaxin-3 by a process of chemical attraction or chemotaxis. It is thought that a process of eotaxin-3 overexpression is responsible for oesophageal tissue damage via activation of the eosinophils and production of further proinflammatory proteins. It is common for immunologists to find food allergy in patients with EoE, especially children, using skin prick testing, food allergy testing and serum food IgE assays but the

clinical utility of these tests is limited as patients are often found to have allergies to many food types. This is the basis of elimination diets in a patient's management.

3.2.6 Dietary effects of disease

In young adults, nutrition is commonly maintained by modification of diet, often supporting themselves with additional liquid nutritional supplements [10]. Although rare, when dysphagia is constant or severe, weight loss and undernutrition may occur and occasionally, some patients require peripheral parenteral nutrition at the time of diagnosis [5].

Often the largest problem faced by these patients is social morbidity. It is common for patients to avoid social occasions involving food and the social exclusion can result in mental health problems.

In children, nutrition commonly poses a larger problem. The presentation of EoE in children may be similar to that of gastro-oesophageal reflux disease and includes abdominal pain, vomiting, eating disturbances and failure to thrive. In younger children, however, the classic presentation is that of behavioural problems related to eating. Some suggest that it arises from a failure to recognise dysphagia as pathological and hence behavioural changes may develop.

3.2.7 Treatment

Treatment of this condition often requires a multidisciplinary approach taking medication, dietary changes and supportive strategies into account. It is generally accepted that dietary changes can help significantly in children but are of less importance in adults. Here pharmacological treatments have a better outcome. Occasionally adults need oesophageal dilation to help relieve symptoms.

Diet

Although allergy seems to play a large role in causation, its value in directing treatment is unreliable. Skin prick testing used in combination with atopy patch testing can guide specific dietary omissions but only in 40–60% of patients [1,11]. The six most common allergens that have been recognised are wheat, eggs, soy, fish/shellfish, dairy and peanuts. It has been proven that elimination of a specific food brought about symptomatic and histological improvement in 77% of patients [12]. Elimination of these common foodstuffs together is now recognised as the six food elimination diet (SFED) which has been proven to be beneficial over more costly and often less well-tolerated amino acid-based elemental enteral nutrition [12]. This study also proved that the use of the SFED without allergy testing showed very high efficacy, with 74% of patients showing improvement both clinically and histologically. Other authors advise adding skin prick test to empirical elimination of milk, but still only report a 77% success rate in symptom resolution [13].

The gold standard for discovering if food allergy is the cause for EoE in children remains the use of elemental enteral nutrition with gradual reintroduction of normal foods. Due to its poor palatability, elemental enteral nutrition may need to be administered by enteral feeding tube and is very costly.

Using the SFED can cause symptom resolution but cessation of this diet and selective reintroduction of foods may not maintain remission [1,14].

Adults tend to be less satisfied with strict elimination diets, and find them difficult to sustain. Although there is evidence that clinical and histological improvement can be brought about with elimination diets in adults, the longer term continuation of these diets (over 1 year) is of unproven value. It is extremely difficult to stay compliant with elimination diets and they often require a drastic social change. Recent work by the Chicago group has shown the feasibility of dietary exclusion in adults over short periods, although in most patients symptoms returned after diets normalised and very few of their initial cohort managed to complete a year on their exclusion diet [15]. Known foods that precipitate symptoms are commonly avoided by adults, with incomplete symptom relief and sometimes dietary deficiencies. Here we hope that the inclusion of dietary professionals will provide better long-term outcomes for our patients by providing support and regular review.

Drugs

Pharmacological treatment of EoE is based on the allergic nature of the condition, with many of the current therapies being similar to those needed for asthma. It has been shown that oral topical steroids, specifically budesonide or fluticasone, can improve EoE after a 15-day course both clinically and histopathologically [16]. This treatment regime, although effective, requires a large amount of education and compliance and relies heavily on the method of administration.

Other pharmacological treatments include montelukast, a leukotriene receptor antagonist which has shown a good symptom resolution in seven of eight patients within a few weeks of treatment, but further assessment is needed [17].

Newer therapies including chemoattractant receptor T-helper cell type 2 (CRTH-2) antagonists which are showing promising results but further studies are needed to fully evaluate their efficacy.

Dilation

Oesophageal dilation has been proven to provide some improvement in symptoms but is associated with procedural risks such as oesophageal tears and perforation.

3.2.8 Conclusion

Eosinophilic oesophagitis is a condition of swallowing difficulty which is underrecognised. In adults, it poses social difficulty and embarrassment and in children, it can cause faltering growth and behavioural changes. It remains difficult to manage but dietary and medical therapies have shown promising results.

With the input of dietitians and allergy specialists, it is hoped that the longer term outcomes for EoE patients are more promising, with lower rates of social morbidity and hospital admissions.

References

1. Liacouras CA, Furuta GT, Hirano I, et al. Eosinophilic esophagitis: updated consensus recommendations for children and adults. *Journal of Allergy and Clinical Immunology* 2011; **98**: 3–20.
2. Attwood SE, Smyrk TC, DeMeester TR, Jones JB. Esophageal eosinophilia with dysphagia. *A distinct clinicopathologic syndrome. Digestive Diseases and Sciences* 1993; **38**(1): 109–116.
3. Kapel RC, Miller JK, Torres C, Aksoy S, Lash R, Katzka DA. Eosinophilic esophagitis: a prevalent disease in the United States that affects all age groups. *Gastroenterology* 2008; **134**(5): 1316–1321.
4. Cherian S, Forbes DA. Rapidly increasing prevalence of eosinophilic oesophagitis in Western Australia. *Archives of Disease in Childhood* 2006; **12**: 1000–1004.
5. Furuta GT. Eosinophilic esophagitis: update on clinicopathological manifestations and pathophysiology. *Current Opinion in Gastroenterology* 2011; **27**(4): 383–388.
6. Straumann A, Grize L, Bucher KA, Beglinger C, Simon HU. Natural history of primary eosinophilic esophagitis: a follow-up of 30 adult patients for up to 11.5 years. *Gastroenterology* 2003; **6**(125): 1660–1669.
7. Liacouras CA, Spergel JM, Ruchelli E, et al. Eosinophilic esophagitis: a 10-year experience in 381 children. *Clinical Gastroenterology and Hepatology* 2005; **12**(3): 1198–1206.
8. Alexander JA, Katzka DA. Therapeutic options for eosinophilic esophagitis. *Gastroenterology and Hepatology* 2011; **7**(1): 59–61.
9. Müller S, Puhl S, Vieth M, Stolte M. Analysis of symptoms and endoscopic findings in 117 patients with histological diagnoses of eosinophilic esophagitis. *Endoscopy* 2007; **39**(4): 339–344.
10. Kanakala V, Lamb C, Haigh C, Stirling RW, Attwood SE. The diagnosis of primary eosinophilic oesophagitis in adults: missed or misinterpreted? *European Journal of Gastroenterology and Hepatology* 2010; **22**(7): 848–855.
11. Spergel JM, Brown-Whitehorn TF, Beausoleil JL, Liacouras CA. Treatment of eosinophilic esophagitis with specific food elimination diet directed by a combination of skin prick and patch tests. *Annals of Allergy, Asthma and Immunology* 2005; **95**(4): 336–344.
12. Kagalwalla AF, Ritz S, Hess T, et al. Effect of six-food elimination diet on clinical and histologic outcomes in eosinophilic esophagitis. *Clinical Gastroenterology and Hepatology* 2006; **4**(9): 1097–1102.
13. Spergel JM, Brown-Whitehorn TF, Cianferoni A, et al. Identification of causative foods in children with eosinophilic esophagitis treated with an elimination diet. *Journal of Allergy and Clinical Immunology* 2012; **130**(2): 461–467.
14. Boyce JA, Assa'ad A, Burks AW, et al. Guidelines for the diagnosis and management of food allergy in the United States: summary of the NIAID-sponsored expert panel report. *Journal of Allergy and Clinical Immunology* 2010; **126**: 1105–1118.
15. Gonsalves N, Yang GY, Doerfler B, Ritz S, Ditto AM, Hirano I. Elimination diet effectively treats eosinophilic esophagitis in adults; food reintroduction identifies causative factors. *Gastroenterology* 2012; **142**: 1451–1459.
16. Straumann A, Degen L, Felder S, et al. Budesonide is effective in adolescent and adult patients with active eosinophilic esophagitis. *Gastroenterology* 2010; **139**(5): 1526–1537.
17. Attwood SE, Lewis CS, Bronder CS, Morris CD, Armstrong GR, Whittam J. Eosinophilic oesophagitis: a novel treatment using Montelukast. *Gut* 2003; **52**(2): 181–185.

Chapter 3.3

Gastro-oesophageal reflux disease and nutrition

Mark Fox[1,2] and Henriette Heinrich[2]
[1]University Hospitals and University of Nottingham, Nottingham, UK
[2]University Hospital Zürich, Zürich, Switzerland

3.3.1 Factors involved in causation of reflux disease

Gastro-oesophageal reflux disease (GORD) is a common disorder affecting at least one in 10 of the population on a weekly basis, that is present when the return of gastric contents into the oesophagus causes symptoms or damages the mucosa [1]. Heartburn and acid regurgitation are typical presenting complaints but GORD can be associated with a variety of other problems, including chest pain, chronic cough and lung diseases. The underlying cause of this condition is most often disruption of the 'reflux barrier' at the gastro-oesophageal junction. The risk of reflux increases as this disruption becomes more severe, particularly in the presence of a hiatus hernia [2]. Additionally, patients with severe GORD clear the oesophagus less efficiently, leading to prolonged acid exposure and complications such as reflux oesophagitis, peptic stricture and Barrett's metaplasia (a premalignant condition). Twin studies have shown that inherited factors are responsible for 20–40% of GORD and acquired factors, such as *Helicobacter pylori* infection, may play a role; however, recent reviews emphasise the importance of lifestyle and dietary factors as a cause of disease [3]. Smokers, workers engaged in strenuous physical activity and individuals with a high body mass reported higher rates of reflux symptoms in epidemiology studies [4,5].

Indeed, the 'epidemic' of obesity may be responsible also for the perceived increase in GORD and its complications [6]. However, this is a complex issue because overweight and obese people also tend to eat larger meals and make food choices that increase the risk of reflux.

It is a common belief among patients and doctors that reflux symptoms may be induced or worsened by certain foods and beverages and published guidelines recommend avoiding 'reflux-inducing foods' as part of the first-line management of GORD [7,8]. Despite this broad-based agreement, the effects of diet on GI function are hotly debated and the efficacy of dietary management for GORD has not been established.

Meal volume and consistency

Physiology studies have shown that distension of the stomach after meals triggers transient lower oesophageal sphincter relaxations (TLOSRs) that open the reflux barrier to release air swallowed with the meal (belching) [2]. A key difference between patients and healthy individuals is that TLOSRs in GORD patients frequently allow 'reflux' not only of air but also gastric acid and semi-digested food, leading to heartburn and regurgitation [9]. Large amounts of food cause more gastric distension and also take a long time to empty from the stomach. Thus larger meal volumes

Advanced Nutrition and Dietetics in Gastroenterology, First Edition. Edited by Miranda Lomer.
© 2014 John Wiley & Sons, Ltd. Published 2014 by John Wiley & Sons, Ltd.

trigger more TLOSRs and lead to more reflux events. On this basis, GORD patients can be advised to avoid large meals and to eat 'little and often'; however, the clinical benefits of this pragmatic approach have never been tested.

Limited data exist on the impact of meal consistency on GORD. Studies that assessed the effect of meal viscosity or compared the effects of liquid and solid meals have shown no change in the frequency of reflux events or acid exposure in the distal oesophagus [10,11]. However, increasing meal viscosity does appear to suppress 'volume regurgitation' and the use of alginate preparations (e.g. Gaviscon) that produce a viscous layer above the meal also reduces reflux and symptoms [12,13]. These effects are useful in clinical practice as regurgitation and also laryngopharyngeal symptoms often persist despite standard acid suppression [2].

Meal composition

In principle, any meal component that delays gastric emptying, stimulates acid secretion, impairs oesophageal function or increases sensitivity of the oesophagus to reflux will worsen the severity of reflux and/or reflux related symptoms [14]. Foods such as chocolate, fried and spicy foods are often mentioned by patients as causing reflux symptoms; however, well-controlled studies reveal little impact of these specific items on objective measurements of acid exposure [15,16]. Further, none of the individual dietary items evaluated was associated with the risk of reflux symptoms in a recent twin study [5]. Thus it seems likely that the effects of food and drink on GORD are most often related to general nutrient composition and not individual ingredients.

The initial findings of a large, cross-sectional study in 951 volunteers suggest that a high-fat diet is an important risk factor for both reflux symptoms and erosive eosophagitis [4]. However, it is difficult to distinguish the effects of fat intake and total energy (i.e. calorie) intake in this work. This was highlighted by the interaction between diet, obesity and reflux such that the effects of fat intake on GORD symptoms became non-significant when adjusted for Body Mass Index [4]. This finding is consistent with other epidemiology and physiology studies that found no consistent effect of fat on TLOSR frequency or acid reflux after a meal when total energy intake is controlled [16–19].

The clinical effects of macronutrient composition and energy intake in GORD were clarified by a study that monitored acid reflux events and symptoms following intake of high-caloric, high-fat (1000 kcal, 50% fat), high-caloric, low-fat (1000 kcal, 25% fat) and low-caloric, low-fat (500 kcal, 25% fat) meals on consecutive days in randomised order [10]. Prolonged, wireless pH monitoring demonstrated that the frequency of reflux events and oesophageal acid exposure was directly related to total energy intake but not to fat content. In contrast, the number of reflux symptoms was 40% higher in the high-fat than the low-fat study day [10]. Thus, similar to its effects on gastric function (see Chapter 1.3), fat does not appear to affect motility but does increase visceral sensitivity to reflux events and so the number and severity of symptoms reported [20,21].

In contrast to fat, there is no evidence that varying the amount of carbohydrate or whole protein in a meal will alter the risk of acid reflux or symptoms. However, it should be noted that aromatic amino acids (e.g. phenylalanine, tryptophan) as well as calcium stimulate gastrin secretion and gastric acid production [22]. Consistent with these data, ingestion of food supplements and test meals containing high concentrations of these micronutrients can cause reflux symptoms even in healthy volunteers [23]. Reflux symptoms are more common also among those who regularly use extra table salt compared with those who never do so, possibly because gastric emptying time increases with osmolality of the meal. Nitrates in the diet mainly derived from the increased use of nitrogenous fertilizers have also been implicated in the aetiology of GORD [4,24]. When saliva, with its high nitrite content derived from the enterosalivary recirculation of dietary nitrate, meets acidic gastric juice, the nitrite is converted to nitrous acid, nitrosative species and nitric oxide. This has been shown to decrease lower oesophageal sphincter (LOS) pressure and increase TLOSR frequency. Moreover, the 'chemical warfare' at the reflux barrier produces chemicals that could be carcinogenic [24,25].

Dietary fibre has been linked to a reduced risk of reflux [4,5]. The mechanism of action is not certain but may include increasing the viscosity of gastric contents and slowing the release of nutrients that exacerbate reflux. However, it is still possible that high fibre intake is simply a marker of a relatively low-fat, low-calorie diet that has not been fully accounted for in the analysis. Indeed, not all effects of fibre are beneficial; one study reported increased TLOSR activity after a high-fibre meal triggered by colonic fermentation and distension [26].

Beverages

Citrus fruit juices, carbonated drinks and other acidic beverages are often avoided by GORD patients as they can aggravate reflux symptoms [27]. This may be due to direct stimulation of acid receptors in the oesophageal mucosa; however, repeated exposure to mildly acidic fluid or other irritants may also impair mucosal integrity, producing wide intracellular spaces that are observed in non-erosive reflux disease and may be responsible for an increase in acid sensitivity [28]. For carbonated drinks these effects are compounded by gross distension of the proximal stomach that reduces LOS pressure and causes repeated TLOSRs that can be accompanied by reflux [29].

Coffee causes reflux symptoms in many GORD patients [30] and direct infusion into the oesophagus can cause heartburn [31]; however, the clinical relevance of these observations has not been confirmed by epidemiology studies [32]. Similarly, although caffeine has several effects on gastric motility and secretory function, physiological studies do not show consistent effects of coffee or caffeine on oesophageal motility or reflux [33,34].

Alcohol may exacerbate GORD in several ways. As a smooth muscle relaxant, it delays gastric emptying, reduces LOS pressure and impairs oesophageal clearance, and as a stimulant for gastrin release, it enhances acid secretion. As a result, alcohol increases the number of reflux events and oesophageal acid exposure in patients and healthy controls (particularly after ingestion of white wine) [35,36]. Despite these findings, epidemiological studies have not consistently confirmed an association between alcohol and GORD symptoms [32]. The inconsistent findings of epidemiological studies that focus on symptoms and physiological studies that measure acid reflux may be explained by the sedative effects of alcohol that reduce sensitivity and vigilance.

Eating behaviour

Not only what we eat but also how and when we eat can affect GORD. The speed of eating has effects on gastric function, with a meal consumed within 5 min causing significantly more reflux than the same meal consumed within 30 min [37]. Similarly, population-based studies in binge eaters showed that heartburn and acid regurgitation are among various GI complaints experienced by these patients [38]. Certain behaviours after the meal can also help to reduce reflux. Chewing sugar-free gum increases saliva production and swallowing frequency. This combination optimises both chemical and mechanical clearance should reflux events occur and has been shown to reduce acid exposure [39]. The flavour is not important. Although peppermint oil has calcium channel-blocking (muscle-relaxing) properties, no effect of mint was observed on the reflux barrier or reflux events in a randomised controlled trial [40].

Avoidance of lying down shortly after meals is often part of the advice given to GORD patients and studies using prolonged, wireless pH monitoring confirmed that GORD patients with hiatus hernia and oesophagitis experienced significantly more supine reflux when consuming a late night meal [41]. Position can also be critical. In patients with severe GORD and hiatus hernia, prolonged reflux events are common in the recumbent position due to passive flow from the stomach and impaired clearance during sleep. In this group, elevating the head of the bed can significantly reduce acid exposure and nocturnal symptoms [42]. In contrast, in patients with mild-to-moderate GORD (i.e. without complete disruption of the reflux barrier), TLOSRs and reflux events are greatly reduced on lying down [43]. Interestingly, this effect is greater in the left relative to the right recumbent position [44]. On this basis, patients with GORD can be recommended to sleep either with the head of the bed elevated or, if recumbent, on their left-hand side.

3.3.2 Dietary effects of disease or its management

Patients with GORD are often overweight or obese. Severe reflux symptoms may reduce oral intake and can lead to weight loss but this is rarely severe.

The mainstay of GORD treatment is medications that either neutralise gastric acid (e.g. calcium carbonate, 'milk of magnesia') or suppress acid secretion (e.g. histamine receptor antagonists such as ranitidine, proton pump inhibitors (PPI), such as omeprazole). This approach is effective because the majority of symptoms in GORD patients are related to acid reflux. However, acid suppression does not prevent reflux itself and some patients experience persistent 'volume regurgitation' or other symptoms related to 'non- or weakly acid' reflux on PPI treatment [2]. These symptoms may respond to preparations that suppress reflux by forming a viscous alginate layer on gastric contents (e.g. Gaviscon) [13] however, if these are not effective then antireflux surgery is an effective option in this group.

Antacids and alginates are rarely taken in quantities that cause side-effects, although large amounts of magnesium salts can cause diarrhoea. Acid suppression by proton pump inhibitors is also safe and well tolerated by the majority of patients in the long term [2]. However, profound acid suppression does impair the digestion and/or absorption of protein and several micronutrients including calcium, iron and vitamin B12 [45]. In the developed world this is unlikely to cause undernutrition but impaired calcium absorption in patients taking PPIs has been linked to an increased risk of osteoporosis and fractures, especially in those already at risk of osteoporosis such as postmenopausal women [46].

Another risk of acid suppression is the loss of protection against food-borne pathogens. Although the absolute risk is low, case–control studies have shown that omeprazole treatment is associated with an increased incidence of *Campylobacter*, *Salmonella* and *Clostridium difficile* [47]. In addition, the lack of gastric acid promotes bacterial colonisation and 'overgrowth' of the small intestine [48], although the clinical impact on nutrient absorption and GI symptoms seems limited. Similarly, there is little evidence for the effect of gastric acid suppression on appetite, nutrient intake and body mass [45]. In animal models caloric intake is often reduced on PPI therapy but in GORD patients the opposite is more likely as symptoms improve [45].

3.3.3 Lifestyle and dietary treatments

Management algorithmns emphasise the importance of lifestyle factors, including weight loss and dietary change, as first-line treatment of GORD [7,8]. These measures may be sufficient to manage mild reflux symptoms in primary care and also to improve the results of medical therapy; however, it is rare for these to remove the need for PPI therapy in more severe cases and a systematic review found just 16 studies of lifestyle and dietary management in GORD and the evidence base was far from conclusive [49]. Recently this evidence was supplemented by a large randomized controlled trial in 332 obese adults that enrolled in a structured weight loss program. One in three of these individuals had reflux symptoms at baseline; however after significant weight loss (average >10kg) this had resolved in over half those affected [50].

Specific interventions that are supported by evidence of improvement in oesophageal acid exposure include weight loss, avoiding lying down/keeping the upper body in an elevated position after a meal,lying down in the right lateral position, not smoking, not consuming alcohol, reduction of meal size and not eating high-calorie, high-fat foods. Of these, only weight loss induced by general dietary advice [50,51,52], head of bed elevation [42] and avoidance of a high-fat diet [10] have been shown also to improve GORD symptoms in at least one study. Absence of evidence does not equal evidence of absence. Indeed, it is very likely that these approaches are not only effective but also cost-efficient. However, there is a pressing need for further, prospective controlled trials ideally complemented by physiological measurement to assess the efficacy and refine the delivery of lifestyle and dietary intervention in the treatment of GORD.

References

1. Vakil N, van Zanten SV, Kahrilas P, Dent J, Jones R. The Montreal definition and classification of gastroesophageal reflux disease: a global evidence-based consensus. *American Journal of Gastroenterology* 2006; **101**: 1900–1920.
2. Fox M, Forgacs I. Gastro-oesophageal reflux disease. *British Medical Journal* 2006; **332**: 88–93.

3. Dent J, El-Serag HB, Wallander MA, Johansson S. Epidemiology of gastro-oesophageal reflux disease: a systematic review. *Gut* 2005; **54**: 710–717.

4. El-Serag, HB, Satia JA, Rabeneck L. Dietary intake and the risk of gastro-oesophageal reflux disease: a cross sectional study in volunteers. *Gut* 2005; **54**: 11–17.

5. Zheng Z, Nordenstedt H, Pedersen NL, Lagergren J, Ye W. Lifestyle factors and risk for symptomatic gastroesophageal reflux in monozygotic twins. *Gastroenterology* 2007; **132**: 87–95.

6. Lagergren J. Adenocarcinoma of oesophagus: what exactly is the size of the problem and who is at risk? *Gut* 2005; **54**(Suppl 1): i1–5.

7. Devault KR, Castell DO. Updated guidelines for the diagnosis and treatment of gastroesophageal reflux disease. *American Journal of Gastroenterology* 2005; **100**: 190–200.

8. Tytgat GN, McColl K, Tack J, et al. New algorithm for the treatment of gastro-oesophageal reflux disease. *Alimentary Pharmacology and Therapeutics* 2008; **27**: 249–256.

9. Trudgill NJ, Riley SA. Transient lower esophageal sphincter relaxations are no more frequent in patients with gastroesophageal reflux disease than in asymptomatic volunteers. *American Journal of Gastroenterology* 2001; **96**: 2569–2574.

10. Fox M, Barr C, Nolan S, Lomer M, Anggiansah A, Wong T. The effects of dietary fat and calorie density on esophageal acid exposure and reflux symptoms. *Clininical Gastroenterology and Hepatology* 2007; **5**: 439–444.

11. Horvath A, Dziechciarz P, Szajewska H. The effect of thickened-feed interventions on gastroesophageal reflux in infants: systematic review and meta-analysis of randomized, controlled trials. *Pediatrics* 2008; **122**: e1268–e1277.

12. Buts JP, Barudi C, Otte JB. Double-blind controlled study on the efficacy of sodium alginate (Gaviscon) in reducing gastroesophageal reflux assessed by 24 h continuous pH monitoring in infants and children. *European Journal of Pediatrics* 1987; **146**: 156–158.

13. Sweis R, Kaufman E, Anggiansah A, et al. Post-prandial reflux suppression by a raft-forming alginate (Gaviscon Advance) compared to a simple antacid documented by magnetic resonance imaging and pH-impedance monitoring: mechanistic assessment in healthy volunteers and randomised, controlled, double-blind study in reflux patients. *Aliment Pharmacol Ther* 2013; **37**: 1093–102.

14. Fox M, Schwizer W. Making sense of oesophageal contents. *Gut* 2008; **57**: 435–438.

15. Nebel OT, Fornes MF, Castell DO. Symptomatic gastroesophageal reflux: incidence and precipitating factors. *American Journal of Digestive Diseases* 1976; **21**: 953–956.

16. Murphy DW, Castell DO. Chocolate and heartburn: evidence of increased esophageal acid exposure after chocolate ingestion. *American Journal of Gastroenterology* 1988; **83**: 633–636.

17. Penagini R, Mangano M, Bianchi PA. Effect of increasing the fat content but not the energy load of a meal on gastro-oesophageal reflux and lower oesophageal sphincter motor function. *Gut* 1998; **42**: 330–333.

18. Pehl C, Waizenhoefer A, Wendl B, Schmidt T, Schepp W, Pfeiffer A. Effect of low and high fat meals on lower esophageal sphincter motility and gastroesophageal reflux in healthy

subjects. *American Journal of Gastroenterology* 1999; **94**: 1192–1196.

19. Ruhl CE, Everhart JE. Overweight, but not high dietary fat intake, increases risk of gastroesophageal reflux disease hospitalization: the NHANES I Epidemiologic Followup Study. *First National Health and Nutrition Examination Survey. Annals of Epidemiology* 1999; **9**: 424–435.

20. Simren M, Abrahamsson H, Bjornsson ES. An exaggerated sensory component of the gastrocolonic response in patients with irritable bowel syndrome. *Gut* 2001; **48**: 20–27.

21. Feinle C, Rades T, Otto B, Fried M. Fat digestion modulates gastrointestinal sensations induced by gastric distention and duodenal lipid in humans. *Gastroenterology* 2001; **120**: 1100–1107.

22. Taylor IL, Byrne WJ, Christie DL, Ament ME, Walsh JH. Effect of individual l-amino acids on gastric acid secretion and serum gastrin and pancreatic polypeptide release in humans. *Gastroenterology* 1982; **83**: 273–278.

23. Goetze O, Fox MR, Treier R, Boesiger P, Fried M, Schwizer W. Effect of gastric secretion on gastric volume responses, emptying and intragastric dilution in humans: a magnetic resonance imaging (MRI) study. *Neurogastroenterology and Motility* 2008; **20**: 1.

24. McColl KE. When saliva meets acid: chemical warfare at the oesophagogastric junction. *Gut* 2005; **54**: 1–3.

25. Manning JJ, Wirz AA, McColl KE. Nitrogenous chemicals generated from acidification of saliva influence transient lower oesophageal sphincter relaxations. *Scandinavian Journal of Gastroenterology* 2007; **42**: 1413–1421.

26. Piche T, des Varannes SB, Sacher-Huvelin S, Holst JJ, Cuber JC, Galmiche JP. Colonic fermentation influences lower esophageal sphincter function in gastroesophageal reflux disease. *Gastroenterology* 2003; **124**: 894–902.

27. Feldman M, Barnett C. Relationships between the acidity and osmolality of popular beverages and reported postprandial heartburn. *Gastroenterology* 1995; **108**: 125–131.

28. Farré R, Fornari F, Blondeau K, et al. Acid and weakly acidic solutions impair mucosal integrity of distal exposed and proximal non-exposed human oesophagus. *Gut* 2010; **59**: 164–169.

29. Hamoui N, Lord RV, Hagen JA, Theisen J, Demeester TR, Crookes PF. Response of the lower esophageal sphincter to gastric distention by carbonated beverages. *Journal of Gastrointestinal Surgery* 2006; **10**: 870–877.

30. Nandurkar S, Locke GR 3rd, Fett S, et al. Relationship between body mass index, diet, exercise and gastro-oesophageal reflux symptoms in a community. *Alimentary Pharmacology and Therapeutics* 2004; **20**: 497–505.

31. Price SF, Smithson KW, Castell D.O. Food sensitivity in reflux esophagitis. *Gastroenterology* 1978; **75**: 240–243.

32. Nilsson M, Johnsen R, Ye W, Hveem K, Lagergren J. Lifestyle related risk factors in the aetiology of gastro-oesophageal reflux. *Gut* 2004; **53**: 1730–1735.

33. Pehl C, Pfeiffer A, Wendl B, Kaess H. The effect of decaffeination of coffee on gastro-oesophageal reflux in patients with reflux disease. *Alimentary Pharmacology and Therapeutics* 1997; **11**: 483–486.

34. Cohen S, Booth GH Jr. Gastric acid secretion and lower-esophageal-sphincter pressure in response to coffee and

caffeine. *New England Journal of Medicine* 1975; **293**: 897–899.

35. Kaufman SE, Kaye MD. Induction of gastro-oesophageal reflux by alcohol. *Gut* 1978; **19**: 336–338.

36. Pehl C, Wendl B, Pfeiffer A.. White wine and beer induce gastro-oesophageal reflux in patients with reflux disease. *Alimentary Pharmacology and Therapeutics* 2006; **23**: 1581–1586.

37. Wildi SM, Tutuian R, Castell DO. The influence of rapid food intake on postprandial reflux: studies in healthy volunteers. *American Journal of Gastroenterology* 2004; **99**: 1645–1651.

38. Cremonini F, Camilleri M, Clark MM, et al. Associations among binge eating behavior patterns and gastrointestinal symptoms: a population-based study. *International Journal of Obesity* 2009; **33**: 342–353.

39. Moazzez R, Bartlett D, Anggiansah A. The effect of chewing sugar-free gum on gastro-esophageal reflux. *Journal of Dental Research* 2005; **84**: 1062–1065.

40. Bulat R, Fachnie E, Chauhan U, Chen Y, Tougas G.. Lack of effect of spearmint on lower oesophageal sphincter function and acid reflux in healthy volunteers. *Alimentary Pharmacology and Therapeutics* 1999; **13**: 805–812.

41. Piesman M, Hwang I, Maydonovitch C, Wong RK. Nocturnal reflux episodes following the administration of a standardized meal. Does timing matter? *American Journal of Gastroenterology* 2007; **102**: 2128–2134.

42. Hamilton JW, Boisen RJ, Yamamoto DT, Wagner JL, Reichelderfer M. Sleeping on a wedge diminishes exposure of the esophagus to refluxed acid. *Digestive Diseases and Sciences* 1988; **33**: 518–522.

43. Schoeman MN, Tippett MD, Akkermans LM, Dent J, Holloway RH. Mechanisms of gastroesophageal reflux in ambulant healthy human subjects. *Gastroenterology* 1995; **108**: 83–91.

44. Van Herwaarden MA, Katzka DA, Smout AJ, Samsom M, Gideon M, Castell DO. Effect of different recumbent positions on postprandial gastroesophageal reflux in normal subjects. *American Journal of Gastroenterology* 2000; **95**: 2731–2736.

45. Pohl D, Fox M, Fried M, et al. Do we need gastric acid? *Digestion* 2008; **77**: 184–197.

46. Yang YX, Lewis JD, Epstein S, Metz DC. Long-term proton pump inhibitor therapy and risk of hip fracture. *Journal of the American Medical Association* 2006; **296**: 2947–2953.

47. Dial S, Delaney JA, Barkun AN, Suissa S. Use of gastric acid-suppressive agents and the risk of community-acquired Clostridium difficile-associated disease. *Journal of the American Medical Association* 2005; **294**: 2989–2995.

48. Thorens J, Froehlich F, Schwizer W, et al. Bacterial overgrowth during treatment with omeprazole compared with cimetidine: a prospective randomised double blind study. *Gut* 1996; **39**: 54–59.

49. Kaltenbach T, Crockett S, Gerson LB. Are lifestyle measures effective in patients with gastroesophageal reflux disease? An evidence-based approach. *Archives of Internal Medicine* 2006; **166**: 965–971.

50. Singh M, Lee J, Gupta N, et al. Weight loss can lead to resolution of gastroesophageal reflux disease symptoms: a prospective intervention trial. *Obesity (Silver Spring)* 2013; **21**: 284–290.

51. Fraser-Moodie CA, Norton B, Gornall C, Magnago S, Weale AR, Holmes GK. Weight loss has an independent beneficial effect on symptoms of gastro-oesophageal reflux in patients who are overweight. *Scandinavian Journal of Gastroenterology* 1999; **34**: 337–340.

52. Mathus-Vliegen EM, van Weeren M, van Eerten PV. Los function and obesity: the impact of untreated obesity, weight loss, and chronic gastric balloon distension. *Digestion* 2003; **68**: 161–168.

Chapter 3.4

Oesophageal cancer and nutrition

Orla Hynes and Saira Chowdhury
Guy's and St Thomas' NHS Trust, London, UK

Oesophageal cancer occurs predominantly in the older population, mainly after the age of 65 years, and is more prevalent in men [1]. It is associated with poor survival rates of up to 14% at 5 years [2]. The morbidity associated with the disease and its treatments, in an ageing population, is high. Disease location, treatment effects and anxiety challenge the nutritional well-being of this group of patients who are recognised to have high supportive care needs. Nutrition interventions play an important role across the cancer journey, from diagnosis through to survivorship and end-of-life care [3–7].

3.4.1 Aetiology

The past 40 years have seen a sharp rise in the incidence of the oesophageal adenocarcinoma subtype within Western countries. This has been linked to rising obesity levels. Principal risk factors for oesophageal adenocarcinoma are obesity, gastro-oesophageal reflux disease and subsequent Barrett's oesophagus. Oesophageal squamous cell carcinoma risk is higher amongst smokers and those with a history of a high alcohol intake. Achalasia, the thermal effect of hot food and beverages, corrosive oesophageal injury, Plummer–Vinson syndrome and tylosis are also influential in the aetiology of the squamous cell carcinoma subtype [8,9].

3.4.2 Effects of disease on nutrition

Oesophageal cancer is usually advanced at diagnosis, with less than 60% having resectable disease [10]. Common presenting symptoms are dysphagia, which arises once less than 1.5 cm of the oesophageal lumen remains, weight loss and odynophagia with incidence at diagnosis of 74%, 57% and 20% respectively [11]. Sarcopenia is present in 57% of patients with oesophagogastric cancer prior to starting curative treatment with chemotherapy before surgery which is further exacerbated by treatment [12]. Advanced oesophageal cancers are associated with a high incidence of loss of appetite, early satiety and pain which may have a negative impact on quality of life and the prognostic indicators weight loss and Performance Status [13,14]. Performance status is a scale used in oncology to assess how well a person is able to undertake ordinary daily activities while living with cancer. It is also used to determine whether someone is fit to proceed with treatment and also as an indicator of how well they may be responding to treatment.

3.4.3 Treatment and nutrition

Multimodality treatment is standard practice in most early-stage cancers. It may last many months, combining chemotherapy, radiotherapy, surgery and oesophageal stenting. The cumulative effects of

Advanced Nutrition and Dietetics in Gastroenterology, First Edition. Edited by Miranda Lomer.
© 2014 John Wiley & Sons, Ltd. Published 2014 by John Wiley & Sons, Ltd.

these treatments increase morbidity and impair quality of life. When combined with symptoms of disease, these result in nutritional compromise, warranting varying levels of nutritional intervention to improve treatment tolerance and preserve performance status.

Chemotherapy

Nutritional side-effects include stomatitis, taste changes, nausea and vomiting, anorexia, altered bowel habit and fatigue. Weight loss before treatment increases the incidence of severe treatment-related dose-limiting toxicities, failure to complete chemotherapy and unplanned hospital admissions [15]. Failure to complete the prescribed treatment can impair its efficacy and influence prognosis. The principles of nutritional management during chemotherapy are to minimise the risk of chemotherapy-related toxicity due to weight loss, enable the patient to complete treatment at the intended dose and regimen, preserve performance status and preserve quality of life. Oral nutritional support is suitable where intake is impaired to the extent that dietary counselling and oral supplements are adequate to maintain nutritional status. Introduction of enteral nutrition (EN) should be considered where significant weight loss has occurred and/or where treatment and disease-related morbidity cause significant difficulty with achieving dietary adequacy [16].

Patients receiving multimodality treatments are at a greater nutritional risk due to the cumulative side-effects and treatment duration. Therefore dietetic interventions should plan for and consider this to preserve performance status and avoid interruption to treatment. A centre placing prophylactic jejunostomy feeding tubes at diagnosis showed that 42% of patients require artificial feeding during neoadjuvant chemotherapy, leading to significant weight gain compared with those who did not feed [17].

Endoscopic gastrostomy tube insertion is not recommended in oesophageal cancer. This is due to the potential presence of an impassable oesophageal tumour, stomach infiltration of oesophagogastric junctional tumours and risk of introducing stoma metastasis. All types of gastrostomy tube placement should be avoided in surgical candidates prior to curative resection as there is a risk of compromising

the use of the stomach as an oesophageal substitute at oesophagectomy [18]. A transnasal feeding tube can be placed safely where needed at any point through treatment. Nutritional difficulties and weight loss are common in the months following oesophageal cancer surgery and this may compromise continuing further treatment. A jejunostomy tube may be placed intraoperatively and has the advantage of providing nutrition support after discharge from hospital.

Radiotherapy

Side-effects of radiotherapy are dependent on treatment dose. High-dose radiotherapy is usually combined with chemotherapy (chemoradiation) with a curative intent. The most common side-effects are oesophagitis causing pain, exacerbation of dysphagia and weight loss. This, combined with the aforementioned side-effects of chemotherapy and the duration of chemoradiation, leads to significant nutritional risk. Australian guidelines on dietetic intervention for radiotherapy recommend the following goals of nutritional intervention: to minimise weight loss, maintain quality of life and provide symptom control [19]. All patients receiving radiotherapy to the GI tract, including the oesophagus, should be referred to the dietitian (Grade A) and should receive at least fortnightly intensive dietary counselling with combined oral supplementation for patients during radiotherapy with follow-up continuing for at least 6 weeks after treatment completion [16,19].

Enteral nutrition (EN) is needed in almost three-quarters of patients undergoing oesophageal chemoradiation [20]. Preservation of nutritional status can improve treatment tolerance and reduce unplanned hospital admission [19]. This may be facilitated by placement of a prophylactic feeding tube [21,22]. Current guidelines recommend EN if an obstructing tumour results in dysphagia and causes difficulty with dietary adequacy [16,19]. Odelli et al. suggest gastrostomy placement prior to embarking on oesophageal chemoradiation in patients with weight loss of at least 10%, a Body Mass Index (BMI) less than 18 or when a patient is only able to swallow a purée consistency or less [22].

The side-effects of dysphagia and oesophagitis may last up to several weeks or a few months after completing treatment and so regular dietetic review remains important. Late effects of this treatment are benign oesophageal stricturing and stenosis due to tissue fibrosis. Management is usually with a series of oesophageal dilations and sometimes oesophageal stent placement with artificial feeding being required in the interim.

Surgery

The surgical resection of the malignant oesophageal tumour remains the principal curative treatment [5,23]. This may be on its own or as part of a multimodality treatment plan. Oesophagectomy is carried out for mid to lower oesophageal cancers and some oesophagogastric junction tumours. It may also be performed in rare cases where definitive chemoradiotherapy has failed.

Enhanced recovery after surgery

The enhanced recovery after surgery (ERAS) approach to pre-, peri- and postoperative care has major benefits for many patients in relation to quicker recovery following major surgery and shorter hospital stay, with no increase in readmission rates. Enhanced recovery after surgery is becoming standard practice for most patients undergoing major surgery in the UK.

Postoperative major surgery-related complications are a predictor of reduced quality of life after oesophageal resection, and any measures that can reduce the risk of complications can decrease the negative impact on quality of life [24].

Early identification and treatment of undernutrition

Preoperative weight loss is an independent risk factor for the onset of postoperative complications in patients with GI cancer [25]. All patients with oesophageal cancer should be screened using a validated nutritional screening tool. Guidelines recommend that patients with severe nutritional risk receive nutritional support, preferably using the enteral route for 10–14 days prior to major surgery, even if surgery has to be delayed [5,26].

Immunonutrition Immunonutrition refers to EN which contains substrates that are postulated to ameliorate the postoperative immune response, modulate the postoperative inflammatory response and upregulate GI microperfusion and oxygen metabolism. An immunonutrition enteral formula commonly used in upper GI malignancies is enriched with omega-3 fatty acids, arginine, ribonucleic acid and soluble fibre. A prospective, randomised, double-blind study was performed on 206 elective surgery patients with cancer of the stomach, pancreas, colon and rectum. Patients receiving perioperative immunonutrition experienced a significantly lower rate of postoperative infections and had a shorter length of stay compared to the control group who received perioperative isonitrogenous, isocaloric liquid feed. Interestingly, the benefits were seen in both well-nourished and undernourished patients [27]. Similar findings are reflected in another study where patients with GI cancer undergoing surgery received pre- and perioperative immunonutrition compared with no nutritional support. Length of hospital stay was shorter in the pre- and perioperative groups. Interestingly, there was no statistical difference between the preoperative and perioperative groups which suggests that preoperative immunonutrition is sufficient in inferring the benefits [28].

Immunonutrition has been shown to be cost-effective in well-nourished patients [29]. A meta-analysis of all randomised clinical trials using immunonutrition identified an optimum dosage of 0.5–1 L/day. Supplementation for 5 days before surgery contributed to reduced morbidity in elective surgical patients, particularly those undergoing GI surgery [30]. European guidelines give a Grade A recommendation for the use of immunonutrition for 5–7 days preoperatively, independent of nutritional risk [26].

Preoperative carbohydrate loading Preoperative carbohydrate loading is recommended in patients undergoing major surgery because of its benefits on postoperative insulin resistance, length of hospital stay and subjective well-being [26,31]. A randomised controlled trial on patients undergoing upper GI surgery failed to show a significant difference in insulin and glucose levels associated with preoperative carbohydrate loading [32]. This may be attributed to the use of less accurate measurements of glucose and insulin compared with other studies which used a hyperinsulinaemic euglycaemic clamp as standard. However, preoperative carbohydrate loading did appear to attenuate the depletion of muscle mass associated with the metabolic stress of surgery and there was an observed trend towards reduced length of stay. The preparation was also shown to be safe to use in this patient group. European guidelines recommend preoperative carbohydrate loading in most patients undergoing major surgery [26].

Postoperative nutrition

After oesophagectomy, oral intake is traditionally avoided to minimise strain on the anastomosis and to reduce the inherent risks of postoperative impaired GI motility. Practice can vary as to the preferred method of nutrition support provided post surgery [33].

Patients undergoing resections for oesophageal, gastric or pancreatic cancer were randomised to receive either postoperative parenteral nutrition (PN) or EN with a jejunostomy [34]. While EN did not improve outcome when compared with PN, it was associated with a significantly shorter length of stay in a subgroup of undernourished patients. This was probably due to the lower complication rate in those given EN. Other studies have demonstrated the following benefits of EN over PN after upper GI surgery: reduced incidence and duration of postoperative complications, shorter length of intensive care unit stay and hospital stay [35,36].

A separate study compared postoperative EN using a nasojejunal tube with intravenous fluids after oesophagectomy. There were no observed differences in complications, ease of reintroduction of oral intake or length of stay. However, a non significant greater loss of weight and lean body mass was seen in patients receiving intravenous fluids [37]. Limitations of this study were a small sample size and nutritional parameters were not measured beyond a week after surgery. More recently, Barlow et al. demonstrated in a prospective, multicentre, randomised controlled trial that early EN after upper GI surgery led to improved morbidity, lower complication rates and reduced length of hospital stay, when compared to intravenous fluids [38].

The benefits of EN over PN and intravenous fluids after GI surgery for cancer were demonstrated in a study involving 1410 patients. Enteral nutrition and PN achieved a benefit on postoperative complications regardless of nutritional status when compared to intravenous fluids. However, EN was the superior feeding modality [25].

European guidance recommends that patients undergoing major upper GI surgery for cancer should receive postoperative EN in the first instance, reserving PN for when complications arise that lead to contraindications to EN [26].

Enteral access after oesophagectomy

Postpyloric feeding using a jejunostomy or nasojejunal feeding tube is recommended by current international guidance for the safe administration of EN [5,26]. The advantage of jejunostomy tube placement arises where patients need to continue EN after their discharge from hospital as it is more discrete, less likely to displace and therefore lends itself to longer term use compared with a nasojejunal tube. Longer term EN after discharge should be considered for patients who are undernourished, fail to progress to sufficient oral intake or if requiring more treatment. Minor complications of jejunostomy and/or nasojejunal feeding include diarrhoea, tube blockages, displacement and entry site infection. Major complications of jejunostomies include dislodgement with subsequent infusion of feed into the peritoneal cavity, jejunostomy-related bowel obstruction requiring relaparotomy and GI necrosis.

Postoesophagectomy complications

Anastomotic leak Conservative management of anastomotic leaks necessitates a prolonged nil-by-mouth status. If enteral tube access distal to the leak is available, feeding can continue until the leak heals and the patient progresses to oral diet. Removable plastic stents may also be used, allowing the patient to return to oral intake.

Chyle leak The leakage of chyle from an injured lymphatic duct is a rare complication with an incidence of 4% after oesophagectomy [39]. Chyle leaks can be sealed by reoperation but clinicians may choose conservative management, in which nutrition plays a central role. If enteral access is available, fat-free or high medium-chain fat and low long-chain fat feed can be used to minimise the leak of lymph fluid through the injured lymphatic duct [40]. For patients who are on oral diet, a very low-fat diet may be used. The use of fat-free oral nutritional supplements can be helpful. Special consideration should be given to the provision of essential fatty acids and fat-soluble vitamins as essential fatty acid deficiency can develop within 5 days [41]. Some clinicians will opt to completely avoid stimulation of the lymphatic system using PN. There are few studies comparing nutritional management strategies of chyle leaks, and clinician preference is usually the determining factor for choice of nutrition support.

Gastric tube necrosis Reoperation is necessary to remove the necrotic gastric tube, to form a cervical oesophagostomy and close off the gastric remnant. These patients will require long-term jejunostomy feeding until they proceed to colonic interposition to restore intestinal continuity.

Dietary advice and quality of life after oesophagectomy

All patients should receive long-term dietary advice. This should focus on the possible side-effects of the surgery which include early satiety, reflux/dyspepsia, diarrhoea and steathorroea, dumping syndrome, regurgitation, dysphagia secondary to anastomotic stricture, delayed gastric emptying, weight loss (and concerns regarding body image) and vitamin and mineral deficiencies.

Side-effects of oesophagectomy significantly impair quality of life [24,42]. Some evidence suggests that quality of life is restored to some extent in patients who survive 2 years after surgery [43,44]. Dietary modification, nutrition support strategies and pharmacology should be employed in the management of side-effects during follow-up.

International guidance on management of upper GI cancer patients highlights the importance of managing nutritional problems after surgery [3,4,7,23].

Oesophageal stenting

This procedure may be used in combination with the above treatments or as a standalone palliative treatment. A stent placement relieves a mechanical obstruction in the oesophagus to restore oral intake. However, underlying nutritional difficulties may remain which require further dietetic management. Advice on eating following an oesophageal stent insertion should aim to minimise risk of stent blockage whilst avoiding unnecessary and excessive dietary restriction.

3.4.4 Nutrition in the palliative setting

The aims of any dietetic intervention are to preserve quality of life and support patients through palliative treatments. Prognosis is an important consideration when managing the nutritional needs of these patients. Interventions should be considered carefully on an individual basis. Disease-related anorexia is a common manifestation in advanced disease. Pharmaceutical measures may be used in the management of this symptom, which include use of a short course of corticosteroids and/or a steroidal progesterone (megestrol acetate) [45]. Complications of advanced disease, which may require enteral nutrition or in some cases parenteral nutrition, include a tracheo-oesophageal fistula, vocal cord palsy and non-stentable obstructing tumours.

The documented incidence of a tracheo-oesophageal fistula in oesophageal cancer varies between 1% and 22% [46,47]. It leads to aspiration of oral intake and saliva into the airways. A nil-by-mouth status is implemented until the fistula is sealed, often with oesophageal and/or tracheal stents. The placement of a transnasal feeding tube in the short term can help maintain nutritional needs until oral intake is safe.

Vocal cord palsy arises from the involvement of tumour infiltrating the recurrent laryngeal nerve within the lung, leading to an unsafe swallowing mechanism. It occurs in 5% of oesophageal cancers, presenting as a hoarse voice, recurrent chest infections or coughing on oral intake [48]. In conjunction with a speech and language therapy assessment, the insertion of a feeding tube may be indicated to safely manage nutritional needs.

A small number of tumours cannot be stented due to their location in the oesophagus and these will require long-term tube feeding. Parenteral nutrition may be needed until an enteral route is established.

References

1. Office for National Statistics (ONS). *Cancer Statistics Registrations: Registrations of Cancer Diagnosed in 2008, England.* Series MB1 no.39. London: Office for National Statistics, 2011.
2. Office for National Statistics (ONS). *Statistical Bulletin. Cancer Survival in England – Patients Diagnosed 2006–2010 and Followed Up to 2011.* London: Office for National Statistics, 2012.
3. Department of Health. *Guidance on Commissioning: Improving Outcomes in Upper Gastrointestinal Cancers: The Manual.* London: Department of Health, 2001.
4. Allum WH, Blazeby JM, Griffin SM, et al. Guidelines for the management of oesophageal and gastric cancer. *Gut* 2011; **60**(11): 1449–1472.
5. Scottish Intercollegiate Guidelines Network. *Management of Oesophageal and Gastric Cancer (A National Guideline).* 2006. Available from: www.sign.ac.uk/pdf/sign87.pdf.
6. National Cancer Peer Review-National Cancer Action Team. *Manual for Cancer Services: Upper GI Measures.* London: Department of Health, 2011.
7. National Comprehensive Cancer Network. *NCCN Clinical Practice Guidelines in Oncology, Esophageal Cancer* 2012. Available from: www.nccn.org/professionals/physician_gls/pdf/esophageal.pdf.
8. Enzinger PC, Mayer RJ. Esophageal cancer. *New England Journal of Medicine* 2003; **349**(23): 2241–2252.
9. Buas MF, Vaughan TL. Epidemiology and risk factors for gastroesophageal junction tumors: understanding the rising incidence of this disease. *Seminars in Radiation Oncology* 2013; **23**(1): 3–9.
10. Ajani JA, Barthel JS, Bentrem DJ, et al. Esophageal and esophagogastric junction cancers. *Journal of the National Comprehensive Cancer Network* 2011; **9**(8): 830–887.
11. Daly JM, Fry WA, Little AG, et al. Esophageal cancer: results of an American College of Surgeons Patient Care Evaluation Study. *Journal of the American College of Surgeons* 2000; **190**(5): 562–572.
12. Awad S, Tan BH, Cui H, et al. Marked changes in body composition following neo-adjuvant chemotherapy for oesophagogastric cancers. *Clinical Nutrition* 2012; **31**(1): 74–77.
13. Deans DAC, Wigmore SJ, de Beaux AC, Paterson-Brown S, Garden OJ, Fearon KC. Clinical prognostic scoring system to aid decision-making in gastro-oesophageal cancer. *British Journal of Surgery* 2007; **94**(12): 1501–1508.
14. Lis CG, Gupta D, Lammersfield CA, Markman, M, Vashi PG. Role of nutritional status in predicting quality of life outcomes in cancer – a systematic review of the epidemiological literature. *Nutrition Journal.* 2012. Available from: www.nutritionj.com/content/pdf/1475-2891-11-27.pdf.
15. Andreyev HJ, Norman AR, Oates J, Cunningham D. Why do patients with weight loss have a worse outcome when undergoing chemotherapy for gastrointestinal malignancies? *European Journal of Cancer* 1998; **34**(4): 503–509.
16. Arends J, Bodoky G, Bozzetti F, et al. for the European Society for Parenteral and Enteral Nutrition). ESPEN guidelines on enteral nutrition: non-surgical oncology. *Clinical Nutrition* 2006; **25**(2): 245–259.
17. Jenkinson AD, Lim J, Agrawal N, Menzies D. Laparoscopic feeding jejunostomy in esophagogastric cancer. *Surgical Endoscopy* 2007; **21**(2): 299–302.
18. Westaby D, Young A, O'Toole P, Smith G, Sanders DS. The provision of a percutaneously placed enteral tube feeding service. *Gut* 2010; **59**(12): 1592–1605.
19. Isenring E, Zabel R, Bannister M, et al. Updated evidence-based practice guidelines for the nutritional management of patients receiving radiation therapy and/or chemotherapy. *Nutrition and Dietetics* 2013. Available from: http://onlinelibrary.wiley.com/doi/10.1111/1747-0080.12013/full.
20. Heath EI, Burtness BA, Heitmiller RF, et al. Phase II evaluation of preoperative chemoradiation and postoperative adjuvant chemotherapy for squamous cell and adenocarcinoma of the esophagus. *Journal of Clinical Oncology* 2000; **18**(4): 868–876.
21. Margolis M, Alexander P, Trachiotis GD, Gharagozloo F, Lipman T. Percutaneous endoscopic gastrostomy before multimodality therapy in patients with esophageal cancer. *Annals of Thoracic Surgery* 2003; **76**(5): 1694–1698.
22. Odelli C, Burgess D, Bateman L, et al. Nutrition support improves patient outcomes, treatment tolerance and admission characteristics in oesophageal cancer. *Clinical Oncology* 2005; **17**(8): 639–645.
23. Department of Health. *National Oesophago-Gastric Cancer Audit: An Audit of the Care Received by People with Oesophago-Gastric Cancer in England and Wales. Annual Report.* 2012. Available from: https://catalogue.ic.nhs.uk/publications/clinical/oesophago-gastric/nati-clin-audi-supp-prog-oeso-gast-canc-2012/clin-audi-supp-prog-oeso-gast-2012-rep.pdf.
24. Viklund P, Wengstrom Y, Rouvelas I, Lindblad M, Lagergren J. Quality of life and persisting symptoms after oesophageal cancer surgery. *European Journal of Cancer* 2006; **42**: 1407–1414.
25. Bozzetti F, Gianotti L, Braga M, di Carlo V, Mariani L. Postoperative complications in gastrointestinal cancer patients: the joint role of the nutritional status and nutritional support. *Clinical Nutrition* 2007; **26**(6): 698–709.
26. Weimann A, Braga M, Harsanyi L, et al for the European Society for Parenteral and Enteral Nutrition. ESPEN guidelines

on enteral nutrition: surgery including organ transplantation. *Clinical Nutrition* 2006; **25**(2): 224–244.

27. Braga M, Gianotti L, Radaelli G, et al. Perioperative immunonutrition in patients undergoing cancer surgery. *Archives of Surgery* 1999; **134**(4): 428–433.

28. Gianotti L, Braga M, Nespoli L, Radaelli G, Beneduce A, di Carlo V. A randomised controlled trial of preoperative oral supplementation with a specialized diet in patients with gastrointestinal cancer. *Gastroenterology* 2002; **122**(7): 1763–1770.

29. Braga M, Gianotti L. Preoperative immunotnutrition: cost benefit analysis. *Journal of Parenteral and Enteral Nutrition* 2005; **29**(Suppl 1): S57–S61.

30. Waitzberg DL, Saito H, Plank LD, et al. Postsurgical infections are reduced with specialised nutrition support. *World Journal of Surgery* 2006; **30**(8): 1592–1604.

31. Noblett S, Watson D, Huong H, Davison B, Hainsworth PJ, Horgan AF. Pre-operative oral carbohydrate loading in colorectal surgery: a randomized controlled trial. *Colorectal Disease* 2006; **8**: 563–569.

32. Yuill K, Richardson R, Davidson H, Garden OJ, Parks RW. The administration of an oral carbohydrate-containing fluid prior to major elective UGI surgery preserves skeletal muscle mass postoperatively – a RCT. *Clinical Nutrition* 2005; **24**: 32–37.

33. Murphy PM, Modi P, Rahamim J, Wheatley T, Lewis SJ. An investigation into the current peri-operative nutritional management of oesophageal carcinoma patients in major carcinoma centres in England. *Annals of the Royal College of Surgeons of England* 2006; **88**: 358–362.

34. Braga M, Gianotti L, Gentilini O, Parisi V, Salis C, di Carlo V. Early postoperative enteral nutrition improves gut oxygenation and reduces costs compared with total parenteral nutrition. *Critical Care Medicine* 2001; **29**: 242–248.

35. Bozzetti F, Braga M, Gianotti L, Gavazzi C, Mariani L. Postoperative enteral versus parenteral nutrition in malnourished patients with gastrointestinal cancer: a randomised multicentre trial. *Lancet* 2001; **358**: 1487–1492.

36. Gabor S, Renner H, Matzi V, et al. Early enteral feeding compared with parenteral nutrition after oesophageal or oesophagogastric resection and reconstruction. *British Journal of Nutrition* 2005; **93**: 509–513.

37. Page RD, Oo AY, Russell GN, Pennefather SH. Intravenous hydration versus naso-jejunal enteral feeding after esophagectomy: a randomised study. *European Journal of Cardiothoracic Surgery* 2002; **22**: 666–672.

38. Barlow R, Price P, Reid TD, et al. Prospective multicentre randomised controlled trial of early enteral nutrition for patients undergoing major upper gastrointestinal surgical resection. *Clinical Nutrition* 2011; **30**: 560–566.

39. Alexiou C, Watson M, Beggs D, Salama FD, Morgan WE. Chylothorax following oesophagogastrectomy for malignant disease. *European Journal of Cardiothoracic Surgery* 1998; **14**: 460–466.

40. Cardenas A, Chopra S. Chylous ascites. *American Journal of Gastoenterology* 2002; **97**: 1896–1900.

41. McCray S, Parrish CR. When chyle leaks: nutrition management options. *Nutrition Issues in Gastroenterology* 2004; **17**: 60–76. Available from: www.bamc.amedd.army.mil/departments/nutritional-medicine/topics/docs/chyle-leaks.pdf.

42. Djärv T, Lagergren J, Blazeby JM, Lagergren P. Long-term health-related quality of life following surgery for oesophageal cancer. *British Journal of Surgery* 2008; **95**: 1121–1126.

43. Blazeby JM, Farndon JR, Donovan J, Alderson D. A prospective longitudinal study examining the quality of life of patients with esophageal carcinoma. *Cancer* 2000; **88**(8): 1781–1787.

44. De Boer AG, Genovesi PI, Sprangers MA, van Sandick JW, Obertop H, van Lanschot JJQuality of life in long-term survivors after curative transhiatal oesophagectomy for oesophageal carcinoma. *British Journal of Surgery* 2000; **87**(12): 1716–1721.

45. Ruiz Garcia V, López-Briz E, Carbonell Sanchis R, Gonzalvez Perales JL, Bort-Marti S. Megestrol acetate for treatment of anorexia-cachexia syndrome. *Cochrane Database of Systematic Reviews* 2013; **3**: CD004310. Available from: http://onlinelibrary.wiley.com/doi/10.1002/14651858.CD004310.pub3/full.

46. Sihoe ADL, Wan IYP, Yim APC. Airway stenting for unresectable esophageal cancer. *Surgical Oncology* 2004; **13**(1): 17–25.

47. Balazs A, Galambos Z, Kupcsulik PK. Characteristics of esophagorespiratory fistulas resulting from esophageal cancers: a single-center study on 243 cases in a 20-year period. *World Journal of Surgery* 2009; **33**(5): 994–1001.

48. Tachimori Y, Kato H, Watanabe H, Ishikawa T, Yamaguchi H. Vocal cord paralysis in patients with thoracic esophageal carcinoma. *Journal of Surgical Oncology* 1995; **59**(4): 230–232.

Chapter 3.5

Gastric cancer and nutrition

Clare Shaw
Royal Marsden NHS Foundation Trust, London, UK

3.5.1 Incidence and aetiology

An estimated 990,000 people were diagnosed with gastric cancer worldwide in 2008, accounting for 8% of the total cancer diagnoses [1]. The incidence of gastric cancer varies around the world with the highest rates occurring in eastern Asia and the lowest rates in northern and southern Africa [1]. The incidence of gastric cancer worldwide is more than double in men than in women (Figures 3.5.1, 3.5.2). Rates of gastric cancer have been declining worldwide for several decades which is thought to be related to improvements in diet, food storage and preservation which may be linked to a decrease in the prevalence of *Helicobacter pylori*.

Over half of gastric cancers are caused by the bacterium *Helicobacter pylori* which was discovered in 1984 by Barry Marshall and Robin Warren [2]. It was initially found to be associated with gastric ulcers and gastritis but has also been identified as a cause of gastric cancer. Particular strains of *H. pylori* predispose to gastric cancer, possibly through a number of mechanisms including inflammation of gastric epithelium, stimulation of inflammatory cells and cellular changes induced by injection of protein products into the epithelial cells of the stomach [3]. These cellular influences in conjunction with environmental factors, including diet, eventually support the growth of malignant cells [4]. There may be a genetic component to these changes with individuals who readily produce cytokines, particularly interleukin-8, being at increased risk of subsequently developing gastric cancer [5].

Other environmental factors that increase the risk of gastric cancer include smoking, with approximately 20% of gastric cancers being attributed to tobacco smoking [6].

Dietary intake also influences the development of gastric cancer. High consumption of salt, as assessed by salt added to food and consumption of processed meat, increases the risk of development of gastric cancer [7]. Other studies have estimated total consumption of salt using a food frequency questionnaire, estimation of salt intake from main food groups and the use of added salt at the table and these too have found an association between higher salt intakes and an increased risk of gastric cancer [8]. High intakes of vegetables may have a protective effect against gastric cancer [9]. Allium vegetables in particular may have a preventive effect, possibly due to a direct action against *H. pylori* [10,11]. Case–control investigations in the European Prospective Investigation into Cancer and Nutrition (EPIC) study examined concentrations of carotenoids, retinol and alpha-tocopherol in individuals in prediagnosis blood samples compared to controls not diagnosed with gastric cancer. The results showed that higher plasma concentrations of some carotenoids, retinol and alpha-tocopherol are associated with reduced risk of gastric cancer [12]. It is thought that the protective effect of carotenoids may be due to their antioxidant properties, limiting DNA damage and oxidative stress. Retinol may have an effect on the control of cellular growth [12].

There is interest in the potential of chemoprevention for gastric cancer although, as yet, the ideas are

Advanced Nutrition and Dietetics in Gastroenterology, First Edition. Edited by Miranda Lomer.
© 2014 John Wiley & Sons, Ltd. Published 2014 by John Wiley & Sons, Ltd.

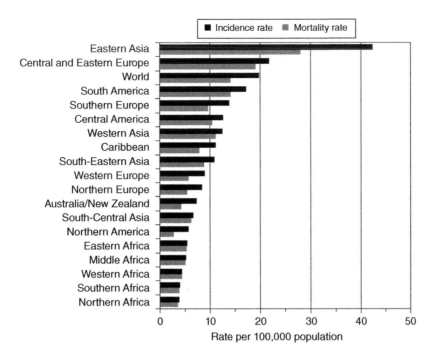

Figure 3.5.1 Stomach cancer: world age-standardised incidence and mortality rates, males, regions of the world, 2008 estimates [1]. Reproduced with permission from Cancer Research UK.

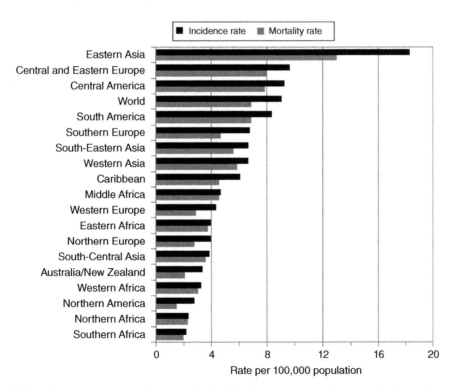

Figure 3.5.2 Stomach cancer: world age-standardised incidence and mortality rates, females, regions of the world, 2008 estimates. Reproduced with permission from Cancer Research UK.

not supported by research evidence [13]. Cyclo-oxygenase-2 (COX-2) is an enzyme responsible for the production of prostaglandins and prostacyclins that are involved in the inflammation cascade, and increased concentrations of COX-2 are present during the progression of atrophic gastritis to intestinal metaplasia and gastric cancer. Environmental factors such as smoking, increased gastric acid production and *H. pylori* are all associated with greater COX-2 expression. Aspirin and other non-steroidal drugs inhibit COX-2 and therefore have been proposed as possible chemopreventive drugs for gastric cancer. There is interest in whether anti-inflammatory fatty acids are also able to modulate this response and work has been carried out in animal models [14]. The results of clinical trials in humans are awaited.

3.5.2 Diagnosis and staging

The presenting symptoms of gastric cancer can range from mild gastritis or indigestion to gastric outflow obstruction, the latter having a significant impact on nutritional status as it causes vomiting and severely impairs adequate dietary intake. Other symptoms may be non-specific and include nausea, anaemia, loss of appetite, fatigue and weight loss [15,16].

All patients with suspected gastric cancer require an endoscopy and, for staging of the disease, all patients should undergo a computed tomography (CT) scan plus a staging laparoscopy. Gastric cancer is staged using the TNM system to describe the size and spread of the tumour and if it has spread to the submucosa or muscle wall or penetrated the stomach wall (T). The N and M denote whether it has spread to lymph nodes (N) and to other parts of the body (M).

3.5.3 Treatment

Treatment of gastric cancer will depend on the stage of the disease and the performance status of the patient which measures general health and ability to perform activities of daily living. Other factors affecting treatment choice include whether any co-morbidities, such as heart disease, are present.

Decisions on the preferred treatment should be made after appropriate staging of the disease and an assessment by members of the multidisciplinary team [13].

Chemotherapy and targeted therapies

Perioperative chemotherapy confers a survival advantage when compared to surgery alone and therefore this is the preferred course of treatment [13]. Some patients may not be suitable for surgery and therefore may benefit from palliative chemotherapy that has been demonstrated to improve health-related quality of life and survival [13]. If cells have human epidermal growth factor receptors (HER2) then the patient may also be treated with trastuzumab, a targeted treatment which has been demonstrated to improve disease-free survival.

Surgery

Surgical resection should only be undertaken in patients who are sufficiently well with a good performance status who are able to withstand a surgical intervention. The resection depends on the site of the tumour and may include a subtotal gastrectomy for distal tumours or a total gastrectomy for proximal tumours. Oesophagogastric junctional tumours require a transhiatal extended total gastrectomy or oeosphagogastrectomy [13]. Additional lymph nodes should be removed, with the extent of this resection depending on the performance status of the patient and the position of the tumour.

Alternatively, surgery may be used with palliative intent to relieve symptoms, such as gastric outflow obstruction, in patients who are not suitable for a curative resection. As with all cancer patients undergoing surgery, nutritional status should be optimised before surgical treatment to reduce morbidity and mortality [17].

Radiotherapy

Radiotherapy may be used in combination with chemotherapy to improve survival and is considered in patients who are at high risk of recurrence and who have not received neoadjuvant therapy, i.e. any form of cancer treatment prior to the main treatment modality. Palliative radiotherapy may be appropriate for some patients depending on their symptoms and performance status. Planning and delivery of such treatment in a palliative setting should always be done in the context of a multidisciplinary team with palliative care support for symptom management.

3.5.4 Nutritional status of gastric cancer patients

Cancer cachexia, a term that describes nutritional and inflammatory changes in the patient, is common in upper GI cancer [16,18]. The relative contributions of changes in dietary intake and inflammation caused by the cancer itself are difficult to ascertain and it is likely that in this group of patients both are contributory factors to changes in body composition.

Weight loss is common at the time of diagnosis of gastric cancer and is influenced by GI symptoms and a reduced dietary intake. In a study of 220 patients with upper GI cancer, 83% had lost weight at the time of diagnosis which amounted to a median loss of 7% of body weight [19]. This equated to a mean weight loss of 2.5% per month prior to diagnosis. In this group of patients 39% had lost more than 10% of their premorbid body weight. In this study, weight loss was associated with advanced disease, difficulty eating and poor dietary intake.

Gastric cancer can have a profound effect on dietary intake that may continue during and after treatment [19]. Symptoms often present in gastric cancer include abdominal pain, anorexia, dysphagia, nausea and vomiting [20]. Gastric outflow obstruction may occur if the tumour is situated near the pylorus. This results in gastric distension, satiety, nausea and vomiting with an inadequate dietary intake.

The metabolic changes of cancer cachexia may influence both protein and fat metabolism. There may be both host and tumour factors that reduce protein synthesis and increase protein degradation, resulting in a preferential loss of skeletal muscle mass [21]. Fat stores in the body are mobilised, possibly as a result of negative energy balance but also due to the action of intermediary metabolites such as lipid-mobilising factor (LMF) or tumour necrosis factor (TNF) alpha.

In gastro-oesophageal cancer patients, high serum C-reactive protein, a measure of inflammation, is also associated with weight loss which indicates that changes in dietary intake and the inflammatory response are both present in patients [19]. Lack of studies specifically measuring metabolic rate in gastric cancer patients prior to treatment makes it difficult to ascertain the relative contribution, if any, of these metabolic changes on energy expenditure and potentially weight loss.

The method of nutritional support is an important consideration for patients in their treatment pathway. If patients are palliative then a pyloric or duodenal stent may be appropriate to manage an obstruction. If patients are being treated with curative intent then they may require nutritional support whilst undergoing chemotherapy, radiotherapy or being prepared for surgery. These decisions should be taken following a full staging of the cancer and a multiprofessional discussion on the treatment plan and support required [13].

Nutritional and performance status can influence treatment options. When both are poor, patients are less able to withstand treatment side-effects. Weight loss is associated with poor tolerance to chemotherapy with increased side-effects, longer breaks during treatment to allow the patient to recover and overall a reduction in the quantity of chemotherapy given to patients [22,23]. Lean body mass is important for the distribution of cytotoxic drugs so increased toxicity to chemotherapy may occur as a result of lower fat-free mass. In a study of patients with lung or GI cancer undergoing 5-FU chemotherapy, those with sarcopenic obesity, and loss of lean body mass, had increased toxicity and poorer survival following chemotherapy [24].

3.5.5 Nutritional support

In the United Kingdom, evidence-based pathways for the provision of nutritional advice to cancer patients can be used by clinicians to ascertain the required clinical input for patients or by commissioners and workforce planners assessing the service that must be provided for a population [25].

Table 3.5.1 European Society of Parenteral and Enteral Nutrition guidelines on enteral nutrition – non-surgical oncology [27]

Subject	Recommendations	Grade of evidence
General	Nutritional assessment of cancer patients should be performed frequently, and nutritional intervention initiated early when deficits are detected.	C
General	Start nutritional therapy if undernutrition already exists or it is anticipated that the patient will be unable to eat for more than 7 days.	C
	Start enteral nutrition if an inadequate food intake (less than 60% of estimated energy expenditure for more than 10 days) is anticipated. It should substitute the difference between actual intake and calculated requirements.	C
	In patients losing weight due to insufficient nutritional intake, enteral nutrition should be provided to improve maintain nutritional status.	B
Perioperative	Patients with severe nutritional risk benefit from nutritional support 10–14 days prior to major surgery even if the surgery has to be delayed.	A
During radiotherapy or radiochemotherapy	Use intensive dietary advice and oral nutritional supplements to increase dietary intake and to prevent therapy-associated weight loss and the interruption of radiation therapy.	A
	Routine enteral nutrition is not indicated in radiation therapy.	C
During chemotherapy	Routine enteral nutrition during chemotherapy has no effect on tumour response to chemotherapy or on chemotherapy-associated unwanted effects and therefore is not considered useful.	C
Application	Use enteral route whenever feasible.	A
Perioperative	Use preoperative enteral nutrition with immune-modulating substrates (arginine, omega-3 fatty acids, nucleotides) for 5–7 days in all patients undergoing major abdominal surgery independent of their nutritional status.	A

Grades of evidence:
A: Meta-analysis of randomised controlled trials (RCT) or at least one RCT.
B: At least once well-designed controlled trial without randomisation or quasi-experimental study or descriptive study.
C: Expert opinion and/or clinical experience of respected authors.
Reproduced with permission from Elsevier.

The provision of good nutritional information, support and monitoring of nutritional status during treatment has been shown to help prevent weight loss and maintain quality of life [26]. This study was undertaken in lower GI cancer patients and demonstrated that dietary counselling during radiotherapy treatment had a sustained effect on patient outcomes of weight and quality of life compared to the provision of oral nutritional supplements or *ad libitum* intake.

Nutritional support before, during and after treatment is crucial to maintain or improve nutritional status and quality of life in this vulnerable group (Table 3.5.1). Studies have demonstrated that dietary advice and/or oral nutritional supplements in patients who are undernourished or at risk of undernutrition can improve nutritional intake and quality of life [28]. However, a comparison of studies looking at oral nutritional interventions and quality of life as measured by the European Organisation for Research and Treatment of Cancer (EORTC) indicated that there was heterogeneity in the studies published, making comparison between them difficult. Lack of a consistent effect of nutrition on the functional and symptom scales and global quality of life makes it difficult to draw firm conclusions about the overall effect of this intervention. Such studies have been unable to demonstrate an impact of oral nutrition interventions on overall survival [28].

Surgery (total or partial gastrectomy)

Patients who are undernourished have poorer outcomes after surgery in terms of morbidity and mortality. It is recommended that all undernourished patients should have nutritional status assessed and managed prior to surgery to optimise outcome. Inadequate dietary intake for 2 weeks prior to surgery is associated with increased mortality, morbidity, length of hospital stay and associated costs [17]. In such patients nutritional support in the form of enteral nutrition should be provided for patients for 10–14 days prior to surgery even if this means delaying the surgery [17]. The provision of such support in undernourished patients has demonstrated improved postoperative outcomes. There appears to be no benefit of routine preoperative nutritional support in patients who are well nourished or mildly undernourished.

However, preoperative immunonutrition has been shown to reduce postoperative infectious complications in both normally nourished and undernourished patients and should be offered 5–7 days preoperatively [29]. Immunonutrition includes the nutrients arginine, ribonucleic acid and omega-3 fatty acids which have been demonstrated to alter eicosanoid synthesis, cytokine production and immune function, thereby modulating the key features of the acute stress response [30]. Patients with gastric outflow obstruction should be considered for preoperative jejunal feeding or alternatively parenteral nutrition (PN) if it is not possible to obtain access to the GI tract to enable maintenance or improvement of nutritional status prior to surgery [17].

The extent of gastric surgery will influence whether enteral nutrition (EN) is required during the postoperative recovery phase. Smaller resections may result in the patient commencing oral fluids 24–48 h post surgery, allowing resumption of normal food intake within approximately 5 days. More extensive gastric resections, including total gastrectomy, will require nutritional support, preferably as jejunostomy tube feeding, to support the patient until oral intake has resumed and the patient is able to meet their nutritional requirements. Supplementary EN can be continued for patients who struggle to eat and drink sufficiently due to early satiety.

Chemotherapy

Cytotoxic chemotherapy agents have an effect on the GI tract, causing inflammation, oedema, ulceration and atrophy. These side-effects influence transit time, absorption and GI permeability, making the patient susceptible to transmural infection [31]. They also cause symptoms such as nausea, vomiting and taste changes which can profoundly influence food intake and quality of life.

3.5.6 Nutritional status and quality of life after treatment

Nutritional status may be difficult to maintain following treatment for gastric cancer due to the number of side-effects and symptoms that affect dietary intake and absorption. Limited gastric resection and minimally invasive surgery may reduce the impact of surgery on dietary intake and nutritional status. In a series of 122 patients undergoing gastric surgery, half of the patients had lost over 10% of their preoperative Body Mass Index at 1 year following treatment. However, just over half still had a normal BMI and 30% were overweight [32]. Many factors may contribute to the weight loss, including reduced dietary intake with some contributory factors being early satiety, taste changes, regurgitation and vomiting [33,34]. Gastric surgery can also have a profound effect on GI functioning with rapid gastric emptying and an early and increased postprandial fullness [35]. The effect on dietary intake can result in inadequate consumption of energy, protein, calcium, iron or vitamin D.

Some patients may require long-term EN, often to supplement an inadequate dietary intake.

Few studies have examined the long-term nutritional status and quality of life of gastric cancer patients. However, studies in oesophagogastric patients have shown that treatment for cancer has a negative impact on the person's quality of life for the first year following surgery [36]. Adaptation to the altered anatomy of the GI tract may occur with time and studies have demonstrated that patients may be able to achieve an adequate dietary intake a number of years following a partial and total gastrectomy [35].

Late effects of treatment

Treatment to the GI tract may result in symptoms that affect food intake, nutrient absorption and GI symptoms in the long term. Gastrointestinal symptoms demonstrated after treatment for gastric cancer may be easily identifiable as being due to the treatment or alternatively some may not initially be attributed to the treatment [31]. Radical surgical resection may cause disturbance in intestinal transit time, altered gastric emptying or emptying of gastric remnant, enzymatic digestion and malabsorption due to a combination of anatomical disruption, intestinal stasis, bacterial overgrowth, bile acid secretion and absorption [31]. Alterations to the nerve supply to the stomach may be primarily responsible but additional factors such as altered GI microbiota are also influential. The prevalence of these symptoms is not well recorded in the literature but increasingly it is recognised that these should be investigated and managed with the aim of improving quality of life [31].

Early dumping, due to a hyperosmolar load being delivered to the intestine postprandially, may occur in up to 68% of patients [37,38]. It causes sweating, palpitations, nausea and upper GI discomfort and significantly impacts on quality of life. The risk of developing dumping may be due to the extent of surgical resection and whether the pylorus is preserved. The development of late dumping has a higher incidence in patients who experience early dumping. Patients may experience rebound hypoglycaemia 1–2 h after eating or after exercise. Dietary advice is crucial to the management of dumping syndrome and patients may find relief of some symptoms by altering the quantity of food eaten, timings of meals and the amount of readily absorbed carbohydrate foods. It is thought that small intestinal bacterial overgrowth may increase the risk of dumping [39].

Vitamin B12 deficiency may develop as early as 1 year after total gastrectomy if vitamin B12 is not administered by intramuscular injection [40]. Loss of parietal cells in the stomach, responsible for the production of intrinsic factor, results in the malabsorption of dietary and enterally supplemented vitamin B12. Regular parenteral vitamin B12 is required in all total gastrectomy patients. Those who have undergone partial gastrectomy will require regular monitoring of vitamin B12 status and appropriate supplementation if concentrations are below the normal range.

Anorexia occurs in 33–38% of patients [41]. When anorexia is experienced following surgical treatment for gastric cancer, it may be partly due to altered plasma ghrelin concentrations. Ghrelin is important in the control of appetite, particularly in the initiation of eating, and is produced by the gastric mucosa. Studies have demonstrated changes in ghrelin concentrations following gastrectomy although these do not correlate directly with weight loss and other anthropometric changes, indicating that other factors may be involved [42].

Early satiety may occur in surgical patients due to a reduced gastric reservoir. It may occur more frequently following pylorus-preserving gastrectomy as demonstrated by an increased presence of gastric food residue at endoscopy in these patients compared to those without pylorus-preserving surgery [43].

All persistent symptoms should be investigated to exclude malignant recurrence and to identify the cause of symptoms, enabling early treatment.

Palliative care

Gastric cancer may be advanced at the time of diagnosis, may not respond to successful treatment or may recur after treatment. In these circumstances, the aim of care is to palliate symptoms which include pain, abdominal discomfort, early satiety and gastric outflow obstruction. Self-expansible metal stents may be used to create an opening of the pylorus or duodenum if the tumour causes an obstruction. These are placed at endoscopy and may allow the patient to eat and drink during the last few weeks of life and ultimately improve quality of life [44]. Late complications, however, are common with 25% of patients experiencing dysphagia due to tumour overgrowth, bolus obstruction and stent migration [13]. Patients with gastric outflow obstruction which is not amenable to stenting may receive some benefit from a venting gastrostomy to relieve gastric distension, thereby enabling them to eat and drink limited amounts.

Survivorship

Improvements in outcomes for many cancer patients have led to increased survival rates following treatment. The management of GI symptoms in patients with gastric cancer is essential to maintain or improve their quality of life [31]. Although the survival rates for gastric cancer have improved in the last 25 years, the rates are still low, with 5-year survival at 15% [45]. It is essential that patients receive timely and appropriate dietary advice and nutritional support with the aim of improving clinical outcomes and quality of life.

References

1. Cancer Research UK. *Stomach cancer*. Available from: http://info.cancerresearchuk.org/cancerstats/world/stomach-cancer-world/, accessed 31 December 2013.
2. Marshall BJ, Warren JR. Unidentified curved Bacilli in the stomach of patients with gastritis and peptic ulceration. *Lancet* 1984; **323**(8390): 1311–1315.
3. Wroblewski LE, Peek RM Jr, Wilson KT. Helicobacter pylori and gastric cancer: factors that modulate disease risk. *Clinical Microbiology Reviews* 2010; **23**(4): 713–739.
4. Woodward M, Tunstall-Pedoe H, McColl K. Helicobacter pylori infection reduces systemic availability of dietary vitamin C. *European Journal of Gastroenterology and Hepatology* 2001; **13**(3): 233–237.
5. Portal-Celhay C, Perez-Perez G. Immune responses to Helicobacter pylori colonization: mechanisms and clinical outcomes. *Clinical Science* 2006; **110**: 305–314.
6. Lagergren J, Bergström R, Lindgren A, Nyrén O. The role of tobacco, snuff and alcohol use in the aetiology of cancer of the oesophagus and gastric cardia. *International Journal of Cancer* 2000; **85**(3): 340–346.
7. Hu J, La Vecchia C, Morrison H, Negri E, Meri L, Canadian Cancer Registries Epidemiology Research Group. Salt, processed meat and the risk of cancer. *European Journal of Cancer Prevention* 2011; **20**(2): 132–139.
8. Peleteiro B, Lopes C, Figueiredo C, Lunet N. Salt intake and gastric cancer risk according to Helicobacter pylori infection, smoking, tumour site and histological type. *British Journal of Cancer* 2011; **104**(1): 198–207.
9. Boffetta P, Couto E, Wichmann J, et al. Fruit and vegetable intake and overall cancer risk in the European prospective investigation into cancer and nutrition (EPIC). *Journal of the National Cancer Institute* 2010; **102**(8): 529–537.
10. World Cancer Research Fund. *Food, Nutrition, Physical Activity and the Prevention of Cancer: A Global Perspective*. Washington, DC: World Cancer Research Fund, 2007.
11. Zhou Y, Zhuang W, Hu W, Liu GJ, Wu TX, Wu XT. Consumption of large amounts of Allium vegetables reduces risk for gastric cancer. *Gastroenterology* 2011; **141**(1): 80–89.
12. Jenab M, Riboli E, Ferrari P, et al. Plasma and dietary carotenoid, retinol and tocopherol levels and the risk of gastric adenocarcinomas in the European prospective investigation into cancer and nutrition. *British Journal of Cancer* 2006; **95**(3): 406–415.
13. Allum WH, Blazeby J, Griffin M, et al. Guidelines for the management of oesophageal and gastric cancer. *Gut* 2011. Available from: www.augis.org/pdf/Gut-2011-Allum-gut-2010-228254.pdf, accessed 31 December 2013.
14. Jostein Christensen B, Berge K, Wergedahl H, et al. Bioactive fatty acids reduce development of gastric cancer following duodenogastric reflux in rats. 12th World Congress of the International Society for Diseases of the Esophagus. *Diseases of the Esophagus* 2011; **23**: 105.
15. Sandgren A, Fridlund B, Nyberg P, Strang P, Petersson K, Thulesius H. Symptoms, care needs and type of cancer diagnosis in palliative cancer patients in acute care hospitals. *European Journal of Cancer* 2009; **7**(2–3): Supplement.
16. Bozzetti F, SCRINIO Working Group. Screening the nutritional status in oncology: a preliminary report on 1,000 outpatients. *Supportive Care in Cancer* 2009; **17**(3): 279–284.
17. Weimann A, Braga M, Harsanyi L, et al. ESPEN Guidelines on Enteral Nutrition: surgery including organ transplantation. *Clinical Nutrition* 2006; **25**(2): 224–244.
18. Fearon KC, Voss AC, Hustead DS. Definition of cancer cachexia: effect of weight loss, reduced food intake, and systemic inflammation on functional status and prognosis. *American Journal of Clinical Nutrition* 2006; **83**(6): 1345–1350.
19. Deans DA, Tan BH, Wigmore SJ, et al. The influence of systemic inflammation, dietary intake and stage of disease on rate of weight loss in patients with gastro-oesophageal cancer. *British Journal of Cancer* 2009; **100**(1): 63–69.
20. Fuchs CS, Mayer RJ. Gastric carcinoma. *New England Journal of Medicine* 1995; **333**(1): 32–41.

21. Tisdale MJ. Cancer cachexia. *Langenbeck's Archives of Surgery* 2004; **389**(4): 299–305.

22. Andreyev HJ, et al. Why do patients with weight loss have a worse outcome when undergoing chemotherapy for gastrointestinal malignancies? *European Journal of Cancer* 1998; **34**(4): 503–509.

23. Ross PJ, Ashley S, Norton A, et al. Do patients with weight loss have a worse outcome when undergoing chemotherapy for lung cancers? *British Journal of Cancer* 2004; **90**(10): 1905–1911.

24. Prado CM, Lieffers JR, McCargar LJ, et al. Prevalence and clinical implications of sarcopenic obesity in patients with solid tumours of the respiratory and gastrointestinal tracts: a population-based study. *Lancet Oncology* 2008; **9**(7): 629–635.

25. National Cancer Action Team. *Living With and Beyond Cancer: Cancer Rehabilitation.* 2010. Available from: http://webarchive.nationalarchives.gov.uk/20130513211237/http://www.ncat.nhs.uk/our-work/living-beyond-cancer/cancer-rehabilitation# , accessed 10 January 2014.

26. Ravasco P, Monteiro Grillo I, Maria C. Cancer wasting and quality of life react to individualised nutritional counselling. *Clinical Nutrition* 2007; **26**(1): 7–15.

27. Arends J, Bodoky G, Bozzetti F, et al. ESPEN Guidelines on Enteral Nutrition: non-surgical oncology. *Clinical Nutrition* 2006; **25**(2): 245–259.

28. Baldwin C, Spiro A, Ahern R, Emery PW. Oral nutritional interventions in malnourished patients with cancer: a systematic review and meta-analysis. *Journal of the National Cancer Institute* 2012; **104**: 371–385.

29. Gianotti L, Braga M, Nespoli L, Radaelli G, Beneduce A, di Carlo V. A randomised controlled trial of preoperative oral supplementation with a specialized diet in patients with gastrointestinal cancer. *Gastroenterology* 2002; **122**: 1763–1770.

30. Cerantola Y, Hübner M, Grass F, Demartines N, Schäfer M. Immunonutrition in gastrointestinal surgery. *British Journal of Surgery* 2011; **98**: 37–48.

31. Andreyev HJ, Davidson S, Gillespie C, Allum WH, Swarbrick E. Practice guidance on the management of acute and chronic gastrointestinal problems arising as a result of treatment for cancer. *Gut* 2011. Available from: http://gut.bmj.com/content/early/2011/11/04/gutjnl-2011-300563.full.pdf, accessed 31 December 2013.

32. Veeramootoo D, et al. The minimally invasive approach to oesophagectomy for cancer may offer a nutritional benefit. *Diseases of the Esophagus* 2010; **23**.

33. Harris AM, Griffin SM. Postoperative taste and smell deficit after upper gastrointestinal cancer surgery – an unreported

34. complication. *Journal of Surgical Oncology* 2003; **82**(3): 147–150.

35. Tian J, Chen JS. Nutritional status and quality of life of the gastric cancer patients in Changle County of China. *World Journal of Gastroenterology* 2005; **11**(11): 1582–1586.

36. Kamiji MM, Troncon LE, Suen VM, de Oliveira RB. Gastrointestinal transit, appetite and energy balance in gastrectomised patients. *American Journal of Clinical Nutrition* 2009; **89**: 231–239.

37. Blazeby JM, Sanford E, Falk SJ, Alderson D, Donovan JL. Health-related quality of life during neoadjuvant treatment and surgery for localised esophageal carcinoma. *Cancer* 2005; **103**: 1791–1799.

38. Delgado del Rey M, Gómez Candela C, Cos Blanco AI, et al. [Nutritional evaluation in patients with total gastrectomy]. *Nutrición Hospitalaria* 2002; **17**(5): 236–239.

39. Mine S, Santo T, Tsutsumi K, et al. Large-scale investigation into dumping syndrome after gastrectomy for gastric cancer. *Journal of the American College of Surgeons* 2010; **211**(5): 628–636.

40. Paik CN, Choi MG, Lim CH, et al. The role of small intestinal bacterial overgrowth in postgastrectomy patients. *Neurogastroenterology and Motility* 2011; **23**(5): e191–e196.

41. Adachi S, Kawamoto T, Otsuka M, Todoroki T, Fukao K. Enteral vitamin B12 supplements reverse postgastrectomy B12 deficiency. *Annals of Surgery* 2000; **2**: 199–201.

42. Khalid U, Spiro A, Baldwin C, et al. Symptoms and weight loss in patients with gastrointestinal and lung cancer at presentation. *Supportive Care in Cancer* 2007; **15**(1): 39–46.

43. An JY, Choi MG, Noh JH, Sohn TS, Jin DK, Kim S. Clinical significance of ghrelin concentration of plasma and tumor tissue in patients with gastric cancer. *Journal of Surgical Research* 2007; **143**(2): 344–349.

44. Yamaguchi T, Ichikawa D, Kurioka H, et al. Postoperative clinical evaluation following pylorus-preserving gastrectomy. *Hepatogastroenterology* 2004; **51**(57): 883–886.

45. Fiocca F, Ceci V, Donatelli G, Moretta MG, Santagati A, Sportelli G. Palliative treatment of upper gastrointestinal obstruction using self-expansible metal stents. *European Review for Medical and Pharmacological Sciences* 2006; **10**(4): 179–182.

46. Cancer Research UK. *Cancer Stats: key facts stomach cancer.* 2010. Available from: http://info.cancerresearchuk.org/prod_consump/groups/cr_common//@nre/@sta/documents/generalcontent/crukmig_1000ast-3130.pdf, accessed 31 December 2013.

Chapter 3.6

Gastroparesis and nutrition

Richard Keld[1] and Simon Lal[2]

[1]Wrightington, Wigan and Leigh NHS Foundation Trust, Wigan, UK
[2]Salford Royal NHS Foundation Trust, Salford, UK

Gastroparesis is defined by delayed gastric emptying in the absence of mechanical obstruction. In health, gastric emptying is governed by rhythmical 'slow waves' of peristaltic contractions of the smooth muscles in the gastric fundus, body and antrum [1]. This activity is initiated in the gastric 'pacemaker cells' or interstial cells of Cajal and is under vagal control. In gastroparesis, perstaltic contractions are reduced by loss of the gastric pacemaker cells [2,3] and/or disruption of the vagus nerve, culminating in one or more abnormalities in gastric motility such as hypomotility, gastric arrhythmia and/or lack of antropyloroduodenal propagation [4]. In the USA, the prevalence of gastroparesis is 1 per 10,000 males and 4 per 10,000 females [5]. However, this may be an underestimate since delayed gastric emptying is thought to occur in up to 50% of patients with diabetes mellitus [6,7] and up to 50% of patients with functional dyspepsia [8] (also known as non-ulcer dyspepsia) or irritable bowel syndrome.

3.6.1 Factors involved in causation

The most common cause of gastroparesis, accounting for up to 50% of cases, is idiopathic [9]. Here the underlying cause is unclear, although a large proportion of patients have a history of viral infections [10,11] and psychological stress [10]; as such, there may be an overlap with functional dyspepsia [8]. The second most common cause of gastroparesis is diabetes mellitus, accounting for up to 30% of cases [9]. Typically, patients also display evidence of an autonomic neuropathy with postural hypotension and cardiac arrhythmias [12]. Postsurgical gastroparesis accounts for up to 13% of all cases of gastroparesis and can occur as a complication of gastric, oesophageal, duodenal or pancreatic surgery following disruption of the vagus nerve [9].

Proton pump inhibitor therapy has significantly reduced the frequency of gastric surgery (for peptic ulcer disease), but this trend is being reversed as a result of the obesity epidemic. The obesity epidemic is accounting for a resurgence of gastric surgery and this is likely to increase the frequency of postsurgical gastroparesis in future years.

Additional causes of gastroparesis are pharmacological, including tricylic antidepressants and opiate analgesics, and multisystem disorders including Parkinson's disease and systemic sclerosis [5].

3.6.2 Dietary effects of disease or its management

Symptoms of gastroparesis typically consist of nausea and/or vomiting, occurring in 74% and 53% of all patients respectively; additional symptoms include abdominal pain, bloating, early satiety, postprandial fullness and weight loss [5]. Of course, this constitution of symptomatology is not specific and is insufficient to clinch a diagnosis of gastroparesis, but in high-risk groups, such as patients with diabetes and those with functional dyspepsia, a low index of suspicion should prevail.

Advanced Nutrition and Dietetics in Gastroenterology, First Edition. Edited by Miranda Lomer.
© 2014 John Wiley & Sons, Ltd. Published 2014 by John Wiley & Sons, Ltd.

Gastroparesis is not only varied in its aetiology but also in severity. Nutritional intake can be significantly compromised, resulting in weight loss, vitamin and mineral loss and dehydration, necessitating hospitalisation in severe cases [13,14]. Gastroparesis is classified by severity according to the Gastroparesis Cardinal Index Score which takes into account all the aforementioned factors and is a useful tool to guide treatment options [15].

3.6.3 Investigations

The diagnosis of gastroparesis can be suspected after normal standard diagnostic endoscopic and radiological investigations that have excluded a mechanical gastric outlet obstruction. Although there are many different modalities for diagnosing gastroparesis (reviewed in Keld et al. [16]), food residue seen on gastroscopy despite a 12-h fast may be an important clue. Scintigraphy is the gold standard to confirm the diagnosis and involves ingestion of a standardised radiolabelled meal containing technetium-99 or indium-111, after an overnight fast. To avoid variation in measurements between laboratories, the Neurogastroenterology and Motility Society and the Society of Nuclear Medicine have recently recommended using a standardised egg-white meal (eggs, two slices of white bread, strawberry jam (30 g), water (120 mL), and technetium-99m sulphur colloid, 0.521 mCi) (Egg Beaters®) [17]. The test is deemed positive if more than 60% residual ingested meal content is detected within the stomach after 2 h, or more than 10% residual content is detected at 4 h [18].

3.6.4 Dietary treatments

Treatment strategies in gastroparesis aim to improve symptoms and reduce nutritional impairment, ideally by improving gastric emptying. Dietary therapy is central to disease management in all cases, although the evidence basis for dietary manipulation solely derives and is extrapolated from research in healthy subjects, not patients with gastroparesis. Alternative treatment strategies include pharmacological therapy, including antiemetics, prokinetics and botulinum toxin (reviewed in Keld et al. [16]), but the evidence basis and response to this approach are also limited [19–22]. Recently, the development of implantable gastric pacemakers shows promise in severe cases of gastroparesis, but this intervention is still under scrutiny and not widely available [23].

A detailed dietary history should focus on the type and consistency of foods tolerated and the timing, content and size of meals in relation to symptoms. Evaluation of nutritional and fluid status (including weight and anthropometric measurements), glycaemic control and the presence of any vitamin and mineral deficiency is also needed.

Food consistency

In health, non-nutrient liquids have fast gastric emptying times of 20 min and, when plotted on a graph, gastric emptying times are exponential [24]. Nutrient-containing liquids have slower emptying times and display a linear plot, and solid foods are slower still due to an initial plateau as a consequence of the grinding of food particles; this is termed the lag phase [24]. Similarly, in patients with gastroparesis, the gastric emptying time for small food particle size (e.g. blended carrots) is quicker than that of a large food particle size (e.g. chopped carrots) [25]. Small food particle sizes have a reduced lag phase of gastric emptying. In view of this change in physiology, simple manipulation of food consistency can be very effective in the management of gastroparesis. In mild cases adequate chewing may be sufficient to reduce food particle size while in moderate to severe cases, a puréed or liquid diet may be required.

Food composition

Manipulation of food content is central to managing gastroparesis. In the diabetic population, maintenance of normoglycaemia is of paramount importance since hyperglycaemia can impair gastric emptying [26]. Alcohol and carbonated drinks are not recommended due to gas production [27,28]. Furthermore, since fats [29] and fibre are known to prolong gastric emptying times in healthy subjects, manipulation of these particular food groups is recommended. Fats are essential to maintain normal metabolism through the provision of energy, so complete dietary omission is clearly not advised and liquid fats are recommended to avoid dietary omission.

Fibre is classified into soluble (gums, pectin and gels) and insoluble forms (cellulose, hemicelluloses). Both forms of fibre are thought to delay gastric emptying but studies to evaluate the effect of fibre have only used artificial fibre supplements and have provided inconsistent results [30,32], with some studies only demonstrating minor effects on emptying times [33]. Furthermore, the effects of fibre on gastric physiology have not been specifically evaluated in gastroparesis; nevertheless, insoluble fibre has been reported to induce bezoar and phytobezoar formation. Phytobezoars are composed of non-digestible food material including cellulose, hemicellulose, lignin and fruit tannins which are often found in raw vegetables, citrus fruits, celery, pumpkins, grapes, prunes and raisins. Currently, albeit on a limited evidence base, insoluble fibre is best avoided in gastroparesis [34].

Food volume

A simple intervention is the adjustment of meal size, as a large volume of food takes more time to empty from the stomach than a small-volume meal [24] and thus a 'regular and often' small-volume meal approach should be adopted. Manipulation of meal consistency, content and size is effective in patients with mild to moderate symptoms and a diet of frequent small-volume meals with low fibre and low fat content and soft to liquid consistency is generally recommended [28].

Enteral nutrition

In severe cases, where patients fail to thrive with oral dietary adjustments, nutritional support may be required. As ever, enteral nutrition (EN) is the preferred route over parenteral nutrition (PN) as this yields a more 'physiological' effect and is associated with fewer complications [35]. The nasogastric route has been suggested by slow pump infusion of a liquid diet [36]. However, in practice, by the nature of the disease, this route is unlikely to meet food energy requirements and of course, there is also the added risk of pulmonary aspiration. The nasojejunal route is preferred due to the lower risk of pulmonary aspiration, and tubes can be placed endoscopically or by the bedside [35]. If nasojejunal feeding is well tolerated, a jejunostomy feeding tube, placed laparoscopically or endoscopically [37], or a percutaneous gastrostomy with jejunal extension (PEG-J) may be sited for comfort as a more permanent route. Compared to jejunostomy tube feeding, PEG-J has the advantage of venting of gastric contents if needed for symptom relief [38], although the occurrence of tube migration back to the stomach is a troublesome complication [39].

Parenteral nutrition

Parenteral nutrition should always be reserved for patients in whom jejunal feeding is not possible due to the high prevalence of serious complications [35,40]. However, small intestinal dysmotility can co-occur with gastroparersis and limit the effectiveness of jejunal feeding. Small intestinal dysmotility can be confirmed by small intestinal manometry studies but this is usually restricted to research centres [41]. A trial of nasojejunal feeding is always advised prior to placement of a definitive feeding tube such as a jejunostomy or PEG-J tube. Where intolerance is shown to occur with jejunal feeding, then PN should be considered as temporary supplemental nutrition or long term in refractory cases.

3.6.5 Conclusion

The diagnosis of gastroparesis can be easily missed so a high index of suspicion should be maintained in patients with suggestive symptoms and no structural cause identified using conventional radiological and endoscopic techniques. Once diagnosed, dietary intervention can have a dramatic effect on the well-being of patients and in the majority, simple manipulation of food content, consistency and volume will have a positive impact on disease management. In severe cases, a structured approach to optimise the feeding route can avoid unnecessary complications and improve nutritional status.

References

1. Sanders KM, Koh SD, Ward SM. Interstitial cells of Cajal as pacemakers in the gastrointestinal tract. *Annual Review of Physiology* 2006; **68**: 307–343.

2. Iwasaki H, Kajimura M, Osawa S, et al. A deficiency of gastric interstitial cells of Cajal accompanied by decreased expression of neuronal nitric oxide synthase and substance P in patients with type 2 diabetes mellitus. *Journal of Gastroenterology* 2006; **41**: 1076–1087.

3. Zarate N, Mearin F, Wang XY, Hewlett B, Huizinga JD, Malagelada JR. Severe idiopathic gastroparesis due to neuronal and interstitial cells of Cajal degeneration: pathological findings and management. *Gut* 2003; **52**: 966–970.

4. Masaoka T, Tack J. Gastroparesis: current concepts and management. *Gut Liver* 2009; **3**: 166–173.

5. Jung HK, Choung RS, Locke GR 3rd, et al. The incidence, prevalence, and outcomes of patients with gastroparesis in Olmsted County, Minnesota, from 1996 to 2006. *Gastroenterology* 2009; **136**: 1225–1233.

6. Horowitz M, O'Donovan D, Jones KL, Feinle C, Rayner CK, Samsom M. Gastric emptying in diabetes: clinical significance and treatment. *Diabetic Medicine* 2002; **19**: 177–194.

7. Jones KL, Russo A, Berry MK, Stevens JE, Wishart JM, Horowitz M. A longitudinal study of gastric emptying and upper gastrointestinal symptoms in patients with diabetes mellitus. *American Journal of Medicine* 2002; **113**: 449–455.

8. Tack J, Bisschops R, Sarnelli G. Pathophysiology and treatment of functional dyspepsia. *Gastroenterology* 2004; **127**: 1239–1255.

9. Feldman M, Corbett DB, Ramsey EJ, Walsh JH, Richardson CT. Abnormal gastric function in longstanding, insulin-dependent diabetic patients. *Gastroenterology* 1979; **77**: 12–17.

10. Soykan I, Sivri B, Sarosiek I, Kiernan B, McCallum RW. Demography, clinical characteristics, psychological and abuse profiles, treatment, and long-term follow-up of patients with gastroparesis. *Digestive Diseases and Sciences* 1998; **43**: 2398–2404.

11. Bityutskiy LP, Soykan I, McCallum RW. Viral gastroparesis: a subgroup of idiopathic gastroparesis – clinical characteristics and long-term outcomes. *American Journal of Gastroenterology* 1997; **92**: 1501–1504.

12. Merio R, Festa A, Bergmann H, et al. Slow gastric emptying in type I diabetes: relation to autonomic and peripheral neuropathy, blood glucose, and glycemic control. *Diabetes Care* 1997; **20**: 419–423.

13. Ogorek CP, Davidson L, Fisher RS, Krevsky B. Idiopathic gastroparesis is associated with a multiplicity of severe dietary deficiencies. *American Journal of Gastroenterology* 1991; **86**: 423–428.

14. Parkman HP, Yates KP, Hasler WL, et al. Dietary intake and nutritional deficiencies in patients with diabetic or idiopathic gastroparesis. *Gastroenterology* 2011; **141**: 486–498.

15. Revicki DA, Rentz AM, Dubois D, et al. Development and validation of a patient-assessed gastroparesis symptom severity measure: the Gastroparesis Cardinal Symptom Index. *Alimentary Pharmacology and Therapeutics* 2003; **18**: 141–150.

16. Keld R, Kinsey L, Athwal V, Lal S. Pathogenesis, investigation and dietary and medical management of gastroparesis. *Journal of Human Nutrition and Dietetics* 2011; **24**(5): 421–430.

17. Abell TL, Camilleri M, Donohoe K, et al. Consensus recommendations for gastric emptying scintigraphy: a joint report of the American Neurogastroenterology and Motility Society and the Society of Nuclear Medicine. *American Journal of Gastroenterology* 2008; **103**: 753–763.

18. Tougas G, Eaker EY, Abell TL, et al. Assessment of gastric emptying using a low fat meal: establishment of international control values. *American Journal of Gastroenterology* 2000; **95**: 1456–1462.

19. Amin K, Bastani B. Intraperitoneal ondansetron hydrochloride for intractable nausea and vomiting due to diabetic gastroparesis in a patient on peritoneal dialysis. *Peritoneal Dialysis International* 2002; **22**: 539–540.

20. Bai Y, Xu MJ, Yang X, et al. A systematic review on intrapyloric botulinum toxin injection for gastroparesis. *Digestion* 2010; **81**: 27–34.

21. Maddern GJ, Kiroff GK, Leppard PI, Jamieson GG. Domperidone, metoclopramide, and placebo. All give symptomatic improvement in gastroesophageal reflux. *Journal of Clinical Gastroenterologyogy* 1986; **8**: 135–140.

22. Erbas T, Varoglu E, Erbas B, Tastekin G, Akalin S. Comparison of metoclopramide and erythromycin in the treatment of diabetic gastroparesis. *Diabetes Care* 1993; **16**: 1511–1514.

23. Soffer E, Abell TL, Lin Z, et al. Review article: gastric electrical stimulation for gastroparesis – physiological foundations, technical aspects and clinical implications. *Alimentary Pharmacology and Therapeutics* 2009; **30**: 681–694.

24. Camilleri M. Integrated upper gastrointestinal response to food intake. *Gastroenterology* 2006; **131**: 640–658.

25. Olausson EA, Alpsten M, Larsson A, Mattsson H, Andersson H, Attvall S. Small particle size of a solid meal increases gastric emptying and late postprandial glycaemic response in diabetic subjects with gastroparesis. *Diabetes Research and Clinical Practice* 2008; **80**: 231–237.

26. Kong MF, Horowitz M, Jones KL, Wishart JM, Harding PE. Natural history of diabetic gastroparesis. *Diabetes Care* 1999; **22**: 503–507.

27. Bujanda L. The effects of alcohol consumption upon the gastrointestinal tract. *American Journal of Gastroenterology* 2000; **95**: 3374–3382.

28. Parkman HP, Hasler WL, Fisher RS. American Gastroenterological Association technical review on the diagnosis and treatment of gastroparesis. *Gastroenterology* 2004; **127**: 1592–1622.

29. Hunt JN, Knox MT. A relation between the chain length of fatty acids and the slowing of gastric emptying. *Journal of Physiology* 1968; **194**: 327–336.

30. Holt S, Heading RC, Carter DC, Prescott LF, Tothill P. Effect of gel fibre on gastric emptying and absorption of glucose and paracetamol. *Lancet* 1979; **1**: 636–639.

31. Schwartz SE, Levine RA, Singh A, Scheidecker JR, Track NS. Sustained pectin ingestion delays gastric emptying. *Gastroenterology* 1982; **83**: 812–817.

32. Schwartz SE, Levine RA, Weinstock RS, Petokas S, Mills CA, Thomas FD. Sustained pectin ingestion: effect on gastric emptying and glucose tolerance in non-insulin-dependent diabetic patients. *American Journal of Clinical Nutrition* 1988; **48**: 1413–1417.

33. Benini L, Castellani G, Brighenti F, et al. Gastric emptying of a solid meal is accelerated by the removal of dietary fibre naturally present in food. *Gut* 1995; **36**: 825–830.

34. Rider JA, Foresti-Lorente RF, Garrido J, et al. Gastric bezoars: treatment and prevention. *American Journal of Gastroenterology* 1984; **79**: 357–359.

35. National Collaborating Centre For Acute Care. *Nutrition Support in Adults: Oral Nutrition Support, Enteral Tube Feeding and Parenteral Nutrition*. London: National Collaborating Centre for Acute Care, 2006.

36. Patrick A, Epstein O. Review article: gastroparesis. *Alimentary Pharmacology and Therapeutics* 2008; **27**: 724–740.

37. Fontana RJ, Barnett JL. Jejunostomy tube placement in refractory diabetic gastroparesis: a retrospective review. *American Journal of Gastroenterology* 1996; **91**: 2174–2178.

38. Kim CH, Nelson DK. Venting percutaneous gastrostomy in the treatment of refractory idiopathic gastroparesis. *Gastrointestinal Endoscopy* 1998; **47**: 67–70.

39. Godbole P, Margabanthu G, Crabbe DC, et al. Limitations and uses of gastrojejunal feeding tubes. *Archives of Disease in Childhood* 2002; **86**: 134–137.

40. Staun M, Pironi L, Bozzetti F, et al. ESPEN Guidelines on Parenteral Nutrition: home parenteral nutrition (HPN) in adult patients. *Clinical Nutrition* 2009; **28**: 467–479.

41. Mahesh V, Unsworth B, Wrightham E, et al. Antroduodenal manometry: impact on clinical management. *Gut* 2010; **59**(Suppl 1): A18.

Chapter 3.7

Pancreatitis and nutrition

Mary Phillips
Royal Surrey County Hospital, Guildford, UK

3.7.1 Acute pancreatitis

Acute pancreatitis is an inflammatory condition which may be mild or severe. In mild cases there are usually few or no long-term effects, and patients do not routinely require any nutritional intervention. However, in severe acute pancreatitis (SAP) there is a risk of developing systemic issues such as adult respiratory distress syndrome (ARDS) and later localised complications including pancreatic necrosis and pseudocysts [1]. Patients with severe disease often have protracted hospital admissions and require intensive nutritional support.

3.7.2 Causes of pancreatitis

The causes of acute pancreatitis are diverse and are summarised in Box 3.7.1; it is estimated that 80% of cases are caused by gallstones or alcohol.

3.7.3 Severity of acute pancreatitis

Acute pancreatitis is mild in 75% of cases but in the remaining 25%, the disease is classified as severe [2]. Severity is predicted by using a scoring system such as the Ranson Score, Atlanta Classification, Acute Physiology and Chronic Health Evaluation (APACHE) II score or the modified Glasgow or Imrie Criteria (Box 3.7.2). In the latter, a score of 3 or more within 48 h of admission is predictive of

SAP. A serum C-reactive protein (CRP) concentration above 150 mg/L may be independently indicative of a severe attack, but this may not become apparent until 48–72 h into the disease process [2].

It is widely accepted that patients predicted to develop SAP require intensive nutritional support. Nutritional assessment, with severity scoring, should occur early in the disease process.

Mild acute pancreatitis

Patients presenting with mild pancreatitis are typically nil by mouth until their pain settles, and they are slowly weaned onto a normal diet over a period of 3–5 days. If the disease aetiology is gallstone related, they will have a laparoscopic cholecystectomy once they are recovered. In others, the cause of the pancreatitis will have to be investigated and treated accordingly.

The European Society of Parenteral and Enteral Nutrition (ESPEN) concluded that there was no evidence that enteral nutrition (EN) administered within the first week of disease onset provided any benefit to patients with mild pancreatitis [3].

Much debate remains over the use of low-fat diets in gallstone pancreatitis, with a paucity of evidence on which to base practice. Where the patient has not had a sphincterotomy and is waiting for a cholecystectomy, it would seem prudent to recommend a low-fat diet until surgery. However, where a sphincterotomy or cholecystectomy has been performed, there appears to be no indication for dietary fat restriction.

Advanced Nutrition and Dietetics in Gastroenterology, First Edition. Edited by Miranda Lomer.
© 2014 John Wiley & Sons, Ltd. Published 2014 by John Wiley & Sons, Ltd.

Box 3.7.1   Causes of pancreatitis [2]

Gallstones
Alcohol
Trauma
Steroids
Mumps
Autoimmune
Scorpion sting
Hypercalcaemia
Hyperlipidaemia
Hypothermia
Endoscopic retrograde cholangiopancreatography
(ERCP)
Drugs (including simvastatin)
Pancreatic cancer
Ischaemia
Postoperative
Infections
Parasites
Idiopathic

Box 3.7.2   Modified Glasgow or Imrie
Criteria [2]

P	Arterial PaO$_2$ <9 kPa
A	Albumin <32 g/L
N	Urea nitrogen >10 mmol/L
C	Calcium <2 mmol/L
R	Raised white cell count >16 mmol/L
E	Enzyme: lactic dehydrogenase (LDH) >600 mmol/L
A	Age >55 years
S	Sugar: glucose >10 mmol/L

Severe acute pancreatitis

Patients with SAP may develop widespread complications including ileus, nausea, vomiting, pain [4], diarrhoea, steatorrhoea (due to exocrine failure), hyperglycaemia (due to endocrine failure), ascites, portal hypertension resulting in gastric varices, and/or the formation of fistulae, pseudocysts and abscesses, all of which affect tolerance of EN and parenteral nutrition (PN).

Patients have increased energy requirements, poor oral intake and reduced nutrient absorption which, in combination with repeated periods of being 'nil by mouth' for investigations and procedures, results in rapid deterioration of nutritional status.

Poor nutritional status results in reduced immune function, which impairs ability to resist nosocomial infections, and these often complicate the disease pathway [4]. Furthermore, higher mortality has been demonstrated in patients with SAP who had persistently negative nitrogen balance, compared to those in positive balance [5].

3.7.4 Enteral nutrition

It is well established that the enteral route is the feeding route of choice for patients with SAP. A meta-analysis comparing EN and PN which identified six randomised controlled trials (RCT) involving 263 patients [6] concluded that there were reductions in the incidence of infections, surgical interventions and length of stay in the EN groups compared to the PN groups. However, there was no difference in mortality or non-infective complications.

Early EN reduces GI atrophy and prevents the loss of villi [7]. Gastrointestinal atrophy is associated with the generation of cytokines and other inflammatory mediators, hypoglycaemia, worsening antioxidant stress and the systemic inflammatory response syndrome [8,9]. Additionally, EN is thought to reduce intestinal permeability. High intestinal permeability permits bacterial translocation and endotoxaemia, and this is hypothesised to be the source of many infectious complications of SAP [10].

Studies examining the effect of EN compared to PN on inflammatory markers did not report any benefit, but were limited by small sample size, unequal disease aetiology and severity in each arm, and with an average length of stay of 10 days, were probably not representative of SAP [11].

The priority in nutrition support has moved to establishing an enteral route early in the treatment pathway. A recent systematic review concluded that establishing EN within 48 h of admission was associated with improvements in mortality, infectious complications and multiorgan failure rates [12].

Nasogastric versus nasojejunal feeding

Increasingly, evidence supports early EN in SAP and research has moved to consider the specifics of enteral tube placement. Studies have shown that jejunal feeding at distances of 40–60 cm beyond the ligament of Treitz prevents stimulation of pancreatic enzymes to the same degree as PN, and also stimulates secretion of plasma glucagon-like peptide 1 and plasma peptide YY which inhibit pancreatic function [13–15]. Whilst postpyloric feeding is beneficial in reducing nausea, duodenal feeding continues to stimulate cholecystokinin and therefore pancreatic function [13,15].

Initial studies examining the use of nasogastric (NG) feeding in SAP suggest this is fairly well tolerated and safe, with 23 of 26 patients tolerating full rate feeding within 36 h [16]. These results led to two randomised controlled studies comparing NG and NJ feeding in SAP. In the first study involving 50 patients, NJ feeding tubes were inserted into the proximal jejunum, although the exact position in relation to the ligament of Treitz was not specified [17]. The authors reported one incidence of cardiac arrest during NJ tube placement in one subject. Although the patient made a full recovery, this serves as a reminder that endoscopic placement of NJ feeding tubes is not without risk. The second study examined data on 31 patients randomised to receive NG or NJ feeds and detailed increased overall mortality in the NG group, although this was not statistically significant [18]. However, the methodology stated that the tube was positioned in the third part of the duodenum, resulting in placement proximal to the ligament of Treitz, and thus excluding the study as a true comparison of NG and NJ feeding.

Despite their limitations, these two studies on 81 patients have been the primary citations in two reviews which conclude that NG feeding may be a safe and effective alternative to NJ feeding in SAP [19,20]. Larger, adequately powered studies are required to confirm the effectiveness of NG feeding in clinical practice and in the interim, NJ feeding remains the enteral route of choice.

Feed formulation

A number of studies comparing EN and PN have used standard polymeric feeds, leading to the hypothesis that these feeds may be well tolerated in this patient group. A small RCT carried out in France compared 15 patients receiving a peptide feed with a standard polymeric feed, and concluded that whilst both feeds were tolerated (in terms of patient-reported abdominal pain, diarrhoea, bloating, steatorrhoea and 24-h stool tests quantifying creatorrhoea, steatorrhoea, stool weight and frequency), weight loss and length of stay were both lower in the peptide feeding group (P=0.01 and P=0.006, respectively), suggesting that peptide feeds are associated with better outcomes [21].

Larger studies are required to examine the use of polymeric feeds, whilst peptide feeds are well established as the feed of choice for feeding beyond the ligament of Treitz [3,22]. Further work is required to establish the efficacy of alternative feed types in gastric and duodenal feeding in SAP.

Probiotics

Initial investigations using probiotics in SAP appeared promising. with *Lactobacillus plantarum* associated with a reduction in disease severity and an improvement in clinical outcome. However, this study compared *L. plantarum*-supplemented EN with PN and as such, the improvement in clinical outcome may be attributable to the use of the enteral route [23].

In a large, multicentre RCT in 296 patients with SAP receiving EN via an NJ tube, a significantly higher incidence of bowel ischaemia was demonstrated in the patients randomised to the probiotic group, with eight patients in the intervention arm dying as a result [24]. There was no difference in infective complications and a significant increase in mortality in the probiotic group. It must be noted that this trial used a novel probiotic that had not undergone extensive animal or human safety testing; in addition, those patients in the intervention arm were experiencing a more severe attack of pancreatitis at the time of randomisation [25]. A number of other trials were abandoned when these results were published, and although the editors of *The Lancet* issued an 'expression of concern' regarding this trial (published March 2010), this appears to be related to study design and reporting procedures, rather than the data collected. At present, there seems to be no reason to doubt the study's findings and as such, probiotics are not recommended in patients with SAP.

3.7.5 Parenteral nutrition

Parenteral nutrition carries a higher risk of sepsis than EN, but with improving multidisciplinary management the risks previously attributed to overfeeding and catheter-related sepsis are falling [26,27]. However, PN does not carry the same benefit to outcome in acute pancreatitis [10] and where PN is indicated it should be used alongside EN wherever possible [28].

Care should be taken with the use of PN in the case of triglyceride-induced pancreatitis where it is necessary to use a lipid-free bag if triglyceride concentrations are in excess of 12 mmol/L [28].

In all patients with pancreatitis it is advisable to monitor triglyceride concentrations weekly while PN is ongoing. Additionally, where the aetiology of pancreatitis is unclear, it is important to check triglyceride concentrations prior to commencing PN.

Glutamine

The ESPEN guidelines recommend that glutamine is added to PN formulae for patients with SAP where PN is indicated [28]. Glutamine is thought to be the primary fuel of enterocytes and as such may reduce bacterial translocation and therefore sepsis. Glutamine has also been linked to the antioxidant defence, where it is used as a fuel by the immune system to produce glutathione [29].

Glutamine, at a dose of 0.4 g/kg, has been shown to reduce the acute inflammatory response, with a reduction in proinflammatory interleukin (IL)-6 and CRP, and an increase in anti-inflammatory IL-10 [30]. In addition, an improvement in immune function was observed in the same group with increased concentrations of CD4 and CD8 lymphocytes and serum IgA. This study examined 44 patients with severe acute pancreatitis randomised to receive 1.5 g/kg amino acids (1.1 g/kg standard amino acid and 0.4 g/kg glutamine in the supplemented group) and 30 kcal/kg. It reported an improvement in biochemical markers (albumin and total protein) and nitrogen balance and a reduction in infectious complications in the glutamine-supplemented group, but no significant reduction in mortality or length of stay [30].

Fish oils

While there are emerging data on the use of fish oils in the general intensive care environment, there are, as yet, few data looking specifically at fish oil in patients with SAP. Omega-3 fish oils have been shown to suppress inflammation and improve the course of infection in patients across multiple disease areas.

A small study examined the effects of fish oils in patients with SAP [31]. Forty patients were randomised to receive a standard soya bean lipid-based PN or PN supplemented with 0.15–0.2 g/kg fish oils. The authors reported a reduction in CRP, fewer days on haemofiltration, better oxygenation index and increased serum eicosapentaenoic acid (EPA) but further studies are required to confirm these benefits in patients with SAP.

3.7.6 Postdischarge care

Patients with mild acute pancreatitis should not require long-term nutrition support. However, in cases of SAP some patients have significant damage to pancreatic parenchyma which may cause exocrine or endocrine failure, resulting in malabsorption and diabetes. In this instance, nutritional management is similar to that used for patients with chronic pancreatitis.

A small number of patients (n=25) were asked about their quality of life following necrotising pancreatitis [32]. Whilst a 'fair' to 'good' quality of life was reported in 77.3 % of cases, abdominal distension (41%), GI symptoms (36.4%), weight loss (31.8%), nausea (31.8%) and vomiting (27.3%) were identified as influencing long-term quality of life.

3.7.7 Chronic pancreatitis

Chronic pancreatitis (CP) is defined as a chronic inflammatory process resulting in fibrosis and destruction of pancreatic exocrine and endocrine tissue. Over time, this causes failure of both these systems, resulting in malabsorption and in many cases diabetes. It is a benign condition which may be attributed to alcohol, autoimmune and genetic factors, or in some cases it may be idiopathic [1].

The most significant symptom is pain, often debilitating, which may be related to eating and leads to depression, opiate dependence and social isolation. Chronic pancreatitis is more prevalent in patients who smoke or have excessive alcohol consumption, and patients are more likely to develop pancreatic cancer. The combination of these physical, psychological and social factors results in patients requiring complex nutritional and psychological management. Patients should be strongly encouraged to give up smoking and alcohol consumption.

Oral nutritional support

Patients with chronic pancreatitis benefit from intensive and regular nutritional support (Box 3.7.3). Low-fat diets are not indicated unless pancreatic enzyme replacement therapy (PERT) is ineffective [33,34]. In these instances, it should be remembered

---

Box 3.7.3 Nutritional recommendations for chronic pancreatitis

- Encourage high-energy diet
- Avoid fat restriction
- Ensure adequate pancreatic enzyme replacement therapy
- Ensure any oral nutritional supplements are taken with pancreatic enzyme replacement therapy
- Annual blood tests to include vitamin A, D, E, selenium, iron studies and parathyroid hormone
- Vitamin and mineral supplements may be required to correct deficiencies; some units use vitamin and mineral supplements routinely
- Regular dietetic assessment to maintain nutritional status and monitor for deficiency symptoms
- Routine DEXA scanning (every 5 years)
- Routine annual screening for diabetes

---

that low-fat diets only manage symptoms but do not compensate for the lack of absorption, and therefore must be used as a last resort under careful nutritional supervision.

High-energy diets with the use of oral supplements must be used in conjunction with enzyme therapy, and patients should be encouraged to adjust their enzyme dose to match changes in oral intake.

Pancreatic exocrine insufficiency

Pancreatic exocrine insufficiency (PEI) usually occurs within 5–10 years of diagnosis of CP [35]. Steatorrhoea is a relatively late symptom of PEI, and optimisation of pancreatic enzyme dosage proves adequate for relieving symptoms in most patients.

Pancreatic enzyme replacement therapy is frequently underused as classic symptoms of steatorrhoea (pale, loose, floating stools) can be masked by the use of constipating opiate-based medication or low-fat diets. PERT products should be given alongside meals in order that they mix with chyme; if more than one capsule is required, the dose may be distributed throughout the meal. PERT should not be swallowed with hot drinks as the enzymes are denatured with excessive heat. All PERT products currently available in the UK are porcine based, and informed consent must be obtained prior to prescription.

The use of a proton pump inhibitor (PPI) alongside PERT can improve efficacy, and advice to manage malabsorption should be individualised, with the early use of oral nutritional supplements and EN where undernutrition is present [36].

Many authors have attempted to quantify the optimal dose of PERT required to manage malabsorption, with results varying from starting doses of 25,000 to 50,000 units per meal [37,38]. However, as exocrine failure is progressive and the dose each patient requires is likely to increase with time, regular dietetic review to ensure adequacy of PERT is crucial.

Antioxidants and pain

Persistent pain in chronic pancreatitis is thought to be multifactorial, and may be attributed to increases in interstitial fluid pressure, active inflammation, irritation of nerve endings or ductal strictures causing ductal hypertension, in addition to stones, masses or cysts within the pancreatic duct itself [39]. Consequently, the pain can be refractory to standard pain relief, and whilst surgical intervention in the form of coeliac nerve block and thoracic splanchnicectomy provides short-term pain relief, pancreatic rest and antioxidant therapy, which are less invasive than pancreatic resection, are commonly used.

Cytochrome C P450 (CYP) mono-oxygenase is a microsomal enzyme that metabolises both endogenous lipophilic substances and exogenous lipids (xenobiotics) using reactive oxygen species and may contribute to pain [39]. Braganza described xenobiotic-mediated injury to the pancreas, and suggested the potential benefit of antioxidant supplements in the management of pain, as removal of free radicals requires antioxidants (vitamin A, C, E and selenium), which are often depleted in chronic pancreatitis [40,41]. Several studies have concluded that antioxidant therapy is beneficial in reducing pain and the frequency of pancreatitis attacks [42–44] but all had small patient numbers (n=28–147), and a recent meta-analysis was unable to analyse the data as pain was recorded differently in the three studies [45]. The authors concluded that further large-scale randomised trials were required, and this is currently under way (EUROPAC2).

Pancreatic rest

Nasojejunal feeding with enteral tube placement at least 40 cm beyond the ligament of Treitz allows for adequate EN whilst preventing pancreatic stimulation, providing pancreatic rest [13–15]. It reduces pancreatic pseudocysts and improves pain control and nutritional status [46]. Enteral nutrition is often given continuously with a peptide formula. To avoid pancreatic stimulation, patients should be counselled to limit all oral intake to clear, caffeine-free fluids at no more than 60 mL per hour.

Parenteral nutrition

Overall, PN is not indicated in chronic pancreatitis in the absence of bowel obstruction. However, the ESPEN guidelines support the use of PN in duodenal stenosis, where the placement of a feeding tube distal to the disease may be difficult [28].

Vitamin and mineral deficiencies

Vitamin A deficiency night blindness has been reported after pancreatic resection and in cystic fibrosis [47,48]. Biochemical deficiencies of other fat-soluble vitamins have been reported in pancreatic resection [49]. While there is a paucity of chronic pancreatitis-specific data, it is reasonable to assume that nutritional data from pancreatic resection and cystic fibrosis may provide a basis for monitoring in chronic pancreatitis.

Bone health

Vitamin D deficiency is associated with the development of osteoporosis in patients with chronic pancreatitis. Adequate concentrations of activated vitamin D (1,25-dihydroxyvitamin D) are required to promote calcium absorption and ensure sufficient supply for bone remodelling [50]. Low concentrations of calcium stimulate parathyroid hormone (PTH) production, which stimulates the synthesis of 1,25-dihydroxyvitamin D to try and restore intestinal calcium absorption. This results in a spiral effect of further depletion of 25-hydroxyvitamin D, and in the absence of supplementation, a further drop in 1,25-dihydroxyvitamin D [51]. It is reasonable to expect poor calcium absorption in patients with ongoing steatorrhoea; thus supplements containing calcium and vitamin D are indicated as first-line treatment of vitamin D deficiency in patients with chronic pancreatitis.

Vitamin D deficiency has been widely documented in patients with pancreatic insufficiency, and is correlated with the degree of insufficiency (faecal elastase-1) to $P<0.01$ [52].

Regular biochemical monitoring and routine dual-energy X-ray absorptiometry (DEXA) scanning in patients with vitamin D deficiency are recommended [53].

Acknowledgements

The authors would like to thank Professor Nariman Karanjia, consultant HPB surgeon, and Clio Myers, HPB dietitian, Regional HPB Unit (Surrey and Sussex), Royal Surrey County Hospital, Guildford, UK.

References

1. Steer ML, Perides G. Pathogenesis: how does acute pancreatitis develop? In: Dominguez-Munoz JE (ed) *Clinical Pancreatology for Practising Gastroenterologists and Surgeons.* Oxford: Blackwell Publishing, 2005.

2. Neoptolemos JP, Bhutani MS. Fast facts. In: Neoptolemos JP (ed) *Diseases of the Pancreas and Biliary Tree.* Oxford: Health Press Ltd, 2006.

3. Meier R, Ockenga J, Pertkiewicz M, et al. ESPEN Guidelines on Enteral Nutrition: pancreas. *Clinical Nutrition* 2006; **25**: 275–284.

4. McClave SA, Ritchie CS. Artificial nutrition in pancreatic disease: what lessons have we learnt from the literature? *Clinical Nutrition* 2000; **19**(1): 1–6.

5. Sitzmann JV, Steinborn PA, Zinner MJ, Cameron LJ. Total parenteral nutrition and alternate energy substrates in treatment of severe acute pancreatitis. *Surgery, Gynecology and Obstetrics* 1989; **168**: 311–317.

6. Marik PE, Zaloga GP. Meta-analysis of parenteral nutrition vs enteral nutrition in patients with acute pancreatitis. *British Medical Journal* 2004; **328**: 1407–1412.

7. Groos S, Hunefeld G, Luciano L. Parenteral versus enteral nutrition: morphological changes in human adult intestinal mucosa. *Journal of Submicroscopic Cytology and Pathology* 1996; **28**: 61–74.

8. Kalfarentzos F, Kehagias J, Mead N, Kokkinis K, Gogos CA. Enteral nutrition is superior to parenteral nutrition in severe acute pancreatitis: results of a randomised prospective trial. *British Journal of Surgery* 1997; **84**: 1665–1669.

9. Windsor AC, Kanwar S, Li AG, et al. Compared with parenteral nutrition, enteral feeding attenuates the acute phase response and improves disease severity in acute pancreatitis. *Gut* 1998; **42**: 431–435.

10. Lehocky P, Sarr MG. Early enteral feeding in severe acute pancreatitis: can it prevent secondary pancreatic (super) infection. *Digestive Surgery* 2000; **17**(6): 571–577.

11. Powell JJ, Murchison JT, Fearon KC, Ross AJ, Siriwardena AK. Randomised controlled trial of the effect of early enteral nutrition on markers of the inflammatory response in predicted severe acute pancreatitis. *British Journal of Surgery* 2000; **87**: 1375–1381.

12. Petrov MS, Pylypchuk RD, Uchugina AF. A systematic review on the timing of artificial nutrition in acute pancreatitis. *British Journal of Nutrition* 2009; **101**: 787–793.

13. Vu MK, van der Veek PP, Frölich M, et al. Does jejunal feeding activate exocrine pancreatic secretion? *European Journal of Clinical Investigation* 1999; **29**: 1053–1059.

14. O'Keefe JS, Lee RB, Anderson FP, et al. Physiological effects of enteral and parenteral feeding on pancreaticobiliary secretion in humans. *American Journal of Physiology – Gastrointestinal and Liver Physiology* 2003; **284**(1): G27–G36.

15. Kaushik N, Pietraszewski M, Holst JJ, O'Keefe SJ. Enteral feeding without pancreatic stimulation. *Pancreas* 2005; **31**: 353–359.

16. Eatock FC, Brombacher GD, Steven A, Imrie CW, McKay CJ, Carter R. Nasogastric feeding in severe acute pancreatitis may be practical and safe. *International Journal of Pancreatology* 2000; **28**(1): 25–31.

17. Eatock FC, Chong P, Menezes N, et al. A randomised study of early nasogastric versus nasojejunal feeding in severe acute pancreatitis. *American Journal of Gastroenterology* 2005; **100**: 432–439.

18. Kumar A, Singh N, Prakash S, Saraya A, Joshi YK. Early enteral nutrition in severe acute pancreatitis: a prospective randomised controlled trial comparing nasojejunal and nasogastric routes. *Journal of Clinical Gastroenterology* 2006; **40**: 431–434.

19. Jiang K, Chen X, Xia Q, Tang W, Wang L. Early nasogastric enteral nutrition for severe acute pancreatitis: a systematic review. *World Journal of Gastroenterology* 2007; **13**(39): 5253–5260.

20. Marik PE. What is the best way to feed patients with pancreatitis? *Current Opinion in Critical Care* 2009; **15**: 131–138.

21. Tiengou L, Gloro R, Pouzoulet J, et al. Semi-elemental formula or polymeric formula: is there a better choice for enteral nutrition in acute pancreatitis? Randomised comparative study. *Journal of Parenteral and Enteral Nutrition* 2006; **30**: 1–5.

22. Silk DB. Formulation of enteral diets for use in jejunal enteral feeding. *Proceedings of the Nutrition Society* 2008; **67**: 270–272.

23. Qin HL, Zheng JJ, Tong DN, et al. Effect of lactobacillus plantarum enteral feeding on the gut permeability and septic complications in the patients with acute pancreatitis. *European Journal of Clinical Nutrition* 2008; **62**: 923–930.

24. Besselink MG, van Santvoort HC, Buskens E, et al, Probiotic prophylaxis in predicted severe acute pancreatitis: a randomised, double blind, placebo-controlled trial. *Lancet* 2008; **371**(9613): 651–660.

25. Reid G, Gibson G, Sanders ME, Guarner F, Versalovic J, for the International Scientific Association for Probiotics and Prebiotics. Probiotic prophylaxis in predicted severe acute pancreatitis. *Lancet* 2008; **372**: 112–113.

26. Dalton MJ, Schepers G, Gee JP, Alberts CC, Eckhauser FE, Kirking DM. Consultative total parenteral nutrition teams: the effect on the incidence of total parenteral nutrition-related complications. *Journal of Parenteral and Enteral Nutrition* 1984; **8**(2): 146–152.

27. Bosonnet L. Total parenteral nutrition: how to reduce the risks. *Nursing Times* 2002; **98**(22): 40.

28. Gianotti L, Meier R, Lobo DN, et al. ESPEN Guidelines on Parenteral Nutrition: pancreas. *Clinical Nutrition* 2009; **28**: 428–435.

29. Haisch M, Fukagawa NK, Matthews DE. Oxidation of glutamine by the splanchnic bed in humans. *American Journal of Physiology – Endocrinology and Metabolism* 2000; **278**: 593–602.

30. Fuentes-Orozco C, Cervantes-Guevara G, Muciño-Hernández I, et al. L-alanyl–L-glutamine-supplemented parenteral nutrition decreases infectious morbidity rate in patients with severe acute pancreatitis. *Journal of Parenteral and Enteral Nutrition* 2008; **32**: 403–411.

31. Wang X, Li W, Li N, Li J. Φ-3 fatty acids-supplemented parenteral nutrition decreased hyperinflammatory response and attenuates systematic disease sequelae in severe acute

pancreatitis: a randomised and controlled trial. *Journal of Parenteral and Enteral Nutrition* 2008; **32**(3): 236–241.

32. Szentkereszley Z, Czimbalmos A, Kotán R, et al. Quality of life following acute necrotising pancreatitis. *Pancreas* 2004; **54**: 1172–1174.

33. Lankisch PG. What to do when a patient with pancreatic exocrine insufficiency does not respond to pancreatic enzyme substitution: a practical guide. *Digestion* 1999; **60**: 97–104.

34. Toouli J, Biankin AV, Oliver MR, et al. Management of pancreatic exocrine insufficiency: Australasian Pancreatic Club recommendations. *Medical Journal of Australia* 2010; **192**(8): 461–467.

35. Dumasy V, Delhaye M, Cotton F, Deviere J. Fat malabsorption screening in chronic pancreatitis. *American Journal of Gastroenterology* 2004; **99**: 1350–1354.

36. Charnley RM, MacDermott C. Case Study 3: Pancreatic enzyme supplementation in chronic pancreatitis. Enzyme supplementation in cystic fibrosis, chronic pancreatitis, pancreatic and periampullary cancer. *Alimentary Pharmacology and Therapeutics* 2010; **32**(suppl 1): 1–25.

37. Imrie CW, Connett G, Hall RI, Charnley RM. Expert commentary: how we do it. Enzyme supplementation in cystic fibrosis, chronic pancreatitis, pancreatic and periampullary cancer. *Alimentary Pharmacology and Therapeutics* 2010; **32**(suppl 1): 1–25.

38. Braganza JM, Lee SH, McCloy RF, McMahon MJ. Chronic pancreatitis. *Lancet* 2011; **377**: 1184–1197.

39. McCloy R. Chronic pancreatitis at Manchester, UK. *Digestion* 1998; **59**(suppl 4): 36–48.

40. Braganza JM. The pancreas. In: Pounder RG (ed) *Recent Advances in Gastroenterology*. London: Churchill Livingstone, 1986, pp. 251–280.

41. Braganza JM. The pathogenesis of chronic pancreatitis. *Quarterly Journal of Medicine* 1996; **89**: 243–250.

42. Uden S, Schofield D, Miller PF, Day JP, Bottiglier T, Braganza JM. Antioxidant therapy for recurrent pancreatitis: biochemical profiles in a placebo-controlled trial. *Alimentary Pharmacology and Therapeutics* 1992; **6**: 229–240.

43. Kirk GR, White JS, McKie L, et al. Combined antioxidant therapy reduces pain and improves quality of life in chronic pancreatitis. *Journal of Gastrointestinal Surgery* 2006; **10**: 499–503.

44. Bhardwaj P, Garg PK, Maulik SK, Saraya A, Tandon RK, Acharya SK. A randomized controlled trial of antioxidant supplementation for pain relief in patients with chronic pancreatitis. *Gastroenterology* 2009; **136**: 149–159.

45. Monfared SS, Vahidi H, Abdolghaffari AH, Nikfar S, Abdollahi M. Antioxidant therapy in the management of acute, chronic and post-ERCP pancreatitis: a systematic review. *World Journal of Gastroenterology* 2009; **15**(36): 4481–4490.

46. Lordan JT, Phillips M, Chun JY, et al. A safe, effective, and cheap method of achieving pancreatic rest in patients with chronic pancreatitis with refractory symptoms and malnutrition. *Pancreas* 2009; **38**(6): 689–692.

47. Livingstone C, Davis J, Marvin V, Morton K. Vitamin A deficiency presenting as night blindness during pregnancy. *Annals of Clinical Biochemistry* 2003; **40**: 292–294.

48. Roddy MF, Greally P, Clancy G, Leen G, Feehan S, Elnazir B. Nightblindness in a teenager with cystic fibrosis. *Nutrition in Clinical Practice* 2011; **26**(6): 718–721.

49. Armstrong T, Strommer L, Ruiz-Jasbon F, et al. Pancreaticoduodenectomy for peri-ampullary neoplasia leads to specific micronutrient deficiencies. *Pancreatology* 2007; **7**(1): 37–44.

50. Mawer EB, Davies M. Vitamin D nutrition and bone disease in adults. *Reviews in Endocrine and Metabolic Disorders* 2001; **2**: 153–164.

51. Mawer EB, Davies M. Bone disorders associated with gastrointestinal and hepatobiliary disease. In: Feldman DG, Glorieux FH, Pike JW (eds) *Vitamin D*. San Diego: Academic Press, 1997, pp. 831–847.

52. Mann ST, Stracke H, Lange U, Klor HU, Teichmann J. Vitamin D3 in patients with various grades of chronic pancreatitis, according to morphological and functional criteria of the pancreas. *Digestive Diseases and Sciences* 2003; **48**(3): 533–538.

53. Duggan S, O'Sullivan M, Feehan S, Ridgway P, Conlon K. Nutrition treatment of deficiency and malnutrition in chronic pancreatitis: a review. *Nutrition in Clinical Practice* 2010; **25**(4): 362–370.

Chapter 3.8

Pancreatic cancer and nutrition

Tanya Klopper

The Royal Surrey County Hospital, Guildford, UK

Pancreatic cancer (PC) represents 2–3% of all cancers, yet it remains the fourth most common cause of death in the world, with a 5-year survival rate of 1–5% [1–4]. The presentation and onset of symptoms are non-specific so the majority of diagnoses are made once the disease is either locally or systemically advanced, thus eliminating curative disease management [5,6].

The incidence of PC has risen and plateaued over the last few decades and correlates with increasing age, peaking in 65–75 year olds. There is an uneven geographical distribution of PC with developed countries having a higher incidence than developing countries. This may be associated with differences in screening practice but also suggests that environmental factors may have a role in the development of the cancer [5,6].

Approximately 95% of tumours develop in the exocrine part of the pancreas. Ductal adenocarcinoma accounts for 80–90% of all pancreatic neoplasms, whilst neuroendocrine tumours and cystic neoplasms are less common [1,6]. Within the pancreas, approximately 75% of tumours are in the head or neck, 15–20% in the body and 5–10% in the tail [1].

As with most cancers, surgical resection is the only curative option. For a pancreatic tumour to be resectable, it must be confined to the pancreas but unfortunately this only comprises 20% of tumours at diagnosis. Successful resection, usually in conjunction with adjuvant treatment, can improve the 5-year survival rate to 10–25% [1,2,7]. For locally advanced tumours and metastatic disease, surgery is not an option so for these patients, chemotherapy and/or radiotherapy are employed. Although not curative, these options can improve symptoms and prolong survival. Median survival is currently 10–12 months [1]. Untreated metastatic and locally advanced disease has a median survival of 3–5 months and 6–10 months respectively [6].

3.8.1 Factors involved in causation

Smoking is the most significant and consistent modifiable risk factor of PC. An estimated 20–30% of cases can be directly attributed to cigarette smoking [8–11]. (The risk correlates with intensity and duration of smoking and smoking cessation does appear to reduce the risk [8,9].

Only 10% of cases result from genetic mutations [12]. Type 2 diabetes and long-standing chronic pancreatitis are associated with an increased risk of developing PC [4,5,10]. Patients with diabetes have a two-fold increased risk independent of alcohol, Body Mass Index (BMI) and smoking-status [13].

Modifiable risk factors associated with diet and lifestyle have attracted a lot of attention for several decades. Despite alcohol being implicated in the aetiology of several other cancers and chronic pancreatitis, the consensus to date is that alcohol is not associated with PC, although one study did

Advanced Nutrition and Dietetics in Gastroenterology, First Edition. Edited by Miranda Lomer.
© 2014 John Wiley & Sons, Ltd. Published 2014 by John Wiley & Sons, Ltd.

suggest that heavy alcohol intake may play a role [14–16].

Red meat and processed meat products have been reported to increase PC risk and preparation methods such as grilling, frying, curing and smoking have been implicated. This could suggest that polycyclic aromatic hydrocarbons, heterocyclic amines and nitrosamines produced during these cooking processes possibly play a role in the etiology of PC [17].

Studies have had varied but inconclusive results and some have attributed the risk to the fat content of the meat products. A study that specifically investigated the different types of fat and PC risk reported positive associations with total, saturated and monounsaturated fats, particularly from red meat and dairy sources, a likely mechanism being that fat promotes pancreatic carcinogenesis. There was, however, no association with fats of plant origins [18]. Other findings include no association between risk of PC and dairy products [17,19].

Several studies have reported either no association or an inverse association existing between fruit and vegetable intake and PC risk [20–22]. Possible mechanisms include antioxidant protection against free radical damage, immune-enhancing properties and inhibition of insulin-like growth factor (IGF) binding to IGF receptors [20].

Cancer-protective effects of flavonols in the prevention of PC were found to be beneficial, particularly for smokers [23]. The Netherlands Cohort Study found no association between the intake of carotenoids and vitamin supplements and PC risk [20].

Uncertainties have existed regarding an association between total sugar intake and PC risk. Previous evidence has been inconclusive, but in the NIH-AARP Diet and Health Study, no association was found between added sugars intake and PC risk [24].

Growing evidence implicates abnormal glucose metabolism and insulin resistance in the development of PC, with an increasing risk in the overweight sedentary population [25–28]. Very overweight people are 20% more likely to develop PC [10]. Further studies confirm that PC risk increases with obesity, with a significant association with central adiposity, especially in women [14,29,30]. Possible mechanisms have been linked to hormonal and inflammatory effects of adipose tissue, increased exposure to carcinogens secondary to increased dietary intake and lack of physical activity [31].

Little or no association has been found with physical activity and PC risk [14,29,30,32].

3.8.2 Dietary effects of disease and treatment

Weight loss is one of the presenting symptoms in PC. It impairs response to cancer treatment and is regarded as an important prognostic factor: the greater the weight loss, the shorter the survival [33,34]. Patients with PC lose 14.2% of their pre-illness weight, increasing to 24.5% prior to death [33].

Cancer cachexia (CC) is characterised by progressive weight loss with or without anorexia. Approximately 80% of patients with PC present with signs of CC at diagnosis and it is one of the main reasons for the decline in nutritional status [35,36].

Pancreatic exocrine insufficiency (PEI) arises from loss of pancreatic parenchyma or from obstruction of the pancreatic duct thus preventing enzymes from reaching the GI tract, causing malabsorption [12,37,38]. Pancreatic exocrine insufficiency presents in 68–92% of PC patients before surgery and in 80% after surgery. It is often overlooked as the main focus is treating the underlying disease [39].

Pancreatic exocrine insufficiency typically presents as excessive foul-smelling flatus, abdominal distension and discomfort, belching and steatorrhoea and ultimately is the other major contributor of the weight loss seen in patients with PC [37,38,40]. Approximately 65% of patients will experience fat malabsorption and 50% will experience protein malabsorption [41]. Fat absorption is further compromised by a reduction in circulating bile salts associated with obstructive jaundice [42]. Deficiencies in fat-soluble vitamins (A, D, E, K), magnesium, calcium and essential fatty and amino acids can also occur [39].

Other presenting symptoms of PC include intractable pain, jaundice, nausea, anorexia, taste changes, early satiety, gastric outlet obstruction and fatigue [35,41]. The development of complications such as glucose intolerance or overt diabetes and pancreatitis has also been reported [43,44]. Understandably these symptoms are distressing and can have an impact on the psychological well-being of patients, with 47–71% of those with PC reported as being depressed [37,41]. This is far greater than in other cancer patients and has a significant impact on morbidity [45]. The combination of these factors can further impact nutritional intake and status which may contribute to the decline in performance status and quality of life.

Standard care for patients with early-stage PC will involve surgical resection followed by adjuvant chemotherapy [43]. Surgery is precluded in those with more advanced disease; instead, these patients are treated with a range of chemotherapy regimes, radiotherapy and new emerging targeted and molecular therapies.

The standard surgical procedures performed will depend on the location and extent of the tumour. Partial pancreaticoduodenectomy with resection of the distal stomach, better known as Whipple's procedure, is performed for tumours of the head of the pancreas. More recently, preservation of the pylorus has become the preferred option for this operation. For tumours of the body and tail of the pancreas, a distal pancreatectomy is performed and for more extensive tumours, a total pancreatectomy is undertaken [7,46].

Gastric outlet obstruction is a late complication of advanced disease that presents in 10–20% of patients, of which 3% are able to undergo a palliative gastrojejunostomy procedure [41,46].

Overall, Gupta and Ihmaidat reported that quality of life after a Whipple's procedure can be excellent [42]. The extent of nutritional complications and their management postoperatively will depend on the procedure performed. The advantages of preserving the pylorus include fewer postgastrectomy complications, less reflux and greater improvement in postoperative nutritional status, weight gain and quality of life [7,46]. Total or partial resection of the pancreas is associated with a combination of exocrine and/or endocrine insufficiency and consequent symptoms of malabsorption and postoperative diabetes [7,47].

Chemotherapy and radiotherapy can have short- and long-term nutritional consequences. This is mainly due to the fact that these treatments cause damage to normal cells, particularly those that divide rapidly and as a result, the ability to ingest, digest and absorb nutrients becomes compromised [48]. The most common side-effects of chemotherapy that affect nutritional status include nausea, vomiting, taste and smell alterations, anorexia, food aversions, diarrhoea, mucositis and early satiety [48,49]. Radiotherapy can damage the GI mucosa, and in patients with PC presents as nausea which directly impacts nutritional intake [49].

3.8.3 Dietary management

Nutritional management of patients with PC can be complex given the myriad factors that can impact nutritional status and the aggressive nature of the disease.

The goals of nutrition support for cancer patients focus on maintaining or improving nutritional status, managing nutrition-related side-effects of treatment and disease as well as aiming to improve quality of life and prognosis [36,37,44].

It is important to set realistic goals depending on diagnosis and prognosis. Although the ideal is weight gain, having a goal of weight maintenance may be a more achievable prospect. Patients who stabilise their weight have more beneficial outcomes, longer survival and improved quality of life than those who continue to lose weight [50,51]. Given the rapid progression of PC and the simultaneous acceleration in weight loss secondary to CC, the goals of maintaining nutritional status eventually become less important and symptom control and palliative management become the priorities [36].

Nutrition assessment is prudent in patients with PC. To facilitate nutrition intervention, the assessment must aim to identify symptoms associated with CC and/or treatment in patients with metastatic and locally advanced disease. For those patients who have already undergone surgery, the type of procedure performed will influence nutritional management [44]. Both patient groups should be screened for symptoms of pancreatic insufficiency.

There are mixed opinions regarding the value of nutritional management in PC patients. These range from there being no positive effect on prognosis to there being an improved quality of life with achievement of an adequate energy intake [36]. Energy expenditure of patients with cancer tends to vary according to treatment and disease stage [50]. As a result, there appear to be variations in the recommendations for energy and protein requirements in this patient group. An energy intake in excess of 28 kcal/kg/day and protein intake in excess of 1.4 g/kg/day has been shown to achieve weight maintenance [50]. A further recommendation is to aim for an energy intake that is 1.2–1.5 times the resting energy expenditure, which can be interpreted as an energy intake of 30–35 kcal/kg/day. The recommended protein requirement is 1.0–1.5 g/kg/day, which is slightly higher than recommendations for the healthy population [36].

Healthy eating guidelines have their role in the prevention of cancer but not in the treatment of cancer-related undernutrition [36]. Similarly, adherence to strict diabetic diet guidelines and cholesterol-lowering diets needs to be modified to overcome the energy deficit between energy intake and requirements. To achieve this on a reduced intake secondary to anorexia, it is recommended that fat intake exceeds the recommended 30% of total energy for healthy individuals [36].

There are currently insufficient data regarding the need for additional vitamin and mineral supplementation in patients with PC. However, given the diminished intake and lack of variety in most patients' diet, a daily multivitamin and mineral supplement at levels of the dietary reference intake (DRI) is recommended [36,37]. For patients who have undergone surgery, there is a greater need for micronutrient supplementation as iron, selenium, vitamin E and vitamin D deficiencies have been reported. It is therefore recommended that a multivitamin and mineral supplement and a calcium and vitamin D supplement are routinely prescribed postoperatively [52].

If adequate energy intake cannot be achieved with diet alone then the use of oral nutritional supplements is recommended. There are a variety of options available, the choice largely being determined by patients' preferences and tolerance. A frequent concern with the use of nutritional supplements is that they may reduce spontaneous food intake. Several studies have, however, shown that compliance with the use of supplements does not have a negative impact on spontaneous food intake [34,50].

If oral strategies are exhausted, then enteral (EN) and parenteral nutrition (PN) support can be considered. Intervention with either of these methods has produced a variety of results.

Several studies suggest that these methods of nutrition support can benefit those patients undergoing pancreatic resections by increasing body weight and reducing anastomotic breakdown rates, wound complications and mortality [42]. PN has been shown to positively influence nutritional indices associated with undernutrition, but further studies either found no benefit or found that complications associated with PN outweighed the benefits [36,42,44]. However, Liu et al. found that EN is superior to PN in improving nutritional status, liver and kidney functions and reducing postoperative complications post pancreaticoduodenectomy [53]. There are limited data with regard to the use of EN and PN in inoperable and/or advanced PC patients but a couple of studies have reported that the use of PN in this patient group can improve their nutritional status and enhance quality of life [35,54].

With regard to novel interventions, eicosapentaenoic acid (EPA) has attracted the most interest for its anti-inflammatory, anticachetic, antitumour and immunomodulating effects. Although EPA, either as capsules or incorporated into oral nutritional supplements and EN, has demonstrated an improvement in performance status and appetite and attenuated weight loss, results are inconsistent [50,55].

Pancreatic enzyme replacement therapy (PERT) is indicated in patients losing weight and presenting with symptoms of malabsorption [47]. It is important to note that not all patients will present with steatorrhoea. Medications, such as pain killers, can cause constipation and mask the diarrhoea associated with malabsorption [56].

Pancreatic enzymes are available in a variety of formulations and dosages. The recommended starting dose is 40,000–50,000 U lipase before meals and 25,000 U lipase before snacks [37,38]. The doses of enzymes are altered and escalated depending on ongoing symptoms and variations in dietary intake. The current upper limit for PERT is 10,000 U/kg/day [57].

Patients are frequently advised to follow a low-fat diet in conjunction with PERT but this is not appropriate for the majority of patients with PC. Patients can continue with a high-fat diet in keeping with high-energy, high-protein diet advice.

Patients with persistent steatorrhoea despite high doses of enzymes could benefit from the addition of loperamide and/or reducing the fat content of the diet [47]. To improve the efficacy of enzymes, a proton pump inhibitor can be prescribed to inhibit gastric secretion [39]. If patients struggle to swallow the capsules, they can be opened and mixed in a small amount of acidic food such as apple sauce [57].

Nutrition counselling to help achieve an adequate energy intake plays a vital role during active treatment and supportive care. Nutrition counselling in conjunction with the implementation of a high-energy, high-protein diet, with or without the use of nutritional supplements, has been shown to increase intake and stabilise weight in a range of cancer patients receiving treatment [36,50]. More specifically, an improvement in weight and appetite has been observed in patients with locally advanced PC following nutrition assessment and counselling [58].

It is important not to forget that there is more to food than its nutritional content. The meaning of food and diet is very individual and can play a very vital part in ensuring that spiritual, psychological and physical needs can be met during active and supportive treatment.

References

1. Saif MW. Pancreatic neoplasm in 2011: an update. *Journal of the Pancreas* 2011; **12**(4): 316–321.
2. Tingstedt B, Weitkamper C, Anderson R. Early onset pancreatic cancer: a controlled trial. *Annals of Gastroenterology* 2011; **24**(3): 1–7.
3. Li J, Saif MW. Advancements in the management of pancreatic cancer. *Journal of the Pancreas* 2009; **10**(2): 109–117.
4. Mössner J (ed). *Clinical Pancreatology for Practising Gastroenterologists and Surgeons.* Oxford: Blackwell Publishing, 2007.
5. Luo J. *Epidemiological Studies of the Etiology of Pancreatic Cancer.* Stockholm, Sweden: Department of Medical Epidemiology and Biostatistics, Karolinska Institutet, 2008.
6. Haraharan D, Saied A, Kocher HM. Analysis of mortality rates for pancreatic cancer across the world. *Journal of the International Hepato Pancreato Biliary Association* 2008; **10**: 58–62.

7. Hackert T, Büchler MW, Werner J. Current state of surgical management of pancreatic cancer. *Cancers* 2011; **3**: 1253–1273.
8. Tranah G, Holly EA, Wang F, Bracci PM. Cigarette, cigar and pipe smoking, passive smoke exposure, and risk of pancreatic cancer: a population-based study in the San Francisco Bay Area. *BMC Cancer* 2011; **11**: 138.
9. Lynch SM, Vrieling A, Lubin JH, et al. Cigarette smoking and pancreatic cancer: a pooled analysis from the pancreatic cancer cohort consortium. *American Journal of Epidemiology* 2009; **170**: 403–413.
10. Gilbert K, Mishra G. Pancreatic cancer: epidemiology and pathology. *Practical Gastroenterology* 2006; **30**(4): 22–32.
11. Lowenfels AB, Maisonneuve P. Epidemiology and risk factors for pancreatic cancer: best practice and research. *Clinical Gastroenterology* 2006; **20**(2): 197–209.
12. Ghaneh P, Costello E, Neoptolemos JP. Recent advances in clinical practice: biology and management of pancreatic cancer. *Gut* 2007; **56**: 1134–1152.
13. Ben Q, Xu M, Ning X, et al. Diabetes mellitus and risk of pancreatic cancer: a meta-analysis of cohort studies. *European Journal of Cancer* 2011; **47**: 1928–1937.
14. Maisonneuve P, Lowenfels AB. Epidemiology of pancreatic cancer. *Digestive Diseases* 2010; **28**: 645–656.
15. Jiao L, Silverman DT, Schairer C, et al. Alcohol use and risk of pancreatic cancer: the NIH-AARP diet and health study. *American Journal of Epidemiology* 2009; **169**(9): 1043–1051.
16. Rohrmann S, Linseisen J, Vrieling A, et al. Ethanol intake and the risk of pancreatic cancer in the European prospective investigation into cancer and nutrition (EPIC). *Cancer Causes and Control* 2009; **20**: 785–794.
17. Nöthlings U, Wilkens LR, Murphy SP, Hankin JH, Henderson BE, Kolonel LN. Meat and fat intake as risk factors for pancreatic cancer: the multiethnic cohort study. *Journal of the National Cancer Institute* 2005; **97**(19): 1458–1465.
18. Thiébaut AC, Jiao L, Silverman DT, et al. Dietary fatty acids and pancreatic cancer in the NIH-AARP diet and health study. *Journal of the National Cancer Institute* 2009; **101**(14): 1001–1010.
19. Chan JM, Wang F, Holly EA. Sweets, sweetened beverages and risk of pancreatic cancer in a large population-based, case–control study. *Cancer Causes and Control* 2009; **20**: 835–846.
20. Heinen MM, Verhage BA, Goldbohm RA, van den Brandt PA. Intake of vegetables, fruits, carotenoids and vitamin C and E and pancreatic cancer risk in The Netherlands Cohort Study. *International Journal of Cancer* 2012; **130**: 147–158.
21. Polesel J, Talamini R, Negri E, et al. Dietary habits and risk of pancreatic cancer: an Italian case–control study. *Cancer Causes and Control* 2010; **21**: 493–500.
22. Chan JM, Wang F, Holly EA. Vegetable and fruit intake and pancreatic cancer in a population-based case–control study in the San Francisco Bay area. *Cancer Epidemiology Biomarkers and Prevention* 2005; **14**: 2093–2097.
23. Nöthlings U, Murphy SP, Wilkens LR, Henderson BE, Kolonel LN. Flavonols and pancreatic cancer risk: the multiethnic

cohort. *American Journal of Epidemiology* 2007; **166**(8): 924–931.

24. Tasevska N, Jiao L, Cross AJ, et al. Sugars in diet and risk of cancer in the NIH-AARP diet and health study. *International Journal of Cancer* 2012; **130**: 159–169.

25. Tsugane S, Inoue M. Insulin resistance and cancer: epidemiological evidence. *Cancer Science* 2010; **101**(5): 1073–1079.

26. Nöthlings U, Murphy SP, Wilkens LR, Henderson BE, Kolonel LN. Dietary glycemic load, added sugars, and carbohydrates as risk factors for pancreatic cancer: the multiethnic cohort study. *American Journal of Clinical Nutrition* 2007; **86**: 1495–1501.

27. Schernhammer ES, Hu FB, Giovannucci E, et al. Sugar-sweetened soft drink consumption and risk of pancreatic cancer in two prospective cohorts. *Cancer Epidemiology, Biomarkers and Prevention* 2005; **14**(9): 2098–2105.

28. Michaud DS, Liu S, Giovannucci E, Willett WC, Colditz GA, Fuchs CS. Dietary sugar, glycemic load, and pancreatic cancer risk in a prospective study. *Journal of the National Cancer Institute* 2002; **94**(17): 1293–1300.

29. Romaguera D, Vergnaud A, Peeters P, et al. Is concordance with World Cancer Research Fund/ American Institute for Cancer Research guidelines for cancer prevention related to subsequent risk of cancer? Results from the EPIC study. *American Journal of Clinical Nutrition* 2012; **96**(1): 150–163.

30. Stolzenberg-Solomon R, Adams K, Leitzmann M, et al. Adiposity, physical activity, and pancreatic cancer in the National Institutes of Health-AARP diet and health cohort. *American Journal of Epidemiology* 2008; **167**(5): 586–597.

31. Bracci PM. Obesity and pancreatic cancer: overview of epidemiologic evidence and biologic mechanisms. *Molecular Carcinogenesis* 2012; **51**: 53–63.

32. Zhang J, Dhakal IB, Gross MD, et al. Physical activity, diet, and pancreatic cancer: a population-based, case–control study in Minnesota. *Nutrition and Cancer* 2009; **61**(4): 457–465.

33. Tisdale MJ. Mechanisms of cancer cachexia. *Physiological Reviews* 2009; **89**: 381–410.

34. Bauer J, Capra S, Battistutta D, Davidson W, Ash S. Compliance with nutrition prescription improves outcomes in patients with unresectable pancreatic cancer. *Clinical Nutrition* 2005; **24**: 998–1004.

35. Pelzer U, Arnold D, Gövercin M, et al. Parenteral nutrition support for patients with pancreatic cancer. Results of a phase II study. *BMC Cancer* 2010; **10**: 86.

36. Ockenga J, Valentini I. Review article: anorexia and cachexia in gastrointestinal cancer. *Alimentary Pharmacology and Therapeutics* 2005; **22**: 583–594.

37. Damerla V, Gotlieb V, Larson H, Saif MW. Pancreatic enzyme supplementation in pancreatic cancer. *Journal of Supportive Oncology* 2008; **6**(8): 393–396.

38. Domínguez-Muñoz JE. Pancreatic enzyme replacement therapy for pancreatic exocrine insufficiency: when is it indicated, what is the goal and how to do it? *Advances in Medical Sciences* 2011; **56**(1): 1–5.

39. Sikkens EC, Cahen DL, van Eijck C, Kuipers EJ, Bruno MJ. The daily practice of pancreatic enzyme replacement therapy

after pancreatic surgery: a Northern European survey. *Journal of Gastrointestinal Surgery* 2012; **16**(8): 1487–1492.

40. Fazal S, Saif MW. Supportive and palliative care of pancreatic cancer. *Journal of the Pancreas* 2007; **8**(2): 240–253.

41. El-Kamar FG, Grossbard M, Kozuch PS. Metastatic pancreatic cancer: emerging strategies in chemotherapy and palliative care. *Oncologist* 2003; **8**: 18–34.

42. Gupta R, Ihmaidat H. Nutritional effects of oesophageal, gastric and pancreatic carcinoma. *European Journal of Surgical Oncology* 2003; **29**(8): 634–643.

43. Stathis A, Moore MJ. Advanced pancreatic carcinoma: current treatment and future challenges. *Nature Reviews Clinical Oncology* 2010; **7**: 163–172.

44. Andersson R, Dervenis C, Haraldsen P, Leveau P. Nutritional aspects in the management of pancreatic cancer. *Annals of Gastroenterology* 2000; **13**(3): 221–224.

45. Makrilia N, Indeck B, Syrigos K, Saif MW. Depression and pancreatic cancer: a poorly understood link. *Journal of the Pancreas* 2009; **10**(1): 69–76.

46. Pancreatric Section, British Society of Gastroenterology; Pancreatic Society of Great Britain and Ireland; Association of Upper Gastrointestinal Surgeons of Great Britain and Ireland; Royal College of Pathologists; Special Interest Group for Gastro-Intestinal Radiology. Guidelines for the management of patients with pancreatic cancer periampullary and ampullary carcinomas. *Gut* 2005; **54**(Suppl 5): 1–16.

47. Domínguez-Muñoz JE. Pancreatic enzyme replacement therapy: exocrine pancreatic insufficiency after gastrointestinal surgery. *Journal of the International Hepato Pancreato Biliary Association* 2009; **11**(Suppl. 3): 3–6.

48. Holmes S. A difficult clinical problem: diagnosis, impact and clinical management of cachexia in palliative care. *International Journal of Palliative Nursing* 2009; **15**(7): 320–326.

49. Van Cutsem E, Arends J. The causes and consequences of cancer-associated malnutrition. *European Journal of Oncology Nursing* 2005; **9**(Suppl 2): S51–S63.

50. Bauer J. Nutritional management and dietary guidelines for cancer cachexia. *European Oncological Disease* 2007; **2**: 12–14.

51. Isenring EA, Capra S, Bauer JD. Nutrition intervention is beneficial in oncology outpatients receiving radiotherapy to the gastrointestinal or head and neck area. *British Journal of Cancer* 2004; **91**(3): 447–452.

52. Armstrong T, Strommer L, Ruiz-Jasbon F, et al. Pancreaticoduodenectomy for peri-ampullary neoplasia leads to specific micronutrient deficiencies. *Pancreatology* 2007; **7**: 37–44.

53. Liu C, Du Z, Lou C, et al. Enteral nutrition is superior to total parenteral nutrition for pancreatic cancer patients who underwent pancreaticoduodenectomy. *Asia Pacific Journal of Clinical Nutrition* 2011; **20**(2): 154–160.

54. Richter E, Denecke A, Klapdor R, Klapdor S. Parenteral nutrition support for patients with pancreatic cancer: improvement of the nutritional condition and the therapeutic outcome. *Anticancer Research* 2012; **31**(5): 1998–1999.

55. Van Bokhorst-de van der Schueren MA. Nutritional support strategies for malnourished cancer patients. *European Journal of Oncology Nursing* 2005; **9**(Suppl 2): S74–S83.

56. Lindsey H. Pancreatic cancer: nutrition, an important element in care. *Oncology Times* 2006; **28**(15): 4–26.

57. Fieker A, Philpott J, Armand M. Enzyme replacement therapy for pancreatic insufficiency: present and future. *Clinical and Experimental Gastroenterology* 2011; **4**: 55–73.

58. Ferruci L, Bell D, Thornton J, et al. Nutritional status of patients with locally advanced pancreatic cancer. *Supportive Cancer Care* 2011; **19**(11): 1729–1734.

Chapter 3.9

Cystic fibrosis and nutrition

Alison Morton
Leeds Teaching Hospital NHS Trust, Leeds, UK

3.9.1 Prevalence

Cystic fibrosis (CF) is the most common, life-threatening, autosomal recessively inherited disease in the UK affecting Caucasians. In the UK, 1 in 25 people (2.3 million people) carry the CF gene and the incidence is approximately 1 in 2500 live births [1]. Ireland has the highest incidence of CF in the world (1 in 1461 live births) [2]. The incidence in non-Caucasians is much lower, and estimated to be 1 in 20,000 in ethnic African populations and 1 in 100,000 in Oriental populations [3].

3.9.2 Life expectancy

Life expectancy, though reduced, has increased dramatically over the last 30 years due to specialist centre care, better nutritional support, introduction of acid-resistant pancreatic enzyme replacement therapy (PERT) and aggressive treatment of respiratory infections. Median survival is currently 34.4 years in the UK [4] and has been predicted to be at least 50 years for children born in 2000 [1]. The UK CF population is over 9000 and more than half are over 16 years of age [4].

3.9.3 Factors involved in causation

Cystic fibrosis is caused by a genetic mutation on the long arm of chromosome 7. The defective gene results in abnormalities in the production and function of a 1480 amino acid protein called the cystic fibrosis transmembrane conductance regulator (CFTR). The protein encoded by the CFTR gene is a chloride channel in the apical membrane of exocrine epithelial cells. In addition to its function as a chloride channel, CFTR modifies the function and properties of other ion transporters including chloride, sodium and potassium channels and the chloride-bicarbonate exchanger [5].

The predominant site of CFTR expression is epithelial cells e.g. sweat glands, pancreas, liver, lungs, etc. though there are increasing numbers of reports describing CFTR expression in non-epithelial tissues [6]. The widespread presence of CFTR throughout the body explains why CF is a complex multisystem disorder, though the main organs affected are the GI tract and respiratory system.

More than 1800 different CFTR mutations have been identified (www.genet.sickkids.on.ca), many of which are rare. Some mutations may not result in clinical signs or symptoms. In the UK, over 85% of the CF population share the same genetic defect (p.Phe508del mutation) [4].

The different CFTR mutations are divided according to their effect on CFTR function into five major classes. Classes I, II and III tend to completely abolish CFTR expression and/or function. Mutations in classes IV and V produce variants of CFTR which have residual expression and/or CFTR channel function [7,8]. The presence of two mutations from class I to III (the more severe mutations) is associated with pancreatic insufficiency. A number of class IV and V mutations are associated with

Advanced Nutrition and Dietetics in Gastroenterology, First Edition. Edited by Miranda Lomer.
© 2014 John Wiley & Sons, Ltd. Published 2014 by John Wiley & Sons, Ltd.

a degree of preservation of both ductular and acinar function and pancreatic sufficiency [9].

The number of patients who will become pancreatic insufficient (PI) depends on the genotype distribution of the population but it is estimated that approximately 90% of people with CF in northern Europe will become PI. This means they have insufficient pancreatic function to achieve normal fat and nitrogen absorption and will require oral PERT. Clinical symptoms of pancreatic insufficiency do not usually occur until duodenal lipase concentrations fall below 5–10% of normal postmeal concentrations [10]. The pathological changes that occur in the pancreas arise in many *in utero*. Duct obstruction occurs due to thick viscous mucus as a result of abnormalities in CFTR and destruction of acinar cells. The pancreas becomes fatty and fibrosed. The exocrine function of secreting digestive enzymes and bicarbonate into the duodenum is impaired. Initially, the endocrine function of the pancreas is preserved, though CF-related diabetes is common later in life [11].

Deficiency of pancreatic enzymes is the major cause of intestinal maldigestion and malabsorption in CF [12]. Multiple factors contribute to intestinal malabsorption in CF (see Chapter 1.4).

3.9.4 Dietary effects of the disease

The main clinical consequence of exocrine pancreatic insufficiency in CF is fat maldigestion and malabsorption, resulting in steatorrhoea and loss of nitrogen in the stool. Carbohydrate malabsorption is minimal [13]. Steatorrhoea is characterised by frothy, foul-smelling, frequent, pale, oily stools that often float in the toilet and are difficult to flush away due to their high fat content. Patients may complain of abdominal pain, severe abdominal cramps and flatulence [14].

Other symptoms include faltering growth in children and weight loss or undernutrition in adults due to faecal energy losses. This is important in CF as nutritional status has important prognostic significance with a positive association being seen between body weight, height, Body Mass Index (BMI) and survival [15,16] and between nutritional status and lung function [17].

Biochemical evidence of fat-soluble vitamin deficiencies occurs early in infants diagnosed with CF by newborn screening [18]. Overt deficiency is reported in people with CF resulting in the classically recognised deficiency symptoms such as night blindness and xerophthalmia [19,20] in vitamin A deficiency, neurological symptoms [21] and haemolytic anaemia [22] in vitamin E deficiency, rickets and osteomalacia [23] in vitamin D deficiency and coagulopathies and severe life-threatening bleeding [24] in vitamin K deficiency. In addition, subclinical vitamin deficiencies may play a significant role in CF.

Essential fatty acid (EFA) deficiency has been reported in CF [25]. Patients have been reported to have low concentrations of the EFA linoleic acid (omega-6) and α-linolenic acid (omega-3). Deficiencies of the omega-3 long-chain polyunsaturated fatty acids are also common [26]. Dietary fat malabsorption contributes to low concentrations of these nutrients [27]. Clinical symptoms of EFA deficiency are rare but suboptimal concentrations may increase the susceptibility to respiratory infections [28].

Increased endogenous faecal losses of calcium [29] and zinc [30] have also been reported.

3.9.5 Dietary management

The involvement of a dietitian to oversee the dietary management of exocrine pancreatic insufficiency is recommended [14]. Pancreatic enzyme replacement therapy is needed to minimise the symptoms and nutritional consequences of malabsorption and to enable a high-fat, high-energy diet to be eaten. Dietary fat restriction is not recommended for people with exocrine pancreatic insufficiency [14] and is inappropriate in CF due to high energy requirements.

Pancreatic insufficient patients with CF require supplementation with the fat-soluble vitamins even when malabsorption is controlled by PERT. There remains some residual malabsorption in these patients. Current recommendations for fat-soluble vitamin supplementation in PI patients are based on historical data and vary between countries. The recommended starting doses per day are summarised in Table 3.9.1.

Table 3.9.1 Recommended starting doses of fat-soluble vitamins in pancreatic insufficient patients with cystic fibrosis

	<1 year	>1 year	<2 years	2–7 years	>7 years	Adults
Vitamin A [67,68]	1500 IU (455 µg)	4000–10,000 IU (1200–3000 µg)				4000–10,000 IU (1200–3000 µg)
Vitamin E [68]	10–50 mg	50–100 mg				100–200 mg
Vitamin D [69]	1000–2000 IU (25–50 µg)	1000–5000 IU (25–125 µg)				1000–5000 IU (25–125 µg)
Vitamin K [70]			300 µg/kg (rounded to nearest mg)	5 mg	10 mg	10 mg

Pancreatic enzyme replacement therapy

There is a strong association between pancreatic phenotype and genotype. Pancreatic enzyme replacement therapy should be started if a patient is known to have two CFTR mutations associated with pancreatic insufficiency [31]. Patients with obvious symptoms of malabsorption should commence PERT as soon as the diagnosis of CF is made [31] and then faecal pancreatic elastase (FPE) should be measured to confirm the diagnosis [31]. This can be done in the presence of exogenous PERT. In the absence of clinical symptoms, FPE should be measured to establish pancreatic status. Pancreatic enzyme replacement therapy should only be commenced if pancreatic insufficiency is diagnosed [12,31]. Faecal pancreatic elastase should be used to monitor the onset of pancreatic insufficiency in patients not previously diagnosed PI annually or if there are symptoms of fat malabsorption [32].

Enzyme preparations

Modern enzymes contain porcine pancreatic extract in microsphere and mini-microspheres with an acid-resistant enteric coat. In the USA, generic and prescribable proprietary PERT are available. Generic products should not be used in CF care [31]. There are several other enzyme preparations in phase I, phase II and phase III trials. Liprotamase is a novel, non-porcine PERT containing a highly purified biotechnologically derived crystalline formulation of lipase, protease and amylase [33]. Liprotamase has been shown to be well tolerated and associated with age-appropriate growth and weight gain or weight maintenance for up to 12 months in PI patients with CF [33]. There is also work under way investigating recombinant human bile salt-stimulated lipase (rBSSL) [34] as an alternative source of PERT.

The aims of PERT are to:

- enable a normal- to high-fat diet to be eaten and achieve optimal fat-soluble vitamin status
- control the signs and symptoms of malabsorption, particularly abdominal pain, abdominal cramps, distension and flatulence
- attain normal stool characteristics and output
- maintain and promote normal nutritional status and growth.

A review of enzyme replacement therapy for pancreatic insufficiency, present and future has been published [35].

Timing of pancreatic enzymes

The timing of enzyme administration can influence the efficacy of PERT. If taken before the meal or with fluids, the mini-microspheres may be emptied from the stomach before they have mixed with food

---

Box 3.9.1 Recommended doses of pancreatic enzyme replacement therapy

Fat-based dosing

Infants: 500–1000 units lipase/g fat
Children/adults 500–4000 units lipase/g fat

The lowest effective dose of enzyme should be used and should not usually exceed 10,000 units lipase/kg/day [39].

Weight-based dosing

Infants: 2000–5000 units lipase/120 mL feed to a maximum of 2500 units lipase/kg body weight/feed
<4 years: 1000–2500 units lipase/kg body weight/meal
>4 years: 500–2500 units lipase/kg body weight/meal

Source: [31,38].

Box 3.9.2 Guidelines for the use of pancreatic enzyme replacement therapy

1. Enzymes should be taken with all fat-containing meals, snacks and drinks; the most appropriate timing may vary but in adults enzymes should be taken with the meal.
2. If meals last longer than 30 minutes, enzymes should be taken during and towards the end of the meal.
3. The dose should be varied according to the fat content of food (see Box 3.9.1) but should not usually exceed 10,000 units lipase/kg/day.
4. Enzymes should not be taken with fat-free snacks and drinks, e.g. soft drinks, fruit, pastilles, boiled or jelly sweets,
5. Enzymes should be taken with all fat-containing enteral nutrition; they should not be added to the feed or administered via the feeding tube.
6. Enzyme capsules should be swallowed whole without being chewed from 3 to 4 years of age (to maintain their efficacy).
7. For infants and young children, the capsules should be opened and the mini-microspheres mixed with a little soft food or fruit purée and administered from a teaspoon. Mini-microsphere enzymes are also available in tubs which avoids the need to open capsules.
8. Mini-microspheres should not be mixed with or sprinkled over a meal.
9. The enzyme dose should be increased slowly (e.g. by 1–2 capsules) if the stools are fatty, loose, offensive or frequent. If this is done too quickly constipation/distal intestinal syndrome can occur.
10. Adequate hydration is important, especially with high-strength PERT.

[36,37]. If taken after the meal, food may leave the stomach before enzymes [37]. In adults, enzymes should be taken with the meal to ensure adequate mixing with chyme [14]. Patients with a poor response to PERT or high dosage requirements may benefit from changing the pattern of PERT administration [36].

Enzyme dosage

The relationship between dose of pancreatic enzymes required and the presence of maldigestion and malabsorption is not linear [14]. There are no studies in infants, children or adults with CF to determine the optimal dose of PERT or whether there is a dose–response association [31,38]. In the USA, dosage is calculated as units of lipase/kg body weight/meal [31,38]. PERT should be taken with all fat-containing food and drinks and the dose should be based on fat intake [39]. Recommendations for PERT dosing are summarised in Box 3.9.1.

Other factors also contribute to intestinal malabsorption in CF, including:

- pancreatic bicarbonate deficiency, causing reduced duodenal pH and inactivation of PERT and precipitation of bile salts [40]
- increased faecal loss of bile salts [41] and altered ratio of glycine:taurine conjugated bile salts
- altered small intestinal transit time and motility [42]
- pharmacological and dissolution characteristics of PERT.

These factors contribute to the large individual variation in enzyme dosage required but doses should not usually exceed 10,000 units lipase/kg body weight/day. If higher intakes are necessary, enzyme efficacy may be improved by reducing gastric acid with H_2 receptor antagonists or proton pump inhibitors [14]. General guidelines for the use of PERT are summarised in Box 3.9.2.

3.9.6 Fibrosing colonopathy

In the early 1990s fibrosing colonopathy (colonic strictures) was reported in a number of children taking high-strength enzymes (>20,000 unit lipase/capsule) [43]. This may be related to the amount of methacrylic acid co-polymer (MAC) coating present in some preparations [44]. As a result, the UK Committee on the Safety of Medicines [45] (CSM, 1995) advised that high-strength enzymes with MAC (Pancrease HL®, Janssen-Cilag, High Wycombe, UK; Nutrizym 22®, Merck Serono, Feltham, UK) should not be used in children with CF under the age of 15 years and total dose of lipase should not usually exceed 10,000 units/kg body weight/day. Other high-strength preparations which do not contain MAC (Creon 25000® and Creon 40000®, Abbott Healthcare Products Ltd, Southampton, UK) continue to be used for many adults and some children.

3.9.7 Assessing efficacy of pancreatic enzyme replacement therapy

The efficacy of PERT can be assessed by measurement of faecal fat and calculation of the coefficient of fat absorption or stool weight. Faecal fat microscopy and steatocrit may also be used. More usually, effectiveness of PERT is monitored by assessment of nutritional status or growth and stool nature and abdominal symptoms.

3.9.8 Distal intestinal obstruction syndrome and constipation

Constipation is common in CF but should not be confused with distal intestinal obstruction syndrome (DIOS) which is caused by the accumulation of intestinal contents and viscous mucus blocking the intestinal lumen. Incomplete or impending DIOS is common and patients present with a short history of abdominal pain and/or distension and a faecal mass in the ileocaecum. Complete DIOS is less common; in addition to the features of incomplete DIOS, the patient has a complete intestinal obstruction with vomiting of bilious material and/or fluid levels on abdominal X-ray in the small intestine [46].

Risk factors include a severe genotype associated with pancreatic insufficiency though it can occur in PS patients (PS patients have sufficient pancreatic function to achieve normal fat and nitrogen absorption), a history of meconium ileus at birth, history of DIOS, ongoing poorly controlled fat absorption or excessive enzyme dose, dehydration and CF-related diabetes (CFRD) [46].

Distal intestinal obstruction syndrome is initially managed medically. Dietetic management includes assessment of PERT and absorption, including knowledge of enzyme doses, titration with fat intake, timing and adherence. Advice about increasing fluid intake is also important. The role of increasing fibre intake is unclear [47] and this should be done with caution.

3.9.9 Other gastrointestinal considerations

The extensive expression of CFTR throughout the GI and hepatobiliary tract results in a number of co-morbidities in CF.

- *Gastro-oesophageal reflux disease* – gastro-oesophageal reflux is common in infants [48], children [49] and adults with CF [50]. It may compromise growth and weight [50], exacerbate respiratory symptoms and have a negative impact on lung function [51]. In the post-transplant patient it is a risk factor for bronchiolitis obliterans syndrome [52].
- *Pancreatitis* – pancreatitis may be a presenting feature in patients diagnosed later in life. Patients with specific CFTR genotypes with mild phenotypes are most at risk of developing pancreatitis [53]; patients have some pancreatic function and are at least partially PS [54].
- *Cystic fibrosis-associated liver disease* – cystic fibrosis-associated liver disease occurs in 27–35% of patients and 5–10% develop multilobular cirrhosis in the first decade of life. Portal hypertension often develops during the second decade. Liver failure usually occurs in adulthood [55].
- *Cholelithiasis* – cholelithiasis is relatively common and occurs in approximately 28% of patients [56].
- *Intestinal inflammation* – a high faecal calprotectin concentration suggestive of mucosal inflammation and observed inflammatory changes in the small intestine have been associated with persistent malabsorption in some patients with CF [57].
- *Small intestinal bacterial overgrowth* – small intestinal bacterial overgrowth has been reported in up to 56% of PI patients [58]. It may contribute to ongoing malabsorption though this improves when patients receive antibiotic therapy for respiratory exacerbations [59].
- *Rectal prolapse* – rectal prolapse was often seen at diagnosis associated with malabsorption [60]. With the introduction of newborn screening and earlier introduction of PERT, it may be less common.
- *Crohn's disease* – an increased incidence of Crohn's disease has been reported [61]. Symptoms of Crohn's disease may be confused with symptoms of uncontrolled malabsorption [62].
- *Gastrointestinal malignancies* – there is an increased risk of both GI and pancreatic malignancies [63,64] which occur at an earlier age [65]. Following lung transplantation, there is an increased risk of all malignancies [66]. Awareness is important as symptoms may be suggestive of malabsorption, e.g. altered stool output.

The management of these conditions is not significantly different from the general population and will be considered in other chapters.

Acknowledgement

The author would like to thank Sue Wolfe, Consultant Paediatric Dietitian, LGI.

References

1. Dodge JA, Lewis PA, Stanton M, Wilsher J. Cystic fibrosis mortality and survival in the UK: 1947–2003. *European Respiratory Journal* 2007; **29**: 522–526.
2. Devaney J, Glennon M, Farrell G, et al. Cystic fibrosis mutation frequencies in an Irish population. *Clinical Genetics* 2003; **63**: 121–125.
3. Corey M, McLaughlin FJ, Williams M, Levison H. A comparison of survival, growth and pulmonary function in patients with cystic fibrosis in Boston and Toronto. *Journal of Clinical Epidemiology* 1988; **41**: 583–591.
4. Cystic Fibrosis Trust. *UK CF* Registry Annual Data Report 2009. *Bromley: Cystic Fibrosis Trust*, 2009.
5. Nissim-Rafinia M, Linde L, Kerem B. The CFTR gene: structure, mutations and specific therapeutic approaches. In: Bush A, Alton EW, Davies J, Griesenbach U, Jaffe A (eds) *Cystic Fibrosis in the 21st Century*. Basel: Karger, 2006, pp. 2–10.
6. Trezise AE. Exquisite and multilevel regulation of CFTR expression. In: Bush A, Alton EW, Davies J, Griesenbach U, Jaffe A (eds) *Cystic Fibrosis in the 21st Century*. Basel: Karger, 2006, pp. 11–20.
7. Welsh MJ, Smith AE. Molecular mechanisms of CFTR chloride channel dysfunction in cystic fibrosis. *Cell* 1993; **73**: 1251–1254.
8. Wilschanski M, Zielenski J, Markiewicz D, et al. Correlation of sweat chloride concentration with classes of the cystic fibrosis transmembrane conductance regulator gene mutations. *Journal of Pediatrics* 1995; **127**: 705–710.
9. Ahmed N, Corey M, Forstner G, et al. Molecular consequences of cystic fibrosis transmembrane regulator (CFTR) gene mutations in the exocrine pancreas. *Gut* 2003; **52**: 1159–1164.

10. DiMagno EO, Go VL, Summerskill WH. Relations between pancreatic enzyme outputs and malabsorption in severe pancreatic insufficiency. *New England Journal of Medicine* 1973; **288**: 813–815.

11. Moran A, Dunitz J, Nathan B, Saeed A, Holme B, Thomas W. Cystic fibrosis-related diabetes: current trends in prevalence, incidence, and mortality. *Diabetes Care* 2009; **32**: 1626–1631.

12. Littlewood JM, Wolfe SP, Conway SP. Diagnosis and treatment of intestinal malabsorption in cystic fibrosis. *Pediatric Pulmonology* 2006; **41**: 35–49.

13. Hoffman RD, Isenberg JN, Powell GC. Carbohydrate malabsorption is normal in school age cystic fibrosis children. *Digestive Diseases and Sciences* 1987; **32**: 1071–1074.

14. Toouli J, Biankin AV, Oliver MR, et al. Management of pancreatic exocrine pancreatic insufficiency: Australasian Pancreatic Club recommendations. *Medical Journal of Australia* 2010; **193**: 461–467.

15. Beker LT, Russek-Cohen E, Fink RJ. Stature as a prognostic factor in cystic fibrosis survival. *Journal of the American Dietetic Association* 2001; **101**: 438–442.

16. Stern M, Wiedemann B, Wenzlaff P, on behalf of the German Cystic Fibrosis Quality Assessment Group. From registry to quality management: the German Cystic Fibrosis Quality Assessment project 1995–2006. *European Respiratory Journal* 2008; **31**: 29–35.

17. Pedreira CC, Robert RG, Dalton V, et al. Association of body composition and lung function in children with cystic fibrosis. *Pediatric Pulmonology* 2005; **39**: 276–280.

18. Sokol RJ, Reardon MC, Accurso FJ, et al. Fat-soluble-vitamin status during the first year of life in infants with cystic fibrosis identified by screening of newborns. *American Journal of Clinical Nutrition* 1989; **50**: 1064–1071.

19. Lindenmuth KA, del Monte M, Marino LR. Advanced xerophthalmia as a presenting sign in cystic fibrosis. *Annals of Ophthalmology* 1989; **21**: 189–191.

20. Joshi D, Dhawan A, Baker AJ, Heneghan MA. An atypical presentation of cystic fibrosis: a case report. *Journal of Medical Case Reports* 2008; **2**: 201–202.

21. Sitrin MD, Lieberman F, Jensen WE, Noronha A, Milburn C, Addington W. Vitamin E deficiency and neurologic disease in adults with cystic fibrosis. *Annals of Internal Medicine* 1987; **107**: 51–54.

22. Swann IL, Kendra JR. Anaemia, vitamin E deficiency and failure to thrive in an infant. *Clinical and Laboratory Haematology* 1998; **20**: 61–63.

23. Elkin SL, Vedi S, Bord S, Garrahan NJ, Hodson ME, Compston JE. Histomorphometric analysis of bone biopsies from the iliac crest of adults with cystic fibrosis. *American Journal of Respiratory and Critical Care Medicine* 2002; **166**: 1470–1474.

24. McPhail GL. Coagulation disorder as a presentation of cystic fibrosis. *Journal of Emergency Medicine* 2010; **38**: 320–322.

25. Aldámiz-Echevarria L, Prieto JA, Andrade F, et al. Persistence of essential fatty acid deficiency in cystic fibrosis despite nutritional therapy. *Pediatric Research* 2009; **66**: 585–589.

26. Strandvik B, Gronowitz E, Enlund F, Martinsson T, Wahlström J. Essential fatty acid deficiency in relation to genotype in patients with cystic fibrosis. *Journal of Pediatrics* 2001; **139**: 650–655.

27. Peretti N, Marcil V, Drouin E, Levy E. Mechanisms of lipid malabsorption in cystic fibrosis: the impact of essential fatty acid deficiency. *Nutrition and Metabolism (London)* 2005; **2**: 11.

28. Lloyd-Still JD. Essential fatty acid deficiency and nutritional supplementation in cystic fibrosis. *Journal of Pediatrics* 2002; **141**: 157–159.

29. Schulze KJ, O'Brien KO, Germain-Lee EL, Baer DJ, Leonard AL, Rosenstein BJ. Endogenous fecal losses of calcium compromise calcium balance in pancreatic-insufficient girls with cystic fibrosis. *Journal of Pediatrics* 2003; **143**: 765–771.

30. Krebs NF, Westcott JE, Arnold TD, et al. Abnormalities in zinc homeostasis in young infants with cystic fibrosis. *Pediatric Research* 2000; **48**: 256–261.

31. Borowitz D, Robinson KA, Rosenfeld M, et al. Cystic Fibrosis Foundation evidence-based guidelines for management of infants with cystic fibrosis. *Journal of Pediatrics* 2009; **155**: S73–S93.

32. Walkowiak J, Nousia-Arvanitakis S, Agguridaki C, et al. Longitudinal follow-up of exocrine pancreatic function in pancreatic sufficient cystic fibrosis patients using the fecal elastase-1 test. *Journal of Pediatric Gastroenterology and Nutrition* 2003; **36**: 474–478.

33. Borowitz D, Stevens C, Brettman LR, et al, for the Liprotamase 726 Study Group. International phase III trial of liprotamase efficacy and safety in pancreatic-insufficient cystic fibrosis patients. *Journal of Cystic Fibrosis* 2011; **10**: 443–452.

34. Strandvik B, Hansson L, Hernell O, et al. Recombinant human bile salt-stimulated lipase improves lipid uptake and reduces the pancreatic enzyme supplementation in patients with cystic fibrosis. *Pediatric Pulmonology* 2004; **27**(Suppl): 333.

35. Fieker A, Philpott J, Armand M. Enzyme replacement therapy for pancreatic insufficiency: present and future. *Clinical and Experimental Gastroenterology* 2011; **4**: 55–73.

36. Taylor CJ, Hillel PG, Ghosal S, et al. Gastric emptying and intestinal transit of pancreatic enzymes in cystic fibrosis. *Archives of Disease in Childhood* 1999; **80**: 149–152.

37. Domínguez-Muñoz JE, Iglesias-García J, Iglesias-Rey M, Figueiras A, Vilariño-Insua M. Effect of the administration schedule on the therapeutic efficacy of oral pancreatic enzyme supplements in patients with exocrine pancreatic insufficiency: a randomized, three-way crossover study. *Alimentary Pharmacology and Therapeutics* 2005; **21**: 993–1000.

38. Stallings VA, Stark LJ, Robinson KA, et al. Evidence-based practice recommendations for nutrition-related management of children and adults with cystic fibrosis and pancreatic insufficiency: results of a systematic review. *Journal of the American Dietetic Association* 2008; **108**: 832–839.

39. Anthony H, Collins CE, Davidson G, et al. Pancreatic enzyme replacement therapy in cystic fibrosis: Australian guidelines. Paediatric Gastroenterological Society and the Dietitians Association of Australia. *Journal of Paediatrics and Child Health* 1999; **35**: 125–129.

40. Robinson PJ, Smith AL, Sly PD. Duodenal pH in cystic fibrosis and its relationship to fat malabsorption. *Digestive Diseases and Sciences* 1990; **35**: 1299–1304.

41. Walters MP, Littlewood JM. Faecal bile acid and dietary residue excretion in cystic fibrosis: age group variation. *Journal of Pediatric Gastroenterology and Nutrition* 1998; **27**: 296–300.

42. Dalzell AM, Freestone NS, Billington D, Heaf DP. Small intestinal permeability and oro-caecal transit time in cystic fibrosis. *Archives of Disease in Childhood* 1990; **65**: 585–588.

43. Smyth RL, van Velzen D, Smyth AR, Lloyd DA, Heaf DP. Strictures of ascending colon in cystic fibrosis and high-strength pancreatic enzymes. *Lancet* 1994; **343**: 85–86.

44. Prescott P, Bakowski MT. Pathogenesis of fibrosing colonopathy: the role of methacrylic acid copolymer. *Pharmacoepidemiological Drug Safety* 1999; **8**: 377–384.

45. Committee on Safety of Medicines. *Report of the Pancreatic Enzyme Working Party.* London: Medicines Control Agency UK, 1995.

46. Columbo C, Ellemunter H, Houwen R, et al, on behalf of the ECFS. Guidelines for the diagnosis and management of distal intestinal obstruction syndrome in cystic fibrosis patients. *Journal of Cystic Fibrosis* 2011; **10**: S24–S28.

47. Van der Doef HP, Kokke FT, van der Ent CK, Houwen RH. Intestinal obstruction syndromes in cystic fibrosis: meconium ileus, distal intestinal obstruction syndrome and constipation. *Current Gastroenterology Reports* 2011; **13**: 265–270.

48. Heine RG, Button BM, Olinsky A, Phelan PD, Catto-Smith AG. Gastro-oesophageal reflux in infants under 6 months with cystic fibrosis. *Archives of Disease in Childhood* 1998; **78**: 44–48.

49. Blondeau K, Pauwels A, Dupont LJ, et al. Characteristics of gastroesophageal reflux and potential risk of gastric content aspiration in children with cystic fibrosis. *Journal of Pediatric Gastroenterology and Nutrition* 2010; **50**: 161–166.

50. Sabati AA, Kempainen RR, Milla CE, et al. Characteristics of gastroesophageal reflux in adults with cystic fibrosis. *Journal of Cystic Fibrosis* 2010; **9**: 365–370.

51. Blondeau K, Dupont LJ, Mertens V, et al. Gastro-oesophageal reflux and aspiration of gastric contents in adult patients with cystic fibrosis. *Gut* 2008; **57**: 1049–1055.

52. Blondeau K, Mertens V, Vanaudenaerde BA, Verleden GM, van Raemdonck DE, Sifrim D. Gastro-oesophageal reflux and gastric aspiration in lung transplant patients with or without chronic rejection. *European Respiratory Journal* 2008; **31**: 707–713.

53. Ooi CY, Dorfman R, Cipolli M, et al. Type of CFTR mutation determines risk of pancreatitis in patients with cystic fibrosis. *Gastroenterology* 2011; **140**: 153–161.

54. Augarten A, Ben Tov A, Madgar I, et al. The changing face of the exocrine pancreas in cystic fibrosis: the correlation between pancreatic status, pancreatitis and cystic fibrosis genotype. *European Journal of Gastroenterology and Hepatology* 2008; **20**: 164–168.

55. Debray D, Kelly D, Houwen R, Strandvik B, Colombo C. Best practice guidance for the diagnosis and management of cystic fibrosis-associated liver disease. *Journal of Cystic Fibrosis* 2011; **10**: S29–S36.

56. Cogliandolo A, Patania M, Currò G, Chillè G, Magazzù G, Navarra G. Postoperative outcomes and quality of life in patients with cystic fibrosis undergoing laparoscopic cholecystectomy: a retrospective study. *Surgical Laparoscopy, Endoscopy and Percutaneous Techniques* 2011; **21**: 179–183.

57. Werlin SL, Benuri-Silbiger I, Kerem E, et al. Evidence of intestinal inflammation in patients with cystic fibrosis. *Journal of Pediatric Gastroenterology and Nutrition* 2010; **51**: 304–308.

58. Fridge JL, Conrad C, Gerson L, Castillo RO, Cox K. Risk factors for small bowel bacterial overgrowth in cystic fibrosis. *Journal of Pediatric Gastroenterology and Nutrition* 2007; **44**: 212–218.

59. Lisowska A, Pogorzelski A, Oracz G, et al. Oral antibiotic therapy improves fat absorption in cystic fibrosis patients with small intestine bacterial overgrowth. *Journal of Cystic Fibrosis* 2011; **10**(6): 418–421.

60. Mascarenhas MR. Treatment of gastrointestinal problems in cystic fibrosis. *Current Treatment Options in Gastroenterology* 2003; **6**: 427–441.

61. Lloyd-Still JD. Crohn's disease and cystic fibrosis. *Digestive Diseases and Science* 1994; **39**: 880–885.

62. Cloney DL, Sutphen JL, Borowitz SM, Frierson H Jr. Crohn's disease complicating cystic fibrosis. *Southern Medical Journal* 1994; **87**: 81–83.

63. Schöni MH, Maisonneuve P, Schöni-Affolter F, Lowenfels AB. Cancer risk in patients with cystic fibrosis: the European data. CF/CSG Group. *Journal of the Royal Society of Medicine* 1996; **89**: 38–43.

64. Maisonneuve P, Marshall BC, Lowenfels AB. Risk of pancreatic cancer in patients with cystic fibrosis. *Gut* 2007; **56**: 1327–1328.

65. Neglia JP, FitzSimmons SC, Maisonneuve P, et al. The risk of cancer among patients with cystic fibrosis. Cystic Fibrosis and Cancer Study Group. *New England Journal of Medicine* 1995; **332**: 494–499.

66. Maisonneuve P, FitzSimmons SC, Neglia JP, Campbell PW 3rd, Lowenfels AB. Cancer risk in nontransplanted and transplanted cystic fibrosis patients: a 10-year study. *Journal of the National Cancer Institute* 2003; **95**: 381–387.

67. Sermet-Gaudelus I, Mayell SJ, Southern KW. Guidelines on the early management of infants diagnosed with cystic fibrosis following newborn screening. *Journal of Cystic Fibrosis* 2010; **9**: 323–329.

68. Cystic Fibrosis Trust Nutrition Working Group. *Nutritional Management of Cystic Fibrosis.* London: Cystic Fibrosis Trust, 2002.

69. Sermet-Gaudelus I, Bianchi ML, Garabedian M, et al. European cystic fibrosis bone mineralisation guidelines. *Journal of Cystic Fibrosis* 2011; **10**: S16–S23.

70. Cystic Fibrosis Trust. *Bone Mineralisation in Cystic Fibrosis.* Bromley, UK: Cystic Fibrosis Trust Bone Mineralisation Working Group, Cystic Fibrosis Trust, 2007.

Chapter 3.10

Lymphangiectasia and nutrition

Anu Paul and Ashish P. Desai

King's College Hospital NHS Foundation Trust, London, UK

Intestinal lymphangiectasia is a rare digestive disease that causes protein loss from the intestine. It is characterised by diffuse or localised dilation of the intestinal lymphatics and stasis of the lymph contained within. This eventually leads to rupture of the lymph vessels, resulting in loss of lymphatic fluid into the lumen of the intestine.

The term 'intestinal lymphangiectasia' was first coined in 1961 by Waldmann and associates. They described 18 cases of idiopathic hypercatabolic hypoproteinemia characterised by low serum albumin and gammaglobulins with high faecal albumin and intestinal biopsies showing dilated lymph vessels [1].

Lymphangiectasia of the intestine may be primary or secondary. Primary intestinal lymphangiectasia is a congenital malformation that usually presents before 3 years of age. Secondary intestinal lymphangiectasia usually occurs as a consequence of increased lymphatic pressure caused by obstruction to the lymphatics or increased venous pressure. It can be seen in syndromes such as Hennekam's syndrome [2], Turner's syndrome, aplasia cutis congenita, von Recklinghausen's syndrome, Klippel–Trenaunay syndrome [3] and Noonan syndrome [4].

3.10.1 Embryology

The progenitors of the lymphatic system are believed to arise from the endothelial cells of the embryonic venous structures [5]. These cells differentiate and express molecular markers that distinguish them from venous cells. These specific cells then attain autonomy from the venous system by budding and peripheral migration. This may be the reason why many lymphatic abnormalities are also associated with malformations of the vascular system.

At a molecular level, the initial signalling molecule responsible for lymphangiogenesis has not been identified. Vascular endothelial growth factor (VEGF) is a key molecular regulator of endothelial proliferation and migration. The VEGF family includes five isotypes: A, B, C, D and E. The isotypes VEGF-C and VEGF-D and their cognate receptor VEGFR-3 represent the first and best studied of the lymphatic specific signalling mechanisms [6].

3.10.2 Functions of the lymphatic system

The lymphatic system provides a system of mass transport parallel to blood circulation in the human body as well as playing a role in water and nutrient absorption. Large biomolecules suchw as enzymes and hormones are transported from their site of synthesis to the blood circulation by means of lymphatic transport. The lymphatic system also ensures absorption of excess fluid and protein from the interstitial space. Thus it is very important for the homeostasis of interstitial fluid [7].

From a nutritional perspective, the main role of the lymphatic system is in the transport of lipids,

Advanced Nutrition and Dietetics in Gastroenterology, First Edition. Edited by Miranda Lomer.
© 2014 John Wiley & Sons, Ltd. Published 2014 by John Wiley & Sons, Ltd.

mainly triglycerides and long-chain fatty acids from the intestine. Ingested lipids are emulsified by bile and digested by lipase to produce monoglycerides and fatty acids. Short- and medium-chain fatty acids can be absorbed directly into the blood circulation. The long-chain fatty acids and monoglycerides are absorbed into enterocytes where they undergo re-esterification to form triglycerides. The triglycerides are aggregated into chylomicrons and actively transported out of the enterocyte into the interstitial space, from where they are passively absorbed in the lacteals and transported in the lymph.

The lymphatic system also has a major role to play in immune trafficking. The lymph nodes strategically placed along the lymph vessels are able to sample the lymph and perform immunological surveillance of the interstitial space [7].

3.10.3 Aetiopathogenesis of intestinal lymphangiectasia

Intestinal lymphangiectasia occurs due to abnormal development of the lymphatic system with dilated lymphatics in the lamina propria of the small intestine [1]. The exact aetiology of intestinal lymphangiectasia is unknown. It is postulated that it may be due to altered expression of the regulator molecules that control lymphangiogenesis such as VEGFR-3. Other regulatory molecules such as Prospero homeobox1 (PROX1), forkhead box C2 (FOXC2) and sex determining region (SRY) Y box 18 (SOX18) may also have a role to play [8].

Nutritional causes

After a meal rich in long-chain fatty acids, lymphatic flow in the lacteals and intestinal lymphatics is known to increase. This promotes further engorgement and dilation of the affected lymphatics in primary intestinal lymphangiectasia, causing them to rupture. Loss of valuable lymph containing proteins and lymphocytes then ensues, leading to protein-losing enteropathy and malabsorption.

3.10.4 Clinical features

Many clinical features of intestinal lymphangiectasia can be attributed to protein-losing enteropathy and malabsorption. The classic triad of features includes lymphocytopenia, hypoalbuminaemia and hypogammaglobulinaemia. This manifests most usually as bilateral lower limb lymphoedema. In extreme cases, oedema may involve the face or scrotum. Effusions may develop in the pleural, pericardial or peritoneal spaces (Figure 3.10.1). This may be accompanied by abdominal pain, inability to gain weight and deficiency of fat-soluble vitamins. Due to impaired fat absorption, steatorrhoea is a presenting feature. Macular oedema can be seen in extreme cases, leading to blindness [9].

Occasionally patients demonstrate Stemmer's sign, i.e. skin fibrosis on the dorsum of the second toe due to chronic lymphoedema. In some cases, a cystic abdominal mass may be felt. Rare cases of intussusception or cutaneous warts have been reported [10].

Lymphocytopenia occurs with B-cell depletion reflected by diminished immunoglobulins IgG, IgA

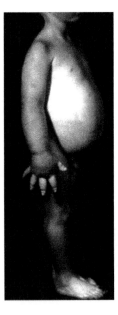

Figure 3.10.1 Patient profile before starting treatment. Reproduced with permission from Dr Babu Vadamalayan, King's College Hospital, London.

and IgM, as well as T-cell depletion, especially in the number of CD4+ T-cells as naïve CD45RA + lymphocytes [11].

Long-term complications of intestinal lymphangiectasia include lymphomas and lymphosarcoma, although this is relatively rare.

3.10.5 Diagnosis

Patients are usually investigated for cause of ascites and hypoalbuminaemia. Investigations will confirm lymphocytopenia, hypoalbuminaemia and hypogammaglobulinaemia. Twenty-four hour stool collection and analysis will show elevated alpha-1 antitrypsin clearance. Currently primary intestinal lymphangiectasia is diagnosed by endoscopy and biopsy. Video capsule endoscopy has been found to be useful in aiding diagnosis and also helps to assess the extent of the disease [12] (Figure 3.10.2).

Fry et al. (2008) reported on the usefulness of double balloon or 'push–pull' enteroscopy in the diagnosis of primary intestinal lymphangiectasia and other types of malabsorption [13]. Ultrasound and computed tomography (CT) scan may demonstrate the presence of lymphangioma with cystic fluid-filled spaces. Historically, lymphangiography,

abdominal lymphoscintigraphy with Tc-99m Sb colloid and 111In-transferrin scanning as well as abdominal scintigraphy with 99mTc-labelled human serum albumin have been used [14].

3.10.6 Nutritional effects

Intestinal lymphangiectasia leads to lymphoedema, fatigue, abdominal pain, weight loss, protein energy malnutrition, diarrhoea, steatorrhoea, and fat-soluble vitamin deficiencies [15]. Hypocalcaemia can develop, secondary to failure to absorb fat and fat-soluble vitamins.

3.10.7 Treatment

Dietary treatment

In the initial phase of treatment, patients may need supplementary parenteral nutrition (PN) to improve nutritional status and decrease symptoms. This should be started while investigations are being undertaken to diagnose intestinal lymphangiectasia and secondary causes of intestinal lymphagiectasia are ruled out. Once diagnosis is confirmed, reducing

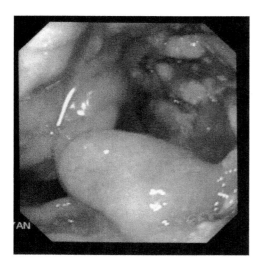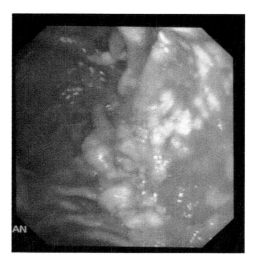

Figure 3.10.2 Enteroscopy picture showing lymphangiectasia-like changes. Reproduced with permission from Dr Babu Vadamalayan, King's College Hospital, London.

dietary fat and supplementing with medium-chain triglycerides (MCT) are the cornerstones of medical management.

The principle behind dietary manipulation is to prevent intestinal lymphatic dilation. Long-chain triglycerides (LCT), with chain length more than 14 carbon atoms, are absorbed into intestinal lacteals, leading to engorgement of intestinal lymphatics. However, MCT, i.e. triglycerides with chain length of 8–10 atoms, are absorbed directly into the portal venous circulation and hence overloading of lacteals is avoided but high-calorie food can still be given.

Diet should consist of 60% carbohydrate, 20% protein and 20% lipids. Total energy intake should be age appropriate. In children above 2 years, it should be continued at 75–80 kcal/kg/day. All lipids should be supplemented by MCT [9].

In a review of literature by Desai et al. (2009), 17 of 27 cases (63%) treated with an MCT diet had complete resolution, with mortality in one case [16]. In another case series by Tang et al. (2011), four patients treated with a low-LCT, high-protein diet supplemented with MCT had a good response [17].

Within 3–4 weeks of starting an MCT diet, patients usually show marked improvement in dependent oedema, diarrhoea and ascites. Nutritional status also improves as demonstrated by anthropometric data as well as biochemical and haematological profile [17,18]. This regimen is also shown to decrease mortality [16].

Most series have shown symptomatic improvement but chronic macronutrient deficiency persists for a long time. All cases need lifelong substitution of LCT to MCT as relapse in symptoms is seen on stopping the dietary treatment.

All patients need long-term vitamin supplements.

Enteral nutrition options include elemental and polymeric formulae which are a better alternative to PN [19]. Elemental diets contain food in easily assimilated forms and are composed of protein as free amino acids, carbohydrate as glucose or short-chain maltodextrins, a small amount of fat as short-chain triglycerides, vitamins and minerals.

Elemental diets are available in various commercially available preparations. They contain varying ratios of LCT to MCT fat. Emsogen is an elemental diet which can be used in children above 5 years and has an MCT:LCT ratio of 83:17. Elemental 028 Xtra can be given to children above 1 year and has a MCT:LCT ratio of 35:65.

Non-dietary treatment

Corticosteroid therapy has proved useful in selected cases. It appears to have benefit where there is an underlying inflammatory process such as lymphangiectasia that is sometimes associated with systemic lupus erythematosus [20]. Antiplasmin tranexamic acid [21] and octreotide [22] have also been reported to produce clinical, biochemical and histological improvement but the mechanism of action of these drugs is unclear.

In extreme cases with severe protein-losing enteropathy, albumin infusions have been administered. However, even this exogenous albumin is ultimately lost through the ruptured lymphatics and the relief provided is only temporary. Supportive treatment for the other physical manifestations of this disease must go hand in hand with drug and diet therapy. Lymphoedema of the limbs will require bandaging and skin care [15].

Surgical management is useful only when lymphangiectasia is localised and segmental in an area of the intestine; resection of that segment has been shown to provide a cure [23]. In resistant cases where dilated lymphatics are demonstrated, ligation of these with fibrin glue application has been attempted.

3.10.8 Conclusion

In summary, intestinal lymphangiectasia is a rare but serious chronic debilitating disease that is best managed by a high-protein, MCT dietary regimen. This regimen needs to be followed for the rest of the patient's life.

Acknowledgement

We would like to thank Dr Babu Vadamalayan for providing patient photographs.

References

1. Shimkin PM, Waldmann TA, Krugman RL. Intestinal lymphangiectasia. *American Journal of Roentgenology, Radium Therapy and Nuclear Medicine* 1970; **110**(4): 827–841.

2. Van Balkom ID, Alders M, Allanson J, et al. Lymphedema-lymphangiectasia-mental retardation (Hennekam) syndrome: a review. *American Journal of Medical Genetics* 2002; **112**(4): 412–421.

3. Thong MK, Thompson E, Keenan R, et al. A child with hemi-megalencephaly, hemihypertrophy, macrocephaly, cutaneous vascular malformation, psychomotor retardation and intestinal lymphangiectasia – a diagnostic dilemma. *Clinical Dysmorphology* 1999; **8**(4): 283–286.

4. Herzog DB, Logan R, Kooistra JB. The Noonan syndrome with intestinal lymphangiectasia. *Journal of Pediatrics* 1976; **88**(2): 270–272.

5. Ribatti D, Crivellato E. The embryonic origins of lymphatic vessels: an historical review. *British Journal of Haematology* 2010; **149**(5): 669–674.

6. Shibuya M, Claesson-Welsh L. Signal transduction by VEGF receptors in regulation of angiogenesis and lymphangiogenesis. *Experimental Cell Research* 2006; **312**: 549–560.

7. Szuba A, Rockson SG. Lymphedema: anatomy, physiology and pathogenesis. *Vascular Medicine* 1997; **2**(4): 321–326.

8. Hokari R, Kitagawa N, Watanabe C, et al. Changes in regulatory molecules for lymphangiogenesis in intestinal lymphangiectasia with enteric protein loss. *Journal of Gastroenterology and Hepatology* 2008; **23**(7 Pt 2): e88–e95.

9. Tift WL, Lloyd JK. Intestinal lymphangiectasia: long-term results with MCT diet. *Archives of Disease in Childhood* 1975; **50**: 269–276.

10. Rao R, Shashidhar H. Intestinal lymphangiectasia presenting as abdominal mass. *Gastrointestinal Endoscopy* 2007; **65**(3): 522–523.

11. Freeman HJ, Nimmo M. Intestinal lymphangiectasia in adults. *World Journal of Gastrointestinal Oncology* 2011; **3**(2): 19–23

12. Chamouard P, Nehme-Schuster H, Simler JM, Finck G, Baumann R, Pasquali JL. Videocapsule endoscopy is useful for the diagnosis of intestinal lymphangiectasia. *Digestive and Liver Disease* 2006; **38**(9): 699–703.

13. Fry LC, Bellutti M, Neumann H, Malfertheiner P, Monkemuller K. Utility of double-balloon enteroscopy for the evaluation of malabsorption. *Digestive Diseases* 2008; **26**(2): 134–139.

14. Burnand KG, McGuinness CL, Lagattolla NR, Browse NL, El-Aradi A, Nunan T. Value of isotope lymphography in the diagnosis of lymphoedema of the leg. *British Journal of Surgery* 2002; **89**(1): 74–78.

15. Vignes S, Bellanger J. Primary intestinal lymphangiectasia (Waldmann's disease). *Orphanet Journal of Rare Diseases* 2008; **3**: 5.

16. Desai AP, Guvenc BH, Carachi R. Evidence for medium chain triglycerides in the treatment of primary intestinal lymphangiectasia. *European Journal of Pediatric Surgery* 2009; **19**(4): 241–245.

17. Tang QY, Wen J, Wu J, Wang Y, Cai W. Clinical outcome of nutrition-oriented intervention for primary intestinal lymphangiectasia. *World Journal of Pediatrics* 2011; **7**(1): 79–82.

18. Koo NH, Lee HJ, Jung JW, Hwan Kim S, Lee KM, Hwang JS. Intestinal lymphangiectasia: a response to medium-chain triglyceride formula. *Acta Paediatrica* 2005; **94**: 982–983.

19. Aoyagi K, Iida M, Matsumoto T, Sakisaka S. Enteral nutrition as a primary therapy for intestinal lymphangiectasia: value of elemental diet and polymeric diet compared with total parenteral nutrition. *Digestive Diseases and Sciences* 2005; **50**(8): 1467–1470.

20. Fleisher TA, Strober W, Muchmore AV, Broder S, Krawitt EL, Waldmann TA. Corticosteroid-responsive intestinal lymphangiectasia secondary to an inflammatory process. *New England Journal of Medicine* 1979; **300**(11): 605–606.

21. Mine K, Matsubayashi S, Nakai Y, Nakagawa T. Intestinal lymphangiectasia markedly improved with antiplasmin therapy. *Gastroenterology* 1989; **96**(6): 1596–1599.

22. Kuroiwa G, Takayama T, Sato Y, et al. Primary intestinal lymphangiectasia successfully treated with octreotide. *Journal of Gastroenterology* 2001; **36**(2): 129–132.

23. Warshaw AL, Waldmann TA, Laster L. Protein-losing enteropathy and malabsorption in regional enteritis: cure by limited ileal resection. *Annals of Surgery* 1973; **178**(5): 578–580.

Chapter 3.11

Coeliac disease and nutrition

Imran Aziz and David S. Sanders
Royal Hallamshire Hospital, Sheffield, UK

Coeliac disease is a common condition affecting up to 1% of the adult population. Delays in diagnosis are common. The average time delay for patients with symptoms prior to the diagnosis being made is 13 years. For every adult case detected, it is estimated that there are eight cases not detected. Patients with coeliac disease have an associated morbidity and mortality. In addition, quality of life studies suggest that the majority of patients benefit from a gluten-free diet (GFD). Furthermore, the GFD reduces or alleviates the risk of associated complications. This chapter will discuss how our conceptual understanding of coeliac disease has evolved over the years and also the impact of a GFD.

3.11.1 Diet and modernisation

Although humankind may have existed in some progressive form for 2.5 million years, it is only in the last 10,000 years that we have been exposed to wheat. Wheat was originally cultivated in the Fertile Crescent (south western Asia) with a farming expansion that lasted from ~9000 BC to 4000 BC. Thus it could be considered that wheat and therefore gluten is a relatively novel introduction to the human diet [1]. Gluten is a high molecular weight heterogeneous compound which occurs in the endosperm of wheat but also in rye and barley, that can be fractionated to produce alpha, beta and gamma peptides.

Prior to 1939 and the outbreak of World War II, the rationing system had already been devised. This led to an imperative to try and increase agricultural production. Thus it was agreed in 1941 that there was a need to establish a Nutrition Society. A meeting of workers interested in nutritional problems was convened by Sir John Orr and held at the Royal Institution [2]. The main objective of the new society was to provide a common meeting place for workers in various fields of nutrition. The very roots of the society were geared towards necessarily increasing the production of wheat [2]. This goal was achieved and by the end of the 20th century, global wheat output had expanded five-fold.

3.11.2 Aetiopathogenesis and prevalence

Coeliac disease, a chronic inflammatory disorder of the small intestine, can be defined as a state of heightened immunological responsiveness to ingested gluten (from wheat, barley or rye) in genetically susceptible individuals [3]. Historically, coeliac disease was felt to be a rare condition with an estimated prevalence of 1 in 8000 [4]. In addition, most clinicians expected to recognise infant or childhood presentations with overt symptoms of malabsorption, in the form of diarrhoea and weight loss (or faltering growth). However, there has been a paradigm shift in our conceptual understanding of coeliac disease. With the advent of endoscopic small intestinal biopsies and new serological assays, the prevalence of this condition is now widely appreciated to be around 1% [5]. Adult presentations are now more

Advanced Nutrition and Dietetics in Gastroenterology, First Edition. Edited by Miranda Lomer.
© 2014 John Wiley & Sons, Ltd. Published 2014 by John Wiley & Sons, Ltd.

frequent than paediatric with a ratio of 9:1[6] with patients most commonly presenting between the ages of 40 and 60 years [7].

3.11.3 Clinical features

It is now recognised that patients do not always have to present with classic GI symptoms of malabsorption, with low Body Mass Index (BMI) accounting for only 5% of all cases diagnosed, with most having normal or overweight BMI [8]. Far more commonly, patients describe non-classic symptoms [9], including atypical GI symptoms consistent with irritable bowel syndrome (such as bloating, abdominal discomfort, gas or altered defaecation [10]), or present insidiously with iron deficiency anaemia [11], osteoporosis [12], ataxia or peripheral neuropathy [13]. Patients who present in this way may be initially overlooked because of the lack of GI symptoms. Finally, some individuals may have the potential to develop coeliac disease (Figure 3.11.1).

3.11.4 Diagnosing coeliac disease

The gold standard diagnosis of coeliac disease requires duodenal biopsies showing villous atrophy (flattened small intestine) [3,14]. There are a number of serological tests that have been reported to be accurate in identifying patients who should then be referred for a duodenal biopsy. Serological testing for coeliac disease has evolved over the years, initially starting with antigliadin antibodies (AGA) followed by endomysial (EMA) and tissue transglutaminase (tTG) antibodies. Due to their poor diagnostic accuracy, as evidenced by their lower sensitivity and specificity, AGA have largely been superseded by EMA and tTG for routine serological testing in coeliac disease. More recently, there has been interest in deamidated gliadin antibodies and point of care tests [15,16].

The human leucocyte antigens (HLA) DQ2 and/ or DQ8 are closely linked with coeliac disease, occurring in up to 98% of cases, but are also present in 25% of the normal population [17,18]. This suggests that other unidentifiable factors, in addition to the correct HLA typing, play a role in the development of coeliac disease. Recent genetics

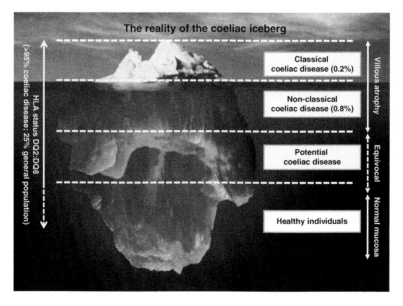

Figure 3.11.1 The coeliac iceberg, model showing the hidden forms of coeliac disease that lie below the waterline. HLA, human leucocyte antigen.

and genome-wide association studies have identified non-HLA loci that may be contributory to the development of coeliac disease [19].

Testing for the HLA DQ2/DQ8 susceptibility genes is not recommended in routine clinical practice as it is an expensive test, not readily available and thus should be reserved for equivocal cases where it can be used as a negatively predictive test [20]. If an individual does not have HLA DQ2 or 8 then it is very unlikely that they have coeliac disease.

There is now growing evidence to suggest that a group of patients may complain of gluten-related symptoms despite the absence of diagnostic markers for coeliac disease, such as negative coeliac serology and normal duodenal biopsies. This is a newly recognised clinical entity, termed non-coeliac gluten sensitivity (NCGS) [21,22]. Currently, we do not fully understand the natural history or indeed the pathophysiology of NCGS. Nevertheless, these individuals do clinically benefit from a GFD.

3.11.5 Dietary causes

There has been recent interest in the effects of feeding practices during infancy on the risk of coeliac disease developing in genetically susceptible individuals. Breast milk seems to have a protective effect although it is not clear whether this is merely delaying or preventing coeliac disease [23]. In order to shed further light on the relationship between breast-feeding, gluten introduction and the prevention of coeliac disease, research is currently under way in 10 European centres studying the influence of infant nutrition, and that of genetic, immunological and environmental factors, on the risk of developing coeliac disease [24]. Current ESPGHAN Committee on Nutrition recommendations and the findings of a recent systematic review suggest that gluten should be introduced into the infant's diet between months 4 to 7 and whilst the infant is being breastfed [25,26].

3.11.6 Dietary and non-dietary effects

Although some patients with coeliac disease may present with iron deficiency anaemia, the non-specific symptom of 'tiredness all the time' is very

common [27,28]; this is attributed to the presence of a low ferritin, folate or vitamin B12. These nutritional deficiencies may occur in up to 50% of coeliac patients at the time of presentation. Generally, these deficiencies correct on a GFD.

Recent population-based studies have described only a modestly increased risk of malignancy and mortality in patients with coeliac disease [29]. Importantly, this risk appears to fall as time from diagnosis increases (in those patients who adhere to a GFD) [30]. Although small intestinal lymphoma may be 50 times more common in an individual with coeliac disease, the annual incidence is low (0.5–1 per million), so the absolute risk for patients with coeliac disease is modest.

Coeliac disease is known to cause metabolic bone disease, with 32–80% of adult coeliac patients having bone mineral density (BMD) measurements more than one standard deviation below the population mean [31]. Corazza et al. demonstrated that those with non-classic disease do not have loss of BMD or metabolic bone derangement to the extent of those with classic disease [32]. Other small studies support this finding [33].

The importance of reduced BMD lies in its translation to fracture risk. In a large population-based cohort study comprising 4732 subjects with coeliac disease, West et al. found a very modest overall increased risk of fracture (hazard ratio 1.3) [34].

Infertility, subfertility and an increased risk of an adverse outcome during pregnancy (miscarriage, low birth weight and intrauterine growth retardation) have all been attributed to undiagnosed coeliac disease. However, these risks may be less than historically described.

Functional hyposplenism has been shown to occur in 30% of patients with coeliac disease. For this reason, *Haemophilus influenzae*, pneumococcal and annual influenza vaccination should be offered to patients with evidence of hyposplenism on blood film [6,35].

Patients with coeliac disease have a reduced quality of life (QOL) and increased likelihood of anxiety and depression in comparison to age- and sex-matched healthy controls, or even those with other organic diseases such as inflammatory bowel disease [36]. Furthermore, it has recently been established that there is an increased prevalence of irritable bowel syndrome and reflux disease in patients with coeliac disease, compared to controls, which accounts for further reductions in QOL and mental status. QOL may therefore be improved if patients with coeliac disease were also assessed and managed for reflux and irritable bowel syndrome [36].

In an obesogenic environment, it has been suggested that undetected coeliac disease may confer a benefit to individuals. It has recently been shown that the mean total cholesterol was 4.84 mmol/L in newly diagnosed adults with coeliac disease (n = 100). Men had 21% lower and women had 9% lower mean total cholesterol in comparison with the general population. There was no change in mean total cholesterol following a GFD. However, there was a small but statistically significant increase of 0.12 mmol/L in the mean HDL cholesterol. Thus there appears to be little benefit conferred to patients with undetected coeliac disease [37].

Recent work pertains to the role of detecting coeliac disease in adult patients with type 1 diabetes. The prevalence of coeliac disease amongst children and adults with type 1 diabetes in the UK has been shown to be 3.3–4.4% [38,39]. At diagnosis, adult type 1 diabetes patients with undetected coeliac disease have worse glycaemic control (8.2% versus 7.5%), lower total cholesterol (4.1 versus 4.9), lower HDL cholesterol (1.1 versus 1.6), and a higher prevalence of retinopathy (58.3% versus 25%), nephropathy (45% versus 5%) and peripheral neuropathy (42.9% versus 15%). After 1 year on a GFD, only the lipid profile improved overall, but in adherent individuals HbA1c and markers for nephropathy also improved. Furthermore, treament with a GFD in this study was safe and there was no difference in QOL after 1 year on a GFD [39]; this suggests that the institution of a GFD in patients with an already complex diabetic diet does not adversely affect QOL [39].

3.11.7 Dietary treatment

The cornerstone of treatment for coeliac disease is lifelong adherence to a strict GFD, which can be a major and initially overwhelming undertaking. For the majority of patients, a GFD leads to clinical and histological remission, normalisation of standardised mortality rate, a reduction in long-term health complications (i.e. osteoporosis) and in some studies, an improvement in psychological well-being

and QOL [40,41]. QOL improves after 1 year on a GFD and may be sustained in the long term. Patients with coeliac disease on a GFD have a reduced QOL compared to healthy controls but this is still an improvement from their undiagnosed state.

Patients with potential coeliac disease, as defined by positive coeliac serology but unremarkable duodenal biopsies (see Figure 3.11.1), may also benefit from a GFD. This is an important group in whom a GFD may be considered without having a clear diagnosis of coeliac disease. A single randomised study suggested an improvement in histology, biochemical parameters, serological titres and symptoms in patients who were EMA positive but had no evidence of villous atrophy on duodenal biopsy [42].

'Gluten' is a generic term encompassing the proteins derived from wheat, rye and barley. Wheat flour is a particularly ubiquitous constituent of a modern diet, being contained in bread, breakfast cereals, pasta, pizza, pastry, biscuits, cakes and sauces. A typical daily diet contains an estimated 10–20 g of gluten, and therefore a GFD necessitates a calculated avoidance of many foods. The Codex standard (used in the UK and Europe), and similarly the Food and Drug Administration in the United States, now suggest that foods containing less than 20 mg/kg of gluten or 20 ppm of gluten can be labelled as 'gluten free' and that foods containing between 21 and 100 ppm of gluten can be labelled as 'very low gluten'.

Oats

Whereas wheat, barley and rye have been shown to be toxic in coeliac individuals, the role of oats remains controversial and a source of continuing debate. It was initially assumed that oats were toxic due to the observation that patients had continued symptoms whilst ingesting oats. However, it became clear that many sources of oats are significantly contaminated with wheat flour during processing.

Recent studies have found pure oats to be safe [43,44] although there is some evidence suggesting that a small number of individuals with coeliac disease may be intolerant to pure oats [45]. Therefore, as a practical guide, it may be helpful to exclude oats in the first 6–12 months of a GFD before reintroduction. This pragmatic approach allows time for patients to settle on their GFD before the introduction of pure oats. If symptoms recur, the first issue to check is that the patient has only been using pure oats and that there is no risk of cross-contamination from wheat. If this is not the case then the most likely cause is intolerance of oats in that individual. In some cases patients may be keen to commence oats from the beginning of their diagnosis of coeliac disease. Given the small risk of developing symptoms, this alternative approach could also be taken but the patient should be encouraged to use gluten-free oats specifically.

Following a gluten-free diet

Following a GFD requires specific education, which should be provided by a dietitian with experience in coeliac disease. This should involve a careful explanation of the principles of a GFD and provision of written information on which foods contain gluten, how to obtain gluten-free products and how to access and use relevant sources of information. Emphasis should be on encouraging adherence to a GFD and the use of alternative products. Further support may be available via a national coeliac disease charity [6]. Most centres ensure that there are at least two separate appointments with a dietitian as it is likely that questions will arise in the first few months of a GFD. However, due to a lack of funding in countries such as the UK, or health insurance issues in the United States, access to specialist dietetic services may be compromised [46,47].

Patient adherence to a GFD has repeatedly been shown to be variable with rates ranging from 42% to 91% depending on how adherence is assessed [48]. Pragmatically, a more realistic level of adherence is probably in the range of 50–70% with 20–80% admitting to either occasional or prolonged lapses. One of the reasons for this is probably a perception that the diet is inconvenient, restrictive and unpalatable. Other factors which may reduce adherence are lack of available information on food content, social stigma (psychosocial issues) and the cost of gluten-free products. Social restrictions related to concerns about eating outside the patient's home may also result in poor adherence [49]. Finally, individuals who do not have many symptoms may believe that adherence is unnecessary. In particular, if lapses do not induce any adverse effects then further indiscretions may be more likely to occur. There is evidence to suggest that membership of an advocacy group (for example, Coeliac UK, Coeliac Australia or Associazione Italiana Celichia, amongst others) and regular follow-up in an outpatient setting improve adherence to a GFD [48,50–52].

It is important that coeliac patients are advised on alternative foods to include in their diet to maintain a healthy and varied intake and to increase the likelihood of adherence. Many ingredients are naturally safe such as fruit, eggs, cheese, vegetables, meat and fish. Bread, breakfast cereals and pasta are staple ingredients of a modern diet. In order to replace these foods and to maintain variety and palatability, manufacturers produce a range of gluten-free substitute products such as bread, pizza and pastry. These are based on gluten-free wheat or other cereals which are safe such as maize, sorghum, rice and oats. Gluten-free wheat is simply wheat starch, separated from wheat flour, and this can be used in cooking or baking as an alternative. Unfortunately, the baking and taste properties of wheat starch are inferior and additionally, small amounts of gluten can remain sufficient to cause intestinal injury in supersensitive patients. Certain individuals are sufficiently sensitive to require a wheat-free diet which entails avoiding any products that are manufactured with wheat.

Patients may require additional nutritional supplementation. In early treatment energy intake may be inadequate and may require augmentation. Calcium supplements may be used to ensure at least 1000–1500 mg daily intake. Non-starch polysaccharide intake is often inadequate and can be increased by rice bran or ispaghula husks [53,54].

3.11.8 Persistent symptoms on a gluten-free diet

In individuals who do not report symptom improvement after starting a GFD, an identifiable cause can be established in 90%. In some cases patients were discovered not to have coeliac disease, and this was the explanation for their failure to improve [55,56]. The validity of the diagnosis of coeliac disease should be checked, which in the majority of cases will involve reviewing the clinical history and the original antibody and biopsy results. It is important to assess the original biopsy, as failure to orientate the mucosa can result in a false diagnosis of villous atrophy. In addition, HLA typing may also be useful – if an individual does not have the HLA DQ2 or DQ8 pattern then it is highly unlikely that they have coeliac disease.

In the remaining group with coeliac disease, the most common cause of persisting symptoms is either deliberate or inadvertent failure to adhere to the GFD. These issues should be explored openly with either a dietitian or a physician who is experienced in coeliac disease. In these cases, small intestinal histology will continue to be abnormal although it may show some improvement if an overall reduction in gluten intake has occurred. Repeat duodenal biopsy can be avoided if patients admit to or are identified as having transgressed and then subsequently report clinical improvement. Coeliac serology may be unreliable as recovery and titres may fall with partial gluten withdrawal [57]. Biopsy remains the gold standard in ambiguous cases where gluten intake is suspected.

A few patients appear to be exquisitely sensitive to trace amounts of gluten in their diet. Products based on wheat starch generally do not cause problems in the majority of coeliac patients but anecdotally symptoms and histology improve after these products are withdrawn from the diet [58]. Dietitians

should also enquire about the possibility of ingestion of non-absorbable sugars, in the form of fermentable oligosaccharides, disaccharides, monosaccharides and polyols (FODMAPs), which can induce abdominal symptoms such as diarrhoea, bloating and abdominal discomfort [59–61]. Exclusion of FODMAPs may lead to clinical improvement.

In those patients who have ongoing symptoms despite having an established diagnosis of coeliac disease and strict adherence to a GFD, the next step would be to exclude other causes that can be associated with coeliac disease – these include microscopic colitis, pancreatic insufficiency, irritable bowel syndrome small intestinal bacterial overgrowth, thyroid dysfunction and secondary intolerances due to mucosal surface damage, such as lactose intolerance [62]. Referral to a gastroenterologist would be advisable to investigate for such conditions. Once these causes of ongoing symptoms have been ruled out, a diagnosis of refractory coeliac disease can be considered. Refractory coeliac disease is a rare but serious clinical entity with potential complications such as severe malabsorption and a high rate of progression to lymphoma [62,63]. Figure 3.11.2 provides an algorithmic approach to patients with persisting symptoms on a GFD.

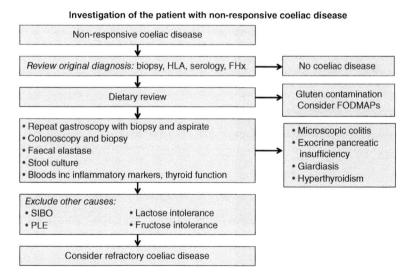

Investigation of the patient with non-responsive coeliac disease

Figure 3.11.2 Investigation of the patient with non-responsive coeliac disease Diagnostic algorithm for non-responsive coeliac disease. FHx, family history; FODMAPs, fermentable oligosaccharides, disaccharides, monosaccharides and polyols; HLA, human leucocyte antigen; SIBO, small intestinal bacterial overgrowth; PLE, protein-losing enteropathy; RCD.

3.11.9 Conclusion

In summary, coeliac disease is a common condition in which the vast majority of patients improve on a GFD. Specialist dietetic services play an essential role in educating patients with coeliac disease and promoting adherence.

References

1. Accomando S, Cataldo F. The global village of celiac disease. *Digestive and Liver Disease* 2004; **36**(7): 492–498.
2. Copping AM. The history of the nutrition society. *Proceedings of the Nutrition Society* 1978; **37**(2): 105–139.
3. AGA Institute. Medical Position Statement on the Diagnosis and Management of Celiac Disease. *Gastroenterology* 2006; **131**(6): 1977–1980.
4. Davidson LS, Fountain JR. Incidence of the sprue syndrome; with some observations on the natural history. *British Medical Journal* 1950; **1**(4663): 1157–1161.
5. West J, Logan RF, Hill PG, et al. Seroprevalence, correlates, and characteristics of undetected coeliac disease in England. *Gut* 2003; **52**(7): 960–965.
6. Coeliac UK. www.coeliac.org.uk.
7. Sanders DS, Hurlstone DP, Stokes RO, et al. Changing face of adult coeliac disease: experience of a single university hospital in South Yorkshire. *Postgraduate Medical Journal* 2002; **78**(915): 31–33.
8. Dickey W, McConnell JB. How many hospital visits does it take before celiac sprue is diagnosed? *Journal of Clinical Gastroenterology* 1996; **23**(1): 21–23.
9. Ludvigsson JF, Leffler DA, Bai JC, et al. The Oslo definitions for coeliac disease and related terms. *Gut* 2013; **62**(1): 43–52.
10. Zipser RD, Patel S, Yahya KZ, Baisch DW, Monarch E. Presentations of adult celiac disease in a nationwide patient support group. *Digestive Diseases and Sciences* 2003; **48**(4): 761–764.
11. Corazza GR, Valentini RA, Andreani ML, et al. Subclinical coeliac disease is a frequent cause of iron-deficiency anaemia. *Scandinavian Journal of Gastroenterology* 1995; **30**(2): 153–156.
12. Kemppainen T, Kröger H, Janatuinen E, et al. Osteoporosis in adult patients with celiac disease. *Bone* 1999; **24**(3): 249–255.
13. Hadjivassiliou M, Gibson A, Davies-Jones GA, Lobo AJ, Stephenson TJ, Milford-Ward A. Does cryptic gluten sensitivity play a part in neurological illness? *Lancet* 1996; **347**(8998): 369–371.
14. Working Group of European Society of Paediatric Gastroenterology and Nutrition. Revised criteria for diagnosis of coeliac disease. *Archives of Disease in Childhood* 1990; **65**(8): 909–111.
15. Lewis NR, Scott BB. Meta-analysis: deamidated gliadin peptide antibody and tissue transglutaminase antibody compared as screening tests for coeliac disease. *Alimentary Pharmacology and Therapeutics* 2010; **31**(1): 73–81.
16. Korponay-Szabó IR, Szabados K, Pusztai J, et al. Population screening for coeliac disease in primary care by district nurses using a rapid antibody test: diagnostic accuracy and feasibility study. *British Medical Journal* 2007; **335**(7632): 1244–1247.
17. Sollid LM, Markussen G, Ek J, Gjerde H, Vartdal F, Thorsby E. Evidence for a primary association of celiac disease to a particular HLA-DQ alpha/beta heterodimer. *Journal of Experimental Medicine* 1989; **169**(1): 345–350.
18. Murdock AM, Johnston SD. Diagnostic criteria for coeliac disease: time for change? *European Journal of Gastroenterology and Hepatology* 2005; **17**(1): 41–43.
19. Romanos J, van Diemen CC, Nolte IM, et al. Analysis of HLA and non-HLA alleles can identify individuals at high risk for celiac disease. *Gastroenterology* 2009; **137**(3): 834–840.
20. National Institute for Health and Clinical Excellence. *Coeliac Disease: Recognition and Assessment of Coeliac Disease.* London: National Institute for Health and Clinical Excellence, 2009. Available at: www.nice.org.uk/CG86.
21. Sapone A, Bai JC, Ciacci C, et al. Spectrum of gluten-related disorders: consensus on new nomenclature and classification. *BMC Medicine* 2012; **10**: 13.
22. Aziz I, Hadjivassiliou M, Sanders DS. Does gluten sensitivity in the absence of coeliac disease exist? *British Medical Journal* 2012; **345**: e7907.
23. Shamir R. Can feeding practices during infancy change the risk for celiac disease? *Israel Medical Association Journal* 2012; **14**(1): 50–52.
24. Hogen Esch CE, Rosén A, Auricchio R, et al. The PreventCD Study design: towards new strategies for the prevention of coeliac disease. *European Journal of Gastroenterology and Hepatology* 2010; **22**(12): 1424–1430.
25. Agostoni C, Braegger C, Decsi T, et al. Breast-feeding: a commentary by the ESPGHAN Committee on Nutrition. *Journal of Pediatric Gastroenterology and Nutrition* 2009; **49**(1): 112–125.
26. Szajewska H, Chmielewska A, Pieścik-Lech M, et al. Systematic review: early infant feeding and the prevention of coeliac disease. *Alimentary Pharmacology and Therapeutics* 2012; **36**(7): 607–618.
27. Sanders DS, Patel D, Stephenson TJ, et al. A primary care cross-sectional study of undiagnosed adult coeliac disease. *European Journal of Gastroenterology and Hepatology* 2003; **15**(4): 407–413.
28. Hin H, Bird G, Fisher P, Mahy N, Jewell D. Coeliac disease in primary care: case finding study. *British Medical Journal* 1999; **318**(7177): 164–167.
29. West J, Logan RF, Smith CJ, Hubbard RB, Card TR. Malignancy and mortality in people with coeliac disease: population based cohort study. *British Medical Journal* 2004; **329**(7468): 716–719.
30. Corrao G, Corazza GR, Bagnardi V, et al. Mortality in patients with coeliac disease and their relatives: a cohort study. *Lancet* 2001; **358**(9279): 356–361.
31. Meyer D, Stavropolous S, Diamond B, Shane E, Green PH. Osteoporosis in a north American adult population with celiac

disease. *American Journal of Gastroenterology* 2001; **96**(1): 112–119.

32. Corazza GR, di Sario A, Cecchetti L, et al. Influence of pattern of clinical presentation and of gluten-free diet on bone mass and metabolism in adult coeliac disease. *Bone* 1996; **18**(6): 525–530.

33. Cellier C, Flobert C, Cormier C, Roux C, Schmitz J. Severe osteopenia in symptom-free adults with a childhood diagnosis of coeliac disease. *Lancet* 2000; **355**(9206): 806.

34. West J, Logan RF, Card TR, Smith C, Hubbard R. Fracture risk in people with celiac disease: a population-based cohort study. *Gastroenterology* 2003; **125**(2): 429–436.

35. Corazza GR, Zoli G, di Sabatino A, Ciccocioppo R, Gasbarrini G. A reassessment of splenic hypofunction in celiac disease. *American Journal of Gastroenterology* 1999; **94**(2): 391–397.

36. Barratt SM, Leeds JS, Robinson K, et al. Reflux and irritable bowel syndrome are negative predictors of quality of life in coeliac disease and inflammatory bowel disease. *European Journal of Gastroenterology and Hepatology* 2011; **23**(2): 159–165.

37. Lewis NR, Sanders DS, Logan RF, Fleming KM, Hubbard RB, West J. Cholesterol profile in people with newly diagnosed coeliac disease: a comparison with the general population and changes following treatment. *British Journal of Nutrition* 2009; **102**(4): 509–513.

38. Goh C, Banerjee K. Prevalence of coeliac disease in children and adolescents with type 1 diabetes mellitus in a clinic based population. *Postgraduate Medical Journal* 2007; **83**(976): 132–136.

39. Leeds JS, Hopper AD, Hadjivassiliou M, Tesfaye S, Sanders DS. High prevalence of microvascular complications in adults with type 1 diabetes and newly diagnosed celiac disease. *Diabetes Care* 2011; **34**(10): 2158–2163.

40. Zarkadas M, Cranney A, Case S, et al. The impact of a gluten-free diet on adults with coeliac disease: results of a national survey. *Journal of Human Nutrition and Dietetics* 2006; **19**(1): 41–49.

41. Mustalahti K, Lohiniemi S, Collin P, Vuolteenaho N, Laippala P, Mäki M. Gluten-free diet and quality of life in patients with screen-detected celiac disease. *Effective Clinical Practice* 2002; **5**(3): 105–113.

42. Kurppa K, Collin P, Viljamaa M, et al. Diagnosing mild enteropathy celiac disease: a randomized, controlled clinical study. *Gastroenterology* 2009; **136**(3): 816–823.

43. Kemppainen T, Janatuinen E, Holm K, et al. No observed local immunological response at cell level after five years of oats in adult coeliac disease. *Scandinavian Journal of Gastroenterology* 2007; **42**(1): 54–59.

44. Sey MS, Parfitt J, Gregor J. Prospective study of clinical and histological safety of pure and uncontaminated Canadian oats in the management of celiac disease. *Journal of Parenteral and Enteral Nutrition* 2011; **35**(4): 459–464.

45. Lundin KE, Nilsen EM, Scott HG, et al. Oats induced villous atrophy in coeliac disease. *Gut* 2003; **52**(11): 1649–1652.

46. Nelson M, Mendoza N, McGough N. A survey of provision of dietetic services for coeliac disease in the UK. *Journal of Human Nutrition and Dietetics* 2007; **20**(5): 403–411.

47. Mahadev S, Simpson S, Lebwohl B, Lewis S, Green P, Tennyson C. Is dietitian use associated with celiac disease outcomes? *Nutrients* 2013; **5**(5): 1585–1594.

48. Hall NJ, Rubin G, Charnock A. Systematic review: adherence to a gluten-free diet in adult patients with coeliac disease. *Alimentary Pharmacology and Therapeutics* 2009; **30**(4): 315–330.

49. Karajeh MA, Hurlstone DP, Patel TM, Sanders DS. Chefs' knowledge of coeliac disease (compared to the public): a questionnaire survey from the United Kingdom. *Clinical Nutrition* 2005; **24**(2): 206–210.

50. Bardella MT, Molteni N, Prampolini L, et al. Need for follow up in coeliac disease. *Archives of Disease in Childhood* 1994; **70**(3): 211–213.

51. Nessman DG, Carnahan JE, Nugent CA. Increasing compliance. Patient-operated hypertension groups. *Archives of Internal Medicine* 1980; **140**(11): 1427–1430.

52. Haines ML, Anderson RP, Gibson PR. Systematic review: the evidence base for long-term management of coeliac disease. *Alimentary Pharmacology and Therapeutics* 2008; **28**(9): 1042–1066.

53. Thompson T, Dennis M, Higgins LA, Lee AR, Sharrett MK. Gluten-free diet survey: are Americans with coeliac disease consuming recommended amounts of fibre, iron, calcium and grain foods? *Journal of Human Nutrition and Dietetics* 2005; **18**(3): 163–169.

54. Kinsey L, Burden ST, Bannerman E. A dietary survey to determine if patients with coeliac disease are meeting current healthy eating guidelines and how their diet compares to that of the British general population. *European Journal of Clinical Nutrition* 2008; **62**(11): 1333–1342.

55. Fine KD, Meyer RL, Lee EL. The prevalence and causes of chronic diarrhea in patients with celiac sprue treated with a gluten-free diet. *Gastroenterology* 1997; **112**(6): 1830–1838.

56. Abdulkarim AS, Burgart LJ, See J, Murray JA. Etiology of nonresponsive celiac disease: results of a systematic approach. *American Journal of Gastroenterology* 2002; **97**(8): 2016–2021.

57. Dickey W, Hughes DF, McMillan SA. Disappearance of endomysial antibodies in treated celiac disease does not indicate histological recovery. *American Journal of Gastroenterology* 2000; **95**(3): 712–714.

58. Biagi F, Campanella J, Martucci S, et al. A milligram of gluten a day keeps the mucosal recovery away: a case report. *Nutrition Reviews* 2004; **62**(9): 360–363.

59. Shepherd SJ, Parker FC, Muir JG, Gibson PR. Dietary triggers of abdominal symptoms in patients with irritable bowel syndrome: randomized placebo-controlled evidence. *Clinical Gastroenterology and Hepatology* 2008; **6**(7): 765–771.

60. Biesiekierski JR, Rosella O, Rose R, et al. Quantification of fructans, galacto-oligosaccharides and other short-chain carbohydrates in processed grains and cereals. *Journal of Human Nutrition and Dietetics* 2011; **24**(2): 154–176.

61. Barrett JS, Gibson PR. Fermentable oligosaccharides, disaccharides, monosaccharides and polyols (FODMAPs) and nonallergic food intolerance: FODMAPs or food chemicals? *Therapeutic Advances in Gastroenterology* 2012; **5**(4): 261–268.

62. Evans KE, Sanders DS. Joint BAPEN and British Society of Gastroenterology Symposium on 'Coeliac disease: basics and controversies'. Coeliac disease: optimising the management of patients with persisting symptoms? *Proceedings of the Nutrition Society* 2009; **68**(3): 242–248.

63. Mooney PD, Evans KE, Singh S, Sanders DS. Treatment failure in coeliac disease: a practical guide to investigation and treatment of non-responsive and refractory coeliac disease. *Journal of Gastrointestinal and Liver Diseases* 2012; **21**(2): 197–203.

Chapter 3.12

Inflammatory bowel disease pathogenesis

Lynnette R. Ferguson[1,2] and Liljana Gentschew[3]
[1]University of Auckland, Auckland, New Zealand
[2]Nutrigenomics, Auckland, New Zealand
[3]University of Kiel, Kiel, Germany

Inflammatory bowel disease (IBD) is the generic name for a group of chronic, relapsing, debilitating disorders of the small or large intestine or both. They typically develop in the teenage years, resulting in adverse symptoms, including abdominal pain and cramping, diarrhoea, rectal bleeding and malabsorption. The two main forms of IBD are Crohn's disease and ulcerative colitis (UC), differing in location and severity. Once the disease begins, Crohn's disease and UC tend to fluctuate between periods of inactivity (remission) and activity (relapse). Crohn's disease can affect any part of the GI tract. However, it predominantly involves the terminal ileum and the beginning of the colon, whereas UC is limited to the rectum and colon. In Crohn's disease, all layers of the intestine are involved. In contrast, UC affects only the superficial layers of the colon. It is believed that the clinicopathological diversity in UC and Crohn's disease may be a reflection of distinct immune-genetic pathways [1,2].

The prevalence and incidence of IBD have been increasing worldwide over the last decades, particularly in industrialised countries [3]. Northern Europe, the UK, North America and New Zealand have shown the highest incidence and prevalence of Crohn's disease [4]. However, these values have also grown in other countries of the world, i.e. southern and central Europe, Asia, Africa and South America [5]. The suggestion is that urbanisation and industrialisation, especially environmental factors such as diet, may be responsible for the changes in incidence [6].

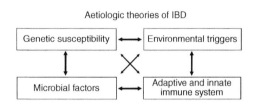

Figure 3.12.1 Interaction of various factors that are known to lead to chronic intestinal inflammation.

Both UC and Crohn's disease have a multifactorial aetiology, with a genetically determined susceptibility [2,7] that is only revealed in the presence of environmental factors such as adverse diet. While dietary factors may act directly on the GI tract, they also appear to act on the GI microbiota, leading to effects on processes that are essential for GI metabolism [8,9]. The nature of the genetics of IBD gives some clues as to disease aetiology, with 163 genes identified thus far [2]. Genetics relates strongly to disease characteristics. A general scheme summarising the interplay of such factors appears in Figure 3.12.1.

3.12.1 Underlying mechanisms of immune dysregulation in inflammatory bowel disease

Several studies implicate that the mucosal immune system and the intestinal epithelium are major factors in the pathogenesis of IBD [1,10,11]. In this

Advanced Nutrition and Dietetics in Gastroenterology, First Edition. Edited by Miranda Lomer.
© 2014 John Wiley & Sons, Ltd. Published 2014 by John Wiley & Sons, Ltd.

context, animal models and human studies including genome-wide association studies (GWAS) have provided important insights into the immune-pathogenesis of IBD [2]. Various components of the mucosal immune system appear to be involved, including luminal antigens, intestinal epithelial cells, cells of the innate and adaptive immune system, and their secreted mediators [12,13]. Thereby, the integrity of barrier organs is maintained by the interplay between epithelial cells, or mucus layer, and the innate and adaptive immune systems [12,14].

Crohn's disease is characterised by abnormal intestinal permeability, defects in mucus production and an inadequate, progressive production of proinflammatory cytokines such as tumour necrosis factor (TNF) alpha, interferon (IFN) gamma and interleukin (IL)-17 that induce intestinal inflammation [12]. Aberrant secretion of several cytokines by epithelial cells may initiate and perpetuate intestinal inflammation. The primary mediators of inflammation in Crohn's disease are the Th1 cytokines IL-12, IFN-gamma and TNF [15,16]. Concerning this, lymphocytes, cytokines and adhesion molecules are dysregulated, resulting in a primary failure of regulatory lymphocytes and cytokines, such as IL-10 and transforming growth factor (TGF) beta. Various other factors have been implicated in the pathogenesis of Crohn's disease, but their mechanism of action is often unknown [15,17,18].

3.12.2 Genetic factors in the development of inflammatory bowel disease

Epidemiological and family studies have provided convincing evidence that genetic factors play an important role in IBD [4,7,19,20]. Compared to UC, Crohn's disease tends to be more common among relatives of patients with Crohn's disease, and family and twin studies support a stronger genetic influence in Crohn's disease than in UC [21–23]. An increasing number of studies demonstrate that Crohn's disease appears more often in first-degree relatives who are not geographically living together, or at the same time [24]. Twin studies have shown that monozygotic twins have a much

higher rate of disease concordance than dizygotic twins [25]. Several family and twin studies indicate that different genetic abnormalities can be broadly characterised as causing defects in mucosal barrier function, immunoregulation or bacterial clearance. Genes that are linked to innate immunity (e.g. NOD2), autophagy (ATG16L1, IRGM, ATG5), defective barrier (including ECM1, CDH1, LAMB1, HNF4A and GNA12), IL-10 signalling (e.g. STAT3, IL10RB, IL22 and IL26) and adaptive immunity (e.g. IL23, IL23R, IL17) have been discovered as key loci in Crohn's disease [2,26].

Genetic and genomics research are rapidly growing areas, and recent studies have lead to advances in understanding of the molecular mechanisms of Crohn's disease. Genome-wide association studies have furthered our understanding of the genetic architecture of IBD by discovering genes and loci that confer susceptibility to Crohn's disease. Susceptibility loci that are associated with Crohn's disease attaining genome-wide significance $(P < 5 \times 10^{-8})$ and statistical power of GWAS are supported by a large sample size. To this point, 163 IBD susceptibility loci have been discovered [2].

There is considerable similarity between IBD and risk factors for other autoimmune diseases. The primary genes are involved in innate and adaptive immunity. Many IBD loci are also implicated in other immune-mediated disorders, most notably with ankylosing spondylitis and psoriasis. Also, there is considerable overlap between susceptibility loci for IBD and mycobacterial infection. The relationships among IBD and related disorders are illustrated in Figure 3.12.2.

3.12.3 Dietary risk factors in inflammatory bowel disease

Diet is a major factor in both the aetiology and progression of the disease [1]. There are a limited number of high-quality studies that have unequivocally associated dietary intake with subsequent development of the disease. These take the form of excessive amounts of certain nutrients, deficiencies in others or excess energy intake with subsequent development of obesity. The literature is also sometimes confused between current diet and pre-illness

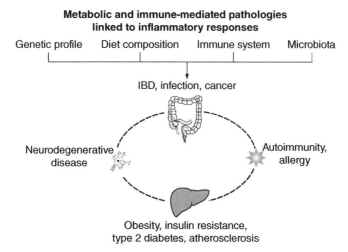

**Metabolic and immune-mediated pathologies
linked to inflammatory responses**

Genetic profile   Diet composition   Immune system   Microbiota

IBD, infection, cancer

Neurodegenerative
disease

Autoimmunity,
allergy

Obesity, insulin resistance,
type 2 diabetes, atherosclerosis

Figure 3.12.2   The link of inflammatory signalling response in various tissues to the development of obesity-related alterations, neurodegenerative disease and autoimmunity that are all influenced by host genetics, diet composition, immune system and microbiota. Modified from Renz et al. [78].

diet of patients with Crohn's disease. For example, Medline and the Cochrane Library were searched for clinical trials and meta-analyses in the scope of diet and nutrition in IBD [27]. These authors identified many studies in small cohorts of patients claiming that intake of Western-type diet constituents, including high saturated fat, refined sugar and low intake of fruits, vegetables and non-starch polysaccharides (NSP), affects the expression of IBD. Unfortunately, however, such studies are often compromised by insufficient data or methodological limitations, and do not provide unequivocal evidence to incriminate any particular dietary factor.

An example of a well-designed study is provided by Sakamoto and co-workers [28] in their Japanese populations. Cases were patients with IBD aged 15–34 years (111 UC and 128 Crohn's disease) within 3 years after diagnosis in 13 hospitals. One control subject was recruited for each case, matched for sex, age and hospital. A semi-quantitative food frequency questionnaire (FFQ) was used to estimate pre-illness intakes of food groups and nutrients. A higher consumption of sweets was positively associated with UC risk and, more generally, the consumption of sugars, sweeteners and sweets was positively associated with Crohn's disease risk. The intakes of total fats, monounsaturated fatty acids

and polyunsaturated fatty acids (whether n-3 or n-6 PUFA) were positively associated with Crohn's disease risk. With respect to micronutrients, the intake of vitamin C was negatively related to UC risk, while the intake of vitamin E was positively associated with Crohn's disease risk. Although this study suffered from the shortcomings of recall bias, the findings reinforced the importance of dietary factors for IBD prevention.

Carbohydrates

Dietary carbohydrates can be divided into three main groups: sugars, in the form of monosaccharides and disaccharides, oligosaccharides such as maltodextrin, and polysaccharides including starches and NSP. The majority of research on the role of carbohydrates in IBD has focused on sugars and NSP.

A case–control study considered the intake of confectionery, preserves, biscuits and cakes 1–3 years prior to the onset of disease. The sample population was a group of 63 German patients with Crohn's disease, using a validated postal questionnaire [29]. Intakes were significantly higher in the patients compared with those of 63 matched controls who recorded their current diet. Other workers

[30–33] also studied pre-illness diet to show that patients with IBD consumed more sugar than age- and sex-matched population groups. Geerling et al. [34] studied pre-illness diet and found a significantly higher carbohydrate intake in patients with Crohn's disease compared with controls and a tendency toward higher sugar intake. Sakamoto et al. [28] in Japan used a semi-quantitative FFQ to compare pre-illness diet in 108 patients with Crohn's disease and 126 patients with UC with the diets of 211 controls. Increasing consumption of sugars, sweeteners and sweets was positively associated with increased risk of Crohn's disease. Higher consumption of sweets was also positively associated with UC risk. In contrast to the other studies mentioned, this study adjusted for total energy intake. More generally, it seems that high intakes of mono- and disaccharides consistently increase the risk of developing either form of IBD.

High vegetable intake and increased fruit, possibly through increased NSP intake, appear to reduce the risk of both forms of the disease. Several case–control studies have more specifically investigated an association between NSP intake and IBD risk. Persson et al. [35] found that the relative risk of Crohn's disease decreased with a high intake of NSP but this was defined as >15 g/day, a relatively low intake. In contrast, Thornton et al. [30,31] and Sakamoto et al. [28] found no difference between the NSP intake of patients with IBD and controls.

Fats and oils

The bulk (c. 95%) of edible fats and oils consist of triglycerides, whose structure is described as three fatty acids on a glycerol backbone. The predominant fatty acid will determine whether this is classified as a saturated, monounsaturated or polyunsaturated fat. The ratios of saturated and unsaturated fatty acids in the structure also determine physical characteristics, including melting point and stability. Technically, if a triglyceride is solid at room temperature, it is termed a fat, while if it is liquid at this temperature, it is termed an oil.

The most important natural sources of dietary fat are meats and dairy products. However, a major source of these in the current diet is provided by oils derived from vegetable sources, various spreads and associated products, including baked goods and confectionery products. Historically, the vegetable oil industry has relied heavily on hydrogenation in order to produce the types of stable fats used for frying, baking and table spreads, including margarines. In parallel with this, major human dietary sources have moved away from predominantly animal sources such as butter, ghee, tallow and lard.

The introduction of margarine in Europe coincided with the first reports of Crohn's disease, and a causal relationship was proposed. The study by Sakamoto et al. found a significantly positive association between consumption of margarine and development of UC [28]. Sonnenberg linked data on margarine consumption obtained in five countries from 1962 to 1982 with mortality data for Crohn's disease over the same period, but found no statistically significant association between them [36]. As mortality associated with Crohn's disease is low and data on the incidence of the disease were not reported, the results should be viewed with caution.

A case–control study design was used to study pre-illness changes in Italian diet as a risk factor for IBD [37]. The study considered 83 new cases of IBD (41 UC, 42 Crohn's disease) in comparison with 160 healthy controls. A validated questionnaire was used to record portions per week of 34 foods and beverages, before onset of symptoms was recorded. The study also recorded duration of symptoms before IBD diagnosis, presence of specific symptoms and their impact on subjective changes in usual dietary habits. In patients with IBD who did not change dietary habits, moderate and high consumption of margarine was associated with increased risk of UC, while high consumption of red meat and cheese was associated with increased risk of Crohn's disease. The authors concluded that more than one-third of patients with IBD changed their dietary habits before diagnosis. However, high intakes of margarine, red meat and cheese increased the risk of both forms of IBD in this population group. These are good sources of both saturated and trans fats.

The association between the incidence of Crohn's disease and dietary changes in Japan between 1966 and 1985 was examined by Shoda et al. [38]. An increased incidence of Crohn's disease was strongly correlated with increased intake of total fat, animal fat and n-6 polyunsaturated fatty acids, and a relatively decreased intake of n-3 fatty acids. There is evidence that n-3 polyunsaturated fatty acids (PUFAs), particularly eicosapentaenoic acid (EPA) and docosahexaenoic acid (DHA), antagonise the production of inflammatory eicosanoid mediators from arachidonic acid, suppress production of some inflammatory cytokines and downregulate the expression of a number of genes involved in inflammation [39,40]

Dietary linoleic acid is an n-6 polyunsaturated fatty acid, which is metabolised to arachidonic acid, a component of colonocyte membranes. Metabolites of arachidonic acid have proinflammatory properties and are increased in the mucosa of patients with UC. In 2009, the IBD in EPIC study investigators considered the intake of linoleic acid as a factor in the aetiology of UC [41]. They utilised a nested case–control study within the EPIC European prospective cohort study. The data showed that a high dietary intake of linoleic acid, as assessed from food frequency questionnaires, significantly increased the risk of developing UC.

Asakura and co-workers reviewed the relationship of the daily consumption of dietary animal meat and fats, dairy products, sugar and other factors that may be linked to the occurrence of Crohn's disease and UC, from the literature and Japanese epidemiological data [42]. They also considered intestinal microbes and other factors contributing to the occurrence of IBD from epidemiological data and case–control studies of IBD in the literature that appeared on Medline, and assessed the reports of intestinal microbes involved in the occurrence of IBD. They found several papers describing the positive association of animal meat and sweets and sugar with the occurrence of Crohn's disease and UC. An analysis of Japanese epidemiological data suggested that the registered number of patients with Crohn's disease or UC started to increase more than 20 years after an increased daily consumption of dietary animal meat and fats, and milk and dairy products, and after a decreased consumption of rice.

Protein

Major sources of dietary protein are meat, cheese, milk, fish, nuts and eggs. Unfortunately, most of these are also good sources of fats, especially saturated fats, making it difficult to pull apart the influence of fats from that of proteins in most of the reported studies. Milk, cheese, eggs and meats, together with cruciferous vegetables and sulphite-preserved foods, provide GI microbiota with sulphate and sulphite. These are fermented to produce hydrogen sulphide, which inhibits butyrate oxidation and has been associated with mucosal hyperproliferation in UC [43]. As described above, an analysis of Japanese epidemiological data [42] suggested that the registered number of patients with Crohn's disease or UC started to increase more than 20 years after an increased daily consumption of dietary animal meat and fats, and milk and dairy products, and after a decreased consumption of rice. Whether protein or animal fat consumption is the causal agent is unclear.

A number of more recent studies have investigated protein intake and IBD. Tragnone et al. [44] found that patients with UC consumed more protein than controls but there was no difference in relation to patients with Crohn's disease. In their case–control study, Reif et al. [45] found no association between risk of IBD and protein intake. In contrast, Shoda et al.'s epidemiological analysis showed a correlation between the incidence of Crohn's disease and the increased consumption of animal and milk protein in Japan [38]. A prospective cohort study carried out by Jowett et al. [46] in patients with UC in remission found that meat, protein and alcohol increased the likelihood of relapse. Dairy products have been suggested as a risk factor, since IBD is more common in 'dairy-based' countries than in 'soy-based' ones [47]. Similarly, Crohn's disease risk has been shown to be associated with dairy food consumption [38,48].

Despite the small number of studies, there appears to be some evidence of a relationship between protein intake and IBD, the proposed mechanism being via the action of intestinal bacteria.

Micronutrients

Low concentrations of certain micronutrients, such as zinc and vitamin D, may also increase the IBD risk. Dietary patterns may also affect disease susceptibility [1].

A high prevalence of inadequate micronutrient concentrations in patients with IBD, including vitamins A, C, D and E, calcium (23%), folate (19%) and iron (13%) has been found [49,50]. Several biochemical deficiencies were also observed. The prevalence of subnormal serum concentrations was haemoglobin (40%), ferritin (39.2%), vitamin B6 (29%), carotene (23.4%), vitamin B12 (18.4%), vitamin D (17.6%), albumin (17.6%) and zinc (15.2%). Dietary intake was not correlated with serum concentrations in all instances, although there was a highly significant correlation between diet and serum values of vitamin B12, folate and vitamin B6 for all IBD subjects, independent of disease activity. This may reflect a high incidence of genetic polymorphisms for uptake, absorption and/or efficacy of these nutrients.

Cantorna reported that vitamin D availability, whether due to sunshine exposure or diet, is likely to play a significant role in the development of IBD [51]. The evidence points to the direct and indirect regulation of T-cell development and function by vitamin D. In the absence of vitamin D and signals delivered through the vitamin D receptor, autoreactive T-cells develop. The presence of active vitamin D (1,25(OH)2D3) and a functional vitamin D receptor redresses the balance in the T-cell response.

3.12.4 Role of obesity in inflammatory bowel disease aetiology

There is evidence that the inflammatory signalling response is linked to insulin resistance, glucose intolerance and endothelial dysfunction, which are all known as obesity-related alterations [52–54]. This is supported by Bregenzer and co-workers [55], showing that insulin resistance is elevated in patients with Crohn's disease compared to healthy subjects. Insulin signalling may be a dominant metabolic pathway in energy homeostasis and Crohn's disease development. It has been shown that fatty acids are able to activate inflammatory pathways through pattern recognition receptors of the innate immune system [56]. These results indicate that key pathways characteristic for a specific disease affect other physiological and pathological mechanisms, suggesting that pathways need to be seen as a part of a complex network system. Any changes of key driver of chronic disease initiation and perpetuation may therefore suppress or activate inflammatory pathways. However, the exact mechanisms and pathways are still unknown, and it needs to be investigated which of these characteristic disease processes come first to predict a risk for developing IBD.

There is more general evidence that a Western dietary pattern may be associated with an increased risk of IBD [57]. This review of studies in migrant populations revealed an increased consumption of several factors of a Western-style diet before diagnosis of UC. Obesity is becoming more prevalent in IBD, and may be associated with higher disease activity [58]. In practice, regular physical activity, prudent diet and maintenance of Body Mass Index (BMI) <25 may help to prevent IBD. Maternal obesity, however, appears to predispose children towards IBD [59]. Chapman-Kiddell and co-workers [60] concluded that the major constituents of a standard 'Western' diet may contribute to intestinal inflammation through several different mechanisms, including obesity. This detailed review critically assessed the evidence for the role of diet in the development of IBD, and examined the evidence for obesity as a contributing factor to IBD pathogenesis. Particular attention was focused on methodological issues including suitability of cases and controls, as well as confounders such as smoking, and total energy expenditure.

No well-designed studies have investigated an association between the increase in obesity and the rising incidence of IBD. Indeed, in a sizeable group of American paediatric patients with IBD, the incidence of obesity and overweight was comparable to that of the general population [60,61]. However, there are some data suggesting that obesity prior to disease onset may be a risk factor for Crohn's disease in older patients [57].

3.12.5 Role of the gastrointestinal microbiota

There is evidence that GI microbiota have an essential role in the pathogenesis of Crohn's disease [1,2,62]. Clinical evidence for bacteria in the pathogenesis of Crohn's disease is supported by the observations of several *in vitro* and *in vivo* studies [63,64]. This argument is confirmed by a number of IBD animal models that showed that intestinal inflammation fails to develop when they are kept in a germ-free environment [17,65,66].

The intraluminal microbiota affects the intestinal immune system and GI development, provides key nutrients and modifies energy metabolism. Imbalances in bacterial functions, defective sensing and clearance of bacteria, impaired autophagy and alpha-defensin and beta-defensin production may have a role in the initiation of Crohn's disease [67,68]. Compositional and functional changes in GI microbiota lead to invasion of epithelial cells of pathogenic bacteria, cytopathic effects, stimulation of proinflammatory cytokines, dysregulated immune response and damage to the intestinal barrier [17,65,69]. However, chronic inflammation is not only caused by compositional changes in GI microbiota but can also be seen as an initiation factor favouring the growth of certain bacteria [70]. In addition, antimicrobial microbes such as intestinal secretory IgA (sIgA), that acts as a defence mechanism against intestinal microorganisms, have an impact on the composition of commensal bacteria [71]. Furthermore, pattern recognition receptors of the innate immune system such as Toll-like receptors (TLRs) and antimicrobial peptides (e.g. NOD2, ATG16L1, XBP-1) secreted by Paneth cells affect the composition and function of commensal bacteria, and may drive the onset of disease by stimulating the production of proinflammatory cytokines [18,67,72]. These results indicate that defective sensing of bacteria may be associated with Crohn's disease.

Composition and distribution of microbial communities are affected by innate and adaptive immune response, environmental factors, antimicrobial peptides and host genetic factors [64]. The commensal microbiota is shaped by structure of the GI tract and changes in lifestyle conditions such as hygiene, nutrition and antibiotics whereas changes are observed also in the bacterial metagenome in IBD. In addition, polymorphisms in genes involved in Crohn's disease pathogenesis may alter interactions between host and microbiota. However, micro-organisms that directly interact with the intestinal mucosa are poorly understood. Improvement in the understanding of the role of the GI microbiota has considerable public health implications by providing new therapeutic targets for the treatment of Crohn's disease.

Although the role of the GI microbiota is not yet fully understood, genetic susceptibility, immune system and environmental triggers that highlight the dynamics of bacterial–host interactions need to be considered when discussing the functional consequences of the GI microbiota or their by-products. To date, detection and quantification of commensal bacteria are still limited due to the complexity of GI mucosal microbiota and lack of sufficient and precise analytical methods. Inconsistent findings might be due to study design, limitations of analytical techniques, interactions of the microbiota with the immune system, environmental factors and host genetic factors that have an impact on certain pathogens in Crohn's disease aetiology. Nevertheless, large-scale analysis of 16S rRNA genes and metagenomic approaches provided new insights into analysis of the intestinal microbiota that may help explain IBD pathogenesis, and improve disease diagnosis and treatment approaches [73]. Recent theory has suggested a breakdown in the balance between putative species of 'protective' versus 'harmful' intestinal bacteria; this concept has been termed dysbiosis resulting in decreased bacterial diversity [74].

Studies by several groups indicate that luminal components might control dysbiosis [17,75]. The bacterial fermentation product n-butyrate has been identified as a critical molecule. Apart from its essential nutritional function for colonocytes, an anti-inflammatory activity of this short-chain fatty acid has been recognised *in vitro* and *in vivo*. Regarding its molecular mode of action, an interference with transcription factors critical for the production of proinflammatory cytokines has been found.

3.12.6 Conclusion

Evidence for a major role of dietary factors that may induce or modify IBD is limited. As identified, some studies suggested that refined sugar consumption,

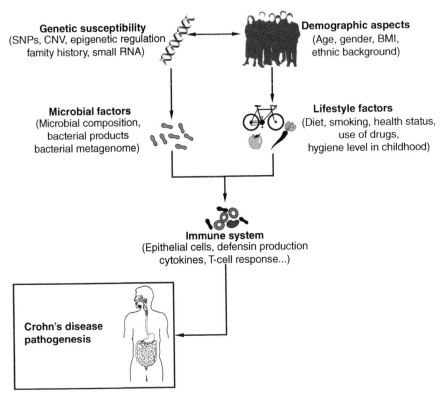

Genetic and non-genetic factors that influence individual susceptibility to Crohn's disease development

Figure 3.12.3 Possible genetic and non-genetic factors that are involved in Crohn's disease pathogenesis. BMI, Body Mass Index; CNV, copy number variant; SNP, single nucleotide polymorphism.

a high-energy diet and processed fat might be risk factors for Crohn's disease, whereas fruit, vegetables and NSP consumption seems to decrease the risk of IBD, but these associations are less certain [5,27,69,76,77]. It is possible that nutritional factors suggested as risk factors for IBD may be merely an expression of a Westernised lifestyle, involving other risk factors that modify the pathogenesis of IBD.

Finally, IBD is caused by combined effects of genetic, microbial, immunological and environmental factors (Figure 3.12.3). Thereby, commensal bacteria , innate and adaptive immune responses, environmental factors and host genetic factors interact with each other [17]. Imbalances or broad changes in one of these factors in turn may lead to functional consequences for other factors in the

network, resulting in chronic inflammatory intestinal conditions. Host genetic factors determine microbiota profile whereas environmental influences alter the intestinal commensal composition. In this context, polymorphisms in genes involved in the pathogenesis of IBD may modify the risk of developing IBD by leading to an aggressive T-cell response [74]. The intestinal microbiota provides antigens and adjuvants that stimulate pathogenic or protective immune responses. A better understanding of these factors may lead to improved treatments and prevention of the disease. Thereby, the impact of the genotype, the GI microbiota and associated conditions such as obesity becomes increasingly important for preventive nutrition in reducing the risks of IBD.

Acknowledgement

Nutrigenomics New Zealand is a collaboration between the University of Auckland, Plant and Food Research Ltd and AgResearch Ltd, with funding through the Ministry of Business, Innovation and Environment.

References

1. Gentschew L, Ferguson LR. Role of nutrition and microbiota in susceptibility to inflammatory bowel diseases. *Molecular Nutrition and Food Research* 2012; **56**(4): 524–535.
2. Jostins L, Ripke S, Weersma RK, et al. Host-microbe interactions have shaped the genetic architecture of inflammatory bowel disease. *Nature* 2012; **491**(7422): 119–124.
3. Bernini P, Bertini I, Luchinat C, et al. Individual human phenotypes in metabolic space and time. *Journal of Proteome Research* 2009; **8**(9): 4264–4271.
4. Bernstein CN. Epidemiologic clues to inflammatory bowel disease. *Current Gastroenterology Reports* 2010; **12**(6): 495–501.
5. Ravikumara M, Sandhu BK. Epidemiology of inflammatory bowel diseases in childhood. *Indian Journal of Pediatrics* 2006; **73**(8): 717–721.
6. Keijer J, van Helden YG, Bunschoten A, van Schothorst EM. Transcriptome analysis in benefit-risk assessment of micronutrients and bioactive food components. *Molecular Nutrition and Food Research* 2010; **54**(2): 240–248.
7. Hedin CR, Stagg AJ, Whelan K, Lindsay JO. Family studies in Crohn's disease: new horizons in understanding disease pathogenesis, risk and prevention. *Gut* 2012; **61**(2): 311–318.
8. Mow WS, Vasiliauskas EA, Lin YC, et al. Association of antibody responses to microbial antigens and complications of small bowel Crohn's disease. *Gastroenterology* 2004; **126**(2): 414–424.
9. Neuman MG, Nanau RM. Inflammatory bowel disease: role of diet, microbiota, life style. Translational Research. *Journal of Laboratory and Clinical Medicine* 2012; **160**(1): 29–44.
10. Adamson S, Leitinger N. Phenotypic modulation of macrophages in response to plaque lipids. *Current Opinion in Lipidology* 2011; **22**(5): 335–342.
11. Jantchou P, Morois S, Clavel-Chapelon F, Boutron-Ruault MC, Carbonnel F. Animal protein intake and risk of inflammatory bowel disease: the E3N prospective study. *American Journal of Gastroenterology* 2010; **105**(10): 2195–2201.
12. Sartor RB. Mechanisms of disease: pathogenesis of Crohn's disease and ulcerative colitis. *Nature Clinical Practice. Gastroenterology and Hepatology* 2006; **3**(7): 390–407.
13. Yu Y, Sitaraman S, Gewirtz AT. Intestinal epithelial cell regulation of mucosal inflammation. *Immunologic Research* 2004; **29**(1-3): 55–68.
14. Duchmann R, Kaiser I, Hermann E, Mayet W, Ewe K, Meyer zum Büschenfelde KH. Tolerance exists towards resident intestinal flora but is broken in active inflammatory bowel disease (IBD). *Clinical and Exprimental Immunology* 1995; **102**(3): 448–455.
15. Sartor RB, Hoentjen F. Proinflammatory cytokines and signaling pathways in intestinal innate immune cells. In: Mestecky J, Lamm ME, Strober W, Bienenstock J, McGhee JR, Mayer L (eds) *Mucosal Immunology*. London: Elsevier Academic Press, 2005, pp. 681–701.
16. Bamias G, Nyce MR, de la Rue SA, Cominelli F, American College of Physicians, American Physiological Society. New concepts in the pathophysiology of inflammatory bowel disease. *Annals of Internal Medicine* 2005; **143**(12): 895–904.
17. Hansen J, Gulati A, Sartor RB. The role of mucosal immunity and host genetics in defining intestinal commensal bacteria. *Current Opinion in Gastroenterology* 2010; **26**(6): 564–571.
18. Sartor RB. Genetics and environmental interactions shape the intestinal microbiome to promote inflammatory bowel disease versus mucosal homeostasis. *Gastroenterology* 2010; **139**(6): 1816–1819.
19. Willing BP, Dicksved J, Halfvarson J, et al. A pyrosequencing study in twins shows that gastrointestinal microbial profiles vary with inflammatory bowel disease phenotypes. *Gastroenterology* 2010; **139**(6): 1844–1854.
20. Ott C, Obermeier F, Thieler S, et al. The incidence of inflammatory bowel disease in a rural region of Southern Germany: a prospective population-based study. *European Journal of Gastroenterology and Hepatology* 2008; **20**(9): 917–923.
21. Halfvarson J, Jess T, Magnuson A, et al. Environmental factors in inflammatory bowel disease: a co-twin control study of a Swedish–Danish twin population. *Inflammatory Bowel Diseases* 2006; **12**(10): 925–933.
22. Orholm M, Binder V, Sørensen TI, Rasmussen LP, Kyvik KO. Concordance of inflammatory bowel disease among Danish twins. Results of a nationwide study. *Scandinavian Journal of Gastroenterology* 2000; **35**(10): 1075–1081.
23. Spehlmann ME, Begun AZ, Burghardt J, Lepage P, Raedler A, Schreiber S. Epidemiology of inflammatory bowel disease in a German twin cohort: results of a nationwide study. *Inflammatory Bowel Diseases* 2008; **14**(7): 968–976.
24. Halme L, Paavola-Sakki P, Turunen U, Lappalainen M, Farkkila M, Kontula K. Family and twin studies in inflammatory bowel disease. *World Journal of Gastroenterology* 2006; **12**(23): 3668–3672.
25. Schreiber S, Rosenstiel P, Albrecht M, Hampe J, Krawczak M. Genetics of Crohn disease, an archetypal inflammatory barrier disease. *Nature Reviews. Genetics* 2005; **6**(5): 376–388.
26. Lees CW, Barrett JC, Parkes M, Satsangi J. New IBD genetics: common pathways with other diseases. *Gut* 2011; **60**(12): 1739–1753.
27. Yamamoto T, Nakahigashi M, Saniabadi AR. Review article: diet and inflammatory bowel disease – epidemiology and treatment. *Alimentary Pharmacology and Therapeutics* 2009; **30**(2): 99–112.
28. Sakamoto N, Kono S, Wakai K, et al. Dietary risk factors for inflammatory bowel disease: a multicenter case-control study in Japan. *Inflammatory Bowel Diseases* 2005; **11**(2): 154–163.

29. Martini GA, Brandes JW. Increased consumption of refined carbohydrates in patients with Crohn's disease. *Klinische Wochenschrift* 1976; **54**(8): 367–371.

30. Thornton JR, Emmett PM, Heaton KW. Diet and Crohn's disease: characteristics of the pre-illness diet. *British Medical Journal* 1979; **2**(6193): 762–764.

31. Thornton JR, Emmett PM, Heaton KW. Diet and ulcerative colitis. *British Medical Journal* 1980; **280**(6210): 293–294.

32. Matsui T, Iida M, Fujishima M, Imai K, Yao T. Increased sugar consumption in Japanese patients with Crohn's disease. *Gastroenterologia Japonica* 1990; **25**(2): 271.

33. Kasper H, Sommer H. Dietary fiber and nutrient intake in Crohn's disease. *American Journal of Clinical Nutrition* 1979; **32**(9): 1898–1901.

34. Geerling BJ, Stockbrugger RW, Brummer RJ. Nutrition and inflammatory bowel disease: an update. *Scandinavian Journal of Gastroenterology* 1999; **230**(Suppl): 95–105.

35. Persson PG, Ahlbom A, Hellers G. Diet and inflammatory bowel disease: a case-control study. *Epidemiology* 1992; **3**(1): 47–52.

36. Sonnenberg A. Geographic and temporal variations of sugar and margarine consumption in relation to Crohn's disease. *Digestion* 1988; **41**(3): 161–171.

37. Maconi G, Ardizzone S, Cucino C, Bezzio C, Russo AG, Bianchi Porro G. Pre-illness changes in dietary habits and diet as a risk factor for inflammatory bowel disease: a case-control study. *World Journal of Gastroenterology* 2010; **16**(34): 4297–4304.

38. Shoda R, Matsueda K, Yamato S, Umeda N. Epidemiologic analysis of Crohn disease in Japan: increased dietary intake of n-6 polyunsaturated fatty acids and animal protein relates to the increased incidence of Crohn disease in Japan. *American Journal of Clinical Nutrition* 1996; **63**(5): 741–745.

39. Belluzzi A, Brignola C, Campieri M, Pera A, Boschi S, Miglioli M. Effect of an enteric-coated fish-oil preparation on relapses in Crohn's disease. *New England Journal of Medicine* 1996; **334**(24): 1557–1560.

40. Danesi F, Philpott M, Huebner C, Bordoni A, Ferguson LR. Food-derived bioactives as potential regulators of the IL-12/IL-23 pathway implicated in inflammatory bowel diseases. *Mutation Research* 2010; **690**(1-2): 139–144.

41. IBD in EPIC Study Investigators, Tjonneland A, Overvad K, et al. Linoleic acid, a dietary n-6 polyunsaturated fatty acid, and the aetiology of ulcerative colitis: a nested case-control study within a European prospective cohort study. *Gut* 2009; **58**(12): 1606–1611.

42. Asakura H, Suzuki K, Kitahora T, Morizane T. Is there a link between food and intestinal microbes and the occurrence of Crohn's disease and ulcerative colitis? *Journal of Gastroenterology and Hepatology* 2008; **23**(12): 1794–1801.

43. Christl SU, Eisner HD, Dusel G, Kasper H, Scheppach W. Antagonistic effects of sulfide and butyrate on proliferation of colonic mucosa: a potential role for these agents in the pathogenesis of ulcerative colitis. *Digestive Diseases and Sciences* 1996; **41**(12): 2477–2481.

44. Tragnone A, Hanau C, Bazzocchi G, Lanfranchi GA. Epidemiological characteristics of inflammatory bowel disease in Bologna, Italy – incidence and risk factors. *Digestion* 1993; **54**(3): 183–188.

45. Reif S, Klein I, Lubin F, Farbstein M, Hallak A, Gilat T. Pre-illness dietary factors in inflammatory bowel disease. *Gut* 1997; **40**(6): 754–760.

46. Jowett SL, Seal CJ, Pearce MS, et al. Influence of dietary factors on the clinical course of ulcerative colitis: a prospective cohort study. *Gut* 2004; **53**(10): 1479–1484.

47. Mishkin S. Dairy sensitivity, lactose malabsorption, and elimination diets in inflammatory bowel disease. *American Journal of Clinical Nutrition* 1997; **65**(2): 564–567.

48. Shrier I, Szilagyi A, Correa JA. Impact of lactose containing foods and the genetics of lactase on diseases: an analytical review of population data. *Nutrition and Cancer* 2008; **60**(3): 292–300.

49. Hwang C, Ross V, Mahadevan U. Micronutrient deficiencies in inflammatory bowel disease: from A to zinc. *Inflammatory Bowel Diseases* 2012; **18**(10): 1961–1981.

50. Tighe MP, Cummings JR, Afzal NA. Nutrition and inflammatory bowel disease: primary or adjuvant therapy. *Current Opinion in Clinical Nutrition and Metabolic Care* 2011; **14**(5): 491–496.

51. Cantorna MT, Zhu Y, Froicu M, Wittke A. Vitamin D status, 1,25-dihydroxyvitamin D3, and the immune system. *American Journal of Clinical Nutrition* 2004; **80**(6 Suppl): 1717S–1720S.

52. Marsollier N, Ferré P, Foufelle F. Novel insights in the interplay between inflammation and metabolic diseases: a role for the pathogen sensing kinase PKR. *Journal of Hepatology* 2011; **54**(6): 1307–1309.

53. Nakamura T, Furuhashi M, Li P, et al. Double-stranded RNA-dependent protein kinase links pathogen sensing with stress and metabolic homeostasis. *Cell* 2010; **140**(3): 338–348.

54. Hotamisligil GS, Erbay E. Nutrient sensing and inflammation in metabolic diseases. *Nature Reviews. Immunology* 2008; **8**(12): 923–934.

55. Bregenzer N, Hartmann A, Strauch U, Schölmerich J, Andus T, Bollheimer LC. Increased insulin resistance and beta cell activity in patients with Crohn's disease. *Inflammatory Bowel Diseases* 2006; **12**(1): 53–56.

56. Shi H, Kokoeva MV, Inouye K, Tzameli I, Yin H, Flier JS. TLR4 links innate immunity and fatty acid-induced insulin resistance. *Journal of Clinical Investigation* 2006; **116**(11): 3015–3025.

57. Cosnes J, Gower-Rousseau C, Seksik P, Cortot A. Epidemiology and natural history of inflammatory bowel diseases. *Gastroenterology* 2011; **140**(6): 1785–1794.

58. Fink C, Karagiannides I, Bakirtzi K, Pothoulakis C. Adipose tissue and inflammatory bowel disease pathogenesis. *Inflammatory Bowel Diseases* 2012; **18**(8): 1550–1557.

59. Franks I. Obesity: maternal obesity may predispose offspring to IBD. *Nature Reviews. Gastroenterology and Hepatology* 2011; **8**(2): 65.

60. Chapman-Kiddell CA, Davies PS, Gillen L, Radford-Smith GL. Role of diet in the development of inflammatory bowel disease. *Inflammatory Bowel Diseases* 2010; **16**(1): 137–151.

61. Long MD, Crandall WV, Leibowitz IH, et al. Prevalence and epidemiology of overweight and obesity in children with inflammatory bowel disease. *Inflammatory Bowel Diseases* 2011; **17**(10): 2162–2168.

62. Baker PI, Love DR, Ferguson LR. Role of gut microbiota in Crohn's disease. *Expert Review of Gastroenterology and Hepatology* 2009; **3**(5): 535–546.

63. Conte MP, Schippa S, Zamboni I, et al. Gut-associated bacterial microbiota in paediatric patients with inflammatory bowel disease. *Gut* 2006; **55**(12): 1760–1767.

64. Elson CO, Cong Y, McCracken VJ, Dimmitt RA, Lorenz RG, Weaver CT. Experimental models of inflammatory bowel disease reveal innate, adaptive, and regulatory mechanisms of host dialogue with the microbiota. *Immunological Reviews* 2005; **206**: 260–276.

65. Sartor RB. Microbial-host interactions in inflammatory bowel diseases and experimental colitis. *Nestlé Nutrition Workshop Series. Paediatric Programme* 2009; **64**: 121–132.

66. Sartor RB. Does Mycobacterium avium subspecies paratuberculosis cause Crohn's disease? *Gut* 2005; **54**(7): 896–898.

67. Man SM, Kaakoush NO, Mitchell HM. The role of bacteria and pattern-recognition receptors in Crohn's disease. *Nature Reviews. Gastroenterology and Hepatology* 2011; **8**(3): 152–168.

68. Sekirov I, Russell SL, Antunes LC, Finlay BB. Gut microbiota in health and disease. *Physiological Reviews* 2010; **90**(3): 859–904.

69. Vijay-Kumar M, Aitken JD, Carvalho FA, et al. Metabolic syndrome and altered gut microbiota in mice lacking Toll-like receptor 5. *Science* 2010; **328**(5975): 228–231.

70. Lin J, McKenna BJ, Appelman HD. Morphologic findings in upper gastrointestinal biopsies of patients with ulcerative colitis: a controlled study. *American Journal of Surgical Pathology* 2010; **34**(11): 1672–1677.

71. Kiyono H, Kweon MN, Hiroi T, Takahashi I. The mucosal immune system: from specialized immune defense to inflammation and allergy. *Acta Odontologica Scandinavica* 2001; **59**(3): 145–153.

72. Garrett WS, Lord GM, Punit S, et al. Communicable ulcerative colitis induced by T-bet deficiency in the innate immune system. *Cell* 2007; **131**(1): 33–45.

73. Greenblum S, Turnbaugh PJ, Borenstein E. Metagenomic systems biology of the human gut microbiome reveals topological shifts associated with obesity and inflammatory bowel disease. *Proceedings of the National Academy of Sciences of the USA* 2012; **109**(2): 594–599.

74. Lakatos PL, Fischer S, Lakatos L, Gal I, Papp J. Current concept on the pathogenesis of inflammatory bowel disease-crosstalk between genetic and microbial factors: pathogenic bacteria and altered bacterial sensing or changes in mucosal integrity take 'toll'? *World Journal of Gastroenterology* 2006; **12**(12): 1829–1841.

75. Ewaschuk JB, Tejpar QZ, Soo I, Madsen K, Fedorak RN. The role of antibiotic and probiotic therapies in current and future management of inflammatory bowel disease. *Current Gastroenterology Reports* 2006; **8**(6): 486–498.

76. Cashman KD, Shanahan F. Is nutrition an aetiological factor for inflammatory bowel disease? *European Journal of Gastroenterology and Hepatology* 2003; **15**(6): 607–613.

77. Rajendran N, Kumar D. Role of diet in the management of inflammatory bowel disease. *World Journal of Gastroenterology* 2010; **16**(12): 1442–1448.

78. Renz H, von Mutius E, Brandtzaeg P, Cookson WO, Autenrieth IB, Haller D. Gene-environment interactions in chronic inflammatory disease. *Nature Immunology* 2011; **12**(4): 273–277.

Chapter 3.13

Inflammatory bowel disease nutritional consequences

Konstantinos Gerasimidis
University of Glasgow, Glasgow, UK

The aetiology of malnutrition in inflammatory bowel disease (IBD) is multifactorial and may present as protein energy malnutrition (PEM), altered body composition, micronutrient deficiencies and poor bone health. In children, growth failure and pubertal development delay can be additional outcomes of poor nutritional status which further complicate disease management. Reduced dietary intake, altered energy/nutrient metabolism, increased GI nutrient losses and drug–nutrient interactions are all implicated in the origins of malnutrition in IBD [1].

3.13.1 Protein energy malnutrition

Protein energy malnutrition is common at the time of diagnosis and the patient's nutritional status fluctuates during the disease course [2]. History of weight loss, underweight and thinness (defined as a low Body Mass Index (BMI)) are common presenting features of the newly diagnosed patient and frequently accompany episodes of disease relapse [3]. Protein energy malnutrition is more common in Crohn's disease compared with ulcerative colitis (UC) and is seen in approximately 60% and 35% of newly diagnosed patients respectively [3]. Apart from the higher prevalence of PEM in Crohn's disease, there is no consistent evidence to link it with other specific disease characteristics (e.g. disease location, diagnosis delay). However, recent data suggest that fewer patients are now seen with PEM compared with previous studies, and a large proportion of patients are overweight or obese at diagnosis, particularly in UC.

In a large North American study of 783 newly diagnosed IBD children, low BMI was seen in 22–24% with Crohn's disease and 7–9% with UC. In contrast, 10% and 20–30% of children with Crohn's disease and UC respectively had a high BMI consistent with being overweight or obese [4]. The obesity epidemic in the general population, combined with earlier disease recognition of IBD nowadays, may explain these secular changes in patterns. There is limited evidence on the progression of undernutrition after diagnosis. In the only study undertaken thus far, a similar proportion of children with Crohn's disease had short stature (height z-score ≤ -2) and 50% fewer children were classified as thin (BMI z-score ≤ -2 SD) at follow-up compared with disease diagnosis. Growth and nutritional retardation at diagnosis, young age, male gender and extraintestinal manifestations at diagnosis were predictors of poor prognosis at follow-up [5].

3.13.2 Body composition

There are several reasons to speculate why body composition in patients with IBD may differ from that of healthy people. Secretion of proinflammatory

Advanced Nutrition and Dietetics in Gastroenterology, First Edition. Edited by Miranda Lomer.
© 2014 John Wiley & Sons, Ltd. Published 2014 by John Wiley & Sons, Ltd.

cytokines may alter energy metabolism, protein turnover and energy substrate utilisation, whereas the use of corticosteroids increases body fat with catabolic effects on lean mass. Physical activity, on the other hand, was reported to be low in adult patients with IBD and correlated inversely with fat mass (FM) [6].

There are few studies that have assessed body composition in IBD. Lean body mass or fat-free mass (FFM) has been consistently reported as significantly lower than healthy control groups whereas occasionally gender-specific associations with FM have been found [7]. Thayu et al., in a well-designed prospective study of newly diagnosed children with Crohn's disease, also reported gender-associated differences with body composition [7]. Fat mass and lean mass for height (adjusted for age, race and pubertal stage) were lower in female than in male patients. Compared with a cohort of healthy controls, body composition in females was more consistent with wasting (low lean and FM) whereas in males there was mostly preservation of FM and deficits in lean mass consistent with cachexia. No consistent associations have been observed between body composition, clinical activity, disease location or diagnosis delay. Interestingly, normalisation of BMI at 2 years follow-up has not been associated with a significant increment in FFM in children with Crohn's disease [8], which implies that changes in body weight or BMI for age are not good proxies for body composition changes in IBD so simple bedside techniques of body composition assessment, for routine use in clinical practice, are required.

Nevertheless, interpretation of body composition data in disease has to be approached with caution since the underlying assumptions about the composition of body compartments may be invalid [9]. Most *in vivo* body composition methods used in previous IBD studies, e.g. dual energy X-ray absorptiometry (DEXA), have been tested and validated in healthy individuals or animal cadavers and their applicability in chronic illness is questionable given the changes that may occur in the hydration level and distribution of fluids within the body compartments [9]. Assessment of the validity of these techniques in an IBD population and replication of these results with the application of more sophisti-

cated methods need to be explored. The use of functional tests (e.g. handgrip strength) has been proposed as a proxy estimate of FFM in patients with IBD but these techniques lack specificity. Wiroth and colleagues found that patients with Crohn's disease in clinical remission have overall lower muscle performance than healthy controls, but this was independent of FFM levels [10].

3.13.3 Bone health

Bone mineralisation is an important aspect in the care of patients with IBD, particularly as peak bone mass, attained during adolescence, was found to be the most important determinant of lifelong skeletal health [11]. Osteopenia and osteoporosis are important extraintestinal manifestations in IBD that may be related to increased risk of fractures [11,12]. In adult studies, a 60–70% higher risk for vertebral and hip fractures incidence was found for patients with IBD compared with healthy controls [12,13] but there is no strong evidence to suggest that in IBD children, bones are more brittle and that they experience more fractures compared with their healthy peers. It is difficult to interpret these discrepancies between adult and paediatric studies but it can mean that children with IBD may be more predisposed to have brittle bones that are at higher risk of fracture in adulthood and may occur earlier than in healthy adults (e.g. before menopause). The use of oral steroids to induce disease remission in adults might explain the higher risk of bone fractures; children are more likely to be treated with enteral nutrition (EN) rather than oral steroids to induce remission. Moreover, it is also possible that vertebral fractures occur in IBD children but these may be asymptomatic and hence remain undiagnosed [14].

A disease-associated effect is well documented, with poor bone health seen more often in Crohn's disease than UC. Disease location, duration and history of disease activity were risk factors in some but not all studies [12,15–18]. Recent data suggest that afflicted children have the potential to improve their bone mineral density by the time they reach early adulthood [19].

Burnham et al. [20] reported that the difference in bone mineral content between Crohn's disease and healthy controls was eliminated when they used a regression model to account for differences in lean mass while Sylvester et al. showed that changes in bone mineral content during a period of 2 years post diagnosis were positively associated with concomitant increments in FFM [8]. These findings suggest that decreased mechanical stress may be an important factor for reduced bone health in Crohn's disease and this opens a treatment opportunity to improve bone mass by optimising lean tissue gain through nutritional support and weight-bearing exercise in patients with IBD [21].

Bone mineralisation in IBD can be negatively affected by undernutrition, low vitamin D status, the effect of proinflammatory cytokines on bone formation, resorption and osteoblast maturation [22] and the long-term use of high steroid doses [23,24]. As delayed skeletal maturation and sexual maturation are commonly seen in IBD, particularly Crohn's disease, it is important to express the results not as z-scores for chronological age but accounting for pubertal staging and bone age [25].

3.13.4 Linear growth and short stature

Short stature and faltering linear growth are commonly encountered in IBD, and frequently precede disease diagnosis. Approximately 23–25% of paediatric patients have presented with deviation from their growth velocity and height for age centiles, or as significantly shorter than their healthy peers [26], and a proportion will fail to attain their genetic potential for linear growth, when their height deficits are compared with their estimated midparental target height [26]. The exact mechanisms by which growth impairment occurs in IBD are unclear but it is believed to be an interplay between undernutrition, delayed puberty, the effect of circulating proinflammatory cytokines and long-term use of steroids [27].

3.13.5 Delayed puberty

Delayed puberty is a frequent feature of young patients, more often in Crohn's disease than UC, and in males than in females [17,23,28]. Mean delays in puberty of 0.7 and 1.5 years were found in Dutch and USA studies, respectively [23]. Delayed pubertal onset may influence linear growth and final adult height and could affect quality of life and self-esteem but the latter aspect has not been addressed prospectively.

Undernutrition has always been thought to be the main reason for delayed puberty in patients with IBD. However, puberty may be delayed despite a normal nutritional status. Observations in animal models of experimental colitis suggested that inflammation may have a direct adverse influence, independent of undernutrition, on the onset and progression of puberty (Figure 3.13.1) but relevant studies in patients with IBD are lacking. *In vitro* studies suggested that proinflammatory cytokines (e.g. tumour necrosis factor (TNF) alpha, interleukin (IL) 1beta, IL-6) can affect sex steroid production at the level of testes and ovaries [29].

3.13.6 Micronutrient status

Although clinical presentation of frank micronutrient deficiencies in IBD is very rare and largely limited to case reports, suboptimal circulating concentrations for virtually every vitamin, mineral and trace element have been reported previously, primarily in adult patients but also evident in the paediatric studies (Table 3.13.1). Antioxidant trace elements (e.g. Zn, Se, Cu) and vitamins (e.g. vitamins A, E, C, carotenoids) were the main nutrients consistently reported at suboptimal circulating concentrations in patients with IBD compared with healthy controls or the normal reference range (see Table 3.13.1). Serum vitamin D has been reported to be low in adult [30] and paediatric studies [31] and is an independent risk factor for poor bone health.

Suboptimal dietary intake, increased utilisation, malabsorption and increased enteric losses have all been postulated as causes of these nutritional deficiencies (see Figure 3.13.1). Some studies have linked nutritional deficiencies with clinical disease activity and inflammatory markers (see Table 3.13.1) but whether micronutrient depletion plays an important role in the

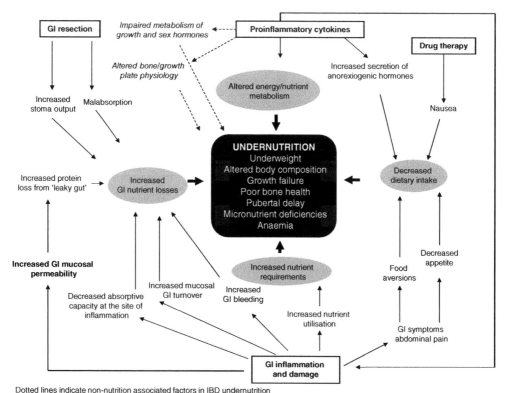

Figure 3.13.1 The aetiology and presentation of malnutrition in IBD. GI, gastrointestinal; IBD, inflammatory bowel disease.

pathogenesis and perpetuation of the mucosal lesions or is the result of these needs remains unknown. However, it must be remembered that changes in the plasma concentrations of many micronutrients and their association with systemic and clinical activity indexes can be an epiphenomenon of the acute phase response in inflammatory conditions like IBD [32]. Although reduced serum concentrations of micronutrients are often used to define deficiency states, these concentrations may better reflect disease activity and inflammation rather than being biomarkers of body tissue deficits [32]. A prime example is the transient decrease in plasma retinol binding protein and accordingly transported vitamin A plasma concentrations in the presence of the acute phase response in inflammatory conditions.

Several experts now propose that assessment of micronutrient body stores using serum concentrations in inflammatory conditions is erroneous and use of other indices of body micronutrient stores which are independent of the effects of the acute phase response, such as red blood cells, is required [33].

3.13.7 Antioxidant status

Inflammatory bowel disease is characterised by aggregation of inflammatory cells (granulocytes, monocytes and neutrophils) at the site of the intestinal lesion and production of reactive oxygen species is part of the normal immune properties of these cells. The damaging action of these free radicals is normally counteracted by the body's defence mechanisms. Uncontrolled production coupled with reduced removal by an impaired endogenous antioxidant defence system may induce tissue damage [34]. There is good evidence that patients with IBD

Table 3.13.1 Major recent studies measured circulating concentrations of multiple micronutrients in patients with inflammatory bowel disease

Study	Participants	Assessed micronutrients	Outcome[†]
Hengstermann et al. 2008 [61]	167 IBD (132 in remission, 35 active); 45 HC	Vitamins: C, E, carotenoids Minerals: Se, Zn, Cu	• Vitamin C and carotenoids were lower in IBD compared with HC • Cu was higher and lycopene lower in active IBD compared with inactive IBD and HC
Filippi et al. 2006 [48]	54 CD in remission	Vitamins: C, A, D, E, B1, B6, B12, E, folate, niacin, beta-carotene Minerals: Fe, Cu, Ca, P, Mg, Zn	• Vitamin C, Cu, niacin, Zn, Fe, B6, B1, B12, folate, beta-carotene, vitamin E were below the reference range for more than 20% of the patients
D'Odorico et al. 2001 [62]	46 UC; 37 CD; 386 HC	Vitamins: A, E, carotenoids	• Vitamins A, E and carotenoids were lower compared with HC • No differences between CD and UC • In active disease several carotenoids were lower compared with patients on remission for both diseases • Malnourished patients had lower vitamins A, E and carotenoids
Wendland et al. 2001 [36]	37 CD; 37 HC	Vitamins: C, E, A, carotenoids Minerals: GSHPx, Se	• Vitamin C and carotenoids were lower compared with HC • No association with clinical disease activity • In patients with systemic inflammation most of the micronutrients were or tended to be lower compared to patients with normal inflammatory markers • Several carotenoids associated with lipid peroxidation
Geerling et al. 2000 [63]	23 CD; 46 UC (newly diagnosed); 69 HC	Vitamins: A, E, C, beta-carotene, B1, B12, folate Minerals: Mg, Cu, Zn, Se, GSHPx	• In UC beta-carotene, Mg, Se, Zn were lower compared with HC • In CD B12 and GSHPx were lower than HC
Geerling et al. 1998 [64]	32 CD in remission; 32 HC	Vitamins: A, E, C, beta-carotene, B1, B12, folate Minerals: Mg, Cu, Zn, Se, GSHPx	• In CD beta-carotene, vitamin C, E, Se, Mg, GSHPx, Zn were lower compared with HC; no difference for vitamin E:cholesterol ratio • Se was positively associated with % body fat • A high proportion of patients had micronutrient concentrations below the reference range
*Ojuawo & Keith 2002 [65]	38 UC; 36 CD (newly diagnosed) IBD; 40 HC	Minerals: Zn, Se, Cu	• Se lower in UC and CD compared with HC • Cu higher in CD compared with UC or HC • Zn in CD was lower than HC
*Levy et al. 2002 [66]	22 CD; 10 HC	Vitamins: retinol, beta-carotene, alpha-tocopherol, gamma-tocopherol	• In CD retinol was lower than HC • No difference between active and inactive disease

Table 3.13.1   Continued

Study	Participants	Assessed micronutrients	Outcome[†]
*Bousvaros et al. 1998 [67]	61 CD; 36 UC (plus young adults); 23 HC	Vitamins: A, E	• 14.4% low vitamin A and 6.2% low vitamin E compared to reference range • 'Deficiencies' more prevalent in active CD
*Hoffenberg et al. 1997 [68]	12 CD; 12 UC; 23 HC	Vitamins: C, A, E, beta-carotenoid, gamma-tocopherol, retinol binding protein Minerals: Se, GSHPx	• As an IBD group vitamin C lower but GSHPx, vitamin E and vitamin E/ cholesterol higher compared with HC • In UC vitamin A was lower than CD • Antioxidants inversely correlated with anthropometry

[†]Nutrients which were assessed but are not presented in the outcome column did not differ between groups. CD, Crohn's disease; GSHPx, cellular glutathione peroxidase; HC, healthy controls; IBD, inflammatory bowel disease; UC, ulcerative colitis.
*Paediatric study.

have increased oxidative stress [35,36] which may cause damage to biological macromolecules [36] and possibly intestinal lesions.

Wendland et al. found that lipid peroxidation, a feature of oxidative stress, was higher in adult patients with Crohn's disease compared with healthy controls [36]. Plasma antioxidant vitamins were low despite no profound difference in the dietary intake of antioxidants between patients with Crohn's disease and healthy controls, although this can be explained simply by the effect of the acute phase response on micronutrient plasma concentrations in some patients with active disease. Following these observations, clinical trials found a reduction in markers of oxidative stress and improved antioxidant status after supplementation with antioxidant micronutrients [37]. Nevertheless, a positive association between improvement of disease activity and restoration of oxidative status has not been established.

3.13.8 Anaemia

Overt or occult intestinal bleeding is a major symptom and a drop in haemoglobin occurs with almost every flare in Crohn's disease and UC. The prevalence of anaemia in IBD varies significantly depending on the characteristics of the population studied and definition used [38]. In a systematic review by Wilson et al., the prevalence of anaemia in patients with inflammatory bowel disease ranged from 8.8% to 73.7% depending on the patient population characteristics [38]. Clinical disease severity was a strong predictor of anaemia in some but not all studies, as was the type of disease, gender, upper GI involvement, nutritional status, and growth [38].

Two predominant types of anaemia have been identified in the context of IBD. Iron deficiency anaemia and the anaemia of chronic disease account for the majority of cases, with the first being more common in children and the latter in adults [39]. Iron deficiency anaemia is a major cause of anaemia in IBD, ascribed to a negative iron balance from excessive iron loss through GI bleeding, increased epithelial sloughing, reduced dietary intake [40] and impairment of iron absorption in active [41] but not in mild or quiescent disease [42]. Similarly, in anaemia of chronic disease, the production of inflammatory cytokines in chronic inflammation has significant systemic effects on iron absorption [41], the proliferation of erythroid progenitor cells, the production of erythropoietin and the life span of red blood cells [43]. Anaemia associated with vitamin B12 and folate deficiency and drug-associated anaemia due to the long-term use of medication to manage IBD have occasionally been reported but these are uncommon. Patients treated with methotrexate, an antagonist of folate metabolism, need background prophylactic supplementation with oral folate. Of utmost importance are also patients whose terminal ileum has been resected since vitamin B12 absorption takes place at this site [44]. Regular monitoring of the vitamin B12 blood concentration and adequate dietary intake in these patients is recommended [44].

As many of the serological markers of the iron body stores are influenced by the acute phase response, their diagnostic value in IBD is poor and can be misleading. Decrease in serum iron and downregulation of transferrin are part of the acute phase response, causing functional iron deficiency, a state that can be misinterpreted as iron deficiency in a patient with active inflammation. On the other hand, inflammation can cause false elevation of ferritin concentrations, bringing them into the normal range in patients with true iron deficiency [45]. As a result, higher cut-offs and evaluation in conjunction with other haematological parameters to detect iron-depleted anaemic patients have been recommended for ferritin in active IBD [44]. Determination of serum transferrin receptor has been proposed as a potential diagnostic marker to distinguish anaemia of chronic disease from other types of anaemia in IBD [46].

For the treatment of anaemia, it is not only important to identify the type and severity of the anaemia but also its origin so that therapy can be targeted at the underlying mechanism and tailored to the patient's needs. Treatment options can vary from oral iron salt preparations to the use of intravenous iron and erythropoietic agents [44].

3.13.9 Aetiology of malnutrition

The aetiology of undernutrition in IBD is multifactorial, as are its manifestations [1]. The inflammatory response, with the activation of the proinflammatory cascade and clinical manifestations of the disease, medical and surgical therapeutic interventions can all affect determinants of nutritional balance (see Figure 3.13.1). These include poor nutritional intake, increased energy and/or nutrient requirements and altered metabolism, malabsorption, excessive GI losses and nutrient–drug interactions (see Figure 3.13.1). Beyond these major nutrition-associated determinants of undernutrition, there are other non-nutrition-associated factors, such as the direct effect of proinflammatory cytokines on bone, growth and pubertal development which can also interact independently (see Figure 3.13.1).

Reduced dietary intake

Results from studies that investigated the energy and/or nutrient intake of adults with IBD have been inconsistent [47,48], whereas in children with Crohn's disease energy intake was reported to be lower than healthy controls and the national recommendations [49], particularly during the active phase of the disease [50]. Children with active Crohn's disease consumed on average 420 kcal/day less than their siblings (matched for height, sex and weight) whereas for 21% of patients, the energy intake was lower than estimated energy requirements compared with 10% of the healthy controls [49]. Perhaps the inconsistent results between adult and paediatric studies are due to misreporting bias and inherent limitations of dietary intake methodology and use of small relatively population samples.

Micronutrient status may also be compromised in patients with IBD compared to national references and healthy controls and for the majority of micronutrients assessed. Most of the evidence comes from adult studies in patients with Crohn's disease. Food aversions and special therapeutic diets to resolve or prevent exacerbation of GI symptoms [51] and anorexia mediated by the interaction of proinflammatory cytokines with appetite hormones may compromise intake in patients with IBD, particularly during the active phase of the disease [52] (see Figure 3.13.1).

Altered energy/nutrient metabolism

Energy intake, resting energy expenditure (REE), physical activity and diet-induced thermogenesis are major components of the energy balance equilibrium and imbalance can cause undernutrition. Higher basal metabolic rate:FFM ratio has regularly been reported in patients with Crohn's disease compared with patients with UC or healthy controls although studies are inconsistent [48,53]. This may indicate that patients with IBD, mainly those with Crohn's disease, have increased energy expenditure per unit of FFM, but low lean body mass.

Moreover, Azcue et al. showed that children with Crohn's disease fail to adapt their REE to their unit of lean mass, in contrast to anorexic adolescents who had significantly lower values than healthy controls, and perhaps this contributed to their undernutrition [53]. The reason why this may happen remains unknown and could be attributed to inflammation and the action of proinflammatory cytokines.

Few studies on the energy metabolism of patients with IBD found that the non-protein respiratory quotient was significantly lower in Crohn's disease compared with UC or healthy controls, suggesting an increased lipid oxidation rate in Crohn's disease that may explain the lower FM found by others [54]. Al-Jaouni et al. [55] also found increased fat oxidation in Crohn's disease that correlated positively with disease activity. Diet-induced thermogenesis, a small component in the energy balance equation, was higher in one study in Crohn's disease [56], which could explain the lower weight and higher risk of undernutrition in IBD. Although there was no difference in the resting metabolic rate between healthy controls and patients with Crohn's disease in remission, diet-induced thermogenesis was higher (6% versus 10% respectively). However, diametrically opposite results were presented by Al-Jaouni et al. [55] who furthermore found that diet-induced thermogenesis was lower in patients with active compared with inactive disease.

Increased gastrointestinal nutrient losses

Nutrient and energy loss due to maldigestion of food or malabsorption, during the active course of the disease, could potentially impact on the maintenance of energy balance, and explain undernutrition in patients with IBD (see Figure 3.13.1). However, apart from some reports on specific micronutrients in patients with ileal resection or with bile acid malabsorption [57], rigorous evidence is lacking to support loss of dietary energy or other micronutri-

ents due to malabsorption. A small study in Israel found that malabsorption is a major contributor to underweight in adult patients with Crohn's disease in remission [58]. The authors found that GI energy excretion was higher in an underweight group with Crohn's disease than in a normal weight group despite no differences between the two groups for dietary energy intake or resting metabolic rate [58]. Similarly, in another study malabsorption and increased faecal fat were observed in severely undernourished patients which was attributed to the impaired gastric acid and pancreatic enzyme secretion in patients with Crohn's disease [59]. Interestingly, gastric acid and pancreatic enzyme secretion were severely impaired in 80% of these patients [59]. Indeed, following nutritional rehabilitation, stool fat output and malabsorption reduced with concomitant improvements in pancreatic enzyme synthesis, stores and secretion.

In theory, the absorption of specific nutrients should be impaired when the disease is located at the site of specific nutrient absorption or if this area has been resected. Patients with ileal Crohn's disease or resection are susceptible to vitamin B12 deficiency due to inadequate absorption [60]. Iron absorption may also be diminished in active Crohn's disease due to the excessive production of hepcidin, a hepatic peptide mediating the absorption of iron at the level of the enterocyte [41].

Apart from malabsorption in IBD, loss of nutrients can occur as a result of excessive intestinal mucosal sloughing, and through protein enteropathy from a ruptured, permeable GI tract.

Drug–nutrient interactions

Several drugs used in IBD management can directly influence nutritional intake or interfere with the absorption, metabolism and excretion of nutrients (see Figure 3.13.1). A prime example is the antagonistic interaction of methotrexate with folate metabolism and its inherent side-effect of nausea. Prophylactic supplementation should be indicated as part of the mainstream management of these patients. Likewise, the long-term effects of steroids on calcium excretion, bone resorption, growth, body composition and nutritional intake are well recognised.

References

1. Gerasimidis K, McGrogan P, Edwards CA. The aetiology and impact of malnutrition in paediatric inflammatory bowel disease. *Journal of Human Nutrition and Dietetics* 2011; **24**(4): 313–326.

2. Lomer MC. Dietary and nutritional considerations for inflammatory bowel disease. *Proceedings of the Nutrition Society* 2011; **70**(3): 329–335.

3. Sawczenko A, Sandhu BK. Presenting features of inflammatory bowel disease in Great Britain and Ireland. *Archives of Disease in Childhood* 2003; **88**(11): 995–1000.

4. Kugathasan S, Nebel J, Skelton JA, et al. Body mass index in children with newly diagnosed inflammatory bowel disease: observations from two multicenter North American inception cohorts. *Journal of Pediatrics* 2007; **151**(5): 523–527.

5. Vasseur F, Gower-Rousseau C, Vernier-Massouille G, et al. Nutritional status and growth in pediatric Crohn's disease: a population-based study. *American Journal of Gastroenterology* 2010; **105**: 1893–1900.

6. Sousa GC, Cravo M, Costa AR, et al. A comprehensive approach to evaluate nutritional status in Crohn's patients in the era of biologic therapy: a case–control study. *American Journal of Gastroenterology* 2007; **102**(11): 2551–2556.

7. Thayu M, Shults J, Burnham JM, Zemel BS, Baldassano RN, Leonard MB. Gender differences in body composition deficits at diagnosis in children and adolescents with Crohn's disease. *Inflammatory Bowel Diseases* 2007; **13**(9): 1121–1128.

8. Sylvester FA, Leopold S, Lincoln M, Hyams JS, Griffiths AM, Lerer T. A two-year longitudinal study of persistent lean tissue deficits in children with Crohn's disease. *Clinical Gastroenterology and Hepatology* 2009; **7**(4): 452–455.

9. Williams JE, Wells JC, Wilson CM, Haroun D, Lucas A, Fewtrell MS. Evaluation of Lunar Prodigy dual-energy X-ray absorptiometry for assessing body composition in healthy persons and patients by comparison with the criterion 4-component model. *American Journal of Clinical Nutrition* 2006; **83**(5): 1047–1054.

10. Wiroth JB, Filippi J, Schneider SM, et al. Muscle performance in patients with Crohn's disease in clinical remission. *Inflammatory Bowel Diseases* 2005; **11**(3): 296–303.

11. Mauro M, Armstrong D. Juvenile onset of Crohn's disease: a risk factor for reduced lumbar bone mass in premenopausal women. *Bone* 2007; **40**(5): 1290–1293.

12. Van Staa TP, Cooper C, Brusse LS, Leufkens H, Javaid MK, Arden NK. Inflammatory bowel disease and the risk of fracture. *Gastroenterology* 2003; **125**(6): 1591–1597.

13. Card T, West J, Hubbard R, Logan RF. Hip fractures in patients with inflammatory bowel disease and their relationship to corticosteroid use: a population based cohort study. *Gut* 2004; **53**(2): 251–255.

14. Stockbrugger RW, Schoon EJ, Bollani S, et al. Discordance between the degree of osteopenia and the prevalence of spontaneous vertebral fractures in Crohn's disease. *Alimentary Pharmacology and Therapeutics* 2002; **16**(8): 1519–1527.

15. Habtezion A, Silverberg MS, Parkes R, Mikolainis S, Steinhart AH. Risk factors for low bone density in Crohn's disease. *Inflammatory Bowel Diseases* 2002; **8**(2): 87–92.

16. Semeao EJ, Jawad AF, Stouffer NO, Zemel BS, Piccoli DA, Stallings VA. Risk factors for low bone mineral density in children and young adults with Crohn's disease. *Journal of Pediatrics* 1999; **135**(5): 593–600.

17. Sentongo TA, Semeao EJ, Piccoli DA, Stallings VA, Zemel BS. Growth, body composition, and nutritional status in children and adolescents with Crohn's disease. *Journal of Pediatric Gastroenterology and Nutrition* 2000; **31**(1): 33–40.

18. Siffledeen JS, Fedorak RN, Siminoski K, et al. Bones and Crohn's: risk factors associated with low bone mineral density in patients with Crohn's disease. *Inflammatory Bowel Diseases* 2004; **10**(3): 220–228.

19. Schmidt S, Mellstrom D, Norjavaara E, Sundh V, Saalman R. Longitudinal assessment of bone mineral density in a population of children and adolescents with inflammatory bowel disease. *Journal of Pediatric Gastroenterology and Nutrition* 2012; **55**(5): 511–518.

20. Burnham JM, Shults J, Semeao E, et al. Whole body BMC in pediatric Crohn disease: independent effects of altered growth, maturation, and body composition. *Journal of Bone and Mineral Research* **2004**; 1912: 1961–1968.

21. Robinson RJ, Krzywicki T, Almond L, et al. Effect of a low-impact exercise program on bone mineral density in Crohn's disease: a randomized controlled trial. *Gastroenterology* 1998; **115**(1): 36–41.

22. Harris L, Senagore P, Young VB, McCabe LR. Inflammatory bowel disease causes reversible suppression of osteoblast and chondrocyte function in mice. *American Journal of Physiology - Gastrointestinal and Liver Physiology* 2009; **296**(5): G1020–G1029.

23. Boot AM, Bouquet J, Krenning EP, de Muinck Keizer-Schrama SM. Bone mineral density and nutritional status in children with chronic inflammatory bowel disease. *Gut* 1998; **42**(2): 188–194.

24. Targownik LE, Leslie WD, Carr R, et al. Longitudinal change in bone mineral density in a population-based cohort of patients with inflammatory bowel disease. *Calcified Tissue International* 2012; **91**(5): 356–363.

25. Hill RJ, Brookes DS, Lewindon PJ, et al. Bone health in children with inflammatory bowel disease: adjusting for bone age. *Journal of Pediatric Gastroenterology and Nutrition* 2009; **48**(5): 538–543.

26. Lee JJ, Escher JC, Shuman MJ, et al. Final adult height of children with inflammatory bowel disease is predicted by parental height and patient minimum height Z-score. *Inflammatory Bowel Diseases* 2010; **16**(10): 1669–1677.

27. Wong SC, Macrae VE, McGrogan P, Ahmed SF. The role of pro-inflammatory cytokines in inflammatory bowel disease growth retardation. *Journal of Pediatric Gastroenterology and Nutrition* 2006; **43**(2): 144–55.

28. Mason A, Malik S, Russell RK, Bishop J, McGrogan P, Ahmed SF. Impact of inflammatory bowel disease on pubertal growth. *Hormone Research in Paediatrics* 2011; **76**(5): 293–299.

29. Terranova PF, Rice VM. Review: cytokine involvement in ovarian processes. *American Journal of Reproductive Immunology* 1997; **37**(1): 50–63.

30. Leslie WD, Miller N, Rogala L, Bernstein CN. Vitamin D status and bone density in recently diagnosed inflammatory bowel disease: the Manitoba IBD Cohort Study. *American Journal of Gastroenterology* 2008; **103**(6): 1451–1459.

31. Alkhouri RH, Hashmi H, Baker RD, Gelfond D, Baker SS. Vitamin and mineral status in patients with inflammatory bowel disease. *Journal of Pediatric Gastroenterology and Nutrition* 2013; **56**(1): 89–92.

32. Galloway P, McMillan DC, Sattar N. Effect of the inflammatory response on trace element and vitamin status. *Annals of Clinical Biochemistry* 2000; **37**(Pt 3): 289–297.

33. Gerasimidis K, Talwar D, Duncan A, et al. Impact of exclusive enteral nutrition on body composition and circulating micronutrients in plasma and erythrocytes of children with active Crohn's disease. *Inflammatory Bowel Diseases* 2012; **18**(9): 1672–1681.

34. Lih-Brody L, Powell SR, Collier KP, et al. Increased oxidative stress and decreased antioxidant defenses in mucosa of inflammatory bowel disease. *Digestive Diseases and Sciences* 1996; **41**(10): 2078–2086.

35. Levy E, Rizwan Y, Thibault L, et al. Altered lipid profile, lipoprotein composition, and oxidant and antioxidant status in pediatric Crohn disease. *American Journal of Clinical Nutrition* 2000; **71**(3): 807–815.

36. Wendland BE, Aghdassi E, Tam C, et al. Lipid peroxidation and plasma antioxidant micronutrients in Crohn disease. *American Journal of Clinical Nutrition* 2001; **74**(2): 259–264.

37. Aghdassi E, Wendland BE, Steinhart AH, Wolman SL, Jeejeebhoy K, Allard JP. Antioxidant vitamin supplementation in Crohn's disease decreases oxidative stress. A randomized controlled trial. *American Journal of Gastroenterology* 2003; **98**(2): 348–353.

38. Wilson A, Reyes E, Ofman J. Prevalence and outcomes of anemia in inflammatory bowel disease: a systematic review of the literature. *American Journal of Medicine* 2004; **116**(Suppl 7A): 44S–49S.

39. Goodhand JR, Kamperidis N, Rao A, et al. Prevalence and management of anemia in children, adolescents, and adults with inflammatory bowel disease. *Inflammatory Bowel Diseases* 2012; **18**(3): 513–519.

40. Lomer MC, Kodjabashia K, Hutchinson C, Greenfield SM, Thompson RP, Powell JJ. Intake of dietary iron is low in patients with Crohn's disease: a case–control study. *British Journal of Nutrition* 2004; **91**(1): 141–148.

41. Semrin G, Fishman DS, Bousvaros A, et al. Impaired intestinal iron absorption in Crohn's disease correlates with disease activity and markers of inflammation. *Inflammatory Bowel Diseases* 2006; **12**(12): 1101–1106.

42. Lomer MC, Cook WB, Jan-Mohamed HJ, et al. Iron requirements based upon iron absorption tests are poorly predicted by haematological indices in patients with inactive inflammatory bowel disease. *British Journal of Nutrition* 2012; **107**(12): 1806–1811.

43. Weiss G, Goodnough LT. Anemia of chronic disease. *New England Journal of Medicine* 2005; **352**(10): 1011–1023.

44. Gasche C, Berstad A, Befrits R, et al. Guidelines on the diagnosis and management of iron deficiency and anemia in inflammatory bowel diseases. *Inflammatory Bowel Diseases* 2007; **13**(12): 1545–1553.

45. Thomson AB, Brust R, Ali MA, Mant MJ, Valberg LS. Iron deficiency in inflammatory bowel disease. Diagnostic efficacy of serum ferritin. *American Journal of Digestive Diseases* 1978; **23**(8): 705–709.

46. Oustamanolakis P, Koutroubakis IE. Soluble transferrin receptor-ferritin index is the most efficient marker for the diagnosis of iron deficiency anemia in patients with IBD. *Inflammatory Bowel Diseases* 2011; **17**(12): E158–E159.

47. Aghdassi E, Wendland BE, Stapleton M, Raman M, Allard JP. Adequacy of nutritional intake in a Canadian population of patients with Crohn's disease. *Journal of the American Dietetic Association* 2007; **107**(9): 1575–1580.

48. Filippi J, Al-Jaouni R, Wiroth JB, Hebuterne X, Schneider SM. Nutritional deficiencies in patients with Crohn's disease in remission. *Inflammatory Bowel Diseases* 2006; **12**(3): 185–191.

49. Thomas AG, Taylor F, Miller V. Dietary intake and nutritional treatment in childhood Crohn's disease. *Journal of Pediatric Gastroenterology and Nutrition* 1993; **17**(1): 75–81.

50. Pons R, Whitten KE, Woodhead H, Leach ST, Lemberg DA, Day AS. Dietary intakes of children with Crohn's disease. *British Journal of Nutrition* 2009; **102**(7): 1052–1057.

51. Gerasimidis K, McGrogan P, Hassan K, Edwards CA. Dietary modifications, nutritional supplements and alternative medicine in paediatric patients with inflammatory bowel disease. *Alimentary Pharmacology and Therapeutics* 2008; **27**(2): 155–165.

52. Moran GW, Leslie FC, McLaughlin JT. Crohn's disease affecting the small bowel is associated with reduced appetite and elevated levels of circulating gut peptides. *Clinical Nutrition* 2013; **32**(3): 404–411.

53. Azcue M, Rashid M, Griffiths A, Pencharz PB. Energy expenditure and body composition in children with Crohn's disease: effect of enteral nutrition and treatment with prednisolone. *Gut* 1997; **41**(2): 203–208.

54. Mingrone G, Greco AV, Benedetti G, et al. Increased resting lipid oxidation in Crohn's disease. *Digestive Diseases and Sciences* 1996; **41**(1): 72–76.

55. Al-Jaouni R, Hebuterne X, Pouget I, Rampal P. Energy metabolism and substrate oxidation in patients with Crohn's disease. *Nutrition* 2000; **16**(3): 173–178.

56. Mingrone G, Capristo E, Greco AV, et al. Elevated diet-induced thermogenesis and lipid oxidation rate in Crohn disease. *American Journal of Clinical Nutrition* 1999; **69**(2): 325–330.

57. Davie RJ, Hosie KB, Grobler SP, Newbury-Ecob RA, Keighley MR, Birch NJ. Ileal bile acid malabsorption in colonic Crohn's disease. *British Journal of Surgery* 1994; **81**(2): 289–290.

58. Vaisman N, Dotan I, Halack A, Niv E. Malabsorption is a major contributor to underweight in Crohn's disease patients in remission. *Nutrition* 2006; **22**(9): 855–859.

59. Winter TA, O'Keefe SJ, Callanan M, Marks T. Impaired gastric acid and pancreatic enzyme secretion in patients with Crohn's disease may be a consequenece of a poor nutritional state. *Inflammatory Bowel Diseases* 2004; **10**(5): 618–625.

60. Duerksen DR, Fallows G, Bernstein CN. Vitamin B12 malabsorption in patients with limited ileal resection. *Nutrition* 2006; **22**(11–12): 1210–1213.

61. Hengstermann S, Valentini L, Schaper L, et al. Altered status of antioxidant vitamins and fatty acids in patients with inactive inflammatory bowel disease. *Clinical Nutrition* 2008; **27**: 571–578.

62. D'Odorico A, Bortolan S, Cardin R, et al. Reduced plasma antioxidant concentrations and increased oxidative DNA damage in inflammatory bowel disease. *Scandinavian Journal of Gastroenterology* 2001; **36**: 1289–1294.

63. Geerling BJ, Badart-Smook A, Stockbrugger RW, Brummer RJ. Comprehensive nutritional status in recently diagnosed patients with inflammatory bowel disease compared with population controls. *European Journal of Clinical Nutrition* 2000; **54**: 514–521.

64. Geerling BJ, Badart-Smook A, Stockbrugger RW, Brummer RJ. Comprehensive nutritional status in patients with longstanding Crohn disease currently in remission. *American Journal of Clinical Nutrition* 1998; **67**: 919–926.

65. Ojuawo A, Keith L. The serum concentrations of zinc, copper and selenium in children with inflammatory bowel disease. *Central Africa Journal of Medicine* 2002; **48**: 116–119.

66. Levy E, Rizwan Y, Thibault L, et al. Altered lipid profile, lipoprotein composition, and oxidant and antioxidant status in pediatric Crohn disease. *American Journal of Clinical Nutrition* 2000; **71**: 807–815.

67. Bousvaros A, Zurakowski D, Duggan C, et al. Vitamins A and E serum levels in children and young adults with inflammatory bowel disease: effect of disease activity. *Journal of Pediatric Gastroenterology and Nutrition* 1998; **26**: 129–135.

68. Hoffenberg EJ, Deutsch J, Smith S, Sokol RJ. Circulating antioxidant concentrations in children with inflammatory bowel disease. *American Journal of Clinical Nutrition* 1997; **65**: 1482–1488.

Chapter 3.14

Inflammatory bowel disease dietary management

Maria O'Sullivan and Tara Raftery
Trinity College Dublin, Dublin, Ireland

3.14.1 Dietary management of Crohn's disease

Enteral nutrition in the treatment of Crohn's disease: active disease

Enteral nutrition (EN), in the form of an elemental diet, was shown to have a primary therapeutic effect in Crohn's disease in the early 1970s. An elemental diet provides nutrients in their simplest form – protein as amino acids, carbohydrate as glucose or short-chain maltodextrins and fat as short-chain triglycerides. Initially, elemental diets were used to nourish patients preoperatively and some of those who had Crohn's disease improved symptomatically, which suggested that this diet may have had a primary therapeutic effect [1,2]. In the 1980s, the first controlled trial confirmed that an elemental diet was as effective as corticosteroids in inducing clinical remission in active Crohn's disease [3]. Several subsequent studies supported this therapeutic effect for elemental diets and, furthermore, that this therapeutic effect could equally be achieved with less expensive and more palatable polymeric (whole protein) EN.

When the goal is primary therapy, EN is generally administered as the sole source of nutrition either orally or by nasogastric tube, ideally for a minimum of 4–6 weeks to allow for mucosal healing, although benefits have been shown from 10 days onwards [4]. Although protocols may differ, generally patients who fail to show a clinical response within 7–10 days are assigned to another therapeutic option [5]. The practicalities of this regimen and the motivation of the patient, who may have other therapeutic options, should be considered. Poor compliance typically results in poor outcome and overcoming the practical challenges of using EN in adults with Crohn's disease is important.

However, the critical question remains – what is the current evidence that EN is an effective therapy in Crohn's disease today? A number of meta-analyses [6,7] and a Cochrane review [8] now show that corticosteroids are more effective than EN in adults. Current guidelines mirror this (Table 3.14.1), recommending that EN is less effective than corticosteroids in inducing remission in Crohn's disease, but that it may be considered as a therapeutic option for adults in special circumstances, for example where other primary therapy may not be feasible [9] or for patients who decline drug therapy [14]. An overview of the guidelines and consensus statements for use of EN as therapy in Crohn's disease is summarised in Table 3.14.1.

The role of EN in the management of adult Crohn's disease in the future remains uncertain, particularly in an era of advanced drug therapies such as the biologics and newer anti-inflammatory agents. Moreover, in adults, guidelines recommend using EN in special circumstances only rather than as a generic therapy. Clearly, the role of EN in managing undernourished patients, or those at risk of undernutrition, is undisputed (Figure 3.14.1).

Advanced Nutrition and Dietetics in Gastroenterology, First Edition. Edited by Miranda Lomer.
© 2014 John Wiley & Sons, Ltd. Published 2014 by John Wiley & Sons, Ltd.

Table 3.14.1 Overview of guidelines for the provision of enteral nutrition as primary therapy in Crohn's disease

Author	Adults	Children
British Society of Gastroenterology 2004 [9]	After detailed discussion, EN may be used in preference to corticosteroids, immune modulators or surgery in any patient with active disease or for those unresponsive to mesalazine or in whom steroids are contraindicated.	EN is appropriate for growth failure in children or adolescents, with active small intestinal CD.
European Society for Clinical Nutrition and Metabolism (ESPEN) 2006 [10]	EN is effective in the treatment of active disease, but in adults corticosteroids are more effective. EN as sole therapy is indicated, therefore, mainly when treatment with corticosteroids is not feasible, e.g. due to intolerance or refusal.	In children with CD, EN is considered as first-line therapy.
Japanese Society for Pediatric Gastroenterology 2006 [11]		EN, in the form of an elemental formula, is indicated as primary therapy for children with CD at onset as well as the active disease (other than serious illness).
World Gastroenterology Global Guideline [12]		Exclusive EN can relieve CD, especially in children.
Guidelines for the Management of Inflammatory Bowel Disease in Children in the United Kingdom, 2010 [13]		Choice of treatment in most cases is between exclusive EN and oral corticosteroids. Exclusive EN is an effective first-line therapy for small and large intestinal disease, inducing remission in 60–80% of cases.
European Crohn's and Colitis Organisation 2010 [14]	Considered appropriate to offer EN as primary therapy only to patients who decline other drug therapy.	
Guidelines for the Management of Inflammatory Bowel Disease in Adults 2011 [15]	EN therapy alters the inflammatory response in CD and may be useful in therapy. There is little evidence to support use of EN as maintenance therapy for CD.	When used in children, EN is effective at inducing remission for small and large intestinal disease in 60–80%.
NICE Clinical Guideline on Crohn's Disease: Management in Children, Adults and Young People 2013 [16]	EN should not be used in adults to maintain remission after surgery.	Consider EN in children where growth or side-effects are a concern and in young people in whom there is a concern about growth.

EN, enteral nutrition (oral nutritional supplements or nasogastric feeding); CD, Crohn's disease.

Enteral nutrition in the treatment of active Crohn's disease in children

In children with Crohn's disease, the rationale for using EN as primary therapy is stronger than in adults. Enteral nutrition appears to have a therapeutic effect comparable to corticosteroids [17] in paediatric Crohn's disease as well as positive effects on growth and development [18–20]. In addition, EN may reduce the requirement for corticosteroids [21] and, consequently, their adverse

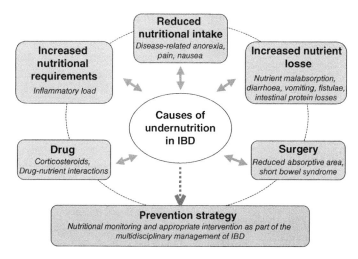

Figure 3.14.1 Causes of undernutrition in IBD, inflammatory bowel disease. Adapted from O'Sullivan [26].

long-term effects such as increased risk of osteoporosis. A meta-analysis [17] concluded that EN had similar efficacy to corticosteroids in children, but cautioned that this outcome was based on limited data. A Cochrane review of treatments for growth failure [19] highlighted the positive effect of EN in promoting growth in children with Crohn's disease. Disease location has been proposed to influence therapeutic response to EN, with paediatric colonic Crohn's disease suggested to respond poorly [22]; however, others have reported no differences in response rates based on disease phenotype [20,22]. Currently, EN is recommended as first-line therapy for active Crohn's disease for children, especially in those with growth failure (see Table 3.14.1).

Enteral nutrition in the treatment of active Crohn's disease: underlying mechanisms

The biological mechanisms underlying a therapeutic response to EN in Crohn's disease are not fully understood. There is evidence that EN promotes mucosal healing and downregulates mucosal pro-inflammatory cytokines [23,24]. Low antigenic load (absence of whole protein) was initially proposed to result in the therapeutic effect but whole protein enteral formulae have been shown to be as effective as the amino acid-based elemental diets [25]. Other

theories [26] suggest immunomodulatory effects of fats in the formula [27], changes in GI microbiota and changes in intestinal permeability. At present, the mechanisms underlying the therapeutic response to EN remain unclear, but there is renewed interest in the potential role of modification of the GI microbiota [28].

In summary, EN arguably offers a safe mode of delivery of potentially immune-modulating substrates directly to the intestinal mucosa. Judged in the context of the best evidence and consensus guidelines, EN is shown to be less effective than corticosteroids in adults but is an effective and important first-line therapy for children.

Enteral nutrition in the treatment of active Crohn's disease: adjunctive therapy for undernutrition

Enteral nutrition has an undisputed role as an adjunct therapy in the prevention and treatment of undernutrition in Crohn's disease. Undernutrition is multifactorial in origin (see Figure 3.14.1) [26] and may be present in over 40% of hospitalised patients with Crohn's disease [29]. Undernutrition is accepted to be associated with significantly higher mortality rates, longer hospital stays and higher healthcare costs. The correction and maintenance of nutritional status, achieved by careful nutritional monitoring and intervention, should be an integral part of the multidisciplinary management throughout all stages of the disease. Nutritional support (including EN, oral nutritional supplements and dietary counselling) is recommended for any malnourished patient with Crohn's disease or for patients with difficulty maintaining normal nutritional status (see Table 3.14.1). In the UK, for example, the IBD Standards Working Group states that all patients with inflammatory bowel disease (IBD) should have access to nutritional support services [30].

Parenteral nutrition in the treatment of active Crohn's disease

Although once advocated as a treatment for Crohn's disease [31], parenteral nutrition (PN) is not recommended as a primary therapy for Crohn's disease. Parenteral nutrition is reserved for use as nutritional support only when feeding into the GI tract is contraindicated or problematic. When the GI tract is functioning, the enteral route is preferred for the provision of nutritional support.

Enteral nutrition in the maintenance of remission in Crohn's disease

In children, the continued use of supplementary EN has been proposed as a strategy to maintain remission. Supplementary EN in addition to normal diet has been shown to prolong remission and improve linear growth in children who have achieved remission by exclusive EN [32].

In adults, data on supplementary EN for maintenance of remission in Crohn's disease are limited. A systematic review [24,33] of 10 studies reported that EN may be useful for maintaining remission in adults; however, the review highlighted that the evidence level was not high and there is a need for randomised controlled trials. An earlier Cochrane review [34] did not support a benefit of supplemental EN for maintaining remission. Current recommendations [14] suggest there is insufficient evidence to support supplementary EN for the maintenance of remission in adult Crohn's disease.

Exclusion diets in the maintenance of remission in Crohn's disease

Exclusion diets [29,35] were previously used as a therapeutic option for maintaining disease remission achieved with an elemental diet. These diets typically comprised limited foods with staged reintroduction of single foods over time. This approach requires considerable nutritional monitoring and input, and while specialist centres reported favourable clinical results, exclusion diets for the maintenance of remission have not become widely used or recommended by consensus guidelines.

An advance on these early exclusion diets for prolonging enteral diet-induced remission is a low-fat, fibre-limited exclusion (LOFFLEX) diet [36]. This diet is based on limiting the intake of both fat and fibre to approximately 50 g of fat and 10 g of non-starch polysaccharide (NSP) per day due to reported reduced tolerability of both in Crohn's disease. For the initial 2 weeks of the diet, foods thought unlikely to cause intolerance are permitted (Table 3.14.2) [36]; this can be increased to 4 weeks if needed [4]. Oral nutritional supplements may be stopped during this period, although they are useful if weight gain is required. Once symptoms are stable on a diet of 'safe' foods', the reintroduction programme begins with a new food introduced every 2–4 days and a nutritionally adequate diet of tolerated foods is built up. Overall, this process is shorter and likely to be more acceptable to patients than the classic elimination diet. However, evidence from well-designed randomised controlled trials (RCTs) of LOFFLEX diets in maintaining disease remission in Crohn's disease is lacking.

Dietary management of functional symptoms in Crohn's disease in remission

Symptoms similar to those experienced in functional bowel disorders, such as irritable bowel syndrome, are reportedly common in IBD in remission. These symptoms include abdominal bloating, abdominal pain, diarrhoea and flatulence, and may be experienced by up to

Table 3.14.2 The LOFFLEX exclusion diet: summary of foods allowed and not allowed

Foods not allowed	Foods allowed
Pork, meat products	All other lean meat and poultry
Fish in batter/crumb/tinned in oil/tomato	All other types of fish/shellfish
Cow/sheep/goat milk, dairy products, eggs, chocolate	Soya milk and products
	Rice, tapioca, sago, arrowroot
Wheat, rye, barley, corn, oats, yeast	Sunflower and olive oils in moderation
Corn and vegetable oil	Potato and all other vegetables, 2 portions a day, no skins/seeds
Pulses, onion, tomato, sweetcorn	
Citrus, apple, banana, dried fruit	All other fruit, 2 portions per day, no skins/seeds
Tea, coffee, alcohol, squash, cola	Fruit/herbal teas, water, Ribena, non-citrus fruit juice

Adapted from Woolner [36].

60% of Crohn's disease patients in remission [37]. It is difficult, however, to determine if such symptoms are functional or are a manifestation of the underlying Crohn's disease. A diet low in fermentable oligosaccharides, disaccharides, monosaccharides and polyols (FODMAP)s has been proposed for the management of functional symptoms in IBD in remission [38,39]. The term 'FODMAP' is used to describe short-chain carbohydrates which are incompletely digested, poorly absorbed and fermentable in the GI tract [38,39]. Consequently, this contributes to increased fluid and gas production in the GI tract which is proposed to lead to, or aggravate, functional symptoms in susceptible individuals [40].

A low FODMAP diet has been more extensively studied in the context of irritable bowel syndrome, where there is RCT evidence of efficacy in symptom control [41] (see Chapter 3.19). Proposed benefits in Crohn's disease have been suggested [38,39] but currently the evidence is limited. In a retrospective study, Gearry et al. reported that approximately one in two patients described improvements in abdominal pain, bloating and diarrhoea [38]. Benefit, however, was significantly associated with compliance and a reported 70% of patients were able to comply with the low FODMAP diet [38]. Further evidence is required to determine the efficacy and role of a low FODMAP diet in managing symptoms in Crohn's disease during remission.

Other dietary treatments of Crohn's disease

Probiotics

Treatments targeted at manipulating the microbiota such as pro-, pre- and symbiotics have been investigated in IBD [42], often with a view to maintaining remission. In a Cochrane review, Rolfe et al. reported no significant benefit of probiotics for maintaining either surgically or medically induced remission in Crohn's disease [43]. Although probiotics remain a strong area of interest, based on the current evidence they are not considered an effective treatment in Crohn's disease [44] to induce [45] or maintain remission [43,46] or to prevent postoperative disease recurrence [47]. Similarly, there is no evidence to support the efficacy of prebiotics [48]. Interestingly, there is emerging evidence relating to symbiotics (combined use of probiotics and prebiotics) in active Crohn's disease, with a RCT suggesting significant improvement in clinical symptoms in patients taking the symbiotic [49] but these findings have yet to be confirmed.

To date, there is insufficient evidence to support the efficacy of prebiotics, probiotics or symbiotic as therapies for Crohn's disease in clinical practice [14,50]. Given the strong research and commercial interest in manipulating the microbiome, this is likely to continue to be an area of research into the future.

Omega-3 fatty acids

Anti-inflammatory effects of omega-3 (n-3) polyunsaturated fatty acids, including fish oils, have been demonstrated in animal models of IBD [51]. Several studies have investigated the therapeutic effects of omega-3 fatty acids in Crohn's disease, but report inconsistent findings. A Cochrane review [52] and further pooled analyses [53,54], however, do not support their use either for maintaining remission or for treating active disease. Although safe for use in Crohn's disease [52], current guidelines do not recommend the use of omega-3 fatty acids for the treatment of this disease [14].

Emerging treatments

The potential anti-inflammatory effects of vitamin D are emerging across several chronic diseases, including Crohn's disease [55,56]. A RCT showed a non-significant reduction in relapse rates in patients with Crohn's disease treated with 1200 IU vitamin D compared with placebo (relapse 13% versus 29%, P=0.06) [57]. This finding remains inconclusive and requires investigation in further large RCTs.

Malnutrition and maintenance of remission

While weight loss and undernutrition during active Crohn's disease may be expected, the nutritional status of patients in disease remission is less clear. It would appear, however, that an increase in Body Mass Index (BMI) and the presence of overweight are the major forms of malnutrition in adults in remission [58,59]. In children with Crohn's disease, a similar picture is emerging, with most (68%) classed with a BMI in the normal range and 10% as overweight or at risk for overweight [60]. Whether this presence of overweight and obesity in Crohn's disease is associated with more severe disease [61,62] or, in contrast, is a reflection of well-controlled disease [59] is unclear. How this adiposity interacts with a background of inflammation and contributes to long-term co-morbidity and complications remains to be seen, but one may expect implications for obesity-related diseases such as cardiovascular disease and colorectal cancer. Thus,

in the future, managing excess body weight may need to be considered in the context of managing malnutrition in Crohn's disease in remission.

The patient perspective of dietary treatments in Crohn's disease

There is often considerable confusion among people living with IBD about the role of diet and nutrition in the management of their condition. Not surprisingly, foods or even eating a meal may aggravate symptoms, yet have no role in either the initiation or treatment of Crohn's disease. Some people may exclude foods and follow unnecessarily restricted diets with the risk of an adverse effect on nutritional status. A recent study confirmed that patients consider dietary issues as important, with 63% rating diet as either 'important' or 'extremely important' in their experience of IBD [63]. While the majority (82%) reported issues with food and nutrition, fewer than half had seen a dietitian for tailored nutritional counselling to address these issues and concerns.

Dietary management in complex Crohn's disease

Patients with intractable Crohn's disease, disease complications, surgical resections or short bowel syndrome will typically have more complex nutritional needs. This may include more complex EN and PN strategies as well as more complex medical and surgical management. Nutritional intervention and support are essential in the presence of short bowel syndrome [64] (see Chapters 3.16 and 3.17). The UK IBD Standards Group recommends that a multidisciplinary nutrition support team should be available for those patients who may require more complex EN and/or PN and for comprehensive assessment, management and ongoing support [30].

Diet may provide symptomatic relief from some Crohn's disease complications. For example, in stricturing disease, limiting fibrous foods is useful to minimise the risk of mechanical obstruction and to reduce pain. Bile acid malabsorption and bile acid-induced diarrhoea may occur after resection of the terminal ileum; in these cases patients may benefit from a reduction in long-chain fatty acids and the use of bile salt-binding agents such as cholestyramine.

3.14.2 Dietary management of ulcerative colitis

In contrast to Crohn's disease, there is limited evidence that dietary approaches are successful in inducing or maintaining remission in ulcerative colitis (UC). The role of diet and nutrition, therefore, is essential to prevent and treat malnutrition and promote optimal nutritional status in this disease.

Enteral and parenteral nutrition in the treatment of ulcerative colitis

Enteral nutrition does not have a primary therapeutic role in UC, either in inducing or maintaining remission (see Table 3.14.1). Enteral nutrition continues to have a role in the provision of nutritional support and the management and prevention of undernutrition (see Figure 3.14.1) as appropriate. Similarly, there is no role for PN as a primary therapy for UC; its use is for nutritional support

where indicated, and then only in cases where feeding into the GI tract is contraindicated.

Beyond primary treatment, EN has an important adjunctive role in the prevention and treatment of undernutrition in UC. Nutritional support is recommended for any undernourished patient with UC or for patients who have difficulty maintaining normal nutritional status (Table 3.14.3), and access to appropriate nutritional support services is recommended [30].

Diet in the maintenance of remission in ulcerative colitis

Strategies that may have a role in maintaining remission in Crohn's disease, such as LOFFLEX and exclusion diets, have no proven role in UC. A diet low in FODMAPs has also been proposed for the management of functional symptoms that may occur during inactive UC [38] although evidence supporting this is limited. Gearry et al. have suggested significant improvements in abdominal

Table 3.14.3 Summary of the dietary management of Crohn's disease (CD) and ulcerative colitis (UC)

Therapy	CD	UC	Comments
EN as primary therapy	Yes	No	In CD, a priority treatment in children. Adults, limited to specific cases only.
EN as maintenance therapy	Consider in children	No	In children, because of role in nutrition and growth.
PN as primary therapy	No	No	As nutritional support and only when EN is not possible.
LOFFLEX	Consider	No	Can be considered for maintenance of remission in CD. Further long-term evidence and consensus guidelines required.
Probiotics	No	No+	+Evidence for use in pouchitis which may be a surgical complication of UC.
Low FODMAP diet	Possible	Possible	No therapeutic effect. Possible benefit in managing functional symptoms in CD and UC.
Omega-3 fatty acids	No	No	Conflicting evidence in maintenance of remission in CD. Insufficient evidence to recommend use.
Nutritional support, including EN, as adjunctive therapy	Yes	Yes	Use as appropriate for nutritional support in the prevention and management of undernutrition in adults and children and at all stages of UC and CD.

symptoms for patients with UC in remission but the study included only 20 patients with this disease [38]. In more complex UC, a reduced FODMAP diet appears to improve stool frequency in patients with an ileal pouch [65] and improve output in those with ileostomies [40].

Probiotics in the treatment of ulcerative colitis

The use of probiotics in the treatment of UC remains inconclusive [66,67] but appears to be more promising than in Crohn's disease. There is evidence for their use as an adjunct therapy to decrease disease activity [68] with suggested comparable efficacy to anti-inflammatory drugs for achieving remission [69]. Consensus for the use of probiotics to maintain or induce remission is classed as 'C' rated evidence [70], highlighting that the evidence remains inconsistent.

In pouchitis, which occurs in up to 60% of patients with UC after ileal pouch anal anastomosis, favourable outcomes are reported for the use of probiotics in preventing pouchitis [71] and maintaining remission [72,73]. The probiotic most extensively investigated for pouchitis is VSL#3, a proprietary blend of eight bacterial strains. A recent meta-analysis of probiotics in GI diseases [74] showed convincing evidence in favour of probiotic treatment in pouchitis (risk ratio 0.17, 95% confidence interval (CI) 0.10–0.30). Clinical practice guidelines now include probiotics as a therapeutic option for recurrent and relapsing antibiotic sensitive pouchitis [75].

Dietary treatment of ulcerative colitis: the patient perspective

Although nutrition plays a lesser role as a potential primary therapy in UC than in Crohn's disease, patients consider it important [63] and may restrict specific foods or food groups to control symptoms. Many, however, do not appear to receive specific professional nutritional counselling or education to address their dietary concerns and issues [63], a feature similarly reported for Crohn's disease.

3.14.3 Conclusion: role of dietary treatment in inflammatory bowel disease

A therapy such as EN that provides both disease-modifying and nutritional benefits in IBD is an attractive proposition. While EN has the capacity to induce remission in at least some patients with Crohn's disease, other therapeutic strategies are now shown to be superior in adults. But the combined growth and disease-modifying effects confer stronger therapeutic benefits for use of EN in children (see Table 3.14.1) with Crohn's disease. In contrast, EN does not have a proven role as primary therapy in UC.

Newer nutritional approaches may have anti-inflammatory potential in IBD. Developing an evidence base for whole-diet approaches to managing IBD is more complex, but worthy of investigation. Future novel dietary therapies, however, are likely to be combined approaches with drug therapy rather than as monotherapy, and all approaches will require appropriate investigation in well-designed intervention studies.

Irrespective of primary therapy, nutrition has an undisputed role in preventing and treating undernutrition in IBD throughout all stages of the disease.

References

1. Voitk AJ, Echave V, Feller JH, Brown RA, Gurd FN.. Experience with elemental diet in the treatment of inflammatory bowel disease. Is this primary therapy? *Archives of Surgery* 1973; **107**: 329–333.
2. Fischer JE, Foster GS, Abel RM, Abbott WM, Ryan JA. Hyperalimentation as primary therapy for inflammatory bowel disease. *American Journal of Surgery* 1973; **125**: 165–175.
3. O'Moráin C, Segal AW, Levi AJ. Elemental diet as primary treatment of acute Crohn's disease: a controlled trial. *British Medical Journal (Clinical Research Ed)* 1984; **288**: 1859–1862.
4. Lee J, Allen R, Ashley S, et al. *Evidence-based Practice Guidelines for the Dietetic Management of Crohn's Disease in Adults.* Birmingham: British Dietetic Association, 2011.
5. Teahon K, Pearson M, Levi AJ, Bjarnason I. Practical aspects of enteral nutrition in the management of Crohn's disease. *Journal of Parenteral and Enteral Nutrition* 1995; **19**: 365–368.
6. Fernández-Banares F, Cabré E, Esteve-Comas M, Gassull MA. How effective is enteral nutrition in inducing clinical remission in active Crohn's disease? A meta-analysis of the randomized

clinical trials. *Journal of Parenteral and Enteral Nutrition* 1995; **19**: 356–364.

7. Messori A, Trallori G, d'Albasio G, Milla M, Vannozzi G, Pacini F. Defined-formula diets versus steroids in the treatment of active Crohn's disease: a meta-analysis. *Scandinavian Journal of Gastroenterology* 1996; **31**: 267–272.

8. Zachos M, Tondeur M, Griffiths AM. Enteral nutritional therapy for induction of remission in Crohn's disease. *Cochrane Database of Systematic Reviews* 2007; **1**: CD000542.

9. Carter MJ, Lobo AJ, Travis SP, IBD Section. Guidelines for the management of inflammatory bowel disease in adults. *Gut* 2004; **53**(Suppl 5): V1–V16.

10. Lochs H, Dejong C, Hammarqvist F, et al. ESPEN Guidelines on Enteral Nutrition: Gastroenterology. *Clinical Nutrition* 2006; **25**: 260–274.

11. Konno M, Kobayashi A, Tomomasa T, et al. Guidelines for the treatment of Crohn's disease in children. *Pediatrics International* 2006; **48**: 349–352.

12. Bernstein CN, Fried M, Krabshuis JH, et al. *Inflammatory Bowel Disease: A Global Perspective*. Milwaukee, WI: World Gastroenterology Organisation Global Guidelines, 2009.

13. Sandhu B, Fell J, Beattie R, Mitton SG, Wilson D, Jenkins H. Guidelines for the management of inflammatory bowel disease in children in the United Kingdom. *Journal of Pediatric Gastroenterology and Nutrition* 2010; **50**: 1–13.

14. Dignass A, van Assche G, Lindsay JO, et al. The second European evidence-based consensus on the diagnosis and management of Crohn's disease: current management. *Journal of Crohn's and Colitis* 2010; **4**: 28–62.

15. Mowat C, Cole A, Windsor A, et al. Guidelines for the management of inflammatory bowel disease in adults. *Gut* 2011; **60**: 571–607.

16. Mayberry JF, Lobo A, Ford AC, Thomas A. NICE clinical guideline (CG152): the management of Crohn's disease in adults, children and young people. *Alimentary Pharmacology and Therapeutics* 2013; **37**: 195–203.

17. Dziechciarz P, Horvath A, Shamir R, Szajewska H. Meta-analysis: enteral nutrition in active Crohn's disease in children. *Alimentary Pharmacology and Therapeutics* 2007; **26**: 795–806.

18. Day AS, Whitten KE, Sidler M, Lemberg DA. Systematic review: nutritional therapy in paediatric Crohn's disease. *Alimentary Pharmacology and Therapeutics* 2008; **27**: 293–307.

19. Newby EA, Sawczenko A, Thomas AG, Wilson D. Interventions for growth failure in childhood Crohn's disease. *Cochrane Database of Systematic Reviews* 2005; **20**(3): CD003873.

20. Buchanan E, Gaunt WW, Cardigan T, Garrick V, McGrogan P, Russell RK. The use of exclusive enteral nutrition for induction of remission in children with Crohn's disease demonstrates that disease phenotype does not influence clinical remission. *Alimentary Pharmacology and Therapeutics* 2009; **30**: 501–507.

21. Knight C, El-Matary W, Spray C, Sandhu BK. Long-term outcome of nutritional therapy in paediatric Crohn's disease. *Clinical Nutrition* 2005; **24**: 775–779.

22. Afzal NA, Davies S, Paintin M, et al. Colonic Crohn's disease in children does not respond well to treatment with enteral

nutrition if the ileum is not involved. *Digestive Diseases and Sciences* 2005; **50**: 1471–1475.

23. Fell JM, Paintin M, Arnaud-Battandier F, et al. Mucosal healing and a fall in mucosal pro-inflammatory cytokine mRNA induced by a specific oral polymeric diet in paediatric Crohn's disease. *Alimentary Pharmacology and Therapeutics* 2000; **14**: 281–289.

24. Yamamoto T, Nakahigashi M, Umegae S, Kitagawa T, Matsumoto K. Impact of long-term enteral nutrition on clinical and endoscopic recurrence after resection for Crohn's disease: a prospective, non-randomized, parallel, controlled study. *Alimentary Pharmacology and Therapeutics* 2007; **25**: 67–72.

25. Verma S, Brown S, Kirkwood B, Giaffer MH. Polymeric versus elemental diet as primary treatment in active Crohn's disease: a randomized, double-blind trial. *American Journal of Gastroenterology* 2000; **95**: 735–739.

26. O'Sullivan M. Symposium on 'The challenge of translating nutrition research into public health nutrition'. Session 3: Joint Nutrition Society and Irish Nutrition and Dietetic Institute Symposium on 'Nutrition and autoimmune disease'. Nutrition in Crohn's disease. *Proceedings of the Nutrition Society* 2009; **68**: 127–134.

27. Gassull MA, Fernández-Banares F, Cabré E, et al. Fat composition may be a clue to explain the primary therapeutic effect of enteral nutrition in Crohn's disease: results of a double blind randomised multicentre European trial. *Gut* 2002; **51**: 164–168.

28. Levine A, Wine E. Effects of enteral nutrition on Crohn's disease: clues to the impact of diet on disease pathogenesis. *Inflammatory Bowel Diseases* 2013; **19**(6): 1322–1329.

29. Pirlich M, Schutz T, Kemps M, et al. Prevalence of malnutrition in hospitalized medical patients: impact of underlying disease. *Digestive Diseases* 2003; **21**: 245–251.

30. IBD Standards Working Group. *Quality Care: Service Standards for the Healthcare of People who have Inflammatory Bowel Disease (IBD)*. St Albans: IBD Standards Working Group, 2009.

31. Greenberg GR, Fleming CR, Jeejeebhoy KN, Rosenberg IH, Sales D, Tremaine WJ. Controlled trial of bowel rest and nutritional support in the management of Crohn's disease. *Gut* 1988; **29**: 1309–1315.

32. Wilschanski M, Sherman P, Pencharz P, Davis L, Corey M, Griffiths A. Supplementary enteral nutrition maintains remission in paediatric Crohn's disease. *Gut* 1996; **38**: 543–548.

33. Yamamoto T, Nakahigashi M, Umegae S, Matsumoto K. Enteral nutrition for the maintenance of remission in Crohn's disease: a systematic review. *European Journal of Gastroenterology and Hepatology* 2010; **22**: 1–8.

34. Akobeng AK, Thomas AG. Enteral nutrition for maintenance of remission in Crohn's disease. *Cochrane Database of Systematic Reviews* 2007; **18**(3): CD005984.

35. Riordan AM, Hunter JO, Cowan RE, et al. Treatment of active Crohn's disease by exclusion diet: East Anglian multicentre controlled trial. *Lancet* 1993; **342**: 1131–1134.

36. Woolner JT, Parker TJ, Kirby JA, et al. The development and evaluation of a diet for maintaining remission in Crohn's disease. *Journal of Human Nutrition and Dietetics* 1998; **11**(1): 1–11.

37. Keohane J, O'Mahony C, O'Mahony L, O'Mahony S, Quigley EM, Shanahan F. Irritable bowel syndrome-type symptoms in patients with inflammatory bowel disease: a real association or reflection of occult inflammation? *American Journal of Gastroenterology* 2010; **105**: 1788, 1789–1794.

38. Gearry RB, Irving PM, Barrett JS, Nathan DM, Shepherd SJ, Gibson PR. Reduction of dietary poorly absorbed short-chain carbohydrates (FODMAPs) improves abdominal symptoms in patients with inflammatory bowel disease – a pilot study. *Journal of Crohn's and Colitis* 2009; **3**: 8–14.

39. Gibson PR, Shepherd SJ. Personal view: food for thought – western lifestyle and susceptibility to Crohn's disease. The FODMAP hypothesis. *Alimentary Pharmacology and Therapeutics* 2005; **21**: 1399–1409.

40. Barrett JS, Gearry RB, Muir JG, et al. Dietary poorly absorbed, short-chain carbohydrates increase delivery of water and fermentable substrates to the proximal colon. *Alimentary Pharmacology and Therapeutics* 2010; **31**: 874–882.

41. Staudacher HM, Lomer MC, Anderson JL, et al. Fermentable carbohydrate restriction reduces luminal bifidobacteria and gastrointestinal symptoms in patients with irritable bowel syndrome. *Journal of Nutrition* 2012; **142**: 1510–1518.

42. Xavier RJ, Podolsky DK. Unravelling the pathogenesis of inflammatory bowel disease. *Nature* 2007; **448**: 427–434.

43. Rolfe VE, Fortun PJ, Hawkey CJ, Bath-Hextall F. Probiotics for maintenance of remission in Crohn's disease. *Cochrane Database of Systematic Reviews* 2006; **18**(4): CD004826.

44. Jonkers D, Penders J, Masclee A, Pierik M. Probiotics in the management of inflammatory bowel disease: a systematic review of intervention studies in adult patients. *Drugs* 2012; **72**: 803–823.

45. Butterworth AD, Thomas AG, Akobeng AK. Probiotics for induction of remission in Crohn's disease. *Cochrane Database of Systematic Reviews* 2008; **16**(3): CD006634.

46. Rahimi R, Nikfar S, Rahimi F, et al. A meta-analysis on the efficacy of probiotics for maintenance of remission and prevention of clinical and endoscopic relapse in Crohn's disease. *Digestive Diseases and Sciences* 2008; **53**: 2524–2531.

47. Doherty G, Bennett G, Patil S, Cheifetz A, Moss AC. Interventions for prevention of post-operative recurrence of Crohn's disease. *Cochrane Database of Systematic Reviews* 2009; **7**(4): CD006873.

48. Benjamin JL, Hedin CR, Koutsoumpas A, et al. Randomised, double-blind, placebo-controlled trial of fructo-oligosaccharides in active Crohn's disease. *Gut* 2011; **60**: 923–929.

49. Steed H, Macfarlane GT, Blackett KL, et al. Clinical trial: the microbiological and immunological effects of synbiotic consumption – a randomized double-blind placebo-controlled study in active Crohn's disease. *Alimentary Pharmacology and Therapeutics* 2010; **32**: 872–883.

50. Shanahan F, Collins SM. Pharmabiotic manipulation of the microbiota in gastrointestinal disorders, from rationale to reality. *Gastroenterology Clinics of North America* 2010; **39**: 721–726.

51. Liu Y, Chen F, Odle J, et al. Fish oil enhances intestinal integrity and inhibits TLR4 and NOD2 signalling pathways in weaned pigs after LPS challenge. *Journal of Nutrition* 2012; **142**: 2017–2024.

52. Turner D, Zlotkin SH, Shah PS, Griffiths AM. Omega 3 fatty acids (fish oil) for maintenance of remission in Crohn's disease. *Cochrane Database of Systematic Reviews* 2009; **1**: CD006320.

53. Cabré E, Manosa M, Gassull MA. Omega-3 fatty acids and inflammatory bowel diseases – a systematic review. *British Journal of Nutrition* 2012; **107**(Suppl 2): S240–S252.

54. Marion-Letellier R, Savoye G, Beck PL, Panaccione R, Ghosh S. Polyunsaturated fatty acids in inflammatory bowel diseases: a reappraisal of effects and therapeutic approaches. *Inflammatory Bowel Diseases* 2013; **19**: 650–661.

55. Cantorna MT. Vitamin D, multiple sclerosis and inflammatory bowel disease. *Archives of Biochemistry and Biophysics* 2012; **523**: 103–106.

56. Raftery T, O'Morain CA, O'Sullivan M. Vitamin D: new roles and therapeutic potential in inflammatory bowel disease. *Current Drug Metabolism* 2012; **13**: 1294–1302.

57. Jorgensen SP, Agnholt J, Glerup H, et al. Clinical trial: vitamin D3 treatment in Crohn's disease – a randomized double-blind placebo-controlled study. *Alimentary Pharmacology and Therapeutics* 2010; **32**: 377–383.

58. Sousa Guerreiro C, Cravo M, Costa AR, et al. A comprehensive approach to evaluate nutritional status in Crohn's patients in the era of biologic therapy: a case–control study. *American Journal of Gastroenterology* 2007; **102**: 2551–2556.

59. Nic Suibhne T, Raftery TC, McMahon O, Walsh C, O'Morain C, O'Sullivan M. High prevalence of overweight and obesity in adults with Crohn's disease: associations with disease and lifestyle factors. *Journal of Crohn's and Colitis* 2012; **7**(7): e241–e248.

60. Kugathasan S, Nebel J, Skelton JA, et al. Body mass index in children with newly diagnosed inflammatory bowel disease: observations from two multicenter North American inception cohorts. *Journal of Pediatrics* 2007; **151**: 523–527.

61. Blain A, Cattan S, Beaugerie L, Carbonnel F, Gendre JP, Cosnes J.. Crohn's disease clinical course and severity in obese patients. *Clinical Nutrition* 2002; **21**: 51–57.

62. Hass DJ, Brensinger CM, Lewis JD, Lichtenstein GR. The impact of increased body mass index on the clinical course of Crohn's disease. *Clinical Gastroenterology and Hepatology* 2006; **4**: 482–488.

63. Prince A, Whelan K, Moosa A, Lomer MC, Reidlinger DP. Nutritional problems in inflammatory bowel disease: the patient perspective. *Journal of Crohn's and Colitis* 2011; **5**: 443–450.

64. O'Keefe SJ, Buchman AL, Fishbein TM, Jeejeebhoy KN, Jeppesen PB, Shaffer J. Short bowel syndrome and intestinal failure: consensus definitions and overview. *Clinical Gastroenterology and Hepatology* 2006; **4**: 6–10.

65. Croagh C, Shepherd SJ, Berryman M, Muir JG, Gibson PR. Pilot study on the effect of reducing dietary FODMAP intake on bowel function in patients without a colon. *Inflammatory Bowel Diseases* 2007; **13**: 1522–1528.

66. Sang LX, Chang B, Zhang WL, Wu XM, Li XH, Jiang M. Remission induction and maintenance effect of probiotics on ulcerative colitis: a meta-analysis. *World Journal of Gastroenterology* 2010; **16**: 1908–1915.

67. Naidoo K, Gordon M, Fagbemi AO, Thomas AG, Akobeng AK. Probiotics for maintenance of remission in ulcerative

colitis. *Cochrane Database of Systematic Reviews* 2011; **7**(12): CD007443.

68. Mallon P, McKay D, Kirk S, Gardiner K. Probiotics for induction of remission in ulcerative colitis. *Cochrane Database of Systematic Reviews* 2007; **17**(4): CD005573.

69. Zigra PI, Maipa VE, Alamanos YP. Probiotics and remission of ulcerative colitis: a systematic review. *Netherlands Journal of Medicine* 2007; **65**: 411–418.

70. Floch MH, Walker WA, Madsen K, et al.. Recommendations for probiotic use – 2011 update. *Journal of Clinical Gastroenterology* 2011; **45**(Suppl): S168–S171.

71. Elahi B, Nikfar S, Derakhshani S, Vafaie M, Abdollahi M. On the benefit of probiotics in the management of pouchitis in patients underwent ileal pouch anal anastomosis: a meta-analysis of controlled clinical trials. *Digestive Diseases and Sciences* 2008; **53**: 1278–1284.

72. Gionchetti P, Rizzello F, Helwig U, et al. Prophylaxis of pouchitis onset with probiotic therapy: a double-blind, placebo-controlled trial. *Gastroenterology* 2003; **124**: 1202–1209.

73. Shen B, Brzezinski A, Fazio VW, et al. Maintenance therapy with a probiotic in antibiotic-dependent pouchitis: experience in clinical practice. *Alimentary Pharmacology and Therapeutics* 2005; **22**: 721–728.

74. Ritchie ML, Romanuk TN.. A meta-analysis of probiotic efficacy for gastrointestinal diseases. *PLoS One* 2012; **7**: e34938.

75. Pardi DS, d'Haens G, Shen B, Campbell S, Gionchetti P. Clinical guidelines for the management of pouchitis. *Inflammatory Bowel Diseases* 2009; **15**: 1424–1431.

Chapter 3.15

Lactose malabsorption and nutrition

Pascale Gerbault, Anke Liebert, Dallas M. Swallow and Mark G. Thomas
University College London, London, UK

The consumption of milk and dairy products varies considerably in different regions of the world. Indeed, according to the statistics of the Food and Agriculture Organization of the United Nations (FAO), in 2007 the consumption of milk and dairy products averaged 240 kg and 360 kg per capita in the UK and Sweden, respectively, while in China it was about 29 kg per capita. Milk is a complex and nutrient-dense food [1] that may have positive or negative effects on adult health [2]. The major carbohydrate component in milk is lactose, a disaccharide whose concentration in bovine milk has been reported to range between 45 and 55 g/L [2–4]. Lactose needs to be digested by the small intestinal enzyme lactase into its constituent monosaccharides, glucose and galactose, before transport across the epithelial cell membranes.

Lactase activity is therefore essential for the development of young mammals, since their sole source of nourishment is their mother's milk. In most mammals, including most humans, lactase expression decreases after the weaning period is over [5]. In humans, this condition is termed lactase non-persistence and is observed in around 65% of adults worldwide [6,7]. Lactase non-persistent individuals are sometimes described as having primary adult hypolactasia and are lactose maldigesters, while adults who have the genetically determined trait of lactase persistence (LP) and continue to produce lactase throughout life are termed lactose digesters.

The range of timing of lactase downregulation varies from one population to another; for example, most Chinese and Japanese become lactase non-persistent between 1 and 5 years old, while on average lactase non-persistence does not manifest in Finns and Estonians until somewhat later [8]. Even though the mechanisms of developmental lactase downregulation are not well understood, it is clear that it is not reversible [9,10]. Lactase production can also be lost through non-genetic mechanisms; this is called secondary hypolactasia and it can occur, for example, after any condition that damages the small intestinal mucosa brush border [11]. Adults with either primary or secondary hypolactasia are lactose malabsorbers and may exhibit symptoms of lactose intolerance after ingestion of lactose. Genetically determined lactase non-persistence is quite normal in the majority of humans worldwide and is distinct from congenital alactasia, the absence of lactase from birth. This, in contrast, is an extremely rare and potentially fatal condition. A number of mutations that affect the structure of the protein, and consequently its function, have been identified in Finnish patients suffering from this condition [12,13].

Two types of tests are available for determining lactase production status at the phenotypic level. Duodenal or jejunal biopsies can be taken by endoscopy and allow direct determination of lactase activity. A lactase assay is usually combined with routine histology and an assay of another enzyme such as sucrase, so that secondary deficiency of lactase can be readily identified. This procedure is the most accurate available, but it is invasive and performed routinely only if a pathological condition such as coeliac disease is indicated. Other methods

Advanced Nutrition and Dietetics in Gastroenterology, First Edition. Edited by Miranda Lomer.
© 2014 John Wiley & Sons, Ltd. Published 2014 by John Wiley & Sons, Ltd.

involve lactose ingestion after an overnight fast to inform indirectly on lactase activity [14]. For the glucose test, an increase in blood glucose is indicative of LP as lactase cleaves lactose into glucose and galactose. Although less commonly used for identifying LP, a urinary galactose test can also be performed, which also involves giving alcohol to block galactose uptake by the liver. Alternatively, the breath hydrogen test measures hydrogen production by colonic bacteria; in lactase non-persistent individuals, undigested lactose reaches the colon and hydrogen is released after fermentation by hydrogen-producing colonic bacteria, while in persistent individuals lactose is cleaved before reaching the colon. These tests require a baseline measurement of glucose, galactose or breath hydrogen before ingestion of the lactose load, and further measurements of the same at about 30-min intervals for 2–3 h. It should be noted that these indirect tests are not 100% accurate (error rates are discussed in Mulcare et al. [15]) and cannot distinguish primary from secondary hypolactasia. For example, there are some individuals who do not have colonic bacteria that produce hydrogen, and therefore do not show a hydrogen rise irrespective of their lactase production status.

The passage of lactose into the colon in non-lactase producers can lead to GI symptoms, such as bloating, flatulence, abdominal pain and diarrhoea. These symptoms are described as 'lactose intolerance'. Lactose intolerance should be distinguished from milk allergy; while the former is a non-toxic and non-immune adverse reaction to undigested lactose, milk allergy involves an immune response, usually to milk protein.

After an individual has been diagnosed as lactase non-persistent, dairy products are often removed from the diet. This may have serious nutritional disadvantages, such as reducing the intake of calcium, phosphorus and vitamins, and may be associated with decreased bone mineral density [2,16,17], while lactose-free milk products intake would avoid symptoms and be nutritious. In contrast, milk powder (which does contain lactose) has been used for famine relief in undernourished populations where the frequency of LP is often very low [18,19] and for whom symptoms of intolerance can potentially exacerbate diarrhoeal disease and mineral deficiency [18,20,21].

3.15.1 Lactase persistence

This section briefly summarises what is known about the genetics and evolution of the LP trait, but further details and references can be found in Gerbault et al. [22] and on the global lactase persistence database website (www.ucl.ac.uk/mace-lab/resources/glad).

The global distribution of lactase persistence

Figure 3.15.1 shows an interpolated map of the frequency of LP in indigenous populations worldwide. LP is particularly common in northern Europe, with frequencies of around 89–96% in the British Isles and southern Scandinavia; a declining gradient towards the south and east is seen in the rest of Europe. On other continents LP is not evenly distributed geographically. Indeed, in Africa and the Middle East it is often found at very different frequencies in neighbouring populations, such as 64% in the Beni Amir (pastoralists) and 23% in the Dounglawi (non-pastoralists) in Sudan. LP frequency has been shown to correlate strongly with a tradition of pastoralism [23].

The genetics of lactase persistence

Lactase persistence is inherited in an autosomal dominant manner. A single gene (*LCT*) codes for lactase. Several single nucleotide changes have been found in a lactase gene regulatory region (so-called enhancer, which is located in the adjacent gene *MCM6*), one of which occurs at high frequency in Europe. Estimates of the age of these changes range between 2,188 and 20,650 years ago [24] and between 7,450 and 12,300 years ago [25] for the *−13,910*T* allele associated with LP in Europe and southern Asia, and between 1200 and 23,200 years ago for the *−14,010*C* allele, one of the major LP-associated variants in Africa [26]. These date estimates bracket those for the domestication of milkable animals and the spread of agriculture and herding obtained from archaeological data (cave paintings, distributions of animal bones and dairy fat residues in pots).

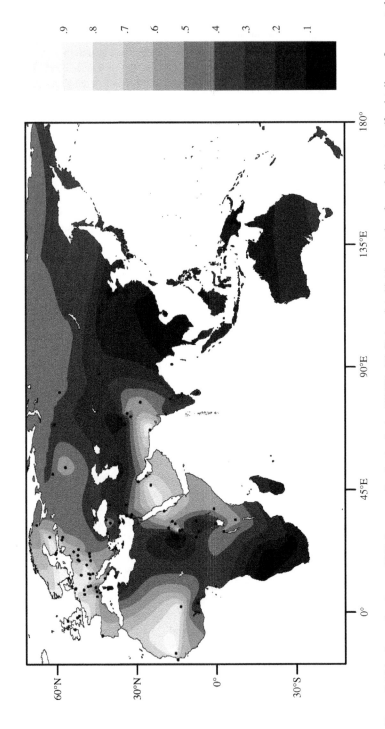

Figure 3.15.1 Interpolated map of LP phenotype distribution in the 'Old World'. Data points (dots) were taken from the literature (for details see Ingram et al. [6]). The key shows the frequency of the LP phenotype, black being used for the lowest frequency while white is used for the highest. Source: Itan et al. [7]. Reproduced with permission from BioMed Central Ltd.

Natural selection and evolution of lactase persistence in humans

A low frequency or absence of −*13,910*T* in early Neolithic central European farmers [27] and early Neolithic farmers from north-east Iberia [28], middle Neolithic Scandinavian hunter-gatherers [29] and late Neolithic farmers from southern France [30] suggests that dairying was practised before LP arose or became common. The age estimates for the LP-associated variants are remarkably young for alleles found at such high frequencies in multiple populations, suggesting that their spread has been boosted by natural selection. The strength of natural selection estimated for the LP-associated alleles is very high (1.4–19% [23] and 5.2–15.9% [31] for −*13,910*T*, and 1–15% for −*14,010*C* [26]), amongst the highest for any human genes in the last 30,000 years.

Several lines of evidence (genetics, anthropology and archaeology) suggest that LP would not have provided a selective advantage without a supply of dairy products containing lactose to adults, implying that these traits evolved as the result of a co-evolutionary process involving both genes and culture. A spatially-explicit computer simulation study of this gene–culture co-evolutionary process in Europe indicate that LP and dairying began between 6856 and 8283 years ago in a region around modern-day Hungary [31].

3.15.2 Implications for diet today

Variable symptoms of hypolactasia in adults

Symptoms of lactose intolerance can arise after an individual with hypolactasia has ingested lactose. Firstly, when undigested lactose passes into the colon it creates an osmotic gradient across the GI wall, driving an influx of water to re-equilibrate the osmotic imbalance, which can lead to diarrhoea. Secondly, the fermentation of lactose by colonic bacteria can lead to the production of fatty acids and various gases as by-products (including hydrogen), potentially causing discomfort, bloating and flatulence

(reviewed in (Hammer et al. [32]). These symptoms usually manifest within 1–2 h of ingestion, but vary greatly from one individual to another.

The symptoms of lactose intolerance are a function of (1) the amount of lactose ingested at one time, (2) gut transit time, which itself is influenced by factors such as the presence and consistency of solid foods and the temperature of the food [33], and (3) the quantity of residual lactase expressed in the small intestine and, (4) the spectrum of microbiota present in the colon. In fact, most lactase non-persistent individuals can consume small amounts of fresh milk (such as in coffee or tea) without symptoms, and some can consume considerably larger quantities. It has variously been reported that lactose-intolerant individuals can tolerate daily amounts of lactose ranging from no more than 12–15 g of lactose – the equivalent of a cup of milk [34,35] – up to 40–70 g of lactose [19,36]. Also, a controlled double-blind study showed a strong placebo effect in the production of symptoms [37]. It thus appears that lactase non-persistent individuals should not be warned off fresh milk, except like all people, while experiencing diarrhoea, but rather need to find their own lactose tolerance threshold. Lactose is often used as a bulking agent in pills. It is relevant to note that administration of capsules containing either 400 mg of lactose or a placebo failed to show any changes in H_2 in breath exhalation or GI symptoms [33].

Some interindividual variation in lactose intolerance symptoms can be explained by the composition of the GI microbiota. Lactase is not an inducible enzyme [10] but it has been suggested that adaptation can come from the GI microbiota when lactose is continuously consumed [33]. The microbial community within the human GI tract is diverse and dynamic in species composition, large in mass and complex in ecology [38]. Furthermore, its equilibrium composition can be shaped by diet [38]. Indeed, both an alteration of the composition of the microbiota and an increase in fecal beta-galactosidase activity have been observed after daily milk feeding and in association with a reduction in lactose intolerance symptoms [34,36]. There are also differences in the production of gases (such as hydrogen), which cause much of the discomfort in lactose intolerance. This highlights the fact that milk and lactose-containing products can often be consumed without provoking symptoms of intolerance, and that dietary tolerance, rather than lactase expression, can be adaptive, as has been observed in lactase non-persistent Somali camel herders who often consume large quantities of milk [19].

Dietary strategies

Many dairy products contain only small amounts of lactose (Table 3.15.1), allowing their consumption by most lactase non-persistent individuals. Bacteria and yeast fermentation convert the lactose in milk into various by-products, reducing the content of lactose by 25–50% [33,39]. For example, yoghurt is made of milk incubated with micro-organisms that contribute to lactose hydrolysis both during the fermentation process and sometimes after ingestion (discussed in Montalto et al. [33]). Such micro-organisms are also called probiotics, i.e. live micro-organisms that are said to confer health benefits to the host when taken in adequate quantities. Even though different microbial species ferment lactose to different extents depending on their morphological and physiological character-istics [2,33], fermented dairy products ultimately contain less lactose, allowing consumption of dairy products without ill effects [39,40].

Should people wish to consume more milk prod-ucts than they can tolerate, exogenous beta-galac-tosidase represents a possible therapy for primary lactase deficiency. Enzymes can be added in a liq-uid or solid (capsules or tablets) form together with milk and dairy products. The efficacy of enzymes extracted from distinct species has been assessed and compared [33,40]. For example, the beta-D-galactosidase from *Aspergillus oryzae* has shown good properties in decreasing symptoms of lactose intolerance for a relatively low dose of enzyme [41]. Pretreated lactose-free products, which were first introduced in Finland and the USA, are now becoming more widely available.

As an alternative approach, Ritter Pharmaceuticals has recently announced the successful completion of a phase II trial of a potential treatment for lactose intolerance, RP-G28, which is an orally adminis-trated proprietary oligosaccharide that is claimed to stimulate the growth of certain colonic lactose-metabolising bacteria (www.ritterpharmaceuticals.com/product-platform/rpg28).

Table 3.15.1 Lactose content in different type of products (adapted from Holland et al. [53], with permission from the Royal Society of Chemistry)

Product	Type	Lactose content in g per 100 g product
Milk	Cattle (whole milk, pasteurised)	4.6
	Cattle (semi-skimmed milk, pasteurised)	4.7
	Cattle (skimmed milk, pasteurised)	4.8
	Human	7.2
	Sheep	5.1
	Goat	4.4
Yoghurt	Whole milk, plain	4.7
	Greek style, plain	3.5
Cream	Single	2.2
	Double	1.7
	Crème fraiche	2.1
Cheese	Cheese spread	4.4
	Fromage frais	4
	Cottage cheese	3.1
	Feta	1.4
	Parmesan	0.9
	Cheddar	0.1
	Stilton	0.1
	Cream cheese	Trace
	Brie/Camembert	Trace
	Edam/Gouda	Trace
	Mozzarella	Trace
Butter		0.6
Chocolate	Milk	10.1
	Plain	0.2
Ice cream	Dairy, vanilla	5.2

Pros and cons of dairy intakes for lactose malabsorbers

Many studies have investigated both the benefits and increased risks to health of dairy product consumption among LP and lactase non-persistent individuals, such as the risk of developing metabolic syndrome compo-nents [42–45], osteoporosis [46–49] and various can-cers [50–52]. Results from these studies should be treated with caution since confounding effects such as mixed ancestry, cryptic population structure or differences in diets are not always accounted for and can yield contradictory results.

The concentration of calcium in bovine milk is about 1 g/L and calcium intake from milk and yoghurt accounts for about 50% of the total calcium intake in Dutch people, though it accounts for only about 15% of the total calcium intake in Austrians [16,17]. This shows the importance of milk as a calcium source but also that other dietary sources of calcium can be used. It is nevertheless important to be aware that lactose malabsorbers need not avoid all milk and dairy products unnecessarily, and if they do, they should not do so without adequate advice.

3.15.3 Conclusion

Far from being a disease or a dysfunctional disorder, lactase non-persistence – causing lactose intolerance – is the norm and it is the adult consumption of milk that is the novel (cultural) variant. Nutritional epidemiology studies, and the staggering selective advantages that have favoured LP-associated alleles over the last 10,000 years, clearly show that adult milk consumption can be highly beneficial.

Lactase non-persistent individuals may or may not exhibit symptoms of lactose intolerance after consumption of lactose, whose intensity depends on both internal (amount of lactase still expressed in the small intestine, GI microbiota, gut transit times) and external factors (food consistency, the lactose content of the food, whether it contains probiotics or not, and if so what probiotics they are). An individual's threshold of lactose intolerance should be assessed before deciding to avoid dairy products, and alternative lactose intolerance management strategies exist, including potential oligosaccharide-based treatments and bacterial beta-galactosidase activity.

References

1. Drewnowski A. The contribution of milk and milk products to micronutrient density and affordability of the U.S. diet. *Journal of the American College of Nutrition* 2011; **30**(5 Suppl 1): 422S–428S.

2. Haug A, Hostmark AT, Harstad OM. Bovine milk in human nutrition – a review. *Lipids in Health and Disease* 2007; **6**: 25.

3. Malacarne M, Martuzzi F, Summer A, Mariani P. Protein and fat composition of mare's milk: some nutritional remarks with reference to human and cow's milk. *International Dairy Journal* 2002; **12**: 869–877.

4. Walsh JP, Rook JAF, Dodd FH. The measurement of the effects of inherent and environmental factors on the lactose content of the milk of individual cows and of the herd bulk milk in a number of commercial herds. *Journal of Dairy Research* 1968; **35**: 107–125.

5. Troelsen JT. Adult-type hypolactasia and regulation of lactase expression. *Biochimica et Biophysica Acta* 2005; **1723**(1–3): 19–32.

6. Ingram CJ, Mulcare CA, Itan Y, Thomas MG, Swallow DM. Lactose digestion and the evolutionary genetics of lactase persistence. *Human Genetics* 2009; **124**(6): 579–591.

7. Itan Y, Jones BL, Ingram CJ, Swallow DM, Thomas MG. A worldwide correlation of lactase persistence phenotype and genotypes. *BMC Evolutionary Biology* 2010; **10**: 36.

8. Sahi T. Genetics and epidemiology of adult-type hypolactasia. *Scandinavian Journal of Gastroenterology* 1994; **202**(Suppl): 7–20.

9. Gutierrez I, Espinosa A, Garcia J, Carabano R, de Blas JC. Effect of levels of starch, fiber, and lactose on digestion and growth performance of early-weaned rabbits. *Journal of Animal Science* 2002; **80**(4): 1029–1037.

10. Keusch GT, Troncale FJ, Thavaramara B, Prinyanont P, Anderson PR, Bhamarapravathi N. Lactase deficiency in Thailand: effect of prolonged lactose feeding. *American Journal of Clinical Nutrition* 1969; **22**(5): 638–641.

11. Villako K, Maaroos H. Clinical picture of hypolactasia and lactose intolerance. *Scandinavian Journal of Gastroenterology* 1994; **202**(Suppl): 36–54.

12. Jarvela I, Torniainen S, Kolho KL. Molecular genetics of human lactase deficiencies. *Annals of Medicine* 2009; **41**(8): 568–575.

13. Kuokkanen M, Kokkonen J, Enattah NS, et al. Mutations in the translated region of the lactase gene (*LCT*) underlie congenital lactase deficiency. *American Journal of Human Genetics* 2006; **78**(2): 339–344.

14. Grant JD, Bezerra JA, Thompson SH, Lemen RJ, Koldovsky O, Udall JN Jr. Assessment of lactose absorption by measurement of urinary galactose. *Gastroenterology* 1989; **97**(4): 895–899.

15. Mulcare CA, Weale ME, Jones AL, et al. The T allele of a single-nucleotide polymorphism 13.9 kb upstream of the lactase gene (*LCT*) (C-13.9kbT) does not predict or cause the lactase-persistence phenotype in Africans. *American Journal of Human Genetics* 2004; **74**(6): 1102–1110.

16. Gugatschka M, Dobnig H, Fahrleitner-Pammer A, et al. Molecularly-defined lactose malabsorption, milk consumption and anthropometric differences in adult males. *Quarterly Journal of Medicine* 2005; **98**(12): 857–863.

17. Koek W, van Meurs J, van der Eerden B, et al. The T-13910C polymorphism in the lactase phlorizin hydrolase gene is associated with differences in serum calcium levels and calcium

intake. *Journal of Bone and Mineral Research* 2010; **25**(9): 1980–1987.

18. Habte D, Sterky G, Hjalmarsson B. Lactose malabsorption in Ethiopian children. *Acta Paediatrica Scandinavica* 1973; **62**(6): 649–654.

19. Ingram CJ, Raga TO, Tarekegn A, et al. Multiple rare variants as a cause of a common phenotype: several different lactase persistence associated alleles in a single ethnic group. *Journal of Molecular Evolution* 2009b; **69**(6): 579–588.

20. Reddy V, Pershad J. Lactase deficiency in Indians. *American Journal of Clinical Nutrition* 1972; **25**(1): 114–119.

21. Scrimshaw NS, Murray EB. The acceptability of milk and milk products in populations with a high prevalence of lactose intolerance. *American Journal of Clinical Nutrition* 1988; **48**(4 Suppl): 1079–1159.

22. Gerbault P, Liebert A, Itan Y, et al. Evolution of lactase persistence: an example of human niche construction. *Philosophical Transactions of the Royal Society of London. Series B, Biological Sciences* 2011; **366**(1566): 863–877.

23. Holden C, Mace R. 1997. Phylogenetic analysis of the evolution of lactose digestion in adults. *Hum Biol.* 69:605–628.

24. Bersaglieri T, Sabeti PC, Patterson N, et al. Genetic signatures of strong recent positive selection at the lactase gene. *American Journal of Human Genetics* 2004; **74**(6): 1111–1120.

25. Coelho M, Luiselli D, Bertorelle G, et al. Microsatellite variation and evolution of human lactase persistence. *Human Genetics* 2005; **117**(4): 329–339.

26. Tishkoff SA, Reed FA, Ranciaro A, et al. Convergent adaptation of human lactase persistence in Africa and Europe. *Nature Genetics* 2007; **39**(1): 31–40.

27. Burger J, Kirchner M, Bramanti B, Haak W, Thomas MG. Absence of the lactase-persistence-associated allele in early Neolithic Europeans. *Proceedings of the National Academy of Sciences USA* 2007; **104**(10): 3736–3741.

28. Lacan M, Keyser C, Ricaut FX, et al. Ancient DNA suggests the leading role played by men in the Neolithic dissemination. *Proceedings of the National Academy of Sciences USA* 2011b; **108**(45): 18255–18259.

29. Malmström H, Gilbert MT, Thomas MG, et al. Ancient DNA reveals lack of continuity between neolithic hunter–gatherers and contemporary Scandinavians. *Current Biology* 2009; **19**(20): 1758–1762.

30. Lacan M, Keyser C, Ricaut FX, et al. Ancient DNA reveals male diffusion through the Neolithic Mediterranean route. *Proceedings of the National Academy of Sciences USA* 2011; **108**(24): 9788–9791.

31. Itan Y, Powell A, Beaumont MA, Burger J, Thomas MG. The origins of lactase persistence in Europe. *PLoS Computational Biology* 2009; **5**(8): e1000491.

32. Hammer HF, Petritsch W, Pristautz H, Krejs GJ. Evaluation of the pathogenesis of flatulence and abdominal cramps in patients with lactose malabsorption. *Wiener Klinische Wochenschrift* 1996; **108**(6): 175–179.

33. Montalto M, Curigliano V, Santoro L, et al. Management and treatment of lactose malabsorption. *World Journal of Gastroenterology* 2006; **12**(2): 187–191.

34. Ito M, Kimura M. Influence of lactose on faecal microflora in lactose maldigestors. *Microbial Ecology in Health and Disease* 1993; **6**: 73–76.

35. Johnson AO, Semenya JG, Buchowski MS, Enwonwu CO, Scrimshaw NS. Adaptation of lactose maldigesters to continued milk intakes. *American Journal of Clinical Nutrition* 1993; **58**(6): 879–881.

36. Hertzler SR, Savaiano DA. Colonic adaptation to daily lactose feeding in lactose maldigesters reduces lactose intolerance. *American Journal of Clinical Nutrition* 1996; **64**(2): 232–236.

37. Briet F, Pochart P, Marteau P, Flourie B, Arrigoni E, Rambaud JC. Improved clinical tolerance to chronic lactose ingestion in subjects with lactose intolerance: a placebo effect? *Gut* 19974; **1**(5): 632–635.

38. Dunne C. Adaptation of bacteria to the intestinal niche: probiotics and gut disorder. *Inflammatory Bowel Diseases* 2001; **7**(2): 136–145.

39. Lomer MC, Parkes GC, Sanderson JD. Review article: lactose intolerance in clinical practice – myths and realities. *Alimentary Pharmacology and Therapeutics* 2008; **27**(2): 93–103.

40. De Vrese M, Stegelmann A, Richter B, Fenselau S, Laue C, Schrezenmeir J. Probiotics –compensation for lactase insufficiency. *American Journal of Clinical Nutrition* 2001; **73**(2 Suppl): 421S–429S.

41. Portincasa P, di Ciaula A, Vacca M, Montelli R, Wang DQ, Palasciano G. Beneficial effects of oral tilactase on patients with hypolactasia. *European Journal of Clinical Investigation* 2008; **38**(11): 835–844.

42. Almon R, Alvarez-Leon EE, Engfeldt P, Serra-Majem L, Magnuson A, Nilsson TK. Associations between lactase persistence and the metabolic syndrome in a cross-sectional study in the Canary Islands. *European Journal of Nutrition* 2009; **49**(3): 141–146.

43. Corella D, Arregui M, Coltell O, et al. Association of the *LCT*-13910C>T polymorphism with obesity and its modulation by dairy products in a Mediterranean population. *Obesity (Silver Spring)* 2011; **19**(8): 1707–1714.

44. Enattah NS, Forsblom C, Rasinpera H, Tuomi T, Groop PH, Jarvela I. The genetic variant of lactase persistence C (−13910) T as a risk factor for type I and II diabetes in the Finnish population. *European Journal of Clinical Nutrition* 2004; **58**(9): 1319–1322.

45. Meloni GF, Colombo C, La Vecchia C, et al. High prevalence of lactose absorbers in Northern Sardinian patients with type 1 and type 2 diabetes mellitus. *American Journal of Clinical Nutrition* 2001; **73**(3): 582–585.

46. Agueda L, Urreizti R, Bustamante M, et al. Analysis of three functional polymorphisms in relation to osteoporosis phenotypes: replication in a Spanish cohort. *Calcified Tissue International* 2010; **87**(1): 14–24.

47. Enattah N, Pekkarinen T, Valimaki MJ, Loyttyniemi E, Jarvela I. Genetically defined adult-type hypolactasia and self-reported lactose intolerance as risk factors of osteoporosis in Finnish postmenopausal women. *European Journal of Clinical Nutrition* 2005; **59**(10): 1105–1111.

48. Enattah NS, Sulkava R, Halonen P, Kontula K, Jarvela I. Genetic variant of lactase-persistent C/T-13910 is associated

with bone fractures in very old age. *Journal of the American Geriatrics Society* 2005; **53**(1): 79–82.

49. Obermayer-Pietsch BM, Bonelli CM, Walter DE, et al. Genetic predisposition for adult lactose intolerance and relation to diet, bone density, and bone fractures. *Journal of Bone and Mineral Research* 2004; **19**(1): 42–47.

50. Larsson SC, Orsini N, Wolk A. Milk, milk products and lactose intake and ovarian cancer risk: a meta-analysis of epidemiological studies. *International Journal of Cancer* 2006; **118**(2): 431–441.

51. Meloni GF, Colombo C, La Vecchia C, et al. Lactose absorption in patients with ovarian cancer. *American Journal of Epidemiology* 1999; **150**(2): 183–186.

52. Shrier I, Szilagyi A, Correa JA. Impact of lactose-containing foods and the genetics of lactase on diseases: an analytical review of population data. *Nutrition and Cancer* 2008; **60**(3): 292–300.

53. Holland B, Welch AA, Unwin ID, Buss DH, Paul AA, Southgate DA. *McCance and Widdowson's The Composition of Foods*. Cambridge, UK: Royal Society of Chemistry and Ministry of Agriculture, Fisheries and Food, 1991.

Chapter 3.16

Intestinal failure and nutrition

Alison Culkin
St Mark's Hospital, Harrow, UK

Intestinal failure (IF) results from obstruction, dysmotility, surgical resection, congenital defect or disease-associated loss of absorption and is characterised by the inability to maintain protein-energy, fluid, electrolyte or micronutrient balance [1]. It is classified using a combination of severity, type and length of nutrition support required [2,3].

- *Type 1* – self-limiting, usually <28 days duration and includes postoperative ileus or small bowel obstruction requiring short-term parenteral nutrition (PN).
- *Type 2* – lasting >28 days and includes complex Crohn's disease, trauma, intestinal fistula or abdominal sepsis. These patients are severely ill with major GI resections plus septic, metabolic and nutritional complications requiring multidisciplinary intervention with metabolic and nutritional support to permit recovery.

Types 1 and 2 are often referred to as *acute intestinal failure*. The prevalence is currently unknown but estimates range from 10% to 15% of patients undergoing intestinal surgery [3]. The introduction of enhanced recovery after surgery (ERAS) programmes may minimise the likelihood of developing type 1 in the future. The Association of Surgeons of Great Britain and Ireland has published good principles on the management of patients with acute IF which includes information on prevention and treatment. The detection and management of abdominal sepsis are a priority for patients as this is the most common cause of death if left untreated [3].

The judgement on whether to instigate nutritional support in type 1 IF is often fraught with indecision. The 'wait and see' approach or the assessment of 'bowel sounds' is misleading and can result in significant periods without adequate nutrition in those who are likely to benefit from PN. In a pragmatic study, patients with inadequate GI function were allocated to PN (n=267) and those with adequate GI function to enteral nutrition (EN) (n=231). Where genuine uncertainty existed, patients were randomised to either PN (n=32) or EN (n=32). In the non-randomised arm, patients receiving EN had a significantly higher mortality and were more likely to receive <80% of their target nutrition compared to PN. In the randomised group there was no difference in mortality between the two routes of nutrition and the authors concluded that if in doubt, PN is superior [4].

- *Type 3* – generally irreversible and therefore known as *chronic intestinal failure*, resulting from massive GI resection, leading to short bowel (e.g. mesenteric infarct/thrombosis, intestinal volvulus, inflammatory bowel disease, chronic radiation enteritis). Patients with failure of intestinal motility (e.g. chronic idiopathic intestinal pseudo-obstruction, visceral myopathy/neuropathy and scleroderma) are included in this group and usually require long-term home parenteral nutrition (HPN).

The incidence of type 3 is unknown but estimations can be made based on the number of patients requiring HPN. A recent UK survey reported a prevalence of 7 per million although it is recognised that this may be an underestimate [5]. The reasons for dependency on HPN are short bowel (55.4%), malabsorption (14.8%), fistula (10.1%) and obstruction (7.5%). Crohn's disease (30.4%), mesenteric ischaemia (18.8%), chronic

Advanced Nutrition and Dietetics in Gastroenterology, First Edition. Edited by Miranda Lomer.
© 2014 John Wiley & Sons, Ltd. Published 2014 by John Wiley & Sons, Ltd.

intestinal pseudo-obstruction (12.8%) and surgical complications (14.2%) represent the major diagnoses responsible for HPN [5].

3.16.1 Consequences of intestinal failure and short bowel

Short bowel is a subcategory of IF and is defined as short bowel syndrome-intestinal failure which results from surgical resection, congenital defect or disease-associated loss of absorption and is characterised by the inability to maintain protein-energy, fluid, electrolyte or micronutrient balances when on a conventionally accepted, normal diet [1]. All patients with short bowel will have problems with fluid and electrolyte balance, particularly in the immediate postoperative period, with nutritional requirements increased as a result of malabsorption.

The consequences of intestinal resection are dependent on four factors:

- extent of resection
- site of resection
- integrity of the remaining bowel
- adaptation in the remaining bowel.

Due to the variability in length of the small intestine, the outcome post resection depends on the length of bowel remaining rather than the length resected. A residual small intestine length of <200 cm is deemed short bowel and can lead to nutritional, fluid and electrolyte depletion if not adequately managed. The loss of the ileum and some of the jejunum considerably impairs digestive and absorptive function. When the absorptive function of the colon is no longer available, more fluid and electrolytes will be lost [6]. It has been shown that the following lengths of small intestine are *inadequate* to be managed on diet alone, and parenteral support of some form is required [7].

- <100 cm jejunum will need long-term parenteral fluid and electrolyte replacement.
- <75 cm jejunum will need long-term PN, fluid and electrolytes.
- <50 cm jejunum plus colon will need long-term PN, fluid and electrolytes.

Citrulline is an intermediary product of glutamine metabolism, mainly occurring in the enterocytes of the small intestine, and therefore citrulline production reflects enterocyte mass. A study of 82 patients with <200 cm of small intestine 2 years post resection found that plasma citrulline concentration correlated with length of small intestine (r=0.83, P<0.0001) with plasma concentration of <20 µmol/L being prognostic of patients with IF who continued to require HPN [8].

Studies in healthy volunteers have shown that approximately 4 litres of fluid pass the duodenojejunal flexure daily, including saliva, gastric and pancreatic secretions and bile. The upper jejunum secretes fluid as part of normal digestion. This process contributes to the high intestinal losses experienced by patients with short bowel, especially those with a jejunostomy. The ingestion of food and fluid further dilutes these secretions [9], exacerbating losses. Balance studies undertaken on 15 jejunostomy patients demonstrated that in patients with <100 cm of jejunum, the intestinal output exceeded the oral intake. These patients, known as 'secretors', are in a constant negative fluid and sodium balance and thus parenteral support is required. Conversely, in patients with >100 cm of jejunum, the intestinal output was less than oral intake. These patients, known as 'absorbers', were able to avoid parenteral support using oral electrolyte supplements (glucose-saline solution or sodium chloride tablets) to maintain fluid and sodium balance. However, these lengths were based on healthy bowel and longer lengths are required if disease is present [10]. In patients with a jejunocolic anastomosis (JCA), the problems of fluid and sodium depletion are reduced as the colon is able to reabsorb fluid and sodium efficiently and intestinal transit time is usually unaffected as the colon acts as a 'brake', increasing transit time [11].

3.16.2 Fluid and electrolyte management in short bowel

The focus of treatment is to reduce intestinal losses, thereby preventing dehydration and electrolyte disturbances. Restricting oral fluids to <1500 mL per day reduced intestinal losses by 23% [12]. The sodium content of jejunostomy effluent averages 88 mmol/L (range 60–118) and when fluids containing <90 mmol/L of sodium are consumed, the jejunum secretes fluid and sodium from the plasma into the lumen of the intestine which is then lost from the body, resulting in dehydration and sodium depletion [10]. The ingestion of 500 mL of water or tea resulted in negative sodium and fluid balance whereas 500 mL of an oral rehydration solution containing 90 mmol/L led to positive sodium and fluid balance [13]. Jejunal absorption of sodium occurs against a small concentration gradient, dependent on water movement and coupled to glucose and amino acids. Therefore, to optimise sodium and fluid absorption in the jejunum, patients are encouraged to consume an oral rehydration solution which has a sodium content of 90 mmol/L (20 g of glucose, 3.5 g of sodium chloride and 2.5 g of sodium bicarbonate). Compliance can be poor due to palatability and the use of overnight infusions via a gastrostomy tube has enabled patients to become independent from HPN.

3.16.3 Pharmaceutical management

The aim of pharmaceutical intervention is to reduce intestinal losses and increase intestinal transit, allowing an increase in the time that nutrients and fluid are in contact with the GI lumen. Post resection, increased gastric acid production and reduced intestinal transit time exacerbate the problems of dehydration and sodium depletion. Gastric antisecretory drugs, such as proton pump inhibitors and H_2 antagonists, have been shown to reduce intestinal losses by 1.5 kg /day [14]. Patients who fail to absorb oral proton pump inhibitors may benefit from parenteral administration [15].

The somatostatin analogue octreotide reduces gastric, pancreatic and biliary secretions but research using a long-acting somatostatin in short bowel confirmed a lack of efficacy [16]. Others have demonstrated that while the treatment can reduce jejunostomy output, its use is associated with the suppression of serum concentrations of gut hormones including insulin, gastrin, glucagon and peptide tyrosine tyrosine (PYY) and could therefore interfere with intestinal adaptation [17]. In practice, octreotide is usually reserved for patients with uncontrollable intestinal losses which are refractory to conventional treatment.

Antimotility agents such as loperamide and codeine phosphate increase GI transit time, decrease intestinal output and reduce electrolyte losses [18]. High doses are normally required in order to achieve the desired outcome. Clonidine, an alpha-2 adrenergic agonist, has been investigated as an antimotility agent. The benefit of this treatment is transdermal application, removing the potential for malabsorption via the GI tract. Clinically significant reductions in intestinal volume, weight and sodium and increased urine production equating to improved hydration were demonstrated in eight jejunostomy patients [19].

Removal of the terminal ileum may cause bile acid depletion, resulting in high intestinal losses. Cholylsarcosine, a synthetic bile acid, has been shown to improve fat absorption in patients with and without a colon although the overall energy gain was poor (6%) with no other benefits demonstrated [20].

Magnesium deficiency is common and can usually be corrected with an oral magnesium preparation. Most magnesium salts result in an increased intestinal output and therefore high doses are required. If oral supplements are ineffective then magnesium sulphate can be added to normal saline and given subcutaneously or intravenously to maintain plasma concentrations [21]. Vitamin D increases intestinal and renal absorption of magnesium so concentrations should be monitored.

Further research is required to establish efficacy and optimum dosage of all medications used in the management of short bowel.

3.16.4 Adaptation

In the postoperative period, spontaneous intestinal adaptation occurs in an attempt to minimise the consequences of intestinal resection. The presence of nutrients in the GI lumen is essential to take advantage of this process so patients should not remain nil by mouth for prolonged periods. Adaptation reaches a plateau 2 years post resection and the optimum diet to stimulate human intestinal adaptation is not yet known as most data come from animal models. Complex diets were found to exert a more potent effect than elemental diets in pigs, suggesting that a polymeric formula is superior [22]. The soluble fibre pectin is fermented by colonic bacteria into short-chain fatty acids which are known to contribute significantly to energy balance in patients with a JCA. A recent study in humans failed to demonstrate improvements in macronutrient or fluid absorption [23].

Non-nutritional interventions include the use of growth hormone and glucagon-like peptide (GLP-2). Studies in humans have investigated the effects of growth hormone in conjunction with glutamine supplementation and dietary manipulation to promote intestinal adaptation and absorption and reduce HPN dependence. However, results remain inconclusive due to variations in the quality and design of studies. Many trial subjects were not optimally managed with regard to oral food and fluid restrictions, antimotility and antisecretory medication and therefore, positive outcomes could reflect improved short bowel management rather than a treatment benefit as reductions in HPN have been shown with structured patient education in isolation [24]. When well-conducted double-blind randomised controlled trials (RCTs) are considered, no sustainable improvements in macronutrient absorption or body composition are observed. Case series and studies with a less robust design have shown improvements in intestinal absorption, enabling either reduction or complete withdrawal of HPN. A Cochrane systematic review concluded that the evidence is inconclusive to recommend growth hormone and glutamine for patients with short bowel [25]. In conclusion, further studies with a robust design and adequate length of follow-up need to be completed in order to ensure that it is the combined effect of these treatments rather than adherence to a suitable short bowel regimen or the spontaneous process of intestinal adaptation that allows patients to reduce dependency or withdraw from HPN.

More promising results have been shown with the administration of teduglutide, an analogue of GLP-2, a peptide secreted from enteroendocrine L-cells in the distal small intestine. A randomised placebo-controlled study of teduglutide at 0.05 mg/kg/day demonstrated improvements in fluid balance resulting in reductions in parenteral support [26].

3.16.5 Nutritional management

The management of IF is a dynamic process which involves overlap or transition between oral, EN and PN as the patient's condition changes or in response to intestinal adaptation. The effect of intestinal resection is best understood by considering where nutrients are normally absorbed. Most nutrients are absorbed within the first 100–150 cm of jejunum. Exceptions include vitamin B12 and bile salts which are absorbed at specific receptor sites in the terminal ileum. Resection of the small intestine will therefore affect absorption but the outcome for the patient will depend on the type, length and quality of the remaining small intestine and the presence or absence of a functioning colon.

Balance studies demonstrate that patients absorb two-thirds of their oral energy and protein intake [27–29], supporting the recommendation of a hyperphagic diet containing 30–60 kcal/kg and 0.2–0.25 gN_2/kg/day in order to compensate for nutrient malabsorption. The composition of the diet is crucial and depends on intestinal anatomy in order to optimise the effects of oral diet (Table 3.16.1).

Table 3.16.1 Recommendations for the dietary treatment of patients with short bowel

	Jejunocolic anastomosis (JCA)	Stoma (jejunostomy)
Total energy	30–60 kcal/kg/day	30–60 kcal/kg/day
Nitrogen	0.2–0.25 g/kg/day	0.2–0.25 g/kg/day
Protein	1.25–1.5 g/kg/day	1.25–1.5 g/kg/day
Fat	20–30% of total energy	30–40% of total energy
– Medium-chain triglyceride	50% of total fat	No proven benefit
Carbohydrate	50–60% of total energy	40–50% of total energy
– Lactose	No need to restrict	No need to restrict
Sodium chloride	Normal	Additions usually required
Enteral nutrition	Polymeric	Polymeric
Oral fluid	No restriction usually required	Restricted

3.16.6 Dietary management of jejunocolic anastomosis

The human colon significantly contributes to the fermentation of polysaccharides delivered unabsorbed from the small intestine resulting in the production of the short-chain fatty acids (SCFA) butyrate, acetate and propionate. These SCFAs are subsequently absorbed into the bloodstream, contributing significantly to energy balance. Danish researchers randomised patients to receive a high-carbohydrate or high-fat diet over a 3-day period to assess the effect of manipulating macronutrient intake on fluid and nutrient absorption [30]. In JCA patients, the high-carbohydrate diet was associated with a reduction in mean faecal energy loss of 478 kcal/day and a higher proportion of absorbed energy compared to the high-fat diet. There was no difference in the mean faecal volume produced between the two diets despite patients on the high-carbohydrate diet consuming an additional ~1000 mL/day more, indicating that the colon is capable of reabsorbing additional fluid or that the high-carbohydrate diet may cause an improvement in fluid absorption. A further study demonstrated that in JCA patients consuming a high-carbohydrate diet, colonic fermentation provided an additional 1000 kcal/day [31].

The role of fat restriction has been controversial with conflicting results from different research groups. Early research demonstrated that a low-fat diet resulted in a reduction in diarrhoea [32] but was undertaken before the benefits of a high-carbohydrate diet were demonstrated and the reduction in fat was accompanied by an increase in carbohydrate which may have been responsible for improvements in absorption observed.

In JCA patients, the substitution of long-chain triglyceride (LCT) with medium-chain triglyceride (MCT) increased fat and energy absorption from 23% to 58% and 46% to 58% respectively with no significant increase in mean faecal volume [33]. MCT may be beneficial in terms of absorption and energy density, being a useful adjunct in patients who struggle to achieve the recommended hyperphagic diet. Further research is required in order to evaluate long-term efficacy and impact on nutritional status, especially as they do not contain essential fatty acids.

The exclusion of lactose is often recommended as it is presumed that lack of intestinal surface area results in reduced lactase production [34]. While this may be true immediately following intestinal resection, the findings from two RCTs [35,36] in stable short bowel patients have refuted this. Both studies demonstrated no clinical signs of intolerance or increase in faecal weight during lactose consumption. Therefore, foods containing lactose should not be excluded from the diet as they provide a valuable source of macro- and micronutrients.

In an observation study, 25% of patients with a JCA developed renal calculae [7] due to increased colonic oxalate absorption resulting in hyperoxaluria. The risk can be minimised by advising patients on a diet low in oxalate, moderate in fat and high in calcium and preventing chronic dehydration.

3.16.7 Dietary management of patients with a jejunostomy

A strong correlation between oral fat ingestion and absorption has been demonstrated in jejunostomy patients [29]. The evidence to date suggests no benefit in following a low-fat diet and as fat provides a concentrated source of energy and essential fatty acids, these patients should be advised to follow a high-fat diet. Despite a lack of evidence supporting a low-fibre diet, patients with a jejunostomy often experience a clinically significant reduction in intestinal losses.

3.16.8 Oral nutritional supplements and enteral nutrition

Some patients require oral nutritional supplements (ONS) or EN and the choice of formula is crucial to success. A comparison between polymeric and semi-elemental formulae showed the polymeric formula was superior regarding both energy absorption and GI transit time [37]. Therefore, it is recommended that if additional nutritional support is required to maintain or improve nutritional status in patients then a polymeric formula is preferable.

An increase in energy, nitrogen and fat absorption without an increase in intestinal output was found during continuous polymeric EN compared to those on diet alone [38]. All commercially available enteral formulae require the addition of strong sodium chloride solutions to reach the optimum concentration of sodium in the jejunum (90 mmol/L).

3.16.9 Micronutrient deficiencies

Several studies have documented a high prevalence of micronutrient deficiencies in patients with short bowel and those on HPN [39,40]. Causes include the underlying condition, increased intestinal losses and inadequate provision. The prevention and treatment of deficiencies are of paramount importance, especially when aiming to reduce dependency on HPN and promote adaptation [41]. Supplementation is essential, often requiring above the recommended doses necessary to take account of malabsorption. The detection of deficiencies can be problematic due to a lack of reliable biochemical assays, especially in the context of the acute phase response. The risk of essential fatty acid deficiency (EFAD) should not be overlooked, especially in patients experiencing severe fat malabsorption maintained on oral diet [42]. The subcutaneous administration of sunflower or safflower oil to prevent EFAD has been recommended [43,44].

Deficiencies and toxicities of micronutrients have been described and can be managed with careful monitoring. The American Gastroenterological Association has published guidelines on the provision of micronutrients in short bowel and states the importance of observing for clinical manifestation of deficiencies, regular monitoring of serum concentrations followed by suitable supplementation [45].

3.16.10 Dietary management of enterocutaneous fistula

Patients can develop an abnormal communication between the GI tract and the skin (enterocutaneous fistula), which functions in a similar way to a jejunostomy. It is common practice for patients who develop an enterocutaneous fistula to be placed nil by mouth and start PN and octreotide in an attempt to heal the fistula. This approach has not been supported by RCTs [46]. In patients where closure is unlikely to occur spontaneously then oral diet can be introduced. Patients with intestinal fistulae who have >75 cm of normal small intestine distal to the fistula may be candidates for fistuloclysis, a technique in which EN is infused into the distal small intestine [47]. For further details on this technique see www.i-rehab.org.uk.

3.16.11 Intestinal transplantation and tissue engineering

Patients with chronic intestinal failure who are considered to be failing on HPN are now being considered for intestinal transplantation. The world-wide experience of intestinal transplantation continues to increase on a yearly basis. Indications for transplantation include life-threatening complications related to intestinal failure or complications of long-term PN. Indications for intestinal transplantation vary between the United States and Europe due to differences in healthcare provision. In the US, HPN is seen as a supportive treatment until a suitable donor can be found whereas in Europe, transplantation is only considered if HPN is failing due to complications such as lack of venous access, severe recurrent catheter sepsis, PN-related severe liver disease or poor quality of life. The 1-year survival data for intestine, intestine and liver and multivisceral transplantation are 78%, 60% and 66% respectively, which decrease after 4 years to 50%, 50% and 62% [48]. Strategies to reduce the indications for transplantation should be a priority. Interventions which can improve liver function are of importance as patients requiring a combined intestinal and liver transplant have a poorer outcome than those requiring intestinal transplant in isolation. Presently, the survival data comparing transplantation to HPN favour HPN as the treatment of choice for patients with chronic intestinal failure, with early referral for those patients with deteriorating liver function [49].

The concept of an 'artificial GI tract' was described 40 years ago. Attempts to create intestinal tissue are still in their infancy and the complexities of creating an organ with all the functions of the human intestine (secretory, peristaltic, digestive, absorptive, hormonal and immunological) have meant that this technology remains at the experimental stage in animal models only. The implantation of a tissue-engineered intestine would prevent all the difficulties which are faced after intestinal transplantation due to graft-versus-host rejection.

References

1. O'Keefe SJ, Buchman AL, Fishbein TM, Jeejeebhoy KN, Jeppesen PB, Shaffer J. Short bowel syndrome and intestinal failure: consensus definitions and overview. *Clinical Gastroenterology and Hepatology* 2006; **4**: 6–10.

2. Lal S, Teubner A, Shaffer JL. Review article: intestinal failure. *Alimentary Pharmacology and Therapeutics* 2006; **24**: 19–31.

3. Carlson G, Gardiner K, McKee R, MacFie J, Vaizey C. *The Surgical Management of Patients with Acute Intestinal Failure.* London: Association of Surgeons of Great Britain and Ireland, 2010.www.asgbi.org.uk/download.cfm?docid=74E316BB-F98D-41D1-854DD3080327CAB0, accessed 20 January 2014.

4. Woodcock NP, Zeigler D, Palmer MD, Buckley P, Mitchell CJ, MacFie J. Enteral verses parenteral nutrition: a pragmatic study. *Nutrition* 2001; **17**: 1–12.

5. Smith T. Adult home parenteral nutrition (HPN). In: Smith T (ed) *Annual BANS Report. Artificial Nutrition Support in the UK 2000–2009.* Redditch: BAPEN, 2010, pp. 40–48.

6. Nightingale JM. Management of a high-output jejunostomy. In: Nightingale JM (ed) *Intestinal Failure.* London: Greenwich Medical Media, 2001, pp. 375–392.

7. Nightingale JM, Lennard-Jones JE, Gertner DJ, Wood, SR, Bartram CI. Colonic preservation reduces the need for parenteral therapy, increases incidence of renal stones, but does not change the high prevalence of gall stones in patients with a short bowel. *Gut* 1992; **33**: 1493–1497.

8. Crenn P, Coudray-Lucas C, Thuillier F, Cynober L, Messing B. Postabsorptive plasma citrulline concentration is a marker of absorptive enterocyte mass and intestinal failure in humans. *Gastroenterology* 2000; **119**: 1496–1505.

9. Borgström B, Dahlqvist A, Lundh G, Sjovall J. Studies of intestinal digestion and absorption in the human. *Journal of Clinical Investigation* 1957; **36**: 1521–1536.

10. Nightingale JM, Lennard-Jones JE, Walker ER, Farthing MJG. Jejunal efflux in short bowel syndrome. *Lancet* 1990; **336**: 765–768.

11. Nightingale JM, Kamm MA, van der Sijp JR, et al. Disturbed gastric emptying in the short bowel syndrome. Evidence for a 'colonic brake'. *Gut* 1993; **34**: 1171–1176.

12. Grischkan D, Steiger E, Fazio V. Maintenance of home hyperalimentation in patients with high-output jejunostomies. *Archives of Surgery* 1979; **114**: 838–841.

13. Newton CR, Gonvers JJ, McIntyre PB, Preston DM, Lennard-Jones JE. Effect of different drinks on fluid and electrolyte losses from a jejunostomy. *Journal of the Royal Society of Medicine* 1985; **78**: 27–34.

14. Nightingale JM, Walker ER, Farthing MJ, Lennard-Jones JE. Effect of omeprazole on intestinal output in the short bowel syndrome. *Alimentary Pharmacology and Therapeutics* 1991; **5**: 405–412.

15. Jeppesen PB, Staun M, Tjellesen L, Mortensen PB. Effect of intravenous ranitidine and omeprazole on intestinal absorption of water, sodium, and macronutrients in patients with intestinal resection. *Gut* 1998; **43**: 763–769.

16. Nehra V, Camilleri M, Burton D, Oenning L, Kelly DG. An open trial of octreotide long-acting release in the management of short bowel syndrome. *American Journal of Gastroenterology* 2001; **96**(5): 1494–1498.

17. O'Keefe SJ, Haymond MW, Bennet WM, Oswald B, Nelson DK, Shorter RG. Long-acting somatostatin analogue therapy and protein metabolism in patients with jejunostomies. *Gastroenterology* 1994; **107**(2): 379–388.

18. King RF, Norton T, Hill GL. A double-blind crossover study of the effect of loperamide hydrochloride and codeine phosphate on ileostomy output. *Australia New Zealand Journal of Surgery* 1982; **52**(2): 121–124.

19. Buchman AL, Fryer J, Wallin A, Ahn CW, Polensky S, Zaremba K. Clonidine reduces diarrhea and sodium loss in patients with proximal jejunostomy: a controlled study. *Journal of Parenteral and Enteral Nutrition* 2006; **30**(6): 487–491.

20. Heydorn S, Jeppesen PB, Mortensen PB. Bile acid replacement therapy with cholylsarcosine for short-bowel syndrome. *Scandinavian Journal of Gastroenterology* 1999; **34**(8): 818–823.

21. Martinez-Riquelme A, Rawlings J, Morley S, Kendall J, Hosking D, Allison S. Self-administered subcutaneous fluid infusion at home in the management of fluid depletion and hypomagnesaemia in gastro-intestinal disease. *Clinical Nutrition* 2005; **24**: 158–163.

22. Tappenden K. Mechanisms of enteral nutrient-enhanced intestinal adaptation. *Gastroenterology* 2006; **130**: S93–S99.

23. Atia A, Girard-Pipau F, Héberterne X, et al. Macronutrient absorption characteristics in humans with short bowel syndrome and jejunocolonic anastomosis: starch is the most important carbohydrate substrate, although pectin supplementation may modestly enhance short chain fatty acid production and fluid absorption. *Journal of Parenteral and Enteral Nutrition* 2011; **35**(2): 229–240.

24. Culkin A, Gabe SM, Madden AM. Improving clinical outcome in patients with intestinal failure using individualised nutritional advice. *Journal of Human Nutrition and Dietetics* 2009; **22**: 290–298.

25. Wales PW, Nasr A, de Silva N, Yamada J. Human growth hormone and glutamine for patients with short bowel syndrome. *Cochrane Database of Systematic Reviews* 2010; **6**: CD006321.

26. Jeppesen PB, Gilroy R, Pertkiewicz M, Allard JP, Messing B, O'Keefe SJ. Randomised placebo-controlled trial of teduglutide in reducing parenteral nutrition and/or intravenous fluid requirements in patients with short bowel syndrome. *Gut* 2011; **60**: 902–914.

27. Woolf GM, Miller C, Kurian R, Jeejeebhoy KN. Nutritional absorption in short bowel syndrome. Evaluation of fluid,

calorie, and divalent cation requirements. *Digestive Diseases and Sciences* 1987; **32**: 8–15.

28. Messing B, Pigot F, Rongier M, Morin MC, Ndeïndoum, Rambaud JC. *Intestinal absorption of free oral hyperalimentation in the very short bowel syndrome. Gastroenterology* 1991; **100**: 1502–1508.

29. Crenn P, Morin MC, Joly F, Penven S, Thuillier F, Messing B. Net digestive absorption and adaptive hyperphagia in adult short bowel patients. *Gut* 2004; **53**: 1279–1286.

30. Nordgaard I, Hansen BS, Mortensen PB. Colon as a digestive organ in patients with short bowel. *Lancet* 1994; **343**: 373–376.

31. Nordgaard I, Hansen BS, Mortensen PB. Importance of colonic support for energy absorption as small-bowel failure proceeds. *American Journal of Clinical Nutrition* 1996; **64**: 222–231.

32. Andersson H, Isaksson B, Sjögren B. Fat-reduced diet in the symptomatic treatment of small bowel disease: metabolic studies in patients with Crohn's disease and in other patients subjected to ileal resection. *Gut* 1974; **15**: 351–359.

33. Jeppesen PB, Mortensen PB. The influence of a preserved colon on the absorption of medium chain fat in patients with small bowel resection. *Gut* 1998; **43**: 478–483.

34. Matarese LE, Steiger E, Seidnber DL. *Intestinal Failure and Rehabilitation. A Clinical Guide.* Boca Raton, FL: CRC Press, 2005.

35. Arrigoni E, Marteau P, Briet F, Pochart P, Rambaud JC. Tolerance and absorption of lactose from milk and yogurt during short bowel syndrome in humans. *American Journal of Clinical Nutrition* 1994; **60**: 926–929.

36. Marteau P, Messing B, Arrigoni E, et al. Do patients with short-bowel syndrome need a lactose-free diet? *Nutrition* 1997; **13**: 13–16.

37. Pironi L, Guidetti M, Agostini F, Pazzeschi C. Intestinal absoprtion and transit time of different liquid diets in type 1 short bowel. *Clinical Nutrition* 2011; **6**(Suppl 1): 38.

38. Joly F, Dray X, Corcos O, Barbot L, Kapel N, Messing B. Tube feeding improves intestinal absorption in short bowel syndrome patients. *Gastroenterology* 2009; **136**: 824–831.

39. Braga CB, Vannucchi H, Freire CM, Marchini JS, Jordão AA Jr, da Cunha SF. Serum vitamins in adult patients with short bowel syndrome receiving intermittent parenteral nutrition. *Journal of Parenteral and Enteral Nutrition* 2011; **35**: 493–498.

40. Buchman AL, Howard LJ, Guenter P, Nishikawa RA, Compher CW, Tappenden KA. Micronutrients in parenteral nutrition: too little or too much? The past, present, and recommendations for the future. *Gastroenterology* 2009; **137**(Suppl 5): S1–S6.

41. Di Baise JK, Materese LE, Messing B, Steiger E. Strategies for parenteral nutrition weaning in adult patients with short bowel syndrome. *Journal of Clinical Gastroenterology* 2006; **40**: S94–S98.

42. Jeppesen PB, Christensen MS, Høy CE, Mortensen PB. Essential fatty acid deficiency in patients with severe fat malabsorption. *American Journal of Clinical Nutrition* 1997; **65**(3): 837–843.

43. Press M, Hartop PJ, Prottey C. Correction of essential fatty acid deficiency in man by the cutaneous application of sunflower oil. *Lancet* 1974; **1**: 597–598.

44. Miller DG, Williams SK, Palombo JD, Griffin RE, Bistrian BR, Blackburn GL. Cutaneous application of safflower oil in preventing essential fatty acid deficiency in patients on home parenteral nutrition. *American Journal of Clinical Nutrition* 1987; **46**: 419–423.

45. Buchman AL, Scolapio J, Fryer J. AGA technical review on short bowel syndrome and intestinal transplantation. *Gastroenterology* 2003; **124**(4): 1111–1134.

46. Lloyd DA, Gabe SM, Windsor AC. Nutrition and management of enterocutaneous fistula. *British Journal of Surgery* 2006; **93**: 1045–1055.

47. Teubner A, Morrison K, Ravishankar HR, Anderson ID, Scott NA, Carlson GL. Fistuloclysis can successfully replace parenteral feeding in the nutritional support of patients with enterocutaneous fistula. *British Journal of Surgery* 2004; **91**: 625–631.

48. Middleton SJ. Is intestinal transplantation now an alternative to home parenteral nutrition? *Proceedings of the Nutrition Society* 2007; **66**: 316–320.

49. Pironi L, Forbes A, Joly F, et al. Survival of patients identified as candidates for intestinal transplantation: a 3-year prospective follow-up. *Gastroenterology* 2008; **135**: 61–71.

Chapter 3.17

Stomas and nutrition

Alison Culkin
St Mark's Hospital, Harrow, UK

A stoma (from the Greek word meaning 'mouth') is an opening, connecting a portion of the GI tract to the outside of the body. Intestinal effluent passes out of the stoma and is collected in an external bag attached to the skin. An ileostomy or colostomy is created when part of the small intestine (ileum) or large intestine (colon) is brought out onto the surface of the abdomen, respectively. A stoma may be temporary or permanent depending on the underlying condition. Several conditions may necessitate the formation of a stoma and some are listed in Table 3.17.1.

There are three types of colostomy [1].

- *Loop colostomy* – often performed in an emergency as a temporary procedure. The colon is sutured to the abdomen and two openings are created in the one stoma: one for intestinal effluent and the other for mucus naturally secreted by the GI tract.
- *End colostomy* – known as a Hartmann's procedure, named after the surgeon who first described it, this involves the removal of the rectosigmoid colon with closure of the rectal stump and formation of an end colostomy.
- *Double barrel colostomy* – the colon is severed and both ends are brought out onto the abdomen with only the proximal stoma functioning.

There are three types of ileostomy [1].

- *Temporary or loop ileostomy* – involves a loop of the small intestine being brought through the skin, and the colon and rectum remain *in situ*,

often performed as the first stage in the surgical construction of an ileo-anal pouch to prevent intestinal effluent entering the pouch until adequate healing has occurred. The ileostomy is then reversed, usually after 8–10 weeks.
- *End ileostomy* – this is often a permanent option where the colon and rectum are removed and the end of the small intestine is brought through the skin.
- *Continent ileostomy* – similar to an end ileostomy but without the need to attach an external bag as a pouch is created internally utilising the end of the small intestine. The stoma is connected to a valve implanted into the skin and can be emptied using a catheter. This option has mainly been

Table 3.17.1 Conditions which may require stoma formation

Colostomy	Ileostomy
Diverticulitis	Crohn's disease
Anal stenosis	Ulcerative colitis
Faecal incontinence	Familial adenomatous polyposis
Pelvic tumours	Hirschsprung's disease
Colorectal cancer	Colorectal cancer
Abdominal trauma	Abdominal trauma
Perianal sepsis	Bowel obstruction
Pseudomembranous enterocolitis	Ischaemic bowel
Radiation enteritis	Radiation enteritis

Advanced Nutrition and Dietetics in Gastroenterology, First Edition. Edited by Miranda Lomer.
© 2014 John Wiley & Sons, Ltd. Published 2014 by John Wiley & Sons, Ltd.

replaced by the ileo-anal pouch although it is still performed in a small minority of patients unable to have this operation.

3.17.1 Preoperative nutritional status

The nutritional status of patients requiring stoma formation will be affected by their underlying medical condition and concurrent treatment such as radiotherapy and chemotherapy. Patients presenting to the outpatient department should be screened for undernutrition using a validated tool, as undernutrition is known to adversely affect clinical outcome. Garth et al. (2010) reported that undernourished GI cancer patients identified using subjective global assessment (SGA) had a longer length of stay (P<0.05) and a greater risk of complications (P<0.01) compared to well-nourished patients [2]. There is currently no agreed international definition of undernutrition and therefore comparisons between centres are problematic. The incidence of undernutrition in colorectal patients varies from 20% to 50% [2–4] depending on the criteria used.

A study in patients with colorectal cancer aimed to examine the associations between different techniques used to assess risk of undernutrition with survival [4]. The risk of undernutrition was assessed using SGA and the nutritional risk screening (NRS-2002) as recommended by the European Society of Parenteral and Enteral Nutrition (ESPEN). Sarcopenia was assessed using computed tomography (CT) scans by calculating the muscle mass cross-sectional area (cm^2). The presence of cachexia was assessed using the Cancer Cachexia Study Group (CCSG) criteria:

- weight loss of ≥10%
- energy intake of ≤1500 kcal/day
- C-reactive protein (CRP) ≥10 mg/L.

The incidence of undernutrition was 34% (SGA) with 42% nutritionally at risk (NRS-2002) and 39% identified as sarcopenic. The authors found that 22% with cachexia (CCSG) had a shorter survival (P=0.005). There was poor agreement between methods but the CCSG cachexia score was the best prognostic factor regarding survival [4].

An international consensus on the definition and classification of cancer cachexia has recently been agreed and includes these parameters [5]:

- Body Mass Index (BMI) <20 kg/m^2 plus weight loss of >2%
- weight loss of >5% in 6 months
- sarcopenia.

It is hoped that after validation, this work will benefit the design of clinical trials and future clinical management.

Patients with inflammatory bowel disease (IBD) requiring surgery and formation of a stoma may be at high risk of undernutrition due to the symptoms associated with acute disease. Weight loss is common and has been estimated to occur in 70–80% of patients during hospital admission and in 20–40% of outpatients [6]. Several studies had determined that patients with IBD are not identified as undernourished when assessed using standard criteria such as SGA or BMI. However, when more sophisticated body composition techniques including bio-impedance, skinfold and muscle circumference plus muscle function measures such as handgrip are used then patients have significant differences from healthy controls [6–8], indicating that standard screening is inadequate.

Guidelines for perioperative care in elective colorectal surgery have identified that a low BMI does not seem to be a risk factor for complications although the presence of sarcopenia is predictive [9]. In a study of 234 patients, 39% were sarcopenic and length of stay was longer (P=0.038), infection risk greater (P=0.025) and inpatient rehabilitation more common (P=0.024) [10]. Therefore screening tools that include BMI may not be sensitive enough to identify patients experiencing the initial stages of sarcopenia, especially those who are overweight and obese.

Micronutrient deficiencies including ferritin, zinc and vitamins B6, B12, D and carotene have been reported in IBD [8]. Therefore screening for deficiencies and appropriate supplementation are recommended perioperatively.

3.17.2 Perioperative nutrition and enhanced recovery after surgery

Patients identified as undernourished are likely to benefit from improvements in nutritional status although evidence in colorectal surgery is lacking. A Cochrane review identified three studies comparing oral and two studies comparing enteral nutrition with standard care and found no difference in complications, infections or length of stay when provided preoperatively [3]. Three trials comparing preoperative parenteral nutrition verses standard care demonstrated a reduction in major complications in undernourished patients (P=0.0048). A meta-analysis of six trials investigating the use of preoperative immune-enhancing formulae versus no or standard nutrition in patients undergoing GI surgery showed a reduction in postoperative (P=0.003) and infective complications (P=0.008) and length of stay (P=0.02). Systematic reviews and meta-analyses are only as good as the data available and the reviewers stated that although benefits in terms of outcome were demonstrated, significant bias was apparent which limits the generalisability to all patients undergoing surgery [3]. In addition, many of the trials were carried out before the implementation of the enhanced recovery after surgery (ERAS) programme and so the results need to be interpreted within the current surgical context.

The ERAS protocol aims to reduce surgical stress, maintain physiological function and encourage early mobilisation. The evidence-based protocol has dramatically altered the perioperative management of surgical patients, resulting in earlier recovery and reduced length of stay [9]. A systematic review and meta-analysis by Lewis et al. (2009) showed that perioperative fasting in GI surgery is no longer recommended [11] and patients are encouraged to eat up to 6 h before surgery and undergo carbohydrate loading by consuming 400 mL of carbohydrate-containing fluids up to 2 h before surgery. Immediately after recovery from anaesthesia, patients are encouraged to drink and on day one can eat normal food, often supplemented with oral nutritional supplements to meet requirements. If patients require nutritional support postoperatively then a polymeric formula is recommended as a study of 12 patients undergoing total colectomy found an elemental diet was not superior to a polymeric in terms of macronutrient and micronutrient absorption [12]. Another study by the same group performed in 16 patients with well-established ileostomies supported the recommendation of a polymeric formula [13].

Postoperative complications cause a prolonged length of hospital stay, resulting in increased healthcare cost. Factors contributing to reduced quality of life for patients include:

- intra-abdominal sepsis which can be life threatening
- inadequate stoma care which can cause excoriated skin
- high intestinal losses resulting in dehydration and electrolyte disturbances
- poor perioperative nutrition support resulting in undernutrition
- immobility
- depression.

All of the above increase the length of rehabilitation during which the patient is unable to return to work and/or family life and therefore all measures should be employed to minimise the risk of these complications [14].

3.17.3 Colostomy

Nutritional consequences of colostomy formation

Formation of a colostomy can occur at any location along the colon, but the most common placement is on the lower left side near the sigmoid where a majority of colon cancers occur. Other locations include the ascending, transverse and descending sections of the colon. The location of the stoma is important as this may affect the risk of complications experienced by the patient due to difficulties absorbing fluid and electrolytes. The formation of a colostomy has minimal impact on the digestion and absorption of fluid and nutrition and most patients will be able to resume a normal healthy diet based on national guidelines such as the 'Eat Well Plate' (UK) or 'Eat Right' (USA) and 'Eating Well with Canada's Food Guide'. Obesity and weight gain have been associated with stoma retraction and therefore maintaining a healthy BMI is important [15].

Dietary management of a colostomy

There are no clinical trials supporting the use of a particular diet after colostomy formation. Immediately after surgery, patients are normally advised to consume a diet low in non-starch polysaccharides (NSP) in order to minimise the risk of obstruction as surgery may result in GI oedema. After surgery, intestinal losses may be liquid and the prevention of dehydration is paramount. Patients will need to consume at least 1.5–2 L of fluid daily. After 6–8 weeks a normal healthy diet can be eaten with foods high in NSP being introduced slowly to assess the effect on GI function. The introduction of ERAS may reduce the requirement for this cautious approach in the future with patients returning to a normal diet much more quickly after laparoscopic versus traditional open surgery.

The current dietary counselling provided to patients on diet and colostomy function comes mainly from patient questionnaires investigating patients with both ileostomies and colostomies. Patients with an ileostomy are much more likely to experience complications than those with a colostomy and therefore future studies would benefit from analysing responses from these different patient groups separately. Ratliff et al. (2005) conducted a prospective review of 220 patients returning for a 2-month follow-up of whom 35% (n=77) had a colostomy [16]. The complication rate was 13% and was due to mechanical or chemical damage related to poor appliance use. None of the patients reported complications due to food and fluid intake. A large survey of 604 patients of whom 83% (n=498) had a colostomy found that only 11.5% (n=69) were following a specific diet. Of those surveyed, 21% (n=125) reported an increase in intestinal output, 14% (n=85) reported odour and 35% (n=215) reported gas in relation to the consumption of certain foods [17].

Diarrhoea

High NSP- and lactose-containing foods are often implicated in causing symptoms of diarrhoea, odour and flatus due to GI microbiota fermentation. Milk and cheese are often avoided plus vegetables including onions, cabbage, peppers, beans, broccoli, lettuce and mushrooms [17,18]. However, these effects are yet to be demonstrated under clinical trial conditions.

Constipation

Constipation is common, especially in cancer patients, due to reduced activity, opiate use, poor food and fluid intake due to anorexia. A thorough medication review by a pharmacist may be useful in identifying drugs which are known to cause this side-effect to ascertain if switching to a different drug may be beneficial. Treatment includes adequate NSP and fluid intake plus suitable laxatives if these measures do not improve GI function [19].

3.17.4 Ileostomy

Nutritional consequences of ileostomy formation

A total colectomy results in considerable loss of absorptive capacity in respect of fluids and electrolytes, most importantly sodium. Postoperatively, considerable quantities of fluid and electrolytes will be lost (1200–2000 mL fluid/day and 120–200 mmol sodium/day) and requirements for both will be increased for at least 6–8 weeks. The ileum then appears to adapt and fluid losses reduce to 400–600 mL/day. While the ileum is adapting and the intestinal output remains liquid, fluid losses should be replaced by the consumption of 1.5–2 L/day of fluid. Additional salt (e.g. up to one teaspoon added to food during the course of a day) may be necessary in hot weather or if losses are particularly high [20]. As stool frequency and consistency improve, losses will decrease but it remains important to ensure adequate fluid and sodium provision. An episode of vomiting or high intestinal losses can rapidly create an electrolyte imbalance and the provision of extra fluid, sodium and potassium is imperative. In severe cases, parenteral therapy may be necessary to prevent dehydration and sodium depletion.

The digestive and absorptive capacity of the small intestine remains, so that no major nutritional deficiencies are to be expected with the exception of vitamin B12 and bile acids as both are absorbed at specific receptor sites in the terminal ileum. Deficiency of vitamin B12 post colectomy has been estimated to occur in 3–9% of patients. Possible causes include reduced absorptive capacity due to ileal involvement, inadequate dietary intake and bacterial overgrowth as GI microbiota utilise vitamin B12, reducing the amount available for absorption [21]. It is usual practice to monitor serum vitamin B12 concentration routinely but Jayaprakash et al. (2004) examined 39 patients who had undergone total colectomy with the formation of an end ileostomy for IBD a mean of 12.5 years ago and were only able to identify deficiency in 5% (n=2) of patients [22]. They concluded that routine screening for vitamin B12 deficiency is not required except in the presence of small intestinal resection or ongoing inflammation.

Dehydration

Several studies have identified dehydration as the most common cause of hospital readmission following ileostomy formation, especially in the elderly [23], those treated with diuretics [24], antidiarrhoeal agents and neo-adjuvant therapy [25]. Recently, concerns have been raised that patients with an ileostomy are chronically dehydrated and have depleted calcium and magnesium stores, putting them at risk of renal impairment, renal stones and bone demineralisation. Ng et al. (2013) identified that patients with an ileostomy (n=60) had significantly lower body weight, BMI, lean body mass and bone mineral density compared to healthy controls [26]. In addition, patients had 24-h urinary volume, calcium and magnesium concentrations significantly lower than controls, with 63% recording a urinary sodium excretion of less than 100 mmol/day. The authors concluded that patients are chronically dehydrated and recommended that routine urinary sodium measurements may detect dehydration and therefore identify patients at risk. Due to the kidneys' attempt to conserve water and sodium, patients are also at greater risk of uric acid stones as a result of producing urine which is low in volume and pH,

and with a high concentration of calcium and oxalate compared with healthy controls [27].

The treatment of dehydration involves adequate provision of fluid and electrolytes. It is of great importance that those experiencing dehydration due to high intestinal losses do not try to restrict oral fluid, as this is likely to exacerbate the situation. The use of an oral rehydration solution is beneficial if the ileostomy output exceeds 1 L/day. Dehydration may be precipitated by several factors including hot weather, strenuous exercise and infection, including food poisoning, medication and, in IBD, recurrence of disease. The introduction of an ileostomy pathway based on patient education and postdischarge monitoring of fluid balance found that readmission rates for dehydration reduced from 15% to zero [28], supporting the importance of patient education in the pre- and postoperative stages. Further information on the management of high-output stomas can be found in Chapter 3.16.

Dietary management of an ileostomy

Following formation of an ileostomy, it may take time before normal appetite is restored. It is therefore important that patients are encouraged to consume small, frequent, nutrient-dense meals and snacks and that additional oral nutritional support measures are instituted when necessary.

There are no randomised controlled trials of the effects of specific foods on ileostomy function. No foods are specifically contraindicated for ileostomy patients but some foods can cause unpleasant symptoms such as odour or flatus. Obstruction with undigested food can occur, particularly if the stoma is tight, and reducing NSP may be required if obstruction occurs frequently and cannot be surgically corrected. However, in most people this is unnecessary and avoidance of the few specific foods which typically cause the problem is sufficient to prevent it [20]. However, it should be borne in mind that individual tolerance may vary considerably so people should be encouraged to discover for themselves on a trial-and-error basis which foods cause repeated and consistent symptoms.

Only two studies to date have aimed to use more objective methods to quantify the effect of food and fluid on the intestinal output of patients with an established ileostomy. McNeil et al. (1982) analysed 7-day

Table 3.17.2 Dietary effects on stoma output

Output effects	Foods identified
Poorly digested foods/ identifiable in output	Grapefruit, lettuce, mushrooms, sweetcorn, lentils, peas, nuts, seeds, tomatoes, coconut, celery, pineapple, Chinese food, pips, pith, seeds, skin of fruits and vegetables, raw cabbage and carrot, dried fruit
Increased stool odour	Onions, garlic, brassica vegetables (Brussels sprouts, cabbage, cauliflower and broccoli), beans, fish, eggs
Increased flatulence/bloating	Baked beans, cabbage, cucumber, turnip, lentils, peas, onions, garlic, brassica vegetables, carbonated drinks, beer and lager.
Increased stool volume	Strawberries*, grapes*, peaches*, raisins*, bananas*, prune juice*, baked beans*, alcohol, Chinese food, whole wheat cereals, sweetcorn, apples, wine, fried and spicy foods, potatoes, bread, pineapple, pears, onions, mushrooms, lettuce, fruit, fruit juice, vegetables, beetroot, rhubarb, fried fish, cabbage
Decreased stool consistency	Beer, wine, fried fish, strawberries, sweetcorn, popcorn, spirits, coleslaw, grapefruit, turnips, raspberries and fruit juice
Peristomal irritation	Spicy foods, citrus fruits, raw carrot, nuts and seeds

*Food identified by Kramer [30] on weighed balance studies.
Data summarised from Thompson et al. [35] (UK), Gazzard et al. [36] (UK), Bingham et al. [37] (UK), Giunchi et al. [18] (Italy) and Floruta [17] (USA).

weighed intakes and 24-h urine and faecal collections in 36 ileostomy patients compared to healthy controls [29]. Most patients were in good nutritional health although 47% (n=17) had an elevated plasma creatinine indicative of mild renal impairment and 25% (n=9) had a raised aldosterone concentration. Aldosterone promotes sodium and fluid water retention and is elevated during dehydration and sodium depletion. Mean stoma volumes of 760 ± 322 g with stomal sodium concentration of 118 mmol/kg were observed, which were highly significantly associated (r=0.98, P=<0.001). Regression analysis identified that the amount of ileum resected was the main determinant of stoma volume and sodium concentration. Patients with Crohn's disease were significantly more likely to be sodium depleted compared to those with ulcerative colitis. Nutritional factors related to increased intestinal losses included total energy, NSP and pentose component of fibre. Foods containing NSP hold water and therefore the physical properties of foods may greatly influence stoma function.

Kramer (1987) conducted balance studies on seven ileostomy patients who were maintained on a self-selected control diet for 3 days and then assessed the effect on ileostomy function of 37 foods over the next 3 days [30]. The findings were of interest, as foods commonly excluded from the diet by patients did not elicit the effects commonly described. Only five out of 12 fruits (grapes, peaches, raisins, strawberries, bananas), one of out five vegetables (baked beans), and one out of seven drinks (prune juice) increased output. Water, alcohol, carbonated drinks, milk, fried foods and spices did not increase output under these controlled conditions. Unlike the relationship found by McNeil et al. [29], no association between amount of NSP and intestinal output could be demonstrated. Thus, many foods and fluids are restricted unnecessarily in patients with an ileostomy. This was further substantiated by a review which found that complications were due to poor stoma formation and poor stoma appliances rather than specific foods [15].

Information acquired from patient questionnaires in Europe and the USA have been used to identify the effect of foods on stoma function as summarised in Table 3.17.2.

It is of interest that many of the foods listed in Table 3.17.2 contain significant sources of poorly absorbed short-chain carbohydrates collectively termed fermentable oligo-, di- and monosaccharides and polyols (FODMAPs). FODMAPs are osmotically active in the GI lumen [31] and result in

Table 3.17.3   Dietary recommendations for colostomy and ileostomy

	Colostomy	Ileostomy
Macronutrients	Healthy eating principles based on a regular meal pattern	Healthy eating principles
Micronutrients	National recommended values	Monitor vitamin B12 in small intestinal disease/resection
Non-starch polysaccharides	↓ Postoperatively aiming for recommended values	↓ Postoperatively aiming for recommended values
Fluid	1.5–2 L/day Additions required if losses ↑	1.5–2 L/day Additions required if losses ↑
Sodium chloride	Normal	Additions usually required
Enteral nutrition support	Polymeric	Polymeric
Functional bowel symptoms	Consider low FODMAP diet	Consider low FODMAP diet

colonic fermentation [32], leading to bloating, flatus and diarrhoea. Therefore reducing these components in the diet offers an interesting new treatment for patients experiencing these symptoms.

A randomised, single-blinded, controlled crossover trial investigated the effect of a high and low FODMAP diet in 10 patients with an ileostomy. Patients were asked to rate on a visual analogue scale (VAS) their perceived change in intestinal volume and consistency. At baseline and after each 4-day diet, patients collected stoma output over 24 h, which was analysed for FODMAP content. Patients perceived a significantly thicker consistency and a non-significant reduction in volume ($p=0.066$) on the low FODMAP diet. The authors reported a significant reduction in the mean total, wet and dry weight on the low FODMAP diet [31]. Although statistically significant, these results may not be clinically significant as the percentage reductions in total (22%), wet (20%) and dry (24%) weight represented a volume reduction of 95 mL (range 28–161 mL), a wet weight reduction of 58 ± 17 mL and a dry weight reduction of 37 ± 15 g. It remains to be determined if these changes would have a clinical benefit in terms of nutritional and hydration status.

Stoma formation may be a relief for many patients as several studies have identified that patients have a less restrictive diet postoperatively. Prince et al. (2011) [33] and Cohen et al. (2013) [34] found that patients without a stoma were more likely to experience food-related difficulties than those with a stoma. A summary of the dietary recommendations for colostomy and ileostomy patients is shown in Table 3.17.3.

Patients should receive regular follow-up to ensure that diet-related problems are remedied, unnecessary food restrictions avoided and that adequate nutritional status is achieved and fluid and electrolyte balance maintained.

References

1. Burch J (ed). *Stoma Care*. Chichester: Wiley-Blackwell, 2008.
2. Garth AK, Newsome CM, Simmance N, Crowe TC. Nutritional status, nutrition practices and postoperative complications in patients with gastrointestinal cancer. *Journal of Human Nutrition and Dietetics* 2010; **23**: 393–401.
3. Burden S, Todd C, Hill J, Lal S. Pre-operative nutrition support in patients undergoing gastrointestinal surgery. *Cochrane Database of Systematic Reviews* 2012; **11**: CD008879.
4. Thoresen L, Frykholm G, Lydersen S, et al. Nutritional status, cachexia and survival in patients with advanced colorectal carcinoma. Different criteria for nutritional status provide unequal results. *Clinical Nutrition* 2013; **32**: 65–77.
5. Fearon K, Strasser F, Anker SD, et al. Definition and classification of cancer cachexia: an international consensus. *Lancet Oncology* 2011; **12**: 489–495.
6. Hartman C, Eliakim R, Shamir R. Nutritional status and nutritional therapy in inflammatory bowel diseases. *World Journal of Gastroenterology* 2009; **15**: 2570–2578.
7. Valentini L, Schaper L, Buning C, et al. Malnutrition and impaired muscle strength in patients with Crohn's disease and ulcerative colitis in remission. *Nutrition* 2008; **24**: 694–702.
8. Vagianos K, Bector S, McConnell J, Bernstein CN. Nutrition assessment of patients with inflammatory bowel disease. *Journal of Parenteral and Enteral Nutrition* 2007; **31**: 311–319.

9. Gustafsson UO, Scott MJ, Schwenk W, et al. for the Enhanced Recovery After Surgery Society. Guidelines for perioperative care in elective colonic surgery: Enhanced Recovery After Surgery (ERAS®) Society recommendations. *Clinical Nutrition* 2012; **31**: 783–800.

10. Lieffers JR, Bathe OF, Fassbender K, Winget M, Baracos VE. Sarcopenia is associated with postoperative infection and delayed recovery from colorectal cancer resection surgery. *British Journal of Cancer* 2012; **107**: 931–936.

11. Lewis SJ, Andersen HK, Thomas S. Early enteral nutrition within 24 h of intestinal surgery versus later commencement of feeding: a systematic review and meta-analysis. *Journal of Gastrointestinal Surgery* 2009; **13**: 569–575.

12. Andersson H, Hultén L, Magnusson O, Sandström B. Energy and mineral utilization from a peptide-based elemental diet and a polymeric enteral diet given to ileostomists in the early postoperative course. *Journal of Parenteral and Enteral Nutrition* 1984; **8**: 497–500.

13. Andersson H, Bosaeus I, Ellegard L, Hallgren B, Hultén L, Magnusson O. Comparison of an elemental and two polymeric diets in colectomized patients with or without intestinal resection. *Clinical Nutrition* 1984; **3**: 183–189.

14. Culkin A. Intestinal failure and Intestinal resection. In: Gandy J (ed) *Manual of Dietetic Practice*, 5th edn. Chichester: Wiley, 2014.

15. Kaidar-Person O, Person B, Wexner SD. Complications of construction and closure of temporary loop ileostomy. *Journal of the American College of Surgeons* 2005; **201**: 759–773.

16. Ratliff CR, Scarano KA, Donovan AM, Colwell JC. Descriptive study of peristomal complications. *Journal of Wound, Ostomy and Continence Nursing* 2005; **32**: 33–37.

17. Floruta CV. Dietary choices of people with ostomies. *Journal of Wound, Ostomy and Continence Nursing* 2001; **28**: 28–31.

18. Giunchi F, Cacciaguerra G, Borlotti ML, Pasini A, Giulianini G. Bowel movement and diet in patients with stomas. *British Journal of Surgery* 1988; **75**: 722.

19. Doughty D. Principles of ostomy management in the oncology patient. *Journal of Supportive Oncology* 2005; **3**: 59–69.

20. Pearson M. Nutrition. In: Burch J (ed) *Stoma Care*. Chichester: Wiley-Blackwell, 2008.

21. Christl SU, Scheppach W. Metabolic consequences of colectomy. *Scandinavian Journal of Gastroenterology* 1997; **222**(Suppl): 20–24.

22. Jayaprakash A, Creed T, Stewart L, et al. Should we monitor vitamin B12 levels in patients who have had end-ileostomy for inflammatory bowel disease? *International Journal of Colorectal Disease* 2004; **19**: 316–318.

23. Åkesson O, Syk I, Lindmark G, Buchwald P. Morbidity related to defunctioning loop ileostomy in low anterior resection. *International Journal of Colorectal Disease* 2012; **27**(12): 1619–1623.

24. Messaris E, Sehgal R, Deiling S, et al. Dehydration is the most common indication for readmission after diverting ileostomy creation. *Diseases of the Colon and Rectum* 2012; **55**: 175–180.

25. Hayden DM, Pinzon MC, Francescatti AB, et al. Hospital readmission for fluid and electrolyte abnormalities following ileostomy construction: preventable or unpredictable? *Journal of Gastrointestinal Surgery* 2013; **17**: 298–303.

26. Ng DH, Pither C, Wootton SA, Stroud MA. The 'Not so short-bowel syndrome': potential health problems in patients with an ileostomy. *Colorectal Disease* 2013; **15**(9): 1154–1169.

27. Christie PM, Knight GS, Hill GL. Comparison of relative risks of urinary stone formation after surgery for ulcerative colitis: conventional ileostomy vs. *J-pouch. A comparative study. Diseases of the Colon and Rectum* 1996; **39**: 50–54.

28. Nagle D, Pare T, Keenan E, Marcet K, Tizio S, Poylin V. Ileostomy pathway virtually eliminates readmissions for dehydration in new ostomates. *Diseases of the Colon and Rectum* 2012; **55**: 1266–1272.

29. McNeil NI, Bingham S, Cole TJ, Grant AM, Cummings JH. Diet and health of people with an ileostomy. 2. Ileostomy function and nutritional state. *British Journal of Nutrition* 1982; **47**: 407–415.

30. Kramer P. Effect of specific foods, beverages, and spices on amount of ileostomy output in human subjects. *American Journal of Gastroenterology* 1987; **82**: 327–332.

31. Barrett JS, Gearry RB, Muir JG, et al. Dietary poorly absorbed, short-chain carbohydrates increase delivery of water and fermentable substrates to the proximal colon. *Alimentary Pharmacology and Therapeutics* 2010; **31**(8): 874–882.

32. Ong DK, Mitchell SB, Barrett JS, et al. Manipulation of dietary short chain carbohydrates alters the pattern of gas production and genesis of symptoms in irritable bowel syndrome. *Journal of Gastroenterology and Hepatology* 2010; **25**(8): 1366–1373.

33. Prince A, Whelan K, Moosa A, Lomer MC, Reidlinger DP. Nutritional problems in inflammatory bowel disease: the patient perspective. *Journal of Crohn's and Colitis* 2011; **5**: 443–450.

34. Cohen AB, Lee D, Long MD, et al. Dietary patterns and self-reported associations of diet with symptoms of inflammatory bowel disease. *Digestive Diseases and Sciences* 2013; **58**: 1322–1328.

35. Thomson TJ, Runcie J, Khan A. The effect of diet on ileostomy function. *Gut* 1970; **11**(6): 482–485.

36. Gazzard BG, Saunders B, Dawson AM. Diets and stoma function. *British Journal of Surgery* 1978; **65**(9): 642–644.

37. Bingham S, Cummings JH, McNeil NI. Diet and health of people with an ileostomy. 1. Dietary assessment. *British Journal of Nutrition* 1982; **47**: 399–406.

Websites

St Mark's Hospital: www.stmarkshospital.org.uk/patient-information-leaflets

Colostomy Association (UK): www.colostomyassociation.org.uk

United Ostomy Associations of America (UOAA): www.ostomy.org

Chapter 3.18

Irritable bowel syndrome pathogenesis

Adam D. Farmer[1,2] and Qasim Aziz[1]
[1]Queen Mary University of London, London, UK
[2]Royal Shrewsbury Hospital, Shrewsbury, UK

Irritable bowel syndrome (IBS) is a chronic fluctuating disorder characterised by recurrent symptoms of abdominal pain or discomfort associated with a change in stool output [1]. IBS has an estimated population prevalence of 40% in Western countries, accounting for up to 60% of outpatient referral to gastroenterological clinics [2,3]. Currently, there is an absence of uniform investigational or treatment strategies for patients despite evidence suggesting that this disorder results in considerable reduction in health-related quality of life [1,4].

The aim of this chapter is to provide the reader with a succinct review of the mechanisms that have been proposed to account for the pathophysiology of IBS, namely genetic and psychological factors, visceral hypersensitivity and inflammatory changes to the milieu within the gastrointestinal (GI) tract. With respect to the latter, we also summarise current understanding of the role of GI microbiota, food hypersensitivity and probiotics.

3.18.1 Genetic factors

Epidemiological studies have suggested that there is a genetic component in the development of IBS with reports of clusters of IBS in families [5,6]. For example, Levy et al. reported that concordance for IBS was significantly greater in monozygotic (17.2%) than in dizygotic twins (8.4%) [7]. Further analysis of this evidence suggests that whilst there is a measureable genetic component to IBS, the effect is, at best, modest [8]. This effect has to be interpreted in the context of the influence of environmental and social factors. For instance, 15.2% of dizygotic twins with IBS have mothers with IBS, yet this is only 6.7% in those whose mothers do not have IBS [7].

These data provide support for the hypothesis that social learning contributes to the development of IBS as mothers share approximately the same number of genes with their children as dizygotic twins share with each other. As such, few diseases display purely Mendelian inheritance with disease phenotypes, such as IBS, actually reflecting a complex interaction between genes and the individual's environment.

Many studies have examined a number of candidate genes in patients with IBS, with genes relating to the serotoninergic system being amongst the most extensively studied. Serotonin that is released from the presynaptic terminal is taken up from the synaptic cleft by the serotonin transporter. Thus the synaptic concentration of serotonin, and serotonin transmission *per se*, are determined by the expression of serotonin transporter protein. The serotonin transporter gene is located on chromosome 17.9, with its gene being located in the promoter region, known as the 5-hydroxytryptamine transporter-linked polymorphic region (5-HTTLPR). The 5-HTTLPR comprises a repetitive sequence with an insertion or deletion variation. The deletion

Advanced Nutrition and Dietetics in Gastroenterology, First Edition. Edited by Miranda Lomer.
© 2014 John Wiley & Sons, Ltd. Published 2014 by John Wiley & Sons, Ltd.

variation comprises a short (*s*) allele, whilst the insertion is known as the long (*l*) allele. The *l* allele produces more serotonin transporter and reuptakes serotonin more efficiently than the *s* allele [9].

Three studies have evaluated this polymorphism in Turkish, American and Korean patients with IBS but did not demonstrate any association with genotype and disease status [10–12]. In addition, a meta-analysis has also concluded that this polymorphism is associated with neither IBS nor its subtypes [13]. However, two studies have found that certain polymorphisms may predict response to therapy. For example, the *LL* genotype has been associated with a better response to alosetron, a 5-HT$_3$ receptor antagonist, and the *s* allele was associated with predicting the response to tegaserod, a 5-HT$_4$ agonist, in those with constipation-predominant IBS [14,15].

Interleukin (IL)-10 is an anti-inflammatory cytokine, where a polymorphism of its gene, 1082G/G, is associated with higher production of IL-10 [16]. Gonsalkorale et al. demonstrated that IBS patients had a reduced frequency of the G/G genotype, thus suggesting that genetically determined immune activity plays a role in the pathophysiology of IBS [17].

In summary, recent evidence does support a modest polygenetic susceptibility in IBS. However, further studies are needed to further delineate clinically important subgroups, or phenotypes, of IBS, which may lead to further insights into its pathophysiology and may facilitate utilisation of the genome-wide association study methodology.

3.18.2 Psychological factors

There has been a considerable degree of controversy in the recent past as to whether psychological factors are related to IBS *per se* or whether they are a sequela of the severity of symptoms. Traditional evidence of the former points to psychological factors influencing fluctuations in symptoms, which thus determines the degree of healthcare-seeking behaviour.

Drossman et al. performed a multivariate analysis of three groups: those with IBS who had sought medical attention, those with IBS who had not sought medical attention, and healthy controls [18]. They demonstrated that psychological factors were associated with healthcare seeking rather than the disorder and these factors may interact with physiological disturbances in the GI tract thus determining how the illness is experienced and acted upon. Furthermore, Whitehead et al. evaluated whether self-selection for treatment accounts for psychological abnormalities in secondary care of patients with IBS [19]. They concluded that the symptoms of psychological distress were not related to IBS status *per se* but did significantly influence consulting behaviour.

However, more recent evidence has begun to challenge this long accepted view. Two studies, conducted in unrelated populations, demonstrated an association between psychological factors and IBS which was unrelated to the degree of healthcare seeking [20,21]. Furthermore, a prospective study by Halder et al. evaluated the factors that may predict the development of abdominal pain, showing that psychological distress, health anxiety and fatigue levels were independent predictors of future onset rather than sequelae of symptoms [22]. Taken together, the exact relationship, and influence, of psychological factors and IBS remain to be fully elucidated although there is little doubt that there is a complex interaction between them.

3.18.3 Visceral hypersensitivity

Visceral pain is a common presenting symptom and a central defining feature of IBS. Many hypotheses have been proposed to explain the origin of this symptom in IBS, but no single factor has achieved primacy in the literature, largely due to the significant heterogeneity of these disorders. However, a common feature of IBS is that patients often display a heightened sensitivity to experimental GI stimulation, termed visceral hypersensitivity. First reported in the early 1970s, it was observed that a proportion of patients with IBS demonstrated rectal hyperalgesia to mechanical distension of their sigmoid colon using an inflatable balloon [23]. Indeed, rectal hypersensitivity to mechanical distension has been proposed to be a clinically useful discriminatory feature between IBS and other GI disorders [24,25]. Nevertheless, visceral hypersensitivity is not a *sine qua non* facet of IBS, with a number of studies not reproducing these initial observations. Whilst the evidence for the role of visceral hypersensitivity in IBS is often conflicting, it should be noted that the positive association between functional symptoms and rectal hypersensitivity was found in the studies with the largest numbers of patients [26,27].

The observation of visceral hypersensitivity has resulted in a considerable research effort from academia and the pharmaceutical industry alike in attempting to identify the culpable molecular mechanisms that are responsible for this epiphenomenon. Therefore, the pathophysiology of visceral hypersensitivity may be conceptualised as being due to aberrant processes that may arise at any level of the visceral nociceptive pathway. Although the pathophysiology of visceral hypersensitivity has not been completely elucidated, several mechanisms have been proposed, including psychosocial stress, nutrient, hormonal, subtle (low-grade) inflammation and changes in the sensorimotor function of the GI tract, including both peripheral and central sensitisation of the visceral afferent neuronal pathways. We will now examine each of these factors in turn.

Psychosocial stress and visceral hypersensitivity

It has been well documented that patients who experience acute severe psychosocial stress are at heightened risk of developing a multitude of functional disorders, including IBS [28]. Up to 86% of patients with IBS report traumatic life experiences [29], with 7.8% fulfilling the criteria for a diagnosis of post-traumatic stress disorder [30]. Interestingly, patients often report that their symptoms are considerably worsened by stress. This has been examined in a number of studies, most notably by Posserud et al. where pain thresholds to rectal distensions were assessed in IBS patients in comparison to healthy controls in response to mental stress [31]. They demonstrated that stress induced an exaggerated neuroendocrine response and an increase in visceral perception, suggesting that stress may exacerbate IBS symptoms.

Nutrient intake and visceral hypersensitivity

Irritable bowel syndrome patients often report a deterioration, or precipitation, in symptoms, in addition to intolerances to one or more food groups [32]. In one study 63% of IBS patients reported that their GI symptoms were exacerbated by foods rich in carbohydrates, as well as fatty food, coffee, alcohol and hot spices [33]. Whilst the role of specific dietary constituents has only been the subject of limited research to date, a number of mechanisms have been postulated to contribute to the escalation of symptoms. Experimental evidence suggests that the physiological response of the intestine to food ingestion may precipitate symptoms in predisposed individuals. For example, Simrén et al. demonstrated that intraduodenal infusion of lipids enhanced rectal sensitivity in IBS patients in comparison to healthy controls [34]. However, this enhancement in rectal sensitivity is nutrient dependent, with fatty meals having a more pronounced effect than carbohydrates [35].

Peripheral sensitisation and visceral hypersensitivity

Noxious stimuli may cause the peripheral release of several inflammatory mediators such as K+, H+, adenosine triphosphate (ATP), 5-hydroxytryptamine (5-HT), bradykinins and prostaglandins [36,37], which may elicit a number of effects including the activation and peripheral sensitisation of nociceptive afferent nerves by reducing their transduction thresholds and by inducing the expression and recruitment of previously silent nociceptors. The main consequence of these inflammatory mediators is an increase in pain sensitivity at the site of injury, known as primary hyperalgesia [38]. A number of ion channels, neurotransmitter receptors and trophic factors have been directly and indirectly implicated in the development of peripheral sensitisation such as transient receptor potential vallinoid (TRPV) receptors 1 and 4, protease activated receptors, cannabinoid receptors, tachykinin receptors, the nitric oxide pathway, mast cells, enterochromaffin cells and 5-hydroxytriptamine, amongst others. Whilst it is beyond the scope of this chapter to examine these in detail, we would refer the reader to the excellent review articles by Anand et al. [39] and Knowles et al. [40].

Central sensitisation and visceral hypersensitivity

Sensitisation is not solely confined to the periphery. When a noxious stimulus is transmitted from the periphery, it induces a complex series of changes at the level of the spinal dorsal horn through the activation of intracellular signalling cascades. This may lead to central sensitisation and amplification of the nociceptive response to the stimuli (secondary hyperalgesia), and previously innocuous stimuli may provoke a nociceptive response (allodynia). Whilst these observations have long been recognised in somatic pain, increasingly central sensitisation is thought to play a central role in the development and maintenance of visceral hypersensitivity [41,42]. Sarkar et al. demonstrated this concept in a reproducible oesophageal model in humans, in which hydrochloric acid was infused into the distal oesophagus [41]. Pain thresholds were reduced not only in the acid-exposed distal region but also in the adjacent proximal unexposed region, thereby suggesting the development of central sensitisation. This effect of central sensitisation was prolonged, lasting up to 5 h after 30 min of acid exposure, suggesting that the duration and magnitude of the central sensitisation of the non-exposed proximal oesophagus were related directly to the intensity of acid exposure in the distal oesophagus.

Prostaglandin (PG) E_2 and the n-methyl d-aspartate (NMDA) receptor have been elucidated as the most important molecular factors in the development of central sensitisation at the spinal dorsal horn [43]. Human pharmacological studies have demonstrated that antagonism of PGE_2 or the NMDA receptor prevents the development of central sensitisation within the oesophagus, and antagonism of the NMDA receptor with ketamine may even reverse established visceral hypersensitivity [44,45]. This concept has also been demonstrated in IBS patients who, following repetitive distension of the sigmoid colon, developed rectal hyperalgesia and increased viscerosomatic referral to experimental rectal distension [27].

3.18.4 Inflammatory mechanisms and dietary components

Previous chronic, or indeed transient, inflammation in the GI tract can potentially result in persistent symptoms. Evidence for this hypothesis emanates from two sources. First, the prevalence of IBS-like symptoms in patients with quiescent inflammatory bowel disease is 2–3 times higher than in the general population [46]. Second, up to 22% of IBS patients report that their symptom onset occurs after an episode of gastroenteritis [47]. Additionally, several studies have identified aberrancies in mucosal T-cell immunity with an increase in enterochromaffin and mast cells being the most frequently reported abnormality [48,49].

3.18.5 Food hypersensitivity

Immune-mediated food hypersensitivity has been proposed to underlie the observation that patients' symptoms may respond to dietary eliminations [50]. These immune-mediated reactions are postulated to be secondary to IgG, IgG4 and to a lesser extent IgE. Generally speaking, tests to predict food sensitivity have lacked the sensitivity and specificity that would make them useful for routine clinical practice. However, the individual tailoring of dietary manipulations has been evaluated by Atkinson et al. where IgG antibodies were measured in a relatively large cohort of patients with IBS [51]. Patients were then randomised to receive either a diet excluding all foods to which they had raised IgG antibodies or a sham diet excluding the same number of foods but not those to which they had antibodies. At 3 months those patients who received the individualised diet had a greater reduction in symptom scores and global rating, with these reductions being more marked in patients who had been fully compliant. This exciting preliminary work warrants further investigation as it may allow for the individualisation of therapy.

3.18.6 Gastrointestinal microbiota

Specific bacterial strains and the composition of intestinal microbiota have been linked to the development of IBS and disturbances of commensal bacteria are thought to maintain low-grade inflammation [52]. Indeed, one leading authority has recently proposed that bacteria are one of many irritants in the GI tract that may lead to persistent long-lasting GI dysfunction and thus symptom generation [53]. In this regard, it is worth highlighting two sources of evidence in particular. First, Pimentel et al. performed a large double-blind clinical trial assessing the efficacy of rifaximin, a poorly absorbed antibiotic, in the treatment of patients with IBS without constipation [54]. It was demonstrated that treatment with 2 weeks' worth treatment of rifaximin provided significant relief of IBS symptoms. Furthermore, these benefits were, to a lesser degree, maintained after a period of 3 months. Second, there are a number of studies showing that, using the lactulose hydrogen breath test, small intestinal bacterial overgrowth is more common in patients with IBS [55,56].

Given the wealth of evidence that intestinal microbiota may be implicated in the genesis and persistence of IBS symptoms, it is not in the least surprising that investigators have attempted to identify specific bacterial species putatively responsible for this epiphenomenon. To a degree, this goal has been hampered by difficulties in culturing anaerobic bacteria using traditional culturing techniques and inadequate sample sizes in many of the published studies. However, Si et al. quantitatively examined the ratio of *Bifidobacterium* to Enterobacteriaceae in both IBS patients in comparison to healthy controls [57]. They reported a relative decrease in the numbers of *Bifidobacterium* and an increase in *Enterobacteriaceae* in IBS patients. Technological advances have facilitated the use of real-time polymerase chain reaction-based quantitative evaluation of bacterial DNA, a method that has been utilised by a number of groups but most notably by Malinen et al. [58]. Whilst considerable variation was observed in the microbiota between IBS patients and healthy controls in this study, the overall analysis suggested differences between *Clostridium coccoides* and *Bifidobacterium catenulatum*.

3.18.7 Conclusion

The clinical observation that patients with functional GI disorders may be hypersensitive to experimental visceral stimulation has had a considerable influence on the direction of research in the field for the last three decades. Great advances have been made in our understanding of the molecular mechanisms that underlie visceral hypersensitivity. Of particular interest has been the implication of inflammation in the genesis of symptoms in IBS and the potential role that the GI microbiota may play accounting for symptom persistence. An intriguing and burgeoning area of research is that of pharmacological manipulation of this microbiota, through either antibiotics or probiotics, which will not doubt increase the clinician's therapeutic armamentarium in the management of IBS.

References

1. Drossman DA. *Rome III: The Functional Gastrointestinal Disorders*, 3rd edn. McLean, VA: Degnon Associates, 2006.
2. Jones R, Lydeard S. Irritable bowel syndrome in the general population. *British Medical Journal* 1992; **304**: 87–90.
3. Talley NJ, Zinsmeister AR, van Dyke C, Melton LJ 3rd. Epidemiology of colonic symptoms and the irritable bowel syndrome. *Gastroenterology* 1991; **101**: 927–934.
4. Drossman DA, Li Z, Andruzzi E, et al. US householder survey of functional gastrointestinal disorders. Prevalence, sociodemography, and health impact. *Digestive Diseases and Sciences* 1993; **38**: 1569–1580.
5. Kalantar JS, Locke GR 3rd, Zinsmeister AR, Beighley CM, Talley NJ. Familial aggregation of irritable bowel syndrome: a prospective study. *Gut* 2003; **52**: 1703–1707.
6. Kanazawa M, Endo Y, Whitehead WE, Kano M, Hongo M, Fukudo S. Patients and nonconsulters with irritable bowel syndrome reporting a parental history of bowel problems have more impaired psychological distress. *Digestive Diseases and Sciences* 2004; **49**: 1046–1053.
7. Levy RL, Jones KR, Whitehead WE, Feld SI, Talley NJ, Corey LA. Irritable bowel syndrome in twins: heredity and social learning both contribute to etiology. *Gastroenterology* 2001; **121**: 799–804.
8. Morris-Yates A, Talley NJ, Boyce PM, Nandurkar S, Andrews G. Evidence of a genetic contribution to functional bowel disorder. *American Journal of Gastroenterology* 1998; **93**: 1311–1317.
9. Lesch KP, Bengel D, Heils A, et al. Association of anxiety-related traits with a polymorphism in the serotonin transporter gene regulatory region. *Science* 1996; **274**: 1527–1531.
10. Pata C, Erdal ME, Derici E, Yazar A, Kanik A, Ulu O. Serotonin transporter gene polymorphism in irritable bowel syndrome. *American Journal of Gastroenterology* 2002; **97**: 1780–1784.
11. Yeo A, Boyd P, Lumsden S, et al. Association between a functional polymorphism in the serotonin transporter gene and diarrhoea predominant irritable bowel syndrome in women. *Gut* 2004; **53**: 1452–1458.
12. Park JM, Choi MG, Park JA, et al. Serotonin transporter gene polymorphism and irritable bowel syndrome. *Neurogastroenterology and Motility* 2006; **18**: 995–1000.

13. Van Kerkhoven LA, Laheij RJ, Jansen JB. Meta-analysis: a functional polymorphism in the gene encoding for activity of the serotonin transporter protein is not associated with the irritable bowel syndrome. *Alimentary Pharmacology and Therapeutics* 2007; **26**: 979–986.

14. Camilleri M, Atanasova E, Carlson PJ, et al. Serotonin-transporter polymorphism pharmacogenetics in diarrhea-predominant irritable bowel syndrome. *Gastroenterology* 2002; **123**: 425–432.

15. Li Y, Nie Y, Xie J, et al. The association of serotonin transporter genetic polymorphisms and irritable bowel syndrome and its influence on tegaserod treatment in Chinese patients. *Digestive Diseases and Sciences* 2007; **52**: 2942–2949.

16. Manicassamy S, Reizis B, Ravindran R, et al. Activation of beta-catenin in dendritic cells regulates immunity versus tolerance in the intestine. *Science* 2010; **329**: 849–853.

17. Gonsalkorale WM, Perrey C, Pravica V, Whorwell PJ, Hutchinson IV. Interleukin 10 genotypes in irritable bowel syndrome: evidence for an inflammatory component? *Gut* 2003; **52**: 91–93.

18. Drossman DA, McKee DC, Sandler RS, et al. Psychosocial factors in the irritable bowel syndrome. A multivariate study of patients and nonpatients with irritable bowel syndrome. *Gastroenterology* 1988; **95**: 701–708.

19. Whitehead WE, Bosmajian L, Zonderman AB, Costa PT Jr, Schuster MM. Symptoms of psychologic distress associated with irritable bowel syndrome. Comparison of community and medical clinic samples. *Gastroenterology* 1988; **95**: 709–714.

20. Weinryb RM, Osterberg E, Blomquist L, Hultcrantz R, Krakau I, Asberg M. Psychological factors in irritable bowel syndrome: a population-based study of patients, non-patients and controls. *Scandinavian Journal of Gastroenterology* 2003; **38**: 503–510.

21. Locke GR 3rd, Weaver AL, Melton LJ 3rd, Talley NJ. Psychosocial factors are linked to functional gastrointestinal disorders: a population based nested case–control study. *American Journal of Gastroenterology* 2004; **99**: 350–357.

22. Halder SL, McBeth J, Silman AJ, Thompson DG, Macfarlane GJ. Psychosocial risk factors for the onset of abdominal pain. Results from a large prospective population-based study. *International Journal of Epidemiology* 2002; **31**: 1219–1225; discussion 1225–1226.

23. Ritchie J. Pain from distension of the pelvic colon by inflating a balloon in the irritable colon syndrome. *Gut* 1973; **14**: 125–132.

24. Wingate DL. The irritable bowel syndrome. *Gastroenterology Clinics of North America* 1991; **20**: 351–362.

25. Bouin M, Plourde V, Boivin M, et al. Rectal distention testing in patients with irritable bowel syndrome: sensitivity, specificity, and predictive values of pain sensory thresholds. *Gastroenterology* 2002; **122**: 1771–1777.

26. Mertz H, Naliboff B, Munakata J, Niazi N, Mayer EA. Altered rectal perception is a biological marker of patients with irritable bowel syndrome. *Gastroenterology* 1995; **109**: 40–52.

27. Munakata J, Naliboff B, Harraf F, et al. Repetitive sigmoid stimulation induces rectal hyperalgesia in patients with irritable bowel syndrome. *Gastroenterology* 1997; **112**: 55–63.

28. Dobie DJ, Kivlahan DR, Maynard C, Bush KR, Davis TM, Bradley KA. Posttraumatic stress disorder in female veterans: association with self-reported health problems and functional impairment. *Archives of Internal Medicine* 2004; **164**: 394–400.

29. Dunphy RC, Bridgewater L, Price DD, Robinson ME, Zeilman CJ 3rd, Verne GN. Visceral and cutaneous hypersensitivity in Persian Gulf war veterans with chronic gastrointestinal symptoms. *Pain* 2003; **102**: 79–85.

30. Cohen H, Jotkowitz A, Buskila D, et al. Post-traumatic stress disorder and other co-morbidities in a sample population of patients with irritable bowel syndrome. *European Journal of Internal Medicine* 2006; **17**: 567–571.

31. Posserud I, Agerforz P, Ekman R, Bjornsson ES, Abrahamsson H, Simren M. Altered visceral perceptual and neuroendocrine response in patients with irritable bowel syndrome during mental stress. *Gut* 2004; **53**: 1102–1108.

32. Morcos A, Dinan T, Quigley EM. Irritable bowel syndrome: role of food in pathogenesis and management. *Journal of Digestive Diseases* 2009; **10**: 237–246.

33. Simrén M, Mansson A, Langkilde AM, et al. Food-related gastrointestinal symptoms in the irritable bowel syndrome. *Digestion* 2001; **63**: 108–115.

34. Simrén M, Abrahamsson H, Bjornsson ES. Lipid-induced colonic hypersensitivity in the irritable bowel syndrome: the role of bowel habit, sex, and psychologic factors. *Clinical Gastroenterology and Hepatology* 2007; **5**: 201–208.

35. Simrén M, Agerforz P, Bjornsson ES, Abrahamsson H. Nutrient-dependent enhancement of rectal sensitivity in irritable bowel syndrome (IBS). *Neurogastroenterology and Motility* 2007; **19**: 20–29.

36. Yu S, Ouyang A. TRPA1 in bradykinin-induced mechano-hypersensitivity of vagal C fibers in guinea pig esophagus. *American Journal of Physiology - Gastrointestinal and Liver Physiology* 2009; **296**: G255–G265.

37. Jones RC 3rd, Xu L, Gebhart GF. The mechanosensitivity of mouse colon afferent fibers and their sensitization by inflammatory mediators require transient receptor potential vanilloid 1 and acid-sensing ion channel 3. *Journal of Neuroscience* 2005; **25**: 10981–10989.

38. Knowles CH, Aziz Q. Visceral hypersensitivity in non-erosive reflux disease. *Gut* 2008; **57**: 674–683.

39. Anand P, Aziz Q, Willert R, van Oudenhove L. Peripheral and central mechanisms of visceral sensitization in man. *Neurogastroenterology and Motility* 2007; **19**: 29–46.

40. Knowles CH, Aziz Q. Basic and clinical aspects of gastrointestinal pain. *Pain* 2009; **141**: 191–209.

41. Sarkar S, Aziz Q, Woolf CJ, Hobson AR, Thompson DG. Contribution of central sensitisation to the development of non-cardiac chest pain. *Lancet* 2000; **356**: 1154–1159.

42. Sarkar S, Hobson AR, Furlong PL, Woolf CJ, Thompson DG, Aziz Q. Central neural mechanisms mediating human visceral hypersensitivity. *American Journal of Physiology - Gastrointestinal and Liver Physiology* 2001; **281**: G1196–G1202.

43. Grundy D, Al-Chaer ED, Aziz Q, et al. Fundamentals of neurogastroenterology: basic science. *Gastroenterology* 2006; **130**: 1391–1411.

44. Sarkar S, Hobson AR, Hughes A, et al. The prostaglandin E2 receptor-1 (EP-1) mediates acid-induced visceral pain hypersensitivity in humans. *Gastroenterology* 2003; **124**: 18–25.

45. Willert RP, Woolf CJ, Hobson AR, Delaney C, Thompson DG, Aziz Q. The development and maintenance of human visceral pain hypersensitivity is dependent on the N-methyl-D-aspartate receptor. *Gastroenterology* 2004; **126**: 683–692.

46. Long MD, Drossman DA. Inflammatory bowel disease, irritable bowel syndrome, or what? A challenge to the functional-organic dichotomy. *American Journal of Gastroenterology* 2010; **105**: 1796–1798.

47. Rhodes DY, Wallace M. Post-infectious irritable bowel syndrome. *Current Gastroenterology Reports* 2006; **8**: 327–332.

48. Wheatcroft J, Wakelin D, Smith A, Mahoney CR, Mawe G, Spiller R. Enterochromaffin cell hyperplasia and decreased serotonin transporter in a mouse model of postinfectious bowel dysfunction. *Neurogastroenterology and Motility* 2005; **17**: 863–870.

49. Lee KJ, Kim YB, Kim JH, Kwon HC, Kim DK, Cho SW. The alteration of enterochromaffin cell, mast cell, and lamina propria T lymphocyte numbers in irritable bowel syndrome and its relationship with psychological factors. *Journal of Gastroenterology and Hepatology* 2008; **23**: 1689–1694.

50. Isolauri E, Rautava S, Kalliomaki M. Food allergy in irritable bowel syndrome: new facts and old fallacies. *Gut* 2004; **53**: 1391–1393.

51. Atkinson W, Sheldon TA, Shaath N, Whorwell PJ. Food elimination based on IgG antibodies in irritable bowel syndrome: a randomised controlled trial. *Gut* 2004; **53**: 1459–1464.

52. Collins S, Verdu E, Denou E, Bercik P. The role of pathogenic microbes and commensal bacteria in irritable bowel syndrome. *Digestive Diseases* 2009; **27**(Suppl 1): 85–89.

53. Ohman L, Simren M. Pathogenesis of IBS: role of inflammation, immunity and neuroimmune interactions. *Nature Reviews Gastroenterology and Hepatology* 2010; **7**: 163–173.

54. Pimentel M, Lembo A, Chey WD, et al. Rifaximin therapy for patients with irritable bowel syndrome without constipation. *New England Journal of Medicine* 2011; **364**: 22–32.

55. Grover M, Kanazawa M, Palsson OS, et al. Small intestinal bacterial overgrowth in irritable bowel syndrome: association with colon motility, bowel symptoms, and psychological distress. *Neurogastroenterology and Motility* 2008; **20**: 998–1008.

56. Ghoshal UC, Kumar S, Mehrotra M, Lakshmi C, Misra A. Frequency of small intestinal bacterial overgrowth in patients with irritable bowel syndrome and chronic non-specific diarrhea. *Journal of Neurogastroenterology and Motility* 2010; **16**: 40–46.

57. Si JM, Yu YC, Fan YJ, Chen SJ. Intestinal microecology and quality of life in irritable bowel syndrome patients. *World Journal of Gastroenterology* 2004; **10**: 1802–1805.

58. Malinen E, Rinttila T, Kajander K, et al. Analysis of the fecal microbiota of irritable bowel syndrome patients and healthy controls with real-time PCR. *American Journal of Gastroenterology* 2005; **100**: 373–382.

Chapter 3.19

Irritable bowel syndrome dietary management

Heidi Staudacher[1] and Gareth Parkes[2]
[1]King's College London and Guy's and St Thomas' NHS Foundation Trust, London, UK
[2]Barts Health NHS Trust, London, UK

3.19.1 Dietary effects of disease or its management

Up to 90% of patients with irritable bowel syndrome (IBS) identify food as having an important role in the generation of symptoms [1–3] and many patients report a preference for dietary management rather than reliance on medical therapy. As a result, self-management is frequently attempted, which almost always involves exclusion of food(s) in the absence of a rationale. Therefore, although IBS does not inherently affect nutritional status, attempts to self-manage symptoms via dietary means may do so.

Up to 50% of patients alter their diet to improve symptoms [4]. Many foods have been reported to trigger symptoms in IBS patients including dairy, grains, fruit, vegetables and egg [1,5]. Commonly reported trigger foods are often rich in important nutrients, so it is unsurprising that nutritional inadequacies become apparent on assessment of dietary intake. Low intake of B vitamins, iron and/or calcium [6–8] has been reported, although not all studies are in agreement [9]. Heterogeneity of studies and the lack of research limit definitive conclusions. However, it is generally well accepted that dietary intake may be at risk, leading to nutritional deficiency.

Guidelines for the management of IBS state that diet and lifestyle should be first-line considerations [10,11]. In most cases, a dietitian will investigate clinical history, anthropometry, symptom profile, dietary pattern, nutritional intake and previously implemented dietary measures prior to providing dietary advice. Determining the level of motivation for dietary modification is important. A diet and symptom diary may help identify poor eating patterns and determine whether food is implicated in symptom provocation, although this is not always a valid measure of identifying problem foods. Various dietary intervention strategies are available for IBS patients and a clinical algorithm for dietary management has been developed (Figure 3.19.1) [10].

Possible underlying pathophysiological mechanisms of IBS include visceral hypersensitivity [12], altered colonic motility [13], altered fermentation [14] or disturbed gas handling [15] and therefore it is not surprising that symptoms are generally induced postprandially [16]. Furthermore, food-related symptoms are more frequent in those with anxiety [16]. Assessment of eating behaviour (e.g. frequency, pattern, the eating environment) is important as symptoms may lead to reduced frequency of meals and greater likelihood of overeating which might exacerbate symptoms. Advice regarding eating at regular intervals and appropriate eating behaviours forms the basis of first-line dietary guidelines [10]. Sitting down to eat and eating slowly, chewing food thoroughly and avoiding eating late at night may be very useful. Explanation

Advanced Nutrition and Dietetics in Gastroenterology, First Edition. Edited by Miranda Lomer.

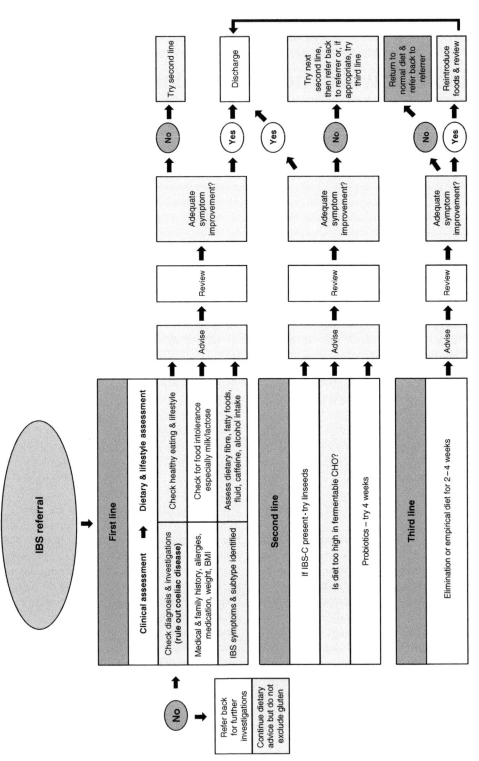

Figure 3.19.1 Algorithm for dietary management of IBS. BMI, Body Mass Index; CHO, carbohydrate; IBS-C, constipation-dominant irritable bowel syndrome.

of the underlying pathophysiology of IBS may reassure patients and prevent unnecessary restriction of foods when poor eating behaviour is suspected as a primary trigger of symptom generation.

3.19.2 Dietary interventions

Lactose

Lactose malabsorption is present in up to 50% of patients with IBS, depending on ethnicity [17]. Lactose hydrogen breath testing can be useful to diagnose lactose malabsorption but may not be available. To assess lactose intolerance, a lactose food challenge using at least 12 g lactose (e.g. 125 mL milk) and a food and symptom diary to identify symptom exacerbation may be useful. Other dietary and lifestyle factors are also often implicated, and therefore exclusion of high-lactose foods may not lead to symptom resolution.

Non-starch polysaccharides

Historically, non-starch polysaccharides (NSP) have been a target for dietary intervention in IBS, particularly in those with constipation or with variable stool output (i.e. alternating constipation and diarrhoea). However, a recent Cochrane review suggested that bulking agents, whether insoluble (e.g. wheat bran) or soluble fibre (e.g. psyllium, ispaghula), are not effective in improving IBS symptoms [18] Indeed, wheat bran may worsen symptoms and the addition of insoluble fibre for patients with IBS is now discouraged [11].

Studies using soluble fibre supplementation indicate that ispaghula husk may be useful in patients with constipation [19] but more recent reviews for its use in IBS present the overall evidence as weak. Studies are often hindered by either the lack of a control group or high placebo response rates. Interpretation of results is difficult due to study heterogeneity. For example, studies differ with respect to patient symptom profiles, the source of supplemental NSP, duration of intervention and outcome measures. Poor study design and high drop-out rates are also common. Furthermore, clinically, supplementation with soluble fibre may induce bloating

and discomfort probably due to its fermentation in the large intestine, although individual symptom response appears to vary markedly.

Constipation-predominant IBS is notoriously difficult to manage via dietary means. The evidence for NSP supplementation is weak but should not be ignored. Supplementation with 50 g/day linseed (flaxseed) increases the number of bowel movements in a healthy population by 30% [20] and 24 g/day linseeds improves constipation more than psyllium over 3–6 months in constipation-predominant IBS patients, although laxative use was not monitored in this study [21]. Recently, a small open-label randomised pilot study showed that intake of ground or whole linseed for 4 weeks was associated with improvement in IBS symptom scores compared to no linseeds in a group of mixed IBS subtypes [22]. This was not statistically significant in the intention-to-treat analysis and further work is needed to verify these results and investigate the effect of linseeds on stool output in constipation-predominant IBS.

Conversely, NSP restriction should reduce stool bulk and frequency and is used to manage diarrhoea-predominant IBS with some good effect. Research on NSP restriction in enterally fed hospital inpatients with diarrhoea and a 2-week NSP-free liquid diet showed an improvement in overall symptom scores in IBS [23]; however, this is impractical to maintain in the long term. Formal investigation into its efficacy, the level of restriction required or nutritional consequences of its implementation has not been performed.

Caffeine

Caffeine is a stimulant of colonic motility in healthy individuals [24] and it is likely that sensitivity and symptom response are exaggerated in those with IBS. There are no randomised controlled trials investigating the effect of restriction of caffeine on symptoms in IBS. However, many patients report symptoms with caffeine consumption [1,5,16] and often limit or avoid it. Exclusion diet studies demonstrate that reintroduction of caffeinated drinks induces symptoms in approximately 30% of patients with IBS [5,25]. Dietary guidelines suggest a trial of caffeine restriction and encourage fluids from non-caffeinated sources.

Alcohol

Alcohol is a perceived symptom trigger in up to 33% of patients with IBS [5,16]. A large cross-sectional study in the community did not find an association with alcohol intake and the incidence of IBS, although an increased likelihood of abdominal pain with moderate intakes of alcohol was found [26]. This does not demonstrate causality and randomised controlled studies on the effects of alcohol in IBS have not been performed. Large individual variation in tolerance is apparent not only to volume but types of alcoholic drinks. It would seem prudent that patients abide within healthy limits for alcohol consumption and specific advice should be given on a case-by-case basis.

Fat

Dietary fat is often a trigger for GI symptoms in patients with IBS, particularly after meals that contain large amounts of cream, oil, butter or foods that are battered or crumbed [1,3,5]. Fat is a stimulant of colonic motility and impairs gas transit in IBS [27]. Furthermore, duodenal lipid infusion results in lower colonic pressure thresholds in IBS patients versus controls, leading to earlier symptoms [28]. However randomised controlled dietary studies are required to confirm that restriction is indeed effective.

Resistant starch

Most dietary starch is completely digested in the small intestine but a fraction, termed 'resistant starch' (RS), survives digestion and contributes to NSP intake [29]. It has similar effects to other NSP in the GI tract, including increased stool bulk [30,31], osmotic pull and fermentative effects leading to increased short-chain fatty acid production [30]. There are a number of classifications, including type 1 which is present in foods where the starch is physically inaccessible, e.g. in seeds. Type 2 RS is found in raw starch granules, e.g. raw potato. Type 3 is formed when amylase and amylopectin are retrograded after heating and subsequent cooling and is present in foods such as bread, cooked and cooled potato and cornflakes. More recently, chemically modified starches have been included in the definition and are classified as type 4 RS and are present in some high-fibre fluids and breads.

Most studies have focused on the physiological effects of RS in healthy individuals and it has been demonstrated that high RS intakes of up to 60 g/day can lead to GI symptoms, including bloating, increased stool frequency and loose stools [32]. This may partly be due to its fermentation in the large intestine. However, the fermentation rate is relatively slow [33] and as a polymerised structure with a high molecular weight, it is usually better tolerated than other indigestible carbohydrates. The effect of RS in patients with IBS has not been investigated. However, anecdotal evidence suggests it might induce symptoms in some patients. Patients reporting symptoms after consumption of foods high in RS (e.g. part-baked breads, pizza, pasta and convenience foods) sometimes respond to avoidance of these foods. However, whether it is the RS or another component that triggers symptoms is unknown and research is warranted to further delineate its role in inducing symptoms.

Fermentable carbohydrates

There is growing interest in the effects of restricting short-chain fermentable carbohydrates, collectively termed FODMAPs (fermentable, oligo-, di- and monosaccharides and polyols), for the management of IBS. Chemical structure, physiological effects in the GI tract and sources of these carbohydrates are described in Chapter 2.2. Many studies have investigated the effect of individual fermentable carbohydrates on GI symptoms in patients with IBS. For example, fructose, sorbitol or fructans, either individually or in combination, are associated with exacerbation of symptoms [34,35,36] and restriction is associated with improvement in functional GI symptoms [37,38]. More recently, research has focused on the effect of avoiding fermentable carbohydrates collectively (i.e. low FODMAP diet) which is effective in improving overall symptoms in up to 70% of patients in randomised controlled trials and up to 94% in patients in uncontrolled work [39]. Gas-related symptoms such as bloating and wind, and urgency and stool frequency appear to be particularly responsive to this type of dietary restriction.

A diet low in FODMAPs involves the avoidance of fructans, galacto-oligosaccharides, polyols, fructose in excess of glucose, and lactose. Poor absorption of fructose and lactose only occurs in a proportion of patients and restriction should occur based on the results of lactose and fructose hydrogen breath testing or clinical suspicion. Dietitian-led education regarding FODMAP restriction should occur with the intervention lasting at least 4 weeks [6]. Although the diet requires substantial effort, recent work has shown that it is no more difficult to follow or understand compared to standard IBS advice [40].

After a period of FODMAP restriction, patients follow a staged reintroduction process, systematically reintroducing foods high in one short-chain fermentable carbohydrate. This helps to determine dose tolerance and ultimately directs long-term dietary habits whilst promoting increased nutritional variety.

Due to the complex nature of the low FODMAP diet, and that foods frequently consumed require restriction (i.e. some breads and cereals, fruits and vegetables, dairy products), it has been suggested that this diet may not be nutritionally adequate, which is always a risk with elimination diets. Indeed, a lower calcium intake was found in patients with IBS following a low FODMAP diet compared to a habitual diet [6]. This is a concern as IBS may be associated with a higher risk of osteoporosis [41]. Emphasis should be placed on inclusion of appropriate portions of high calcium, low lactose foods. Specific instruction on suitable brands of low lactose dairy alternatives.

A low FODMAP diet also affects the GI microbiota and recent work has shown that luminal bifidobacteria are markedly lower after a 4-week low FODMAP diet in patients with IBS [6]. This is probably due to the restriction of prebiotic fructo- and galacto-oligosaccharides. Whether this effect persists long term or affects long-term health is not known and requires further investigation.

Finally, research on the efficacy of FODMAP restriction has thus far been limited to a dietitian-led approach. Compliance, which is influenced by patient motivation but also careful advice from an experienced dietitian who has access to up-to-date lists of suitable and unsuitable foods, is vital to its success. The success of a simpler modified approach when complete restriction is not justified, led either by a dietitian or other health practitioner, is yet to be determined.

Gluten

Gluten has also been proposed as a provoker of GI symptoms, and is often reported as problematic by patients with IBS. A recent double-blind placebo-controlled study has shown that symptoms return when patients previously well controlled on a gluten-free diet are challenged with gluten [42]. No changes in coeliac serology, intestinal permeability or immune markers were found to explain a mechanism supporting this finding and further recent work by the same group did not reproduce the same effect on symptoms [43]. Further work is required before a gluten-free diet becomes a recommended dietary strategy for patients with IBS.

3.19.3 Food allergy

The above dietary interventions assume that symptoms are elicited by the effect of food residue in the GI lumen. Food-provoked GI symptoms are not always caused by underlying IBS. For example, IgE food allergy, diagnosed using skin prick tests or food-specific blood immunoglobulin E (IgE) concentrations, occurs in 1–4% of the adult population [44] and can provoke GI symptoms. Gastrointestinal symptoms may also present as delayed-onset non-IgE-mediated food allergy, although this is less well understood, poorly defined, difficult to diagnose and almost exclusively studied in the paediatric population [45]. It relies dietary elimination and controlled reintroduction, monitoring for allergic response. Pathophysiological studies show that the GI immune system, particularly mast cell activation, might be important in IBS [46]. Furthermore, there is some overlap between IBS and atopic disease [47]. However, whether the primary diagnosis is allergy and not IBS in these patients, or whether IBS truly has a significant inflammatory component needs to be clarified [48]. Both IgE and non-IgE allergies are, of course, distinct conditions in themselves, although they may co-exist with IBS [47].

The use of food-specific IgG antibody concentration as a diagnostic tool for identifying culprit foods in food allergy or any other adverse food reaction has been investigated [49]. Its validity is questionable and a European position paper [50], supported by the national US allergy body [51], has affirmed that this type of testing is not recommended as a diagnostic tool.

3.19.4 Pharmacological food intolerance

Pharmacological food intolerance may also contribute to GI symptoms. Restriction of naturally occurring food chemicals including salicylates and vasoactive amines as well as additives (e.g. colours, preservatives) may be helpful. The literature to date is predominantly dedicated to their effect on non-GI symptoms (e.g. migraine, urticaria) [44,45] although clinically they appear to provoke GI symptoms in some individuals with IBS. Treatment involves dietary exclusion and stepwise food reintroduction.

3.19.5 Other exclusion diets

Various other types of exclusion diets for the management of IBS have been described but the limited data and lack of understanding of the active components in restricted foods make them a final option when other strategies have failed [10].

Strict exclusion diets are difficult to comply with and may be of prolonged duration. The use of food reintroduction to challenge tolerance is more practical than capsule challenges, which are considered the gold standard in diagnosis of food intolerance. However, food composition is complex, and a single challenge food item contains numerous possible constituents that could induce symptoms, leading to erroneous interpretation of food challenge results and increasing the risk of inappropriate long-term food exclusion.

3.19.6 Probiotics

There has been interest in the role that the GI microbiota plays in the aetiology of IBS and its potential as a therapeutic target, in particular through the use of probiotics and to a lesser extent prebiotics

[52]. Probiotics have been shown to have several mechanisms of action, which may be important in the treatment of IBS.

- *Anti-inflammatory* – in the pilot trial of the probiotic bacteria *Bifidobacterium infantis* 35624, patients randomised to *B. infantis* 35624 demonstrated a reduction in systemic inflammatory cytokines which was not seen in either the placebo or a second probiotic strain [53]. These findings correlated with clinical benefit.
- *Modulate visceral hypersensitivity* – *Lactobacillus acidophilus* has been shown to upregulate mu-opioid and cannabinoid receptors in colonic epithelial cell lines and in the colonic epithelium in pretreated rats and mice [54]. Similarly, *L paracasei* attenuated abdominal pain and mucosal inflammation in an antibiotic-induced murine model of visceral hypersensitivity [55].
- *Small intestinal permeability* – a probiotic drink containing *Streptococcus thermophilus*, *Lactobacillus bulgaricus*, *L acidophilus* and *Bifidobacterium longum* in patients with IBS-D led to a significant decrease in small intestinal permeability, as well as an improvement in global symptom scores [56].
- *GI transit* – the probiotic mixture VSL#3 (*Lactobacillus casei, L. plantarum, L. acidophilus*, and *L. bulgaricus, Bifidobacterium longum, B. breve, B. infantis* and *Streptococcus thermophilus*) has been shown to significantly decrease intestinal transit in patients with IBS-D although this did not correlate with a reduction in stool frequency [57]. Conversely, *B. animalis* DN 175101 has been shown to increase colonic transit in patients with IBS-C [58].

There have now been numerous clinical trials investigating the therapeutic benefit of probiotics in IBS with heterogeneity in dosing regimens, species used and clinical end-points. Many of the recent RCTs are summarised below.

Lactobacillus plantarum

There are three small single-centre studies using a liquid form of *L. plantarum* with two studies showing some benefit [59,60] and one with no benefit although this was significantly underpowered [61].

These initial results have never been followed up in larger multicentred studies.

Bifidobacterium infantis 35624

In a trial of 77 patients with IBS randomised to *B. infantis* 35624 or *Lactobacillus salivarius* or placebo, *B. infantis* 35624 significantly reduced pain, bloating and symptom satisfaction scores in comparison to placebo as well as composite scores [53]. A second multicentre dose-finding trial of *B. infantis* 35624 in 362 female patients with IBS found that the group taking *B. infantis* 10^8 cfu per day scored significantly better than placebo in all symptom groups, including a global assessment of IBS relief [62].

Bifidobacterium animalis DN 173010

A multicentre trial of *B. animalis* DN 173010 in 274 primary care patients with IBS-C did not demonstrate significant benefit over placebo [63]. However, subgroup analysis of patients with less than three bowel motions a week (n = 19) at baseline showed a significant rise in stool frequency compared to controls.

Escherichia coli DSM 17252

A primary care-based, placebo-controlled trial of *E. coli* DSM 17252 in 298 patients with IBS found that the treatment arm achieved complete remission in significantly more cases than placebo [64]. Data from primary rather than secondary care are particularly useful given that the majority of IBS patients are treated by primary care physicians.

VSL#3

A combination probiotic, VSL#3, has been used in two small trials of patients with IBS by the same group [57,65]. Both trials failed to meet their primary end-point of reduction in GI transit [57] or reduction in bloating scores [65]. However, there was a significant reduction in flatulence in the latter trial and the combination probiotic significantly retarded colonic transit although without a corresponding change in stool frequency or form. Thus there is only weak evidence supporting the use of this combination probiotic in IBS at present.

Bifidobacterium bifidum MIMBb75

A single 4-week controlled trial of *B. bifidum* MIMBb75, in which 122 patients with IBS were randomised to either probiotic or placebo, demonstrated that it was superior to placebo in reducing global symptom scores [66]. This improvement was maintained over a 2-week washout period. In addition, the probiotic strain significantly reduced subscores of abdominal pain, bloating/distension and satisfaction with stool output.

Escherichia coli Nissle 1917

This probiotic strain has been shown to be clinically effective in the treatment of ulcerative colitis [67,68]. A trial in 120 patients with IBS demonstrated only a modest benefit in reduction of global symptom score, requiring 11 weeks of treatment prior to reaching significance [69]. However, in a subgroup analysis of 17 patients in whom the symptoms of IBS followed either an episode of acute gastroenteritis or a course of antibiotics, response rates were significantly superior in the *E. coli* Nissle 1917 group compared to placebo. This is the first trial in which patients with postinfective IBS have been studied as a subgroup and further work is required to validate these results.

The probiotics with the best efficacy data in treating IBS are *B. infantis* 35624 and *E. coli* DSM 17252. Both of these probiotics have had initial successful trials supported by larger multicentre studies [53,62,64,70]. In particular, *B. infantis* 35624 has *in vitro* and human data supporting a putative mechanism of action. Clinical guidelines recommend that individuals choosing to try probiotics should select one product at a time and monitor the effects. They should try it for a minimum of 4 weeks at the dose recommended by the manufacturer [10,11].

3.19.7 Prebiotics

There have been very few trials of prebiotics in IBS. A randomised placebo-controlled trial of transgalacto-oligosaccharide in 44 patients with IBS found that at a dose of 7 g/day, there was a significant improvement in a subjective global score (SGA) over placebo [71]. This corresponded with a significant rise in bifidobacteria and a significant reduction in *Bacteroides-Prevotella* spp in the prebiotic group compared to controls.

3.19.8 Conclusion

In conclusion, a number of dietary components have been reported to trigger symptoms in IBS. Good-quality evidence exists for the effectiveness of FODMAP restriction in a majority of IBS patients, and this should be implemented when removal of basic IBS triggers is not effective. Further data are required to unearth the full potential of other dietary regimens. Reliable identification of food chemical and gluten sensitivity and a better understanding of the role of the GI immune system will be vital for optimising the dietetic IBS treatment pathway.

References

1. Hayes P, Corish C, O'Mahony E, Quigley EM. A dietary survey of patients with irritable bowel syndrome. *Journal of Human Nutrition and Dietetics* 2013; May 9 (epub ahead of print).
2. Lacy BE, Weiser K, Noddin L, et al. Irritable bowel syndrome: patients' attitudes, concerns and level of knowledge. *Alimentary Pharmacology and Therapeutics* 2007; **25**: 1329–1341.
3. Halpert A, Dalton CB, Palsson O, et al. What patients know about irritable bowel syndrome (IBS) and what they would like to know. National Survey on Patient Educational Needs in IBS and development and validation of the Patient Educational Needs Questionnaire (PEQ). *American Journal of Gastroenterology* 2007; **102**: 1972–1982.
4. Faresjo A, Johansson S, Faresjo T, Roos S, Hallert C. Sex differences in dietary coping with gastrointestinal symptoms. *European Journal of Gastroenterology and Hepatology* 2010; **22**: 327–333.
5. Nanda R, James R, Smith H, Dudley CR, Jewell DP. Food intolerance and the irritable bowel syndrome. *Gut* 1989; **30**: 1099–1104.
6. Staudacher HM, Lomer MC, Anderson JL, et al. Fermentable carbohydrate restriction reduces luminal bifidobacteria and gastrointestinal symptoms in patients with irritable bowel syndrome. *Journal of Nutrition* 2012; **142**: 1510–1518.
7. Ligaarden SC, Farup PG. Low intake of vitamin B6 is associated with irritable bowel syndrome symptoms. *Nutrition Research* 2011; **31**: 356–361.
8. Prescha A, Pieczynska J, Ilow R, et al. Assessment of dietary intake of patients with irritable bowel syndrome. *Roczniki Państwowego Zakładu Higieny* 2009; **60**: 185–189.
9. Williams EA, Nai X, Corfe BM. Dietary intakes in people with irritable bowel syndrome. *BMC Gastroenterology* 2011; **11**: 9.
10. McKenzie YA, Alder A, Anderson W, et al. British Dietetic Association evidence-based guidelines for the dietary management of irritable bowel syndrome in adults. *Journal of Human Nutrition Dietetics* 2012; **25**: 260–274.
11. National Institute for Health and Clinical Excellence (NICE). Irritable bowel syndrome in adults. Diagnosis and management of irritable bowel syndrome in primary care. 2008. www.nice.org.uk/nicemedia/live/11927/39622/39622.pdf, accessed 7 January 2014.
12. Camilleri M, McKinzie S, Busciglio I, et al. Prospective study of motor, sensory, psychologic, and autonomic functions in patients with irritable bowel syndrome. *Clinical Gastroenterology and Hepatology* 2008; **6**: 772–781.
13. Manabe N, Wong BS, Camilleri M, Burton D, McKinzie S, Zinsmeister AR. Lower functional gastrointestinal disorders: evidence of abnormal colonic transit in a 287 patient cohort. *Neurogastroenterology and Motility* 2010; **22**: 293–e82.
14. King TS, Elia M, Hunter JO. Abnormal colonic fermentation in irritable bowel syndrome. *Lancet* 1998; **352**: 1187–1189.
15. Serra J, Azpiroz F, Malagelada JR. Impaired transit and tolerance of intestinal gas in the irritable bowel syndrome. *Gut* 2001; **48**: 14–19.
16. Simrén M, Mansson A, Langkilde AM, et al. Food-related gastrointestinal symptoms in the irritable bowel syndrome. *Digestion* 2001; **63**: 108–115.
17. Lomer MC, Parkes GC, Sanderson JD. Review article: lactose intolerance in clinical practice – myths and realities. *Alimentary Pharmacology and Therapeutics* 2008; **27**: 93–103.
18. Ruepert L, Quartero AO, de Wit NJ, van der Heijden GJ, Rubin G, Muris JW. Bulking agents, antispasmodics and antidepressants for the treatment of irritable bowel syndrome. *Cochrane Database of Systematic Reviews* 2011; **8**: CD003460.
19. Prior A, Whorwell PJ. Double blind study of ispaghula in irritable bowel syndrome. *Gut* 1987; **28**: 1510–1513.
20. Cunnane SC, Hamadeh MJ, Liede AC, Thompson LU, Wolever TM, Jenkins DJ. Nutritional attributes of traditional flaxseed in healthy young adults. *American Journal of Clinical Nutrition* 1995; **61**: 62–68.
21. Tarpila S, Tarpila A, Grohn P, Silvennoinen T, Lindberg L. Efficacy of ground flaxseed on constipation in patients with irritable bowel syndrome. *Current Topics in Nutraceutical Research* 2004; **2**: 119–125.
22. Cockerell KM, Watkins AS, Reeves LB, Goddard L, Lomer MC. Effects of linseeds on the symptoms of irritable bowel syndrome: a pilot randomised controlled trial. *Journal of Human Nutrition Dietetics* 2012; **25**: 435–443.
23. Dear KL, Elia M, Hunter JO. Do interventions which reduce colonic bacterial fermentation improve symptoms of irritable bowel syndrome? *Digestive Diseases and Sciences* 2005; **50**: 758–766.
24. Brown SR, Cann PA, Read NW. Effect of coffee on distal colon function. *Gut* 1990; **31**: 450–453.
25. Parker TJ, Naylor SJ, Riordan AM, Hunter JO. Management of patients with food intolerance in irritable bowel syndrome – the

development and use of an exclusion diet. *Journal of Human Nutrition Dietetics* 1995; **8**: 159–166.

26. Halder SL, Locke GR 3rd, Schleck CD, Zinsmeister AR, Talley NJ. Influence of alcohol consumption on IBS and dyspepsia. *Neurogastroenterology and Motility* 2006; **18**: 1001–1008.

27. Serra J, Salvioli B, Azpiroz F, Malagelada JR. Lipid-induced intestinal gas retention in irritable bowel syndrome. *Gastroenterology* 2002; **123**: 700–706.

28. Simrén M, Abrahamsson H, Bjornsson ES. Lipid-induced colonic hypersensitivity in the irritable bowel syndrome: the role of bowel habit, sex, and psychologic factors. *Clinical Gastroenterology and Hepatology* 2007; **5**(2): 201–208.

29. Cummings JH, Macfarlane GT. The control and consequences of bacterial fermentation in the human colon. *Journal of Applied Bacteriology* 1991; **70**: 443–459.

30. Jenkins DJ, Vuksan V, Kendall CW, et al. Physiological effects of resistant starches on fecal bulk, short chain fatty acids, blood lipids and glycemic index. *Journal of the American College of Nutrition* 1998; **17**: 609–616.

31. Maki KC, Sanders LM, Reeves MS, Kaden VN, Rains TM, Cartwright Y. Beneficial effects of resistant starch on laxation in healthy adults. *International Journal of Food Sciences and Nutrition* 2009; **60**(Suppl 4): 296–305.

32. Storey D, Lee A, Bornet F, Brouns F. Gastrointestinal responses following acute and medium term intake of retrograded resistant maltodextrins, classified as type 3 resistant starch. *European Journal of Clinical Nutrition* 2007; **61**: 1262–1270.

33. Achour L, Flourie B, Briet F, et al. Metabolic effects of digestible and partially indigestible cornstarch: a study in the absorptive and postabsorptive periods in healthy humans. *American Journal of Clinical Nutrition* 1997; **66**: 1151–1159.

34. Olesen M, Gudmand-Hoyer E. Efficacy, safety, and tolerability of fructooligosaccharides in the treatment of irritable bowel syndrome. *American Journal of Clinical Nutrition* 2000; **72**: 1570–1575.

35. Fernández-Bañares F, Esteve-Pardo M, de Leon R, et al. Sugar malabsorption in functional bowel disease: clinical implications. *American Journal of Gastroenterology* 1993; **88**: 2044–2050.

36. Shepherd SJ, Parker FC, Muir JG, et al. Dietary triggers of abdominal symptoms in patients with irritable bowel syndrome: randomized placebo-controlled evidence. *Clinical Gastroenterolology & Hepatolology* 2008; **6**: 765–771.

37. Fernández-Bañares F, Rosinach M, Esteve M, Forne M, Espinos J, Viver JM. Sugar malabsorption in functional abdominal bloating. *Gastroenterology* 2005; **128**: A331–A332.

38. Ledochowski M, Widner B, Bair H, Probst T, Fuchs D. Fructose- and sorbitol-reduced diet improves mood and gastrointestinal disturbances in fructose malabsorbers. *Scandinavian Journal of Gastroenterology* 2000; **35**: 1048–1052.

39. Staudacher HM, Irving PM, Lomer MC, et al. Mechanisms and efficacy of dietary FODMAP restriction in IBS. *Nature Reviews Gastroenterology and Hepatology* 2014; **11**: 256–66.

40. Staudacher HM, Whelan K, Irving PM, Lomer MC. Comparison of symptom response following advice for a diet low in fermentable carbohydrates (FODMAPs) versus standard dietary advice in patients with irritable bowel syndrome. *Journal of Human Nutrition Dietetics* 2011; **24**: 487–495.

41. Stornbaugh DJ, Deepak P, Ehrenpreis ED. Increased risk of osteoporosis-related fractures in patients with irritable bowel syndrome. *Osteoporosis International* 2013; **24**: 1169–1175.

42. Biesiekierski JR, Newnham ED, Irving PM, et al. Gluten causes gastrointestinal symptoms in subjects without celiac disease: a double-blind randomized placebo-controlled trial. *American Journal of Gastroenterology* 2011; **106**: 508–514.

43. Biesiekierski JR, Peters SL, Newnham ED, Rosella O, Muir JG, Gibson PR. No effects of gluten in patients with self-reported non-celiac gluten sensitivity after dietary reduction of low-fermentable, poorly absorbed, short-chain carbohydrates. *Gastroenterology* 2013; **145**(2): 320–328.

44. Bischoff S, Crowe SE. Gastrointestinal food allergy: new insights into pathophysiology and clinical perspectives. *Gastroenterology* 2005; **128**: 1089–1113.

45. Skypala I. Adverse food reactions – an emerging issue for adults. *Journal of the American Dietetic Association* 2011; **111**: 1877–1891.

46. Ohman L, Simrén M. Pathogenesis of IBS: role of inflammation, immunity and neuroimmune interactions. *Nature Reviews Gastroenterology and Hepatology* 2010; **7**: 163–173.

47. Tobin MC, Moparty B, Farhadi A, Demeo MT, Bansal PJ, Keshavarzian A. Atopic irritable bowel syndrome: a novel subgroup of irritable bowel syndrome with allergic manifestations. *Annals of Allergy Asthma and Immunology* 2008; **100**: 49–53.

48. Sampson HA, Sicherer SH, Birnbaum AH. AGA technical review on the evaluation of food allergy in gastrointestinal disorders. *Gastroenterology* 2001; **120**: 1026–1040.

49. Zar S, Benson MJ, Kumar D. Food-specific serum IgG4 and IgE titers to common food antigens in irritable bowel syndrome. *American Journal of Gastroenterology* 2005; **100**: 1550–1557.

50. Stapel SO, Asero R, Ballmer-Weber BK, et al. Testing for IgG4 against foods is not recommended as a diagnostic tool: EAACI Task Force Report. *Allergy* 2008; **63**: 793–796.

51. Bock SA. AAAAI support of the EAACI Position Paper on IgG4. *Journal of Allergy and Clinical Immunology* 2010; **125**: 1410.

52. Parkes GC, Brostoff J, Whelan K, Sanderson JD. Gastrointestinal microbiota in irritable bowel syndrome: their role in its pathogenesis and treatment. *American Journal of Gastroenterology* 2008; **103**: 1557–1567.

53. O'Mahony L, McCarthy J, Kelly P, et al. Lactobacillus and bifidobacterium in irritable bowel syndrome: symptom responses and relationship to cytokine profiles. *Gastroenterology* 2005; **128**: 541–551.

54. Rousseaux C, Thuru X, Gelot A, et al. Lactobacillus acidophilus modulates intestinal pain and induces opioid and cannabinoid receptors. *Nature Medicine* 2007; **13**: 35–37.

55. Verdu EF, Bercik P, Verma-Gandhu M, et al. Specific probiotic therapy attenuates antibiotic induced visceral hypersensitivity in mice. *Gut* 2006; **55**: 182–190.

56. Zeng J, Li YQ, Zuo XL, Zhen YB, Yang J, Liu CH. Clinical trial: effect of active lactic acid bacteria on mucosal barrier function in patients with diarrhoea-predominant irritable bowel syndrome. *Alimentary Pharmacology and Therapeutics* 2008; **28**: 994–1002.

57. Kim HJ, Camilleri M, McKinzie S, et al. A randomized controlled trial of a probiotic, VSL#3, on gut transit and symptoms in diarrhoea-predominant irritable bowel syndrome. *Alimentary Pharmacology and Therapeutics* 2003; **17**: 895–904.

58. Agrawal A, Houghton LA, Morris J, et al. Clinical trial: the effects of a fermented milk product containing Bifidobacterium lactis DN-173 010 on abdominal distension and gastrointestinal transit in irritable bowel syndrome with constipation. *Alimentary Pharmacology and Therapeutics* 2009; **29**: 104–114.

59. Nobaek S, Johansson ML, Molin G, Ahrne S, Jeppsson B. Alteration of intestinal microflora is associated with reduction in abdominal bloating and pain in patients with irritable bowel syndrome. *American Journal of Gastroenterology* 2000; **95**: 1231–1238.

60. Niedzielin K, Kordecki H, Birkenfeld B. A controlled, double-blind, randomized study on the efficacy of Lactobacillus plantarum 299V in patients with irritable bowel syndrome. *European Journal of Gastroenterology and Hepatology* 2001; **13**: 1143–1147.

61. Sen S, Mullan MM, Parker TJ, Woolner JT, Tarry SA, Hunter JO. Effect of Lactobacillus plantarum 299v on colonic fermentation and symptoms of irritable bowel syndrome. *Digestive Diseases and Sciences* 2002; **47**: 2615–2620.

62. Whorwell PJ, Altringer L, Morel J, et al. Efficacy of an encapsulated probiotic Bifidobacterium infantis 35624 in women with irritable bowel syndrome. *American Journal of Gastroenterology* 2006; **101**: 1581–1590.

63. Guyonnet D, Chassany O, Ducrotte P, et al. Effect of a fermented milk containing Bifidobacterium animalis DN-173 010 on the health-related quality of life and symptoms in irritable bowel syndrome in adults in primary care: a multicentre, randomized, double-blind, controlled trial. *Alimentary Pharmacology and Therapeutics* 2007; **26**: 475–486.

64. Enck P, Zimmermann K, Menke G, Klosterhalfen S. Randomized controlled treatment trial of irritable bowel syndrome with a probiotic E-coli preparation (DSM17252) compared to placebo. *Zeitschrift fur Gastroenterologie* 2009; **47**: 209–214.

65. Kim HJ, Vazquez Roque MI, Camilleri M, et al. A randomized controlled trial of a probiotic combination VSL# 3 and placebo in irritable bowel syndrome with bloating. *Neurogastroenterology and Motility* 2005; **17**: 687–696.

66. Guglielmetti S, Mora D, Gschwender M, Popp K. Randomised clinical trial: Bifidobacterium bifidum MIMBb75 significantly alleviates irritable bowel syndrome and improves quality of life – a double-blind, placebo-controlled study. *Alimentary Pharmacology and Therapeutics* 2011; **33**: 1123–1132.

67. Kruis W, Fric P, Pokrotnieks J, et al. Maintaining remission of ulcerative colitis with the probiotic Escherichia coli Nissle 1917 is as effective as with standard mesalazine. *Gut* 2004; **53**: 1617–1623.

68. Kruis W, Schutz E, Fric P, Fixa B, Judmaier G, Stolte M. Double-blind comparison of an oral Escherichia coli preparation and mesalazine in maintaining remission of ulcerative colitis. *Alimentary Pharmacology and Therapeutics* 1997; **11**: 853–858.

69. Kruis W, Chrubasik S, Boehm S, Stange C, Schulze J. A double-blind placebo-controlled trial to study therapeutic effects of probiotic Escherichia coli Nissle 1917 in subgroups of patients with irritable bowel syndrome. *International Journal of Colorectal Disease* 2012; **27**: 467–474.

70. Enck P, Zimmermann K, Menke G, Muller-Lissner S, Martens U, Klosterhalfen S. A mixture of Escherichia coli (DSM 17252) and Enterococcus faecalis (DSM 16440) for treatment of the irritable bowel syndrome – a randomized controlled trial with primary care physicians. *Neurogastroenterology and Motility* 2008; **20**: 1103–1109.

71. Silk DB, Davis A, Vulevic J, Tzortzis G, Gibson GR. Clinical trial: the effects of a trans-galactooligosaccharide prebiotic on faecal microbiota and symptoms in irritable bowel syndrome. *Alimentary Pharmacology and Therapeutics* 2009; **29**: 508–518.

Chapter 3.20

Diverticular disease and nutrition

Santhini Jeyarajah
Kings College Hospital NHS Foundation Trust, London, UK

3.20.1 Dietary factors involved in causation

Diverticula of the colon are acquired herniations of colonic mucosa, protruding through the circular muscle at the points where the blood vessels (vasa recta) penetrate through the colonic wall. They tend to occur in rows between the strips of longitudinal muscle, sometimes partly covered by appendices epiploicae. They most commonly involve the sigmoid colon but can be pancolonic. As the rectum has a complete muscle layer it is not affected [1].

It is important to differentiate between diverticulosis and the presence of diverticula which may be asymptomatic, and clinical diverticular disease (DD) where the diverticula are causing symptoms due to disordered colonic function resulting in distension, pain and altered stool output. There are several terms used in the modern description of DD that must be clearly understood. Diverticular disease is an all-encompassing term including symptomatic and asymptomatic disease. The most commonly used terms are defined in Table 3.20.1. The evolution of normal colon to symptomatic DD is summarised in Figure 3.20.1.

Dietary fibre/non-starch polysaccharides

Dietary fibre is not a chemically defined material, unlike NSP, and will be used throughout this chapter (see Chapter 2.1 for definitions). Fibre is the part of fruit, grains or vegetables not digested in the GI tract and contributes to stool bulk. Restriction of fibre results in a reduction in the size and number of stools.

Lack of dietary fibre results in slower gut transit, greater water resorption and production of smaller firmer stools which are implicated in formation of diverticula. It is proposed that a low-fibre diet results in exaggerated contractions of the colonic circular muscle, dividing the lumen into a series of segments, raising the intracolonic pressure and leading to mucosal herniation [5,6]. Decreasing these effects is thought to decrease the likelihood of developing both diverticula and symptoms of DD [5,7].

When measurements are obtained from within the true sigmoid colon, there appears to be a link between exaggerated colonic motility, increased pressures and symptomatic DD [8,9] as well as abnormal motor and propulsive activities confined to the regions affected by DD [10]. However, there is considerable heterogeneity within these studies due to methodological factors that lead to scepticism about the link between altered colonic motility and DD and whether these findings play a role in pathogenesis or are simply related to diverticular symptoms.

Low-fibre diets and increased DD prevalence have also been shown to exist in non-Western populations in South Africa where the urban black population with higher dietary fibre intake (mean daily dietary fibre intake of 32.5 ± 11.4 g) than the local whites (mean daily dietary fibre intake of 22.4 ± 6.0 g) had an increased prevalence of DD compared to non-urban blacks with significantly

Advanced Nutrition and Dietetics in Gastroenterology, First Edition. Edited by Miranda Lomer.
© 2014 John Wiley & Sons, Ltd. Published 2014 by John Wiley & Sons, Ltd.

Table 3.20.1 Definition of terms in diverticular disease

Term	Definition
Diverticular disease	The entire spectrum of asymptomatic to symptomatic disease associated with colonic diverticula
Diverticulosis	The presence of one diverticulum or, more commonly, multiple diverticula that are not inflamed
Diverticulitis	Diverticulosis with clinical symptoms and evidence of inflammation
Complicated diverticulitis	Disease state of diverticulitis including abscess, fistula, obstruction or free perforation

Source: Rodkey [2], Stollman [3].

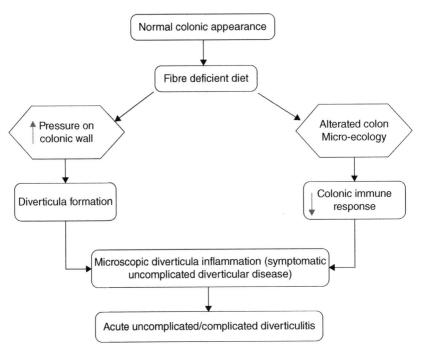

Figure 3.20.1 Pathogenetic events leading from diverticulosis to diverticular disease. Source: Tursi and Papagrigoriadis [4].

higher dietary fibre intake [11]. It has to be noted, however, that this is a small population study and it is difficult to draw firm conclusions from it. In right-sided colonic DD commonly seen in the Asian populations of the Far East, similar increased risk is seen in urban populations with lower fibre intakes [12,13] with decreasing intake over time from 25.0 g/day per capita in 1946 to 14.5 g/day in 1991 [14] coinciding with increased prevalence and daily dietary fibre intake of 17.4±5.1 g in patients compared to 21.1±6.6 g in controls [15].

Evidence exists that high-meat diets change bacterial metabolism in the colon [16]. It is possible that the interaction of red meat and bacteria results in production of a 'toxic metabolite' which promotes bowel wall spasm, resulting in weakening of the colon wall and diverticula formation [17]. Studies have revealed that a high intake of either red or processed meat correlates with a 2–4-fold increase in the risk of developing DD [18,19]. When compared to vegetarians, meat eaters were three times more likely to develop DD with diets containing half the dietary fibre of that in a vegetarian diet (21.4 g/day versus 41.6 g/day) [20]. A lifetime vegetarian diet, with a fibre intake of 42 g/day over 45 years, has been shown to be protective from DD compared to a meat eater's diet of 21 g/day of fibre with a 20-fold difference in prevalence [21]. In a more recent UK study over a mean follow-up time of 11.6 years, vegetarians (22 g/day fibre intake in men and 21 g/day in women) had a 31% lower risk of DD compared with meat eaters (18 g/day fibre intake in men and women). The cumulative probability of admission to hospital or death from DD between the ages of 50 and 70 for meat eaters was 4.4% compared with 3.0% for vegetarians. Vegetarians also have faster colonic transit times and less disease, again probably due to the higher dietary fibre intakes [22].

A prospective study examining the relationship between red meat consumption and DD found age and energy-adjusted relative risk (RR) were significant for certain servings of meat, such as beef, pork and lamb as a main dish (RR 3.23); in sandwiches or mixed dishes (RR 1.98); processed meat (RR 1.90); bacon (RR 1.07); and hot dogs (RR 1.38). When further adjusted for dietary fibre intake and physical activity, consumption of red meat, as a single category, was still positively associated with risk of DD (RR 1.48) but did not reach statistical significance. Further analysis showed that the association of red meat with DD was not related to its protein or fat content. There was little association between DD and intake of chicken and fish or dairy fat [18].

The relationship between high-meat diets and DD extends to Asian patients as well, where the risk of right-sided disease may be increased by nearly 25 times compared with patients with low overall meat consumption [12].

Fat

A systematic review of dietary factors which were potential risk factors for the development of DD found that other than low fibre intake, high fat intake and high meat intake were associated [23]. Positive associations were found between DD and saturated, monounsaturated, trans-saturated and polyunsaturated fats, particularly in the presence of low fibre intake. A weak inverse association was observed for omega-3 fatty acids and DD. When adjusted for physical activity and dietary fibre, however, the association of DD with total fat and various types of fat was no longer significant [18].

3.20.2 Dietary effects of disease or its management

Diverticular disease is a disease of the West where decreased fibre intake, increased fat intake and sedentary lifestyles are major health issues resulting in obesity, cardiovascular disorders and diabetes. Management includes increasing dietary fibre and fluid intake. However, this blanket approach to managing DD can sometimes result in diarrhoea and flatulence in patients and there is a need to balance individual dietary requirements and sensitivities in order to satisfactorily manage the condition in different patients. This is a problem also because of the overlap with irritable bowel syndrome in these symptomatic patients. Although irritable bowel syndrome is considered a diagnosis of exclusion, the symptoms of variable stool output and abdominal pain can commonly co-exist alongside uncomplicated DD where diverticulosis is present with no evidence of inflammation, making a clear differentiation difficult.

3.20.3 Dietary management

Dietary fibre and colonic physiology

High-fibre diets are commonly recommended as part of the preventive and treatment regimen for symptomatic uncomplicated DD. In particular, fibre which is incompletely or slowly fermented by microbiota in the large intestine promotes normal laxation, provides relief from constipation and ultimately prevents the development of DD and diverticulitis by accelerating the faecal transit time and reducing the intraluminal pressure.

Dietary fibre can be classified according to its water solubility. The structural fibres which consist of cellulose, lignin and some hemicelluloses are insoluble and the natural gel-forming fibres, which are the pectins, gums, mucilages and remaining hemicelluloses, are soluble [24]. Insoluble fibre, such as wheat bran, is primarily important for GI health, while soluble fibre, such as oat bran, has been thought to reduce risk of chronic disease. Fruit and vegetable fibre has been found to be inversely associated with risk of DD. The relative risk associated with fruit fibre was 0.62 and that for vegetable fibre was 0.55. The insoluble component of fibre, particularly cellulose, was strongly associated with decreased risk of DD. Cereal fibre, however, was not associated with decreased risk of DD [24].

Several controlled clinical trials tested the efficacy of wheat bran and bulking agents in the relief of GI dysfunction in symptomatic DD patients [25–28]. The most commonly used supplements are wheat bran and ispaghula husk. However, high-level evidence to support this recommendation is lacking.

Dietary fibre and symptoms

Painter was the first to advocate fibre supplementation in symptomatic DD [29] and over time the positive effect of increased fibre on symptom relief has been repeatedly seen. The treatment found to be most effective was 24 g/day of wheat bran for at least 6 months resulting in symptomatic relief, accelerated transit times, increased stool weight and decreased postprandial intracolonic high pressure waves, especially during and after eating [30]. Fibre supplementation has also retrospectively been shown not only to provide symptom relief with less pain and constipation but also required less surgery [31].

Symptom relief from fibre supplementation is reported to last over 6 years in more than half of patients undertaking it [32–34]. Constipation is the symptom which is most consistently relieved by fibre supplementation; the effect on other symptoms can be more variable although a lower relative risk of abdominal pain, bleeding and change in stool output has been shown to be inversely related to a low-fibre diet [18].

Prospective comparison of treatment over 12 weeks with the laxative lactulose or a high-fibre diet found a similar improvement in bowel frequency, stool consistency, frequency and severity of pain on bowel movement and abdominal pain [35].

However, despite the evidence for the positive effect of fibre supplementation, a recent systematic review [36] concluded that compared with placebo, wheat bran and ispaghula husk may be no more effective at 16 weeks at relieving symptoms of uncomplicated DD, based on one cross-over randomised controlled trial (RCT) [37]. Methylcellulose may be no more effective at 3 months at reducing mean symptom scores in people with uncomplicated DD compared with placebo based on one RCT [38].

It is therefore difficult to conclusively recommend the use of fibre supplementation or laxative use to improve outcomes in symptomatic DD. However, as the benefits outweigh the very minimal risks of this relatively benign dietary modification, advocating it to patients does not cause apparent harm. In the United States, fibre recommendations for an individual with DD are 6–10 g/day higher than the normally recommended 25–35 g/day [39]. And although there are some recommendations to avoid nuts, seeds and popcorn there appears to be no real evidence to support this [40].

A vegetarian diet has also been shown to have beneficial effects on disease prevention, but this is a very much more difficult lifestyle change to make. A case-by-case view needs to be taken in order to adjust treatment for patients with overlapping irritable bowel syndrome symptoms who can react negatively to increased dietary fibre.

Medical management

The management of DD takes a staged approach in which symptomatic uncomplicated disease where patients present with pain, bloating, constipation or diarrhoea is treated mainly with a change in diet to high fibre, low fat and the recommendation of exercise. As the disease gets more complicated to involve inflammation as an attack of acute diverticulitis, antibiotics become the mainstay of treatment, orally where the attack is mild, parenterally where the attack involves phlegmon or abscess. Treatment then progresses to radiological or surgical intervention where necessary [4].

The anti-inflammatory role of 5-aminosalicylic acid (5-ASA) has been applied to DD in the form of mesalazine. It has been shown to be effective in improving symptoms in patients with symptomatic uncomplicated DD [41]. Combining it with a broad-spectrum antibiotic such as rifaximin has shown synergy thus preventing disease recurrence and improving symptoms in patients with symptomatic, uncomplicated diverticulitis and mild-to-moderate colonic obstruction, rather than using rifaximin on its own [42].

Probiotics

Probiotics are living micro-organisms that, if consumed in sufficient numbers, can alter the host microbiota and exert specific health benefits without increasing the risk of antibiotic resistance [43]. The addition of non-pathogenic *E. coli* (Nissle strain) to antibiotic therapy (dichlorchinolinol) and an intestinal absorbent (active coal tablets) resulted in greater symptomatic improvement and longer periods of disease quiescence than with the antibiotic with absorbent regimen alone [44].

The probiotic *Lactobacillus casei* DG and the high-potency probiotic mixture VSL#3 in combination with 5-ASA or balsalazide in patients with symptomatic, uncomplicated DD in remission found the probiotic with 5-ASA combination performed better in preventing disease relapses and improving symptoms than the single-agent regimens [45,46].

Studies on the use of mesalazine and probiotics are, however, limited and their use in the treatment of DD is yet to become clearly established.

References

1. Mortensen NJ. *The Small and Large Intestine.* London: Edward Arnold, 2000.
2. Rodkey GW, Welch JP. *Diverticular Disease. Management of the Difficult Surgical Case. An overview.* Philadelphia, PA: Lippincott Williams and Wilkins, 1998.
3. Stollman N, Raskin JB. *Diverticular Disease.* New Jersey: Slack, Inc., 2002.
4. Tursi A, Papagrigoriadis S. Review article: the current and evolving treatment of colonic diverticular disease. *Alimentary Pharmacology and Therapeutics* 2009; 30: 532–546.
5. Painter NS, Truelove SC, Ardran GM, Tuckey M. Segmentation and the localization of intraluminal pressures in the human colon, with special reference to the pathogenesis of colonic diverticula. *Gastroenterology* 1965; 49: 169–77.

6. Arfwidsson S, Knock NG, Lehmann L, Winberg T. Pathogenesis of multiple diverticula of the sogmoid colon in diverticular disease. *Acta Chirurgica Scandinavica* 1964; 63(Suppl 342): 1–68.
7. Painter NS, Truelove SC. The intraluminal pressure patterns in diverticulosis of the colon. I. Resting patterns of pressure. II. The effect of morphine. *Gut* 1964; 5: 201–213.
8. Cortesini C, Pantalone D. Usefulness of colonic motility study in identifying patients at risk for complicated diverticular disease. *Diseases of the Colon and Rectum* 1991; 34: 339–342.
9. Trotman IF, Misiewicz JJ. Sigmoid motility in diverticular disease and the irritable bowel syndrome. *Gut* 1988; 29: 218–222.
10. Bassotti G, Battaglia E, Spinozzi F, Pelli MA, Tonini M. Twenty-four hour recordings of colonic motility in patients with diverticular disease: evidence for abnormal motility and propulsive activity. *Diseases of the Colon and Rectum* 2001; 44: 1814–1820.
11. Segal I, Walker AR. Diverticular disease in urban Africans in South Africa. *Digestion* 1982; 24: 42–46.
12. Lin OS, Soon MS, Wu SS, Chen YY, Hwang KL, Triadafilopoulos G. Dietary habits and right sided colonic diverticulosis. *Diseases of the Colon and Rectum* 2000; 43: 1412–1418.
13. Nakaji S, Danjo K, Munakata A, et al. Comparison of etiology of right-sided diverticula in Japan with that of left-sided diverticula in the West. *International Journal of Colorectal Disease* 2002; 17: 365–373.
14. Nakaji S, Sugawara K, Saito D, et al. Trends in dietary fiber intake in Japan over the last century. *European Journal of Nutrition* 2002; 41: 222–227.
15. Ohta M, Ishiguro S, Iwane S, et al. [An epidemiological study on relationship between intake of dietary fiber and colonic diseases]. *Nihon Shokakibyo Gakkai Zasshi* 1985; 82: 51–57.
16. Cummings JH, Hill MJ, Bone ES, Branch WJ, Jenkins DJ. The effect of meat protein and dietary fiber on colonic function and metabolism. *II.* Bacterial metabolites in feces and urine. *American Journal of Clinical Nutrition* 1979; 32: 2094–2101.
17. Heaton KW. Diet and diverticulosis – new leads. *Gut* 1985; 26: 541–543.
18. Aldoori WH, Giovannucci EL, Rimm EB, Wing AL, Trichopoulos DV, Willett WC. A prospective study of diet and the risk of symptomatic diverticular disease in men. *American Journal of Clinical Nutrition* 1994; 60: 757–764.
19. Manousos O, Day N, Tzonou A, et al. Diet and other factors in the aetiology of diverticulosis: an epidemiological study in Greece. *Gut* 1985; 26: 544–549.
20. Miettinen TA, Tarpila S. Fecal beta-sitosterol in patients with diverticular disease of the colon and in vegetarians. *Scandinavian Journal of Gastroenterology* 1978; 13: 573–576.
21. Gear JS, Ware A, Fursdon P, et al. Symptomless diverticular disease and intake of dietary fibre. *Lancet* 1979; 1: 511–514.
22. Gear JS, Brodribb AJ, Ware A, Mann JI. Fibre and bowel transit times. *British Journal of Nutrition* 1981; 45: 77–82.
23. Aldoori W, Ryan-Harshman M. Preventing diverticular disease. Review of recent evidence on high-fibre diets. *Canadian Family Physician* 2002; 48: 1632–1637.
24. Aldoori WH, Giovannucci EL, Rockett HR, Sampson L, Rimm EB, Willett WC. A prospective study of dietary fiber

types and symptomatic diverticular disease in men. *Journal of Nutrition* 1998; **128**: 714–719.

25. Brodribb AJ. Treatment of symptomatic diverticular disease with a high-fibre diet. *Lancet* 1977; **1**: 664–666.

26. Ewerth S, Ahlberg J, Holmstrom B, Persson U, Uden R. Influence on symptoms and transit-time of Vi-SiblinR in diverticular disease. *Acta Chirurgica Scandinavica: Supplementum* 1980; **500**: 49–50.

27. Ornstein MH, Littlewood ER, Baird IM, Fowler J, Cox AG. Are fibre supplements really necessary in diverticular disease of the colon? *British Medical Journal (Clinical Research Ed)* 1981; **282**: 1629–1630.

28. Weinreich J. Treatment of diverticular disease. *Scandinavian Journal of Gastroenterology* 1982; **79**: 128–129.

29. Painter NS, Almeida AZ, Colebourne KW. Unprocessed bran in treatment of diverticular disease of the colon. *British Medical Journal* 1972; **2**: 137–140.

30. Brodribb AJ, Humphreys DM. Diverticular disease: three studies. Part II – Treatment with bran. *British Medical Journal* 1976; **1**: 425–428.

31. Leahy AL, Ellis RM, Quill DS, Peel AL. High fibre diet in symptomatic diverticular disease of the colon. *Annals of the Royal College of Surgeons of England* 1985; **67**: 173–174.

32. Hyland JM, Taylor I. Does a high fibre diet prevent the complications of diverticular disease? *British Journal of Surgery* 1980; **67**: 77–79.

33. Parks TG. Natural history of diverticular disease of the colon. A review of 521 cases. *British Medical Journal* 1969; **4**: 639–642.

34. Parks TG, Connell AM. The outcome in 455 patients admitted for treatment of diverticular disease of the colon. *British Journal of Surgery* 1970; **57**: 775–778.

35. Smits BJ, Whitehead AM, Prescott P. Lactulose in the treatment of symptomatic diverticular disease: a comparative study with high-fibre diet. *British Journal of Clinical Practice* 1990; **44**: 314–318.

36. Unlu C, Daniels L, Vrouenraets BC, Boermeester MA. A systematic review of high–fibre dietary therapy in diverticular disease. *International Journal of Colorectal Disease* 2012; **27**: 419–427.

37. Ornstein MH, Littlewood ER, Baird IM, Fowler J, North WR, Cox AG. Are fibre supplements really necessary in diverticular disease of the colon? A controlled clinical trial. *British Medical Journal (Clinical Research Ed)* 1981; **282**: 1353–1356.

38. Hodgson WJ. The placebo effect. Is it important in diverticular disease? *American Journal of Gastroenterology* 1977; **67**: 157–162.

39. Marlett JA, McBurney MI, Slavin JL. Position of the American Dietetic Association: health implications of dietary fiber. *Journal of the American Dietetic Association* 2002; **102**: 993–1000.

40. Tarleton S, Dibaise JK. Low-residue diet in diverticular disease: putting an end to a myth. *Nutrition in Clinical Practice* 2011; **26**: 137–142.

41. Trespi E, Panizza P, Colla C, Bottani G, de Vecchi P, Matti C. [Efficacy of low dose mesalazine (5-ASA) in the treatment of acute inflammation and prevention of complications in patients with symptomatic diverticular disease. Preliminary results]. *Minerva Gastroenterologica e Dietologica* 1997; **43**: 157–162.

42. Tursi A, Brandimarte G, Daffina R. Long-term treatment with mesalazine and rifaximin versus rifaximin alone for patients with recurrent attacks of acute diverticulitis of colon. *Digestive and Liver Disease* 2002; **34**: 510–515.

43. Guarner F, Schaafsma GJ. Probiotics. *International Journal of Food Microbiology* 1998; **39**: 237–238.

44. Fric P, Zavoral M. The effect of non-pathogenic Escherichia coli in symptomatic uncomplicated diverticular disease of the colon. *European Journal of Gastroenterology and Hepatology* 2003; **15**: 313–315.

45. Tursi A, Brandimarte G, Giorgetti GM, Elisei W. Mesalazine and/or Lactobacillus casei in preventing recurrence of symptomatic uncomplicated diverticular disease of the colon: a prospective, randomized, open-label study. *Journal of Clinical Gastroenterology* 2006; **40**: 312–316.

46. Tursi A, Brandimarte G, Giorgetti GM, Elisei W, Aiello F. Balsalazide and/or high-potency probiotic mixture (VSL#3) in maintaining remission after attack of acute, uncomplicated diverticulitis of the colon. *International Journal of Colorectal Disease* 2007; **22**: 1103–1108.

Constipation and nutrition

Yolande M. Causebrook and Chris Speed
Newcastle University, Newcastle upon Tyne, UK

Constipation in adults is often trivialised. However, it is a frequent (2–34% of the population in Western countries) and often debilitating medical problem, generating many medical visits and having a considerable impact on individual physical and emotional well-being [1–3].

3.21.1 Definitions and types

Functional constipation (primary or idiopathic) is chronic constipation with an unknown cause [4]. Several physiological subtypes have been described.

- *Colonic inertia or slow transit constipation* – when movement of GI contents through the colon is slowed.
- *Outlet delay constipation (or obstructed defaecation)* – which can be caused by pelvic floor dyssynergia (the pelvic floor muscles contract or fail to relax during attempted defaecation) and by anismus (the external anal sphincter contracts instead of relaxing during attempted defaecation).
- *Normal transit constipation (without delays in colonic transit or outlet delay)* – the least clearly defined and most common subgroup.

Secondary constipation (organic constipation) is caused by a drug or medical condition. Faecal loading/impaction is retention of faeces resulting in difficulty in evacuation. Retained faeces are usually palpable on abdominal examination, and may be felt on internal rectal examination or by external palpation around the anus.

Although constipation means different things to different people, frequency, consistency and normal bowel movements are considered as important criteria to clinicians and patients; it is how these criteria are perceived that differs. The Rome Criteria are considered as the gold standard for constipation and are useful in clinical practice and research [5,6].

Rome III defines functional constipation as a functional bowel disorder that presents as persistently difficult, infrequent or seemingly incomplete defaecation, which does not meet irritable bowel syndrome criteria and includes the criteria shown in Box 3.21.1 [6]. These can be used with the Bristol Stool Form Scale, which helps define stool types and evaluate transit time, to provide a comprehensive clinical definition.

A patient's perception of constipation may include the objective observation of infrequent defaecation patterns and the subjective complaints of straining at stooling, incomplete evacuation, abdominal bloating or pain, hard or small stools, or a need for digital manipulation to enable defaecation. Stool frequency, as a measure, is imprecise, as it varies between healthy individuals, let alone constipated patients.

3.21.2 Factors involved in causation

Demographics

Although there is a lack of consensus on the prevalence rates of constipation, many researchers have found that certain demographic and dietary factors

Advanced Nutrition and Dietetics in Gastroenterology, First Edition. Edited by Miranda Lomer.
© 2014 John Wiley & Sons, Ltd. Published 2014 by John Wiley & Sons, Ltd.

Box 3.21.1   Diagnostic criteria* for functional constipation

1. Must include *two or more* of the following:
   a. Straining during at least 25% of defaecations
   b. Lumpy or hard stools in at least 25% of defaecations
   c. Sensation of incomplete evacuation for at least 25% of defaecations
   d. Sensation of anorectal obstruction/blockage for at least 25% of defaecations
   e. Manual maneuvers to facilitate at least 25% of defecations (e.g. digital evacuation, support of the pelvic floor)
   f. Fewer than 3 defaecations per week
2. Loose stools are rarely present without the use of laxatives
3. There are insufficient criteria for irritable bowel syndrome

*Criteria fulfilled for the last 3 months with symptom onset at least 6 months prior to diagnosis.
Source: Longstreth et al. [6]. Reproduced with permission from BMJ.

---

may increase causation. Constipation is reported to be higher in women than men (median female:male ratio of 1.5) [6] and this persists after age adjustment. Age is inversely associated with constipation, with increasing prevalence of constipation affecting the very young or the very old [7]. Constipation among older people could be due to changes in mobility, diet, fluid intake or polypharmacy. The use of laxatives increases with age, with adults over 65 being frequent users, even when bowel movements would be described as 'normal' by clinicians [3,7–9]. Independent living also plays a role in the prevalence of constipation in older people. Healthy, active individuals living in the community are often less likely to experience functional constipation than those in institutions (including hospitals) [3,7,9].

Constipation affects non-white people more than white [6]. Reasons for this are unclear, but it may be linked to dietary differences or genetics. A strong relationship exists between low socioeconomic groups and greater reporting of constipation [3]. This may be related to poor diet and reduced level of physical activity or limited education, as socioeconomic position is often associated with lower attained education level.

Non-starch polysaccharides

It is often said that the prevalence of constipation has increased due to modern food processing methods, resulting in a diet low in non-starch polysaccharides (NSP) [10]. However, a low NSP diet should not be assumed to be the cause of constipation, but possibly a contributory factor [11]. Although evidence is controversial, intake of NSP, mostly insoluble fibre, has been shown to be beneficial [6] and to increase gut transit time, faecal weight and bowel frequency in healthy individuals, but also in some constipated patients [11]. Constipation is often lower among vegetarians [7] and in developing countries, where higher amounts and types of NSP are consumed. Many people with constipation, especially the elderly, report having a low NSP intake because of chewing difficulties and/or denture problems. There are a few cases where high NSP is contraindicated: patients with secondary to slow transit and/or pelvic floor dyssynergia, or where abdominal distension has worsened or resulted in incontinence (mostly in the elderly) [12]. However, these represent a minority.

Fluid

Dehydration is a risk factor [12,13], slowing colonic transit or lowering stool output in healthy adults. This is a problem among the elderly, who tend to drink less in an attempt to control continence. Evidence for increasing fluid intake generally or when NSP is ingested is controversial [14].

3.21.3 Dietary effects of disease or its management

Constipation is common in irritable bowel syndrome and symptomatic diverticulosis or diverticulitis leading to an overlap of risk factors between those diseases and functional constipation.

Reduced NSP intake is believed to be a contributory factor to functional constipation. The greatest effect on constipation seemed to be related to the insoluble fibre component, especially cellulose, found in fruit and vegetables, rather than in cereals [11,15]. Insoluble fibre is known to increase faecal bulk and be a potent stimulus to colon transit [16], which may result in reduced constipation symptoms. Diverticulosis is generally asymptomatic [11,15]. However, when active, NSP should be decreased to reduce pain and bloating sensation, but increased gradually when symptoms lessen. Although symptoms may worsen initially, improvement should follow after a few weeks. Intake of a high-fibre diet is in line with healthy dietary recommendations, but any treatment management should be carefully monitored.

3.21.4 Dietary treatments

A multifaceted approach is preferred to treat patients with functional constipation, with dietary and lifestyle changes being the first step. If unsuccessful, fibre supplements can be used, and if this fails then laxative treatment can be given [1,7]. The latter is currently the most used by health professionals and patients, especially among the elderly population. However, there is little evidence to support either their clinical or cost-effectiveness. Emmanuel designed a draft algorithm for such an approach, which is useful as there is no treatment protocol at present, probably due to the complexity of the condition and the lack of uniformity in defining it [17]. Although toileting time [13], posture [18], physical activity [8] and psychological counselling [2] are important aspects of constipation management, only the dietary aspect of the treatment will be considered here.

Non-starch polysaccharides

Soluble fibre has an effective water-holding capacity to form highly viscous solutions, but has little effect on stool output and colon transit. Whilst insoluble fibre has poor water-holding capacity, it increases faecal bulk and offers potent stimuli to colon transit [16]. Wheat bran and oat bran contain differing amounts of insoluble fibre (>90% and 50–60% respectively) but have similar effects on daily stool output although they work by a different mechanism. Oat bran is higher in soluble fibre than wheat bran and when consumed results in greater bacterial growth, and the insoluble fibre provides more slowly fermentable polysaccharides to maintain the microbial population during transit through the large intestine [19]. Other food plants (prunes and kiwis) have been shown to be effective in improving constipation [20–22]. It is difficult to ascertain which fibres are most effective in these fruits, but probably a combination of both and other components within the fruit.

Adequate fluid intake is recommended when consuming a high NSP diet or fibre supplements [23] but this can be problematic for some individuals, such as the frail and elderly. However, encouraging such practice may increase the beneficial effects of NSP and decrease some of the common side-effects, e.g. increased bloating and flatulence [10,11]. Incremented intake (about 5 g/day weekly until the recommended amount is achieved) and patient monitoring are crucial for compliance, which can be poor [10,11] as some patients believe that high NSP diets make their constipation worse. Patients should be informed that benefits may take from a few days to several weeks to become evident.

In the UK, it is recommended that the healthy adult diet should contain an average of 18 g/day of NSP [24] whilst the US dietary guidelines [25] recommend a NSP intake of 14 g/1000 kcal, which represents around 25–38 g/day for healthy adult women and men respectively.

Probiotics and prebiotics

The GI microbiota comprises 400–500 bacterial species in the colon alone and has many

Table 3.21.1 Probiotic strains and their beneficial effects on constipation

Probiotic	Beneficial effects						Study reference
	↑ Stool frequency	Improved stool consistency*	↓ Bloating	↓ Flatulence	↓ Colonic transit time	Improved defaecation conditions	
Lactobacillus casei Shirota (in a probiotic drink)	√	√	No change	No change	Not studied	Not studied	Koenick et al. 2003 [38]
Escherichia coli Nissle 1917	√	√	Not studied	Not studied	Not studied	Not studied	Mollenbrink and Bruckschen 1994 [39]
Bifidobacterium lactis DN-173010 (in fermented milk)	√	√	Not studied	Not studied	Not studied	√	Yang et al. 2008 [40]
Bifidobacterium animalis SP/ DN-173010					√		Bouvier et al. 2001 [41] Meance et al. 2003 [42] Marteau et al. 2002 [43]

*Less hard or lumpy stool.

important metabolic, trophic and protective functions.

Research evidence for beneficial effects of probiotics in constipation is strain dependent and fairly limited but includes improvements in transit time, faecal frequency and stool consistency [26] (Table 3.21.1). *Bifidobacterium lactis, B. longum* and *Lactobacillus GG* have been shown to normalise stool output in the elderly in nursing homes [27]. The benefits of *Lactobacillus GG* have only been demonstrated when ingested with fibre-rich rye bread [28] and are known to improve stool frequency in constipated children [29].

One issue with probiotics is the quality control of (often milk-based) products (see Chapter 2.3).

Inulin and fructo-oligasaccharides (FOS) are prebiotics fermented by bifodobacteria and lactobacilli within the GI tract (see Chapter 2.4). There is insufficient evidence to fully identify the health benefits of inulin and FOS in patients with constipation. However, they contribute to the increase of microbial mass and the production of short-chain fatty acids [30], and have a laxative effect. Studies using inulin and lactose in the elderly have shown clinical improvements in constipation with 15 g/day [31] or 20–40 g/day of inulin [32]. The greater laxative effect of inulin, combined with an increase in bifidobacteria and a decrease in enterococci and enterobacteria, might explain such improvement. There is no optimum dose recommended for inulin and FOS but daily doses above 20 g/day may cause undesirable effects, such as abdominal pain, and intestinal cramps in some patients with constipation [33]. These effects vary between individuals [32]. Considering the limited strength of evidence, it is difficult to recommend these products to all patients with constipation.

Fluid

Although hydration status may or may not contribute to constipation [14,34], it is well established that being well hydrated is important to health [35,36]. Therefore regular habits of fluid consumption should be started from an early age and continued throughout life. It is recognised that thirst sensation decreases in later life, and dehydration can then become a problem for general health and may lead

to constipation [12–14]. Studies undertaken in controlled environments among elderly patients showed that establishing regular drinking times, with the support of medical staff, improved constipation. A fluid intake of 1.5–2 L/day, excluding caffeinated drinks and depending on NSP intake, decreased constipation. Encouraging oral fluids is essential, but mobility issues should be considered too, particularly in the elderly, as increased fluid consumption results in increased urine output. Close monitoring of fluid intake is particularly important among elderly patients with cardiac and renal disease [9].

The recommended fluid intake is 2 L/day; water is best but the amount will vary for each individual depending on levels of physical activity and consumption of water-containing foods and other liquids (i.e. juices, tea, coffee, soups and fruit and vegetables) [37].

References

1. McCallum IJ, Ong S, Mercer-Jones M. Chronic constipation in adults. *British Medical Journal* 2009; **338**: 763–766.
2. Speed C, Heaven B, Adamson A, et al. LIFELAX – diet and LIFEstyle versus LAXatives in the management of chronic constipation in older people: randomised controlled trial. *Health Technology Assessment* 2010; **14**(52): 1–251.
3. Mugie SM, Benninga MA, di Lorenzo C. Epidemiology of constipation in children and adults: a systematic review. *Best Practice and Research in Clinical Gastroenterology* 2011; **25**(1): 3–18.
4. NHS Evidence. Clinical Knowledge Summaries. Constipation. 2013. http://cks.nice.org.uk/constipation, accessed 20 January 2014.
5. Drossman DA. The functional gastrointestinal disorders and the Rome III process. *Gastroenterology* 2006; **130**: 1377–1390.
6. Longstreth GF, Thompson WG, Chey WD, Houghton LA, Mearin F, Spiller RC. Functional bowel disorders. *Gastroenterology* 2006; **130**(5): 1480–1491.
7. Petticrew M, Watt I, Sheldon T. Systematic review of the effectiveness of laxatives in the elderly. *Health Technology Assessment* 1997; **1**(13): 1–52.
8. Dukas L, Willett WC, Giovannucci EL. Association between physical activity, fiber intake, other lifestyle variables and constipation in a study of women. *American Journal of Gastroenterology* 2003; **98**(8): 1790–1796.
9. Rao SSC, Go JT. Update on the management of constipation in the elderly. *Clinical Interventions in Aging* 2010; **5**: 163–171.
10. Taylor R. Management of constipation: high fibre diets work. *British Medical Journal* 1990; **300**: 1063–1064.
11. Cabré E. Clinical nutrition university: nutrition in the prevention and management of irritable bowel syndrome, constipation

and diverticulosis. *European e-Journal of Clinical Nutrition and Metabolism* 2011; **6**(2): e85–e95. www.e-spenjournal.org/.

12. Muller-Lissner SA, Kamm MA, Scarpignato C, Wald A. Myths and misconceptions about chronic constipation. *American Journal of Gastroenterology* 2005; **100**: 232–242.

13. Imershein N, Linnehan E. Nutrition management in home health and long-term care. Constipation: a common problem of the elderly. *Journal of Nutrition for the Elderly* 2000; **19**(3): 49–54.

14. Arnaud MJ. Mild dehydration: a risk factor of constipation? *European Journal of Clinical Nutrition* 2003; **57**: S88–S95.

15. Stollman NH, Raskin JB. Diverticular disease of the colon. *Lancet* 2004; **363**: 631–639.

16. Spiller RC. Pharmacology of dietary fibre. *Pharmacology and Therapeutics* 1994; **62**(3): 407–427.

17. Emmanuel A. Current management strategies and therapeutics targets in chronic constipation. *Therapeutic Advances in Gastroenterology* 2011; **4**(1): 37–48.

18. Sikirov D. Comparison of straining during defecation in three positions. Results and implications for human health. *Digestive Diseases and Sciences* 2003; **48**(7): 1201–1205.

19. Chen H, Haack VS, Janecky CW, Vollendorf NW, Marlett JA. Mechanism by which wheat bran and oat bran increase stool weight in humans. *American Journal of Clinical Nutrition* 1998; **68**: 711–719.

20. Stacewicz-Sapuntzakis M, Bowen PE, Hussain EA, Damayanti-Wood BI, Farnworth NR. Chemical composition and potential health effects of prunes: a functional food? *Critical Reviews in Food Science and Nutrition* 2001; **41**(4): 251–286.

21. Rush EC, Patel M, Plank LD, Ferguson LR. Kiwifruit promotes laxation in the elderly. *Asia Pacific Journal of Clinical Nutrition* 2002; **11**(2): 164–168.

22. Attaluri A, Donahoe R, Valestin J, Brown K, Rao SSC. Randomised clinical trial: dried plums (prunes) vs psyllium for constipation. *Alimentary Pharmacology and Therapeutics* 2011; **33**: 822–828.

23. Rodrigues-Fisher LC, Bourguignon BV. Good, dietary fiber nursing intervention: prevention of constipation in older adults. *Clinical Nursing Research* 1993; **2**: 464–477.

24. Department of Health. *Dietary Reference Values for Food Energy and Nutrients for the United Kingdom*. London: HMSO, 1991.

25. US Department of Health and Human Services and Department of Agriculture. *Dietary Guidelines for Americans*, 2005. www.health.gov/dietaryguidelines/dga2005/document/pdf/DGA2005.pdf, accessed 20 January 2014.

26. Pathmakanthan S, Meance S, Edwards CE. Probiotics: a review of human studies to date and methodological approaches. *Microbial Ecology in Health and Disease* 2000; **2**: 10–30.

27. Pitkala KH, Strandberg TE, Finne-Soveri UH, et al. Fermented cereal with specific bifidobacteria normalizes bowel movements in elderly nursing home residents. A randomized, controlled trial. *Journal of Nutrition, Health and Aging* 2007; **11**(4): 305–311.

28. Hongisto SM, Paajanen L, Saxelin M, Korpela R. A combination of fibre-rich rye bread and yoghurt containing *Lactobacillus GG* improves bowel function in women with self-reported constipation. *European Journal of Clinical Nutrition* 2006; **60**(3): 319–324.

29. Banaszkeiwicz A, Szajewska H. Ineffectiveness of *Lactobacillus GG* as an adjunct to lactulose for the treatment of constipation in children: a double-blind, placebo-controlled randomized trial. *Journal of Paediatrics* 2005; **146**(3): 364–369.

30. Schneeman BO. Fiber, inulin and oligofructose: similarities and differences. *Journal of Nutrition* 1999; **129**: 1424S–1427S.

31. Gibson GR, Beatty ER, Xin W, Cummings JH. Selective stimulation of bifidobacteria in the human colon by oligofructose and inulin. *Gastroenterology* 1995; **108**: 975–982.

32. Kleesen B, Sykura B, Zunft HJ, Blaut M. Effects of inulin and lactose on fecal microflora, microbial activity, bowel habit in elderly constipated persons. *American Journal of Clinical Nutrition* 1996; **65**: 1397–1402.

33. Tuohy KM, Rouzaud GC, Brück WM, Gibson GR. Modulation of the human gut microflora towards improved health using prebiotics – assessment of efficacy. *Current Pharmaceutical Design* 2005; **11**: 75–90

34. Linderman RD, Romero LJ, Hwa Chi L, Baumgartner RN, Koehler KM, Garry PJ. Do elderly persons need to be encouraged to drink more fluids? *Journal of Gerontology Series A - Biological Sciences and Medical Sciences* 2000; **55A**(7): M361–M365.

35. Kleiner SM. Water: an essential but overlooked nutrient. *Journal of the American Dietetic Association* 1999; **99**(2): 200–206.

36. World Health Organization. *Water for Health – Taking Charge*. Geneva: World Health Organization, 2001.

37. Goldberg G. Water, water. *Nutrition Bulletin* 2001; **26**(3): 197–198.

38. Koenick C, Wagner I, Leitzmann P, Stern U, Zunft HJ. Probiotic beverage containing *Lactobacillus casei shirota* improves gastrointestinal symptoms in patients with chronic constipation. *Canadian Journal of Gastroenterology* 2003; **17**: 655–659.

39. Mollenbrink M, Bruckschen E. Treatment of chronic constipation with physiologic Escherichia coli bacteria. Results of a clinical study of the effectiveness and tolerance of microbiological therapy with the E.coli Nissle 1917 strain (Mutaflor). *Medizinische Klinik (Munich)* 1994; **89**: 587–593.

40. Yang YX, Mei H, Gang H, Wei J, Philippe P, Bourdu-Naturel S. Effect of a fermented milk containing *Bifidobacterium lactis* DN-173010 on Chinese constipated women. *World Journal of Gastroenterology* 2008; **14**(40): 6237–6243.

41. Bouvier M, Meance S, Bouley C, Berta JL, Grimaud JC. Effects of consumption of a milk fermented by the probiotic *Bifidobacterium animalis* DN 173010 on colonic transit time in healthy humans. *Bioscience and Microflora* 2001; **20**(2): 43–48.

42. Meance S, Cayuela C, Raimondi A, Turchet P, Lucas C, Antoine JM. Recent advances in the use of functional foods: effects of the commercial fermented milk with bifidobacterium animalis strain dn-173010 and yoghurt strains on gut transit time in the elderly. *Microbiological Ecology in Health and Disease* 2003; **15**(1): 15–22.

43. Marteau P, Cuillerier E, Meance S, et al. Bifidobacterium animalis strain DN-173010 shortens the colonic transit time in healthy women in a double-blind, randomized, controlled study. *Alimentary Pharmacology and Therapeutics* 2002; **16**(3): 587–593.

Colorectal cancer and nutrition

Rachel Lewis[1] and Sorrel Burden[2]
[1]Glangwili Hospital, Carmarthen, UK
[2]Central Manchester NHS Foundation Trust, Manchester, UK

Colorectal cancer (CRC) is the third most common cancer worldwide after lung and breast cancer with an estimated 1.24 million new cases diagnosed in 2008 [1]. In 2010 there were approximately 40,695 new cases of CRC diagnosed in the UK, around two-thirds in the colon and one-third in the rectum [2].

The incidence of CRC varies between countries and the highest rates are found in Australia, New Zealand (approximately 45 cases per 10,000 population in men and 33 cases per 10,000 in women) and Western Europe, with the lowest rates reported in middle Africa (approximately four cases/10,000 in men and three cases/10,000 in women) [1]. Geographical variation in incidence across the world has been attributed to dietary variations and different levels of physical activity. Epidemiological studies report a rapid increase in risk for CRC in migrants moving from low- to high-risk countries and in countries that have had a rapid 'Westernisation' of diet, such as Japan [3].

Presenting symptoms include an alteration in stool output, rectal bleeding and anaemia with abdominal pain, anorexia and weight loss in more advanced tumours. Worldwide, CRC is the fourth most common cause of cancer death, estimated to be responsible for around 8% of the total (almost 610,000 deaths) in 2008 [1]. Mortality has been falling over the last decade, with the 5-year survival rates for both men and women improving considerably between the early 1970s and early 2000s [2]. Overall, 5-year survival rates average 55% in high-income countries and 39% in middle- to low-income countries [4]. Worldwide, it is estimated that there were 3.26 million CRC patients still alive in 2008, up to 5 years after their diagnosis. These changes can be attributed to screening programmes leading to earlier detection of tumours and substantial advances in treatment options.

Surgical resection with curative intent is the primary treatment for 80% of patients diagnosed with CRC [5]. The extent of intestinal resection and the presence of a stoma may affect the patient's nutritional status.

3.22.1 Factors involved in causation

Colorectal cancer is widely considered to be an environmental disease, with diet strongly influencing risk [6]. In the UK, it has been estimated that approximately 57% of CRC cases in men and 52% in women are linked to lifestyle and environmental factors [7], with incidence of CRC generally higher in populations that consume 'Westernised' diets . Colorectal cancer is one of the main cancers for which modifiable causes have been identified and therefore a large proportion of disease is theoretically preventable. It has been suggested that changes in dietary habits might reduce up to 70% of this cancer burden [6].

The link between diet and cancer is multifaceted and difficult to unravel. Diet may affect GI mucosa either directly from the luminal side or indirectly through whole-body metabolism. Compounds derived from food that are constantly present in the intestine, or the blood content of

Advanced Nutrition and Dietetics in Gastroenterology, First Edition. Edited by Miranda Lomer.
© 2014 John Wiley & Sons, Ltd. Published 2014 by John Wiley & Sons, Ltd.

nutrients, hormones and growth factors, may shift cellular balance toward harmful outcomes [8]. Variation in dietary intake and the complexity of interactions of dietary components, with each other and with metabolites, make it difficult to design studies that accurately identify dietary components that might induce or prevent CRC.

A recent report entitled *Food Nutrition, Physical Activity and the Prevention of Cancer: A Global Perspective* produced by the World Cancer Research Fund (WCRF) in collaboration with the American Institute for Cancer Research (AICR) provided a series of recommendations based on expert judgement, systemic reviews and case studies of the world literature [9]. Based on mainly prospective cohort studies, it was concluded that there is convincing evidence that physical activity can decrease the risk of CRC, while there is a probable reduction in cancer risk associated with foods rich in non-starch polysaccharides (NSP), garlic and calcium. Conversely, processed meat, red meat, alcohol, body fatness and in particular abdominal fatness are associated with cancer risk.

Red and processed meat

Meat consumption, most notably red and processed meat, has been described as a promoter of carcinogenesis. It has been estimated that 21% of CRC in the UK was linked to meat consumption [10], with the positive association stronger for colon cancer than rectal cancer [11]. Over the past three decades a plethora of epidemiological and prospective studies have evaluated this hypothesis. However, the possible role of this food group in CRC is equivocal.

Meta-analysis of the literature has concluded that there was a significantly increased risk of CRC in the highest category of red meat consumption when compared to the lowest category. An intake of 25–50 g/day processed meat was associated with 9–50% increased risk and a 17–30% increased risk of CRC was associated with a red meat intake of 100–120 g/day [11]. In contrast, a pooled analysis of UK case–control studies found no effect of 50 g/day red or processed meat; however, a relatively low amount of meat was consumed and the number of participants was relatively small [12].

The WCRF/AICR report concluded that consumption of red meat is a 'convincing' cause of CRC [9]. There has been much debate on the WCRF/AICR conclusions and a review of prospective epidemiological studies by Alexander et al. suggested that there are limitations to the available data [13]. Specifically, the epidemiological associations across the consortium of studies have been considered as being relatively weak in magnitude, most individual studies have not observed statistically significant associations, evidence of dose–response is unclear and patterns of associations vary by study characteristics. Also it is worth noting that red meat is defined and analysed heterogeneously across studies. The authors concluded that the available evidence is not sufficient to support a clear positive association between red and processed meat consumption and CRC.

Several postulated mechanisms regarding meat consumption and CRC incidence have been examined. Dietary mutagens (e.g. heterocyclic amines, polycyclic aromatic hydrocarbons) or chemical compounds that may develop during cooking at high temperatures have been most intensively studied, but associations from epidemiological analysis have been variable across several specific compounds [14]. Other mechanisms involve the potential role of nitrate and nitrite, commonly used in processed meat as preservation agents, and N-nitroso compounds, which have been shown to be carcinogenic in some laboratory animal studies. Finally, some researchers have suggested that iron may play a role in increasing CRC. However, relatively few studies have evaluated the potential role that this factor may play in cancer risk [14].

Obesity

Obesity, categorised as a Body Mass Index (BMI) >30 kg/m^2, is associated with an increased risk of colon cancer. In 2010 it was estimated that 13% of CRC cases in the UK were associated with an individual being overweight or obese [10].

Meta-analyses have shown that the risk of colon cancer increases by approximately 30% per 5 kg/m^2 increase in BMI for men, increasing to a 53% higher risk in obese men in comparison to healthy weight men (BMI <25 kg/m^2). The data for rectal cancer show a weaker association with BMI and cancer risk; a $5\,kg/m^2$ BMI increase is associated with a 9–12% higher risk in men, with those being obese having a 27% higher risk of developing rectal cancer [15]. The data for women are less clear with a non-significant association for colon cancer risk in one meta-analysis. It is likely that the female sex hormone oestrogen may affect the correlation between risk and BMI but the exact nature of this relationship is unclear.

Alcohol

Alcohol intake has been implicated as a risk factor for CRC, with the greatest risks associated with intakes in excess of 30 g/day. Thirteen cohort studies and 41 case–control studies reported a linear relationship with increased risk of CRC with increasing ethanol intakes. No contrary results were found with statistical significance [9].

A recent systemic review reported a 21% increase in risk for both colon and rectal cancers with an alcohol intake of 1.6–6.2 UK units (12.8–49.6 g) per day when compared to those categorised as non-drinkers or occasional drinkers [16]. Dose–response analysis within this study showed a 7% increase risk for every 10 g/day alcohol consumed. There is a suggestion of sexual dysmorphism, with evidence stronger for men. This is believed to be as a result of fewer data for women [9]. The EPIC study also found a significant positive association between alcohol consumption and CRC risk, with higher risks observed in the rectum compared to the distal colon. Several plausible mechanisms have been reported for this, including the hypothesis that individuals with habitually high alcohol intake have suboptimal intakes of essential nutrients, making them more susceptible to carcinogenesis.

Non-starch polysaccharides

It has been estimated that 12% of CRC could be attributed to poor NSP intakes <23 g/day [7]. Although the WCRF/AICR study noted foods high in NSP as being 'probable' in terms of decreasing the risk of CRC, it was acknowledged that the evidence is conflicting [9].

Studies have reported no correlation between CRC incidence and NSP whereas the EPIC study found a direct link, specifically in populations with low average intakes of NSP. More recently, a meta-analysis of 25 prospective studies with 2 million participants found that CRC risk was reduced by 10% for every 10 g/day total NSP [17]. Conflicting results have been attributed to possible confounding effects which include the overall amount of NSP consumed, the definition of NSP and type of fibre.

3.22.2 Nutritional status of colorectal cancer patients

Impaired nutritional status is a frequent complication in patients with CRC and can negatively affect the outcome of treatment and quality of life The consequences of underlying pathology or disease-associated symptoms such as diarrhoea, nausea or vomiting all contribute to the high incidence of protein energy malnutrition (PEM). All causes of excessive nutrient loss with or without increased metabolic needs will influence nutritional status. The undernourished cancer patient responds poorly to therapeutic interventions, such as chemotherapy, radiotherapy and surgery, with increased morbidity and mortality compared with well-nourished patients.

From early studies, the incidence of PEM in patients with CRC was cited as 37% [18]. More recently, Gupta et al. reported that PEM is observed in up to 41% of patients with advanced CRC [19]. Available data on the prevalence of PEM can vary broadly depending on evaluation criteria, for example tumour site, extension and anticancer treatment. Early identification and treatment of PEM in a patient's cancer journey are crucial in order to achieve favourable outcomes.

Surgical treatment

It is well recognised that patients undergoing GI surgery have an increased risk of developing undernutrition secondary to inadequate nutritional intake and metabolic stress following surgery. Furthermore, undernutrition can increase the incidence of postoperative complications, such as delayed wound healing or anastomosis dehiscence [20].

Surgery induces a catabolic response associated with a rise in stress hormone release and insulin resistance [21]. The generalised 'stress response' takes the form of a widespread endocrinal, biochemical reaction, involving the release of inflammatory markers such as prostaglandins, interleukins, histamine and also vascular endothelial cell products, the magnitude of which is determined by the severity, intensity and duration of the stressor. Cytokine concentration has been shown to have a significant bearing on the development of postoperative complications [22]. It has been reported that the balance between tumour necrosis factor (TNF) alpha and interleukin (IL)-10 seems to determine the occurrence of postoperative complications, particularly after abdominal surgery [23]. This hypermetabolic state, a delay in postoperative feeding coupled with preoperative starvation, often results in significant negative nitrogen balance [24]. The cumulative net nitrogen loss after elective abdominal surgery ranges between 40 and 80 g/day. Furthermore, it has been suggested that complications which delay the use of the GI tract can result in nitrogen losses of up to 150 g/day.

Loss of lean body mass and reduced muscle strength as a result of postoperative protein depletion increases the risk of cardiorespiratory impairment and compromised immune function, increasing the likelihood of infectious complications [24]. This can culminate in prolonged convalescence and increased morbidity The GI tract has a central modulatory role in the inflammatory and immune response to major surgery [25]. Gastrointestinal manipulation and splanchnic hypoperfusion have been shown to downregulate local and systemic immune function and increase intestinal permeability, potentially resulting in bacterial or endotoxin translocation into the systemic circulation, contributing to the systemic inflammatory response syndrome [26].

Studies have shown that measures to reduce the stress of surgery can minimise catabolism and support anabolism throughout surgical treatment, improving time to recovery [27], even after major surgical operations. There is extensive evidence to show that patients undergoing colorectal surgery should be managed within an enhanced recovery after surgery (ERAS) programme. ERAS programmes, first described by Professor Henri Kehlet in 2000, are a patient-centred method of optimising surgical outcomes, integrating a range of perioperative interventions proven to maintain physiological function, attenuate the stress response and facilitate postoperative recovery, especially after colonic resection [28].

A cohort study by Pascal et al. compared mortality, morbidity and length of stay between ERAS patients and carefully matched historical controls [29]. They concluded that ERAS reduces morbidity and length of hospital stay for patients undergoing elective colonic or rectal surgery. ERAS advocates that nutritional management becomes an integral component for all patients undergoing major surgery.

Preoperative nutritional status

Associations between weight loss, poorer outcomes and increased mortality rate have been documented since 1936. Since then, several studies have shown that when patients are undernourished their outcome after surgery is negatively affected. More recently, 66% of preoperative CRC patients were found to have lost weight, and weight loss greater than 10% was reported in 20% of this patient group [30]. It is worth considering whether it would be beneficial to correct preoperative weight loss using oral nutritional supplements (ONS). Standard ONS have been shown to decrease the incidence of wound infections in weight-losing CRC patients [30].

Immune-enhancing nutrition

Several specific substrates have been shown to augment or modulate host immune function. These nutrients include glutamine, arginine, n-3 fatty acids and nucleotides [31]. The mechanism by which supplementation of these nutrients exerts beneficial effects is unclear. All may exert their effects by suppressing inflammation, n-3 fatty acids by direct suppression of the process and glutamine by acting indirectly on antioxidant status. Glutamine and nucleotides exert a direct effect on lymphocyte proliferation [32].

The clinical benefits of these specially supplemented enteral diets, administered to those undergoing major surgical procedures, have been documented in a number of randomised clinical trials. It has been proposed that compared with standard enteral nutrition

(EN), immune-enhancing EN upregulates the immune response, controls the inflammatory response and improves GI function after surgery [33]. To date, there has been a large number of randomised clinical trials and four meta-analyses reporting that perioperative immune-enhancing nutrition is associated with a substantial reduction in both incidences of infection and length of hospital stay. These results have been found in both upper and lower GI patients, regardless of their baseline nutritional status. In a recent meta-analysis preoperative immune-enhancing nutrition was demonstrated to have a positive effect on both total complications and infections in GI surgical patients. However, studies using ONS in unselected GI surgical patients failed to demonstrate a decrease in postoperative complications [34].

Currently there are limited studies on immune-enhancing EN in conjunction with ERAS programmes so immune-enhancing EN has not been fully evaluated with other advances in surgical practice. Also some components of immune-enhancing formulae have been noted to have unfavourable effects in other patient groups. Some unwanted effects have been reported with components of immune-enhancing EN in critical care patients and it is unknown whether there would be detrimental effects by administering immune-enhancing EN to patients who require critical care support after their surgery [35].

Fasting guidelines and carbohydrate loading

Historically, elective surgical patients present in surgery in a catabolic fasted state. Although fasting from midnight has been standard practice to avoid pulmonary aspiration in elective surgery, a review has found no evidence to support this [36]. The typical order of 'nil by mouth after midnight' has been challenged in recent years, so much so that several anaesthetic associations across the world have updated their guidelines.

A Cochrane review of 22 randomised controlled trials (RCTs) in adult patients provides robust evidence that reducing the preoperative fasting period for clear fluids to 2 h does not increase complications [37]. National anaesthesia societies now recommend intake of clear fluids until 2 h before induction of anaesthesia as well as a 6-h fast for solid food. These developments in practice improve patient comfort and reduce adverse outcomes. Despite the change in recommendations, however, patients remain exposed to unnecessary starvation.

The provision of a carbohydrate-rich beverage has been shown to alter metabolic state; ensuring patients undergo surgery in a metabolically fed state. An oral dose of 50 g of carbohydrate results in an insulin and glucose response similar to that following the ingestion of a normal meal, representing a switch from a fasting state to an anabolic metabolic state. This modulates the postoperative insulin response, reducing postoperative insulin resistance [38].

Patients in a more anabolic state have fewer postoperative nitrogen and protein losses [39], as well as better maintained lean body mass and muscle strength. Data from RCTs indicate accelerated recovery and shorter hospital stay in patients receiving preoperative carbohydrate loading in colorectal surgery [21]. Reductions in preoperative thirst, hunger and anxiety have also been well documented, improving patient experience. Practically, carbohydrate solutions should be administered 12 and 2–3 h preoperatively. Preoperative carbohydrate loading has been shown to be safe in patients without type 1 diabetes [40]. Patients with diabetic neuropathy may have delayed gastric emptying, possibly increasing the risk of regurgitation and aspiration [41]. Patients with uncomplicated type 2 diabetes can have normal gastric emptying, and a study of preoperative carbohydrate loading did not find increased aspiration rates in such patients [42] or hyperglycaemia [43]. However, monitoring of blood glucose levels should be carried out at regular intervals.

Postoperative nutrition

There is a growing body of data which proposes that patients undergoing different types of GI surgery could benefit from early postoperative EN. However, the role of early postoperative EN after GI surgery is somewhat controversial. Traditionally, fluids and oral diet have been reintroduced cautiously after colorectal surgery, often rendering the patients nil by mouth or on oral sips only for many days in the postoperative period. This decision is based upon fears that early feeding may lead to postoperative complications if oral intake begins prior to return of GI function.

Enteral nutrition is a key preventive measure to minimise progression of sepsis, maintain mucosal integrity and prevent further deterioration of the immune function of the GI tract [44]. Several RCTs of early EN or oral diet versus 'nil by mouth' conclude that there is no advantage to keeping patients fasted after elective GI resection [45]. Early feeding is associated with a reduced risk of infection and length of hospital stay although it was not associated with an increased risk of anastomotic dehiscence, pneumonia and intra-abdominal abscess [45].

Tolerance to early feeding provides a more objective evaluation of GI function than assessment of bowel sounds or passage of flatus [40]. However, there is an increased risk of vomiting in patients fed early, and early feeding has been associated with bloating, impaired pulmonary function and delayed mobilisation in the absence of multimodal anti-ileus therapy [46]. When used in combination, preoperative oral carbohydrate loading, epidural analgesia and early EN have been shown to result in nitrogen equilibrium without concomitant hyperglycaemia [47].

For optimal benefit, delivery of oral or EN should be commenced within 12 h of surgery [48], considering EN in patients who are unable to achieve adequate nutrition via the oral route alone [49]. The use of ONS is encouraged through ERAS and has been used successfully for at least the first 4 postoperative days to achieve recommended intakes of energy and protein [50]. There is a clear advantage of prescribing postoperative ONS to patients with pre-existing undernutrition, improving nutritional status, protein economy and quality of life. Positive clinical outcomes from ONS given to patients undergoing elective surgery who are not undernourished have also been demonstrated [51].

3.22.3 Medical treatment of colorectal cancer

The role of adjuvant chemotherapy after curative surgery for colon cancer is well established. However, controversies remain surrounding the optimal chemotherapy regimen. Medical treatment of CRC usually focuses on the administration of cytotoxic agents with or without radiation therapy. These modes of treatments can potentially eradicate or reduce tumour size but may have several toxic side-effects that can negatively affect nutritional status. When PEM is established, it can be necessary to reduce the dose of cytotoxic agents and modify the timing of radiation or duration of treatment. Direct associations between the necessity to stop or delay anticancer treatment with time of remission, overall survival and response rates to chemoradiotherapy have been reported [52].

An RCT of patients undergoing pelvic radiation for CRC reported that 32% of patients experienced 5% weight loss prior to starting treatment [53]. A review by McGough et al. complemented the findings of the earlier trial, concluding that the incidence of PEM in patients commencing radiotherapy for pelvic malignancy was 11–33% [54]. Over 70% of patients undergoing pelvic radiation develop acute inflammatory small intestinal changes, leading to GI symptoms during and after treatment [55]. Six percent to 78% of patients may develop symptoms which affect quality of life [56]. These symptoms can include faecal incontinence, diarrhoea, steatorrhoea, tenesmus, pain, constipation and weight loss [53]. Serious complications such as bowel obstruction, fistulation, intractable bleeding or secondary cancer have been seen in 5–10% of patients [57].

A variety of dietary modifications have been studied to help alleviate acute and chronic GI side-effects associated with treatment. Dietary fat and NSP manipulation, elemental diets or supplementation of antioxidant or probiotics may show some benefit but the evidence for the use of nutritional intervention is limited and further research is required [54].

References

1. Ferlay J, Shin HR, Bray F, Forman D, Mathers C, Parkin DM. Estimates of worldwide burden of cancer in 2008: GLOBOCAN 2008. *International Journal of Cancer* 2010; **127**(12): 2893–2917.
2. Cancer Research. CancerStats: Cancer Statistics for the UK, 2013. www.cancerresearchuk.org/cancer-info/cancerstats/, accessed 17 January 2014.

3. Matsumara Y. Nutrition trends in Japan. *Asia Pacific Journal of Clinical Nutrition* 2001; **10**(Suppl): S40–S47.

4. Parkin DM, Bray F, Ferlay J, et al. Global cancer statistics, 2002. *CA Cancer J Clin* 2005; **55**: 74–108.

5. National Institute for Clinical Excellence (NICE). Improving outcomes in colorectal cancer. Manual update, 2012. http://guidance.nice.org.uk/CSGCC, accessed 17 January 2014.

6. Willett W C. Diet and cancer: an evolving picture. *Journal of the American Medical Association*. 2005; **293**(2):233–234

7. Parkin M, Boyd L, Walker LC. The fraction of cancer attributable to lifestyle and environmental factors in the UK in 2010. *British Journal of Cancer* 2011; **105**(Suppl 2): S77–S81.

8. Nystrom M, Mutanen M. Diet and epigenetics in colon cancer. *World Journal of Gastroenterology* 2009; **15**(3): 257–263.

9. World Cancer Research Fund/American Institute for Cancer Research. Continuous Update Project: Colorectal Cancer Report 2010 Summary. Food, Nutrition, Physical Activity, and the Prevention of Colorectal Cancer. www.wcrf.org/PDFs/Colorectal-cancer-report-summary-2011.pdf, accessed 17 January 2014.

10. Parkin DM. Cancers attributable to dietary factors in the UK in 2010. *British Journal of Cancer* 2011; **105**(Suppl 2): S24–S26.

11. Larsson SC, Wolk A. Meat consumption and risk of colorectal cancer: a meta-analysis of prospective studies. *International Journal of Cancer* 2006; **119**(11): 2657–2664.

12. Spencer EA, Key TJ, Appleby PN, et al. Meat, poultry and fish and risk of colorectal cancer: pooled analysis of data from the UK dietary cohort consortium. *Cancer Causes and Control* 2010; **21**(9): 1417–1425.

13. Alexander DD, Cushing CA. Red meat and colorectal cancer: a critical summary of prospective epidemiologic studies. International Association for the Study of Obesity. *Obesity Reviews* 2011; **12**(5): e472–e493.

14. Scientific Advisory Committee on Nutrition (SACN). Draft iron report. Scientific consultation, 2012. www.sacn.gov.uk, accessed 17 January 2014.

15. Harriss DJ, Atkinson G, George K, et al. Lifestyle factors and colorectal cancer risk (1): systematic review and meta-analysis of associations with body mass index. *Colorectal Disease* 2009; **11**(6): 547–563.

16. Fedirko V, Tramacere I, Bagnardi V, et al. Alcohol drinking and colorectal cancer risk: an overall and dose–response meta-analysis of published studies. *Annals of Oncology* 2001; **22**(9): 1958–1972.

17. Aune D, Chan DS, Lau R, et al. Dietary fibre, whole grains, and risk of colorectal cancer: systematic review and dose–response meta-analysis of prospective studies. *British Medical Journal* 2011; **343**: d6617.

18. Rombeau J, Goldman S, Apelgren K, Sanford I, Frey C. Protein-calorie malnutrition in patients with colorectal cancer. *Diseases of the Colon and Rectum* 1978; **21**(8): 587–589.

19. Gupta D, Lis C, Granick J, Grutsch J, Vashi P, Lammersfeld C. Malnutrition was associated with poor quality of life in colorectal cancer: a retrospective analysis. *Journal of Clinical Epidemiology* 2006; **59**(7): 704–709.

20. Capra S, Ferguson M, Ried K. Cancer: impact of nutrition intervention outcome – nutrition issues for patients. *Nutrition* 2001; **17**: 769–772.

21. Noblett SE, Watson DS, Huong H, Davison B, Hainsworth PJ, Horgan AF. Pre-operative oral carbohydrate loading in colorectal surgery: a randomized controlled trial. *Colorectal Disease* 2006; **8**(7): 563–569.

22. Ward N. Nutrition support to patients undergoing gastrointestinal surgery. *Nutrition Journal* 2003; **2**: 18.

23. Dimopoulu I, Aramaganidis A, Douka E. Tumor necrosis factor (TNF) and IL10 are crucial mediators in postoperative systemic inflammatory response and determine the occurrence of complications after major abdominal surgery. *Cytokine* 2007; **37**(1): 55–61.

24. Inui A. Cancer anorexia-cachexia syndrome: are neuropeptides the key? *Cancer Research* 1999; **59**(18): 4493–4501.

25. Holland J, Carey M, Hughes N, et al. Intraoperative splanchnic hypoperfusion, increased intestinal permeability, down-regulation of monocyte class II major histocompatibility complex expression, exaggerated acute phase response, and sepsis. *American Journal of Surgery* 2005; **190**: 393–400.

26. Schietroma M, Carlei F, Cappelli S, et al. Intestinal permeability and systemic endotoxaemia after laparotomic or laparoscopic cholecystectomy. *Annals of Surgery* 2006; **243**(3): 459–463.

27. Weinmann A, Braga M, Harsanyi L, et al. ESPEN guidelines on Enteral Nutrition: surgery including organ transplantation. *Clinical Nutrition* 2006; **2**: 224–244.

28. Khoo CK, Vickery CJ, Forsyth N, Vinall NS, Eyre-Brook IA. A prospective randomized controlled trial of multi-modal perioperative management protocol in patients undergoing elective colorectal resection for cancer. *Annals of Surgery* 2007; **245**(6): 867– 872.

29. Pascal HE, Teeuwen RP, Bleichrodt C, et al. Enhanced Recovery After Surgery (ERAS) versus conventional postoperative care in colorectal surgery. *Journal of Gastrointestinal Surgery* 2010; **14**(1): 88–95.

30. Burden ST, Hill J, Shaffer J, Todd C. Nutritional status of preoperative colorectal cancer patients. *Journal of Human Nutrition and Dietetics* 2010; **23**: 402–407.

31. Saito H. Immunonutrition. *Nippon Geka Gakkai Zasshi* 2004; **105**(2): 213–217.

32. Grimble RF. Nutritional modulation of immune function. *Proceedings of the Nutrition Society* 2001; **60**(3): 389–397.

33. Braga M. Perioperative immunonutrition and gut function. *Current Opinion in Clinical Nutrition and Metabolic Care* 2012; **15**(5): 485–488.

34. Burden S, Todd C, Hill J, Lal S. Pre-operative nutrition support in patients undergoing gastrointestinal surgery. *Cochrane Database of Systematic Reviews* 2012; **11**: CD008879.

35. Rice TW, Wheeler AP, Thompson T, de Boisblanc PB, Steingrub J, Rock P. Enteral omega-3 fatty acid, alfa-linolenic acid, and antioxidant supplementation in acute lung injury. *Journal of the American Medical Association* 2011; **12**: 1574–1581.

36. Ljungqvist O, Søreide E. Preoperative fasting. *British Journal of Surgery* 2003; **90**(4): 400–406.

37. Brady M, Kinn S, Stuart P. Preoperative fasting for adults to prevent perioperative complications. *Cochrane Database of Systematic Reviews* 2003; **4**: CD004423.

38. Nygren J. The metabolic effects of fasting and surgery. *Best Practice and Research in Clinical Anaesthesiology* 2006; **20**(3): 429–438.

39. Svanfeldt M, Thorell A, Hausel J, et al. Randomized clinical trial of the effect of preoperative oral carbohydrate treatment on postoperative whole-body protein and glucose kinetics. *British Journal of Surgery* 2007; **94**(11): 1342–1350.

40. Association of Surgeons of Great Britain and Ireland (ASGBI). Guidelines for Implementation of Enhanced Recovery Protocols, 2008. www.asgbi.org.uk/en/publications/issues_in_professional_practice.cfm, accessed 17 January 2014.

41. Kong MF, Horowitz M. Diabetic gastroparesis. *Diabetic Medicine* 2005; **22**(Suppl 4): 13–18.

42. Breuer JP, von Dossow V, von Heymann C, et al. Preoperative oral carbohydrate administration to ASA III-IV patients undergoing elective cardiac surgery. *Anesthesia and Analgesia* 2006; **103**(5): 1099–1108.

43. Gustafsson UO, Nygren J, Thorell A, et al. Pre-operative carbohydrate loading may be used in type 2 diabetes patients. *Acta Anaesthesiologica Scandinavica* 2008; **52**(7): 946–951.

44. Dervenis C, Smailis D, Hatzitheoklitos E. Bacterial translocation and its prevention in acute pancreatitis. *Journal of Hepatobiliary and Pancreatic Surgery* 2003; **10**(6): 415–418.

45. Lewis SJ, Egger M, Sylvester PA, Thomas S. Early enteral feeding vs "nil by mouth" after gastrointestinal surgery: systematic review and meta-analysis of controlled trials. *British Medical Journal* 2001; **323**(7316): 773–776.

46. Charoenkwan K, Phillipson G, Vutyavanich T. Early vs delayed (traditional) oral fluids and food for reducing complications after major abdominal gynaecologic surgery. *Cochrane Database of Systematic Reviews* 2007; **4**: CD004508.

47. Soop M, Carlson GL, Hopkinson J, et al. Randomized clinical trial of the effects of immediate enteral nutrition on metabolic responses to major colorectal surgery in an enhanced recovery protocol. *British Journal of Surgery* 2004; **91**(9): 1138–1145.

48. Mochizuki H, Trocki O, Dominioni L, et al. Mechanism of prevention of postburn hypermetabolism and catabolism by early enteral feeding. *Annals of Surgery* 1984; **200**(3): 297–310.

49. National Institute for Clinical Excellence (NICE). Nutrition Support in Adults. Guideline 32, 2006. www.nice.org.uk//CG32, accessed 17 January 2014.

50. Fearon KC, Luff R. The nutritional management of surgical patients: enhanced recovery after surgery. *Proceedings of the Nutrition Society* 2003; **62**(4): 807–811.

51. Smedley F, Bowling T, James M, et al. Randomized clinical trial of the effects of preoperative and postoperative oral nutritional supplements on clinical course and cost of care. *British Journal of Surgery* 2004; **91**(8): 983–990.

52. Norman K, Pichard C, Lochs H, Pirlich M. Prognostic impact of disease-related malnutrition. *Clinical Nutrition* 2008; **27**: 5–15.

53. Bye A. The influence of low fat, low lactose diet on diarrhoea during pelvic radiotherapy. *Clinical Nutrition* 1992; **11**: 147–153.

54. McGough C. Role of nutritional intervention in patients treated with radiotherapy for pelvic malignancy. *British Journal of Cancer* 2004; **90**: 2278–2287.

55. Resbeut M, Marteau P, Cowen D, et al. A randomised double blind placebo controlled multicentre study of mesalazine for the prevention of acute radiation enteritis. *Radiotherapy Oncology* 1997; **44**: 59–63.

56. Gami B. How patients manage gastrointestinal symptoms after pelvic radiotherapy. *Alimentary Pharmacology and Therapeutics* 2003; **18**; 987–994.

57. Nostrant TT. Radiation injury. In: Yamada T, Alpers DH, Owyans C, Powell DW, Silverstein FE (eds) *Textbook of Gastroenterology*. Philadelphia: J.B. Lippincott, 1995, pp. 2605–2616.

SECTION 4

Hepatobiliary disorders

Chapter 4.1

Gallbladder disease and nutrition

Angela M. Madden[1] and Emma Currie[2]
[1]University of Hertfordshire, Hatfield, UK
[2]Addenbrooke's Hospital, Cambridge, UK

4.1.1 Gallstones

Gallstones are dense hard structures formed from the precipitation of solids in bile and are usually located within the gallbladder or, less frequently but with potentially greater clinical significance, lodged in a bile duct outside or within the liver. The type of gallstone is defined by its composition and can be divided into two main groups: those which are cholesterol rich and comprise approximately 70% of cases in Western populations and those composed predominantly of bile pigments [1]. Although there are some common features and the clinical consequences are similar between the two groups, the pathogenesis and risk factors differ.

The worldwide prevalence of gallstones varies with stone composition and between countries (Table 4.1.1). Prevalence is generally considered to be increasing as a consequence of nutritional and lifestyle changes, ageing populations, the increasing global prevalence of obesity and improved diagnostic capabilities [9]. Although gallstones are associated with a comparatively low mortality rate of 0.6%, the burden of morbidity and direct and indirect costs are high, estimated in the United States as being approximately $6.2 billion annually [9].

4.1.2 Factors involved in causation

A number of nutritional and other aetiological factors, including demographic, genetic and biliary issues (Table 4.1.2), are associated with increased risk of gallstone formation. Cholesterol supersaturation of bile is the primary requirement for the formation of cholesterol-rich gallstones and this is influenced by dietary intake, eating behaviour and body weight but supersaturation alone does not automatically lead to the production of stones.

Obesity

Carrying excessive body weight, particularly as abdominal fat, is well recognised as a risk factor for developing cholesterol-rich gallstones [18,19]. The relationship is linear in women with least risk associated with Body Mass Index (BMI) $<20 kg/m^2$, and increasing to a relative risk of 1.7 (95% confidence interval (CI) 1.1–2.7) with BMI between 24.0 and $24.9 kg/m^2$ and relative risk of 6.0 (95% CI 4.0–9.0) associated with BMI $>32 kg/m^2$ [18]. Increasing waist circumference is also independently associated with greater risk of developing gallstones in both men and women, with the greatest relative risk in men associated with measurements of 102–106 cm (relative risk 3.9, 95% CI 1.5–10.7 compared to <86 cm) and in women with measurements of 81–86 cm (relative risk 2.9, 95% CI 1.6–5.2 compared to <71 cm) [19]. The risk is mediated by increased cholesterol synthesis and cholesterol secretion into bile associated with raised insulin concentrations in excessive body weight. Counterintuitively, weight reduction increases the risk of cholesterol-rich gallstone formation in the short term as a negative energy balance results in cholesterol mobilisation from adipose stores [20]. Risk

Advanced Nutrition and Dietetics in Gastroenterology, First Edition. Edited by Miranda Lomer.
© 2014 John Wiley & Sons, Ltd. Published 2014 by John Wiley & Sons, Ltd.

Table 4.1.1 Worldwide prevalence* of gallstones

Population (number studied)	Prevalence (%)		Study
	Men	Women	
USA, North American Indians (3296)	29.5	64.1	Everhart et al. 2002 [2]
Italy, Padua (1065)	17	35	Lirussi et al. 1999 [3]
Peru, Lima (1534)	16.1	10.7	Moro et al. 2000 [4]
Taiwan, Taipei (3647)	10.7	11.5	Chen et al. 1998 [5]
USA, Mexican Americans (4174)	8.9	26.7	Everhart et al. 1999 [6]
USA, White Americans (5275)	8.6	16.6	Everhart et al. 1999 [6]
UK, Bristol (1896)	6.9	8.0	Heaton et al. 1991 [7]
India, Uttar Pradesh and Bihar (22861)	2.0	5.6	Unisa et al. 2011 [8]

*Studies vary in the age of participants and diagnostic criteria so direct comparisons between populations should be undertaken with caution.

Table 4.1.2 Non-nutritional factors influencing the formation of gallstones

Risk factor	Explanation
Age	Increased risk with increasing age, especially after 40 years [10]
Gender	Increased risk in women, particularly premenopause [11]
Reproductive history	Increased risk with pregnancy, oral contraceptive use and oestrogen replacement therapy in women [12]
Genetics	Increased risk in people with family history of gallstones; some rare monogenetic defects identified but gallstone formation is probably polygenic disorder [13,14]
Gastrointestinal health	Increased risk associated with disruption to enterohepatic circulation and faecal loss of bile salts and conditions including gastric bypass, pre-existing liver disease, Crohn's disease and malabsorption due to cystic fibrosis [15,16]
Biliary health	Increased risk associated with incomplete gallbladder emptying, impaired gallbladder motility, sphincter of Oddi dysfunction, congenitally misshaped or diseased gallbladder and with biliary infections [1,17]

can be reduced by maintaining a rate of weight loss below 1.5 kg/week [21], minimising weight cycling where body weight is sequentially lost and regained [22,23] and maintaining weight loss <25% of total body weight after bariatric surgery [24].

Dietary fat and cholesterol

Several studies investigating the effects of total dietary fat, monounsaturated and polyunsaturated fatty acids on gallstone formation have provided conflicting results from which no definitive conclusion can be drawn [25]. This equivocal evidence may reflect that although dietary fat is associated with obesity and high cholesterol concentrations, it also stimulates the release of cholecystokinin (CCK) which provokes gallbladder contraction, thus expelling potentially lithogenic bile and reducing stone formation. Studies of dietary cholesterol intake have also yielded no definitive association between intake and gallstone formation. However, examining specific lipid fractions may provide further evidence as epidemiological and experimental investigations into the effects of n-3 fatty acids, i.e. derived from fish oil, have shown that these may have a protective effect [26]. Conversely, long-term consumption of a high intake of trans fatty acids, formed during hydrogenation of lipid in food processing, is associated with a modest but independent increased risk of developing gallstones (comparison of highest and lowest intake quintiles, relative risk 1.23, 95% CI 1.04–1.44) [27]. This is probably mediated via a lowering of serum high-density lipoprotein (HDL) cholesterol which is associated with the reduction of cholesterol saturation in bile [28].

Dietary carbohydrate and fibre

High intakes of refined carbohydrate are associated with increased risk of developing gallstones [29,30]. It has been suggested that this arises because diets containing more carbohydrate usually provide less fat and therefore will provoke less CCK secretion and thus less contraction of the gallbladder. This hypothesis is logical but not supported by any evidence of an association between high intakes of unrefined carbohydrate and increased risk of gallstone formation. It is likely that the lithogenic effects of refined carbohydrate are mediated through increased cholesterol saturation of bile [31] secondary to raised insulin concentrations [32] and through a reduction in sensitivity to CCK in the presence of raised serum triglycerides, which are associated with high refined carbohydrate intake [33].

Studies have identified a protective effect of dietary fibre on cholesterol gallstone formation [18,30,34]. This is probably mediated through the reduction of intestinal transit time by insoluble fibre, thus limiting colonic reabsorption of the bile acid deoxycholic acid (DCA), and so reducing biliary DCA concentrations and increasing the synthesis of bile acids from cholesterol resulting in reduced bile cholesterol saturation [35]. The effects of soluble fibre, which is known to reduce serum cholesterol [36], may be the same but also explained by luminal binding of bile acids or the formation of a physical barrier which reduces bile acid reabsorption [37].

Alcohol

Consumption of alcohol is inversely associated with gallstone development in men and cholecystectomy in women [38]. In a recent study of 2417 adults, the independent relative risk of developing gallstones in those consuming alcohol compared to non-drinkers was 0.67 (95% CI 0.46–0.99) [39]. The EPIC-Norfolk

study of 25,639 adults identified a 3% reduction in risk of developing gallstones associated with every unit of alcohol consumed by men but no effect in women [19]. The effect of alcohol in men is probably mediated via an increase in HDL cholesterol which is associated with the reduction of cholesterol saturation in bile [28,31].

Other dietary factors

A number of other nutrients and foods have been investigated as possible causative agents in gallstone formation, including protein, vitamin C, caffeine and nuts. However, the findings from different studies are conflicting and do not allow firm conclusion to be drawn [25].

Physical activity

Whilst physical activity might not be considered a nutritional variable, it is a potentially modifiable influence on the risk of cholesterol-rich gallstone formation. A number of epidemiological studies have identified the beneficial effects of physical activity in reducing the risk of gallstone disease in men and women [40]. These effects are independent of BMI and probably mediated through an increase in serum HDL cholesterol and reduction in serum insulin [40].

4.1.3 Nutritional management

Optimising nutritional intake may play a role in the prevention of cholesterol-rich but not pigment gallstones. However, few dietary intervention studies have been undertaken to investigate nutritional management and therefore advice should be based on evidence from epidemiology which is supported by a plausible mechanism. It is necessary to consider the stage of the individual's condition as this will influence their dietary intake and the relevance of nutritional advice. Once formed, gallstones may be asymptomatic or lead to chronic or acute cholecystitis when the gallbladder becomes inflamed, causing pain. It is estimated that approximately 10% of the population with asymptomatic gallstones will develop symptoms or require treatment within 5 years [41].

Minimising risk of gallstone formation and management of asymptomatic gallstones

Strategies are based on reducing the cholesterol saturation of bile. This should include consuming an energy intake to achieve or maintain a healthy BMI below 25 kg/m^2, reducing excess body weight at a rate of less than 1.5 kg/week, minimising intake of refined carbohydrate and trans fatty acids, consuming alcohol within safe drinking limits and increasing dietary fibre. This is compatible with current healthy eating guidelines in many countries [42,43]. A supplement of n-3 fatty acid may be of benefit to weight reducers [26]. In addition, it is logical to advise regular food intake, including breakfast, in order to stimulate gallbladder contraction and so reduce the time that bile, particularly lithogenic overnight bile, is retained [44].

Acute cholecystitis

Pain is usually severe in acute cases of cholecystitis and occurs primarily in the epigastric or right upper abdomen and lasts 2–4 h. It is often accompanied by nausea and sometimes pyrexia. Some patients with acute cholecystitis experience loss of appetite. Short-term dietary management may include encouraging intake through offering food 'little and often', food fortification and strategies to address nausea and vomiting. If nutritional requirements cannot be met by consuming food alone, oral nutritional supplements andor enteral nutrition (EN) may be required. When pain subsides, nutritional management compatible with chronic cholecystitis is appropriate.

Chronic cholecystitis

Chronic cholecystitis can occur with or without a previously documented acute episode and is characterised by often vague symptoms including epigastric discomfort, particularly after eating, abdominal distension, nausea, belching and flatulence. Nutritional management should be based on minimising risk of further stone formation and avoiding foods that worsen symptoms in individuals. As symptoms are usually abdominal and sometimes associated with eating, advice or self-preference to avoid specific foods is

common in people with cholecystitis. However, this is often individual and mostly unsupported by evidence from studies [45]. Specifically, there is no logic to avoiding dietary fat with the intention of minimising pain through reducing gallbladder contractions [46]. The gallbladder indeed contracts in response to dietary fat but also does so following consumption of mixed meals, elemental diets [47], protein [48] and medium-chain triglycerides [49] as well as in response to cephalic stimulation [50] and spontaneously [51]. This indicates that minimising dietary fat is unlikely to eliminate pain and may even result in increasing the risk of further cholesterol stone formation [52]. Therefore, it is reasonable to recommend a healthy diet providing less than 35% of food energy from total dietary fat as suitable in chronic cholecystitis [53].

After cholecystectomy

Treatment for symptomatic gallstones is surgical removal of the gallbladder which is undertaken laparoscopically without overnight admission to hospital in 75–95% of cases. The consumption of a carbohydrate-rich drink before laparoscopic cholecystectomy is associated with reduced postoperative nausea and vomiting [54]. Oral nutrition can be initiated, in most cases, immediately after surgery, as neither oesophagogastric decompression [55] nor delayed oral intake has proven beneficial after cholecystectomy. Furthermore, enhanced recovery programmes, which include early postoperative oral feeding, are associated with improved patient outcomes in those undergoing gastrointestinal surgery [56].

Most patients will not require any specific dietetic intervention after surgery. In a small minority of patients who are unable to achieve an adequate intake, postoperative advice should focus on dietary manipulation and food fortification tailored to individual symptoms. EN via a feeding tube may be indicated, and a standard whole protein feed is appropriate for most. In those who are malnourished at the time of surgery and in whom it is anticipated that oral intake will remain inadequate (<60% of estimated requirements) for more than 10 days, tube feeding should ideally be initiated within 24 h after surgery [57]. Postoperative ileus or prolonged gastrointestinal dysfunction may contraindicate oral or EN. In these cases, parenteral nutrition (PN) may be appropriate [58].

Although there is evidence of increased faecal fat excretion after cholecystectomy [59] and some patients continue to experience food-related pain after gallbladder removal [60], weight gain is common following surgery [61]. Therefore, rather than any specific nutritional manipulation, a diet compatible with healthy eating guidelines, as described for minimising risk of gallstone formation and chronic cholecystitis, is recommended after cholecystectomy for patients without complications. Whilst a relatively low fat intake is compatible with a healthy diet, the avoidance of all dietary fat after cholecystectomy is not necessary [62].

Complications following cholecystectomy

Diarrhoea is commonly reported by patients following cholecystectomy and prevalence may vary between 1% and 36% [63]. A number of different causes may contribute.

Exocrine pancreatic function may be impaired in patients with gallstones and following cholecystectomy [64]. Gallstones can lodge in the common bile duct, preventing the normal flow of exocrine pancreatic secretions, including pancreatic enzymes, into the duodenum. This blockage can lead to inflammation of the pancreas, causing gallstone pancreatitis and pancreatic exocrine insufficiency which does not resolve following cholecystectomy. In severe cases, this can result in steatorrhoea. Treatment of pancreatic insufficiency should include pancreatic enzyme replacement therapy (PERT) and consideration of supplementation with fat-soluble vitamins A, D, E and K. Dietary fat restriction is unnecessary as it may compromise energy intake in patients who may already be undernourished (see Chapter 3.16).

Diarrhoea secondary to bile acid malabsorption (BAM) occurs in a number of gastrointestinal tract disorders. Although this has been reported after cholecystectomy, a causal relationship between BAM and postcholecystectomy diarrhoea has not been substantiated [65]. The 75-SeHCAT test can be used to diagnose BAM following gallbladder surgery [66] and limited prevalence data based on this method indicate that BAM is present in approximately 58%

of patients following vagotomy and pyloroplasty with or without cholecystectomy who have chronic or recurrent diarrhoea [67]. Bile acid sequestrants, including cholestyramine, can be used to treat BAM symptoms by binding with bile acids and preventing reabsorption. As these also reduce absorption of fat-soluble vitamins, patients taking bile sequestrants should be checked for deficiencies.

Psychological and psychosomatic factors might also contribute to postcholecystectomy diarrhoea [63].

Common bile duct injury caused during cholecystectomy may result in biliary leaks and fistula formation. The prevalence of injury varies between 0.1–0.4% in open surgery and 0.2–0.7% during laparoscopic procedures [68]. Conservative treatment includes sepsis management, wound care, correction of fluid and electrolyte disturbances and nutritional support [69]. EN should be used in preference to PN with close monitoring of drain output and for evidence of fat malabsorption. Semi-elemental or low-fat EN should be considered if fat malabsorption is present. Complex enterocutaneous fistulae with output exceeding 500 mL/24 h may require advice on oral rehydration solutions, avoidance of hypotonic fluids and possible use of antisecretory or antimotility medications. If fistula output remains high, PN may be beneficial (see Chapter 3.16). If biliary leaks do not heal spontaneously, corrective surgery may be required.

4.1.4 Functional dyskinesia of the gallbladder

Episodic biliary pain that is associated with abnormal gallbladder motility in the absence of gallstones has been described as gallbladder dyskinesia [70]. Although some of the pain described in this condition is related to eating food [71], there is no evidence that dietary modification is helpful in alleviating this. Dyskinesia is associated with impaired gallbladder emptying in many patients, which increases the risk of cholesterol supersaturated bile and microlithiasis (formation of crystals) and then gallbladder inflammation [72]. Dietary advice for minimising gallstone risk is, therefore, appropriate in these cases.

4.1.5 Steatocholecystitis

Lipid deposits that are associated with inflammation in the wall of the gallbladder have been reported in obese patients both with and without gallstones and also in animal models [73,74]. This condition, referred to as steatocholecystitis or cholecystosteatosis, is analogous to non-alcoholic steatohepatitis in the liver. The lipid deposits infiltrating the smooth muscle cells, endothelium of capillaries and fibroblasts in the gallbladder wall provoke a cytokine cascade causing inflammation and impairing the ejection of bile [75]. These, in turn, are likely to increase the risk of gallstone formation and potentially the risk of gallbladder cancer [76]. The treatment to date has focused on pharmacotherapy with ezetimibe, which inhibits intestinal fat absorption, and no studies have investigated dietary interventions. However, as this condition appears to obesity related, it is logical to recommend a healthy, well-balanced diet that is compatible with reducing excessive body weight.

4.1.6 Gallbladder cancer

Gallbladder cancer (ICD-10 code C23) is a relatively rare malignancy with approximately 160 new cases diagnosed per year in the UK and 150,000 worldwide [77,78]. Countries with the highest incidence include areas in Chile, India, Korea and Peru and in most of these, it is more common in women than men [79]. Risk factors include a history of gallstones, primary sclerosing cholangitis, choledochal cysts, obesity, parity and chronic infection with *Salmonella typhi*, *Salmonella paratyphi*, *Helicobacter bilis* and *Helicobacter pylori* [80,81]. A large multicentred case–control study identified high intakes of energy and carbohydrate (refined or unrefined not specified) as independent nutritional risk factors whilst high intakes of vitamins B6, C and E and dietary fibre were protective [82]. Dietary advice to minimise risk of gallbladder cancer is compatible with the international recommendations to prevent cancer [83]. Protein-energy malnutrition is common in those with advanced cancer due to tumour-related catabolism, physical symptoms impairing intake and nutrient absorption, reduced oral intake due to anxiety or depression and the side-effects of treatment. The nutritional management of patients diagnosed with gallbladder cancer should be individualised and planned as an integral part of their care so that nutrient requirements are provided in a format that is acceptable to the patient and compatible with surgery, radiotherapy or other anticancer treatment they are receiving.

References

1. Venneman NG, van Erpecum KJ. Pathogenesis of gallstones. *Gastroenterology Clinics of North America* 2010; **39**: 171–183.
2. Everhart JE, Yeh F, Lee ET, et al. Prevalence of gallbladder disease in American Indian populations: findings from the Strong Heart Study. *Hepatology* 2002; **35**: 1507–1512.
3. Lirussi F, Nassuato G, Passera D, et al. Gallstone disease in an elderly population: the Silea study. *European Journal of Gastroenterology and Hepatology* 1999; **11**: 485–491.
4. Moro P, Checkley W, Gilman R, et al. Gallstone disease in Peruvian coastal natives and highland migrants. *Gut* 2000; **46**: 569–573.
5. Chen CY, Lu CL, Huang YS, et al. Age is one of the risk factors in developing gallstone diseases in Taiwan. *Age and Ageing* 1998; **27**: 437–441.
6. Everhart JE, Khare M, Hill M, Maurer KR. Prevalence and ethnic differences in gallbladder disease in the United States. *Gastroenterology* 1999; **117**: 632–639.
7. Heaton KW, Braddon FEM, Mountford RA, Hughes AO, Emmett PM. Symptomatic and silent gall stones in the community. *Gut* 1991; **32**: 316–320.
8. Unisa S, Jagannath P, Dhir V, Khandelwal C, Sarangi L, Roy TK. Population-based study to estimate prevalence and determine risk factors of gallbladder diseases in the rural Gangetic basin of North India. *HPB (Oxford)* 2011; **13**: 117–125.
9. Stinton LM, Myers RP, Shaffer EA. Epidemiology of gallstones. *Gastroenterology Clinics of North America* 2010; **39**: 157–169.
10. Einarsson K, Nilsell K, Lijd B, Angelin B. Influence of age on secretion of cholesterol and synthesis of bile acids by the liver. *New England Journal of Medicine* 1985; **313**: 277–282.
11. Rome Group for the Epidemiology and Prevention of Cholelithiasis (GREPCO). The epidemiology of gallstone disease in Rome, Italy, part I. Prevalence data in men. *Hepatology* 1988; **8**: 904–906.
12. Cirillo DJ, Wallace RB, Rodabough RJ, et al. Effect of estrogen therapy of gallbladder disease. *Journal of the American Medical Association* 2005; **293**: 330–339.
13. Sarin SK, Negi VS, Dewan R, Sasan S, Saraya A. High familial prevalence of gallstones in the first-degree relatives of gallstone patients. *Hepatology* 1995; **22**: 138–141.
14. Stokes CS, Krawczyk M, Lammert F. Gallstones: environment, lifestyle and genes. *Digestive Diseases* 2011; **29**: 191–201.
15. Jebbink MC, Hiejerman HG, Masclee AA, Lamers CB. Gallbladder disease in cystic fibrosis. *Netherlands Journal of Medicine* 1992; **41**: 123–126.
16. Hutchinson R, Tyrrell PN, Kumar D, Dunn JA, Li JK, Allan R. Pathogenesis of gall stones in Crohn's disease: an alternative explanation. *Gut* 1994; **35**: 94–97.

17. Abayli B, Colakoglu S, Serin M, et al. Helicobacter pylori in the etiology of cholesterol gallstones. *Journal of Clinical Gastroenterology* 2005; **39**: 134–137.

18. Maclure KM, Hayes KC, Colditz GA, Stampfer MJ, Speizer FE, Willett WC. Weight, diet and the risk of symptomatic gallstones in middle-aged women. *New England Journal of Medicine* 1989; **321**: 563–569.

19. Banim PJ, Luben RN, Bulluck H, et al. The aetiology of symptomatic gallstones quantification of the effects of obesity, alcohol and serum lipids on risk. Epidemiological and biomarker data from a UK prospective cohort study (EPIC Norfolk). *European Journal of Gastroenterology and Hepatology* 2011; **23**: 733–740.

20. Everhart JE. Contributions of obesity and weight loss to gallstone disease. *Annals of Internal Medicine* 1993; **119**: 1029–1035.

21. Weinsier RL, Wilson LJ, Lee J. Medically safe rate of weight loss for the treatment of obesity: guidelines based on the risk of gallstone formation. *American Journal of Medicine* 1995; **98**: 115–117.

22. Syngal S, Coakley EH, Willett WC, Byers T, Williamson DF, Colditz GA. Long-term weight patterns and risk for cholecystectomy in women. *Annals of Internal Medicine* 1999; **130**: 471–477.

23. Tsai CJ, Leitzmann MF, Willett WC, Giovannucci EL. Weight cycling and risk of gallstone disease in men. *Archives of Internal Medicine* 2006; **166**: 2369–2374.

24. Li VKM, Pulido N, Fajnwaks P, Szomstein S, Rosenthal R, Martinez-Duartez P. Predictors of gallstone formation after bariatric surgery: a multivariate analysis of risk factors comparing gastric bypass, gastric banding, and sleeve gastrectomy. *Surgical Endoscopy* 2009; **23**: 2488–2492.

25. Méndez-Sánchez N, Zamora-Valdés D, Chávez-Tapia NC, Uribe M. Role of diet in cholesterol gallstone formation. *Clinica Chimica Acta* 2007; **376**: 1–8.

26. Méndez-Sánchez N, González V, Aquavo P, et al. Fish oil (n-3) polyunsaturated fatty acids beneficially affect biliary cholesterol nucleation time in obese women losing weight. *Journal of Nutrition* 2001; **131**: 2300–2303.

27. Tsai CJ, Leitzmann MF, Willett WC, Giovannucci EL. Long-term intake of trans-fatty acids and risk of gallstone disease in men. *Archives of Internal Medicine* 2005; **165**: 1011–1015.

28. Petitti DB, Friedman GD, Klatsky AL. Association of a history of gallbladder disease with a reduced concentration of high-density-lipoprotein cholesterol. *New England Journal of Medicine* 1981; **304**: 1396–1398.

29. Moerman CJ, Smeets FW, Kromhout D. Dietary risk factors for clinically diagnosed gallstones in middle-aged men. A 25-year follow-up study (the Zutphen Study). *Epidemiology* 1994; **4**: 248–254.

30. Misciagna G, Centonze S, Leoci C, et al. Diet, physical activity and gallstones – a population-based, case–control study in southern Italy. *American Journal of Clinical Nutrition* 1999; **69**: 120–126.

31. Thornton J, Symes C, Heaton K. Moderate alcohol intake reduces bile cholesterol saturation and raises HDL cholesterol. *Lancet* 1983; **ii**: 819–822.

32. Tsai CJ, Leitzmann MF, Willett WC, Giovannucci EL. Macronutrients and insulin resistance in cholesterol gallstone disease. *American Journal of Gastroenterology* 2008; **103**: 2932–2939.

33. Smelt AHM. Triglycerides and gallstone formation. *Clinica Chimica Acta* 2010; **411**: 1625–1631.

34. Attili AF, Scafato E, Marchioli R, Marfisi RM, Festi D. Diet and gallstones in Italy: the cross-sectional MICOL results. *Hepatology* 1998; **27**: 1492–198.

35. Heaton KW. Epidemiology of gall-bladder disease – role of intestinal transit. *Alimentary Pharmacology and Therapeutics* 2000; **14**(Suppl 2): 9–13.

36. Brown L, Rosner B, Willett WW, Sacks FM. Cholesterol-lowering effects of dietary fibre: a meta-analysis. *American Journal of Clinical Nutrition* 1999; **69**: 30–42.

37. Theuwissen E, Mensink RP. Water-soluble dietary fibers and cardiovascular disease. *Physiology and Behavior* 2008; **94**: 285–292.

38. Leitzmann MF, Tsai CJ, Stampfer MJ, et al. Alcohol consumption in relation to risk of cholecystectomy in women. *American Journal of Clinical Nutrition* 2003; **78**: 339–347.

39. Walcher T, Haenle MM, Mason RA, et al. for the EMIL Study Group. The effect of alcohol, tobacco and caffeine consumption and vegetarian diet on gallstone prevalence. *European Journal of Gastroenterology and Hepatology* 2010; **22**: 1345–1351.

40. Banim PJ, Luben RN, Wareham NJ, Sharp SJ, Khaw KT, Hart AR. Physical activity reduces the risk of symptomatic gallstones: a prospective cohort study. *European Journal of Gastroenterology and Hepatology* 2010; **22**: 983–988.

41. Halldestam I, Enell EL, Kullman E, Borch K. Development of symptoms and complications in individuals with asymptomatic gallstones. *British Journal of Surgery* 2004; **91**: 734–738.

42. National Health Service. The Eat Well Plate. www.nhs.uk/Livewell/Goodfood/Pages/eatwell-plate.aspx, accessed 15 January 2014.

43. US Department of Agriculture.www.choosemyplate.gov/, accessed 15 January 2014.

44. Metzger AL, Adler, R, Heymsfield S, Grundy SM. Diurnal variation in biliary lipid composition. Possible role in cholesterol gallstone formation. *New England Journal of Medicine* 1973; **288**: 333–336.

45. Mogadam M, Albarelli J, Ahmed SW, Grogan EJ, Mascatello VJ. Gallbladder dynamics in response to various meals: is dietary fat restriction necessary in the management of gallstones? *American Journal of Gastroenterology* 1984; **79**: 745–747.

46. Madden A. The role of low fat diets in the management of gall-bladder disease. *Journal of Human Nutrition and Dietetics* 1992; **5**: 267–273.

47. Hopman WPM, de Jong AJL, Rosenbusch G, Jansen JBMJ, Lamers CBHW. Elemental diet stimulated gallbladder contraction and secretion of cholecystokinin and pancreatic polypeptide in man. *Digestive Diseases and Sciences* 1987; **32**: 45–49.

48. Hopman WPM, Jansen JBMJ, Lamers CBHW. Comparative study of the effects of equal amounts of fat, protein and starch on plasma cholecystokinin in man. *Scandinavian Journal of Gastroenterology* 1985; **20**: 843–847.

49. Hopman WPM, Jansen JBMJ, Rosenbusch G, Lamers CBHW. Effect of equimolar amounts of long-chain triglycerides and medium-chain triglycerides on plasma cholecystokinin and gallbladder contraction. *American Journal of Clinical Nutrition* 1984; **39**: 356–359.

50. Hopman WPM, Jansen JBMJ, Rosenbusch G, Lamers CBHW. Cephalic stimulation of gallbladder contraction in humans: role of cholecystokinin and the cholinergic system. *Digestion* 1987; **38**: 197–203.

51. Behar J, Lee KY, Thompson WR, Biancani P. Gallbladder contraction in patients with pigment and cholesterol stones. *Gastroenterology* 1989; **97**: 1479–1484.

52. Festi D, Colecchia A, Larocca A, et al. Review: Low caloric intake and gall-bladder motor function. *Alimentary Pharmacology and Therapeutics* 2000; **14**(Suppl 2): 51–53.

53. Department of Health. *Dietary Reference Values for Food Energy and Nutrients for the United Kingdom*. Report of the Panel on Dietary Reference Values of the Committee on Medical Aspects of Food Policy (COMA). Report on Health and Social Subjects 41. London: HMSO, 1991.

54. Hausel J, Nygren J, Thorell A, Lagerkranser M, Ljungqvist O. Randomized clinical trial of the effects of oral preoperative carbohydrates on postoperative nausea and vomiting after laparoscopic cholecystectomy. *British Journal of Surgery* 2005; **92**: 415–421.

55. Elmore MF, Gallagher SC, Jones JG, Koons KK, Schmalhausen AW, Strange PS. Esophagogastric decompression and enteral feeding following cholecystectomy: a randomised prospective trial. *Journal of Parenteral and Enteral Nutrition* 1989; **13**: 377–381.

56. Department of Health. *Delivering Enhanced Recovery: Helping Patients to Get Better Sooner After Surgery*. London: Department of Health, 2010.

57. Weimann A, Braga M, Harsanyi L, Laviano A, Ljungqvist O, Soeters P. ESPEN guidelines on enteral nutrition: surgery including organ transplantation. *Clinical Nutrition* 2006; **25**: 224–244.

58. Braga M, Ljungqvist O, Soeters P, Fearon K, Weimann A, Bozzetti F. ESPEN guidelines on parenteral nutrition: surgery. *Clinical Nutrition* 2009; **28**: 378–386.

59. Brydon WG, Ross AH, Anderson JR, Douglas S. Diet and faecal lipids following cholecystectomy in men. *Digestion* 1982; **25**: 248–252.

60. Qureshi MA, Burke PE, Brindley NM, et al. Post-cholecystectomy symptoms after laparoscopic cholecystectomy. *Annals of the Royal College of Surgeons of England* 1993; **75**: 349–353.

61. Houghton PW, Donaldson LA, Jenkinson LR, Crumplin MK. Weight gain after cholecystectomy. *British Medical Journal* 1984; **289**: 1350.

62. Chan HH, Lai KH, Lin CK, et al. Impact of food on hepatic clearance of patients after endoscopic sphincterotomy. *Journal of the Chinese Medical Association* 2009; **72**: 10–14.

63. Fisher M, Spilias D, Tong LK. Diarrhoea after laparoscopic cholecystectomy: incidence and main determinants. *Australia and New Zealand Journal of Surgery* 2008; **78**: 482–486.

64. Hardt PD, Bretz L, Krauss A, et al. Pathological pancreatic exocrine function and duct morphology in patients with cholelithiasis. *Digestive Diseases and Sciences* 2001; **46**: 536–539.

65. Walters JRF, Pattni SS. Managing bile acid diarrhoea. *Therapeutic Advances in Gastroenterology* 2010; **3**: 349–357.

66. Sciarretta G, Fumo A, Mazzoni M, Malaguti P. Post-cholecystectomy diarrhea: evidence of bile acid malabsorption assessed by SeHCAT test. *American Journal of Gastroenterology* 1992; **87**: 1852–1854.

67. Smith MJ, Cherian P, Raju GS, Dawson BF, Mahon S, Bardhan KD. Bile acid malabsorption in persistent diarrhoea. *Journal of the Royal College of Physicians London* 2000; **34**: 448–451.

68. Ou ZB, Li SW, Liu AN, et al. Prevention of common bile duct injury during laparoscopic cholecystectomy. *Hepatobiliary and Pancreatic Diseases International* 2009; **8**: 414–417.

69. Connor S, Garden OJ. Bile duct injury in the era of laparoscopic cholecystectomy. *British Journal of Surgery* 2005; **93**: 158–168.

70. Behar J, Corazziari E, Guelrud M, Hogan W, Sherman S, Toouli J. Functional gallbladder and sphincter of Oddi disorders. *Gastroenterology* 2006; **130**: 1498–1509.

71. Hansel SL, DiBaise JK. Functional gallbladder disorder: gallbladder dyskinesia. *Gastroenterology Clinics of North America* 2010; **39**: 369–379.

72. Francis G, Baillie J. Gallbladder dyskinesia: fact or fiction? *Current Gastroenterology Reports* 2011; **13**: 188–192.

73. Al-Azzawi HH, Nakeeb A, Saxena R, Maluccio MA, Pitt HA. Cholecystosteatosis: an explanation for increased cholecystectomy rates. *Journal of Gastrointestinal Surgery* 2007; **11**: 835–842.

74. Mathur A, Al-Azzawi HH, Lu D, et al. Steatocholecystitis: the influence of obesity and dietary carbohydrate. *Journal of Surgical Research* 2008; **147**: 290–297.

75. Tsai CJ. Steatocholecystitis and fatty gall bladder disease. *Digestive Diseases and Sciences* 2009; **54**: 1857–1863.

76. Gilloteaux J, Tomasello LM, Elgison DA. Lipid deposits and lipo-mucosomes in human cholecystis and epithelial metaplasia in chronic cholecystitis. *Ultrastructural Pathology* 2003; **27**: 313–321.

77. Cancer Research UK. Cancer Stats, Incidence 2008. http://publications.cancerresearchuk.org/downloads/product/cs_pdf_incidence_feb_2008.pdf, accessed 15 January 2014.

78. International Agency for Research on Cancer. http://globocan.iarc.fr/, accessed 15 January 2014.

79. Eslick GD. Epidemiology of gallbladder cancer. *Gastroenterology Clinics of North America* 2010; **39**: 307–330.

80. Randi G, Franceschi S, La Vecchia C. Gallbladder cancer worldwide: geographical distribution and risk factors. *International Journal of Cancer* 2006; **118**: 1591–1602.

81. Rustagi T, Dasanu CA. Risk factors for gallbladder cancer and cholangiocarcinoma: similarities, differences and updates. *Journal of Gastrointestinal Cancer* 2012; **43**: 137–147.

82. Zatonski WA, Lowenfels AB, Boyle P, et al. Epidemiologic aspects of gallbladder cancer: a case–control study of the SEARCH Program of the International Agency for Research for Cancer. *Journal of the National Cancer Institute* 1997; **89**: 1132–1138.

83. World Cancer Research Fund/American Institute for Cancer Research. *Food, Nutrition, Physical Activity and the Prevention of Cancer: A Global Perspective*. Second Expert Report. Washington, DC: American Institute for Cancer Research, 2007.

Chapter 4.2

Primary biliary cirrhosis and primary sclerosing cholangitis and nutrition

Natasha A. Vidas

King's College Hospital NHS Foundation Trust, London, UK

Primary biliary cirrhosis (PBC) is marked by chronic progressive inflammation and destruction, predominantly of the small but also the medium-sized intrahepatic bile ducts. The destruction of the bile ducts leads to reduced bile flow from the liver into the GI tract, known as cholestasis. The consequent build-up of bile in the liver over time causes progressive inflammatory destruction of the hepatocytes leading to fibrosis, then cirrhosis and ultimately liver failure [1]. Patients with advanced PBC and cirrhosis may develop ascites, hepatic encephalopathy and portal hypertension. The latter may develop in patients before cirrhosis is established, in contrast to other liver diseases [2]. The pathogenesis is thought to be autoimmune with a complex interplay of environmental triggers such as bacteria and viruses, combined with a genetic predisposition [2].

Primary sclerosing cholangitis (PSC) is a chronic progressive disorder defined by inflammation, fibrosis and stricture formation of the whole biliary tree, both intra- and extrahepatic bile ducts, mostly medium and large bile ducts [3]. The hepatic injury that ensues is as for PBC; cirrhosis, portal hypertension and liver failure usually follow [4]. The pathogenesis is less clear but evidence suggests involvement of autoimmune, genetic and infectious factors [5].

4.2.1 Factors involved in causation

Fatigue is debilitating and affects quality of life and normal daily activities in PBC and PSC [6]. Tyrosine and tryptophan are involved in the pathogenesis of fatigue and Borg et al. (2005) found that patients with PBC and increased tyrosine concentrations had less fatigue [6]. However, further studies are required to evaluate the effect of tyrosine and tryptophan supplementation before recommendations can be made.

4.2.2 Nutritional consequences

Malnutrition

Malnutrition has been reported in patients with PBC with and without established cirrhosis [7,8] and in most patients with cirrhosis irrespective of disease aetiology, including PSC [9,10]. Contributing factors include reduced oral intake, particularly in patients with ascites, fat malabsorption and increased metabolic rate. The latter has been found to increase as liver disease progresses [11].

Metabolic bone disease in liver disease (hepatic osteodystrophy)

Hepatic osteodystrophy, seen predominantly in cholestatic liver disease but also in other chronic liver diseases, includes osteoporosis, the dominant form of hepatic bone disease [12], and osteomalacia, which is more frequent in severe malabsorption and advanced liver disease [13]. Both may affect quality of life and morbidity [13]. Osteoporosis has been found to increase with worsening liver disease in both PBC and PSC [14]. The reported incidence of osteoporosis is 30% in PBC [2] and 4–10% in

PSC [15]. The pathogenesis of this disorder is complex and multifactorial [13]. Suggested causes in PBC include raised bilirubin inhibiting osteoblast function; increased bone resorption; deficiencies of calcium, magnesium, vitamin D and vitamin K; reduced muscle mass; increased duration of cholestasis; and medication side-effects (e.g. corticosteroids and cholestyramine that are sometimes used to treat the disease process) [13,16,17]. The causes of osteoporosis in PSC are similar to those in PBC [14].

Biochemical indices frequently guide treatment of osteomalacia as bone biopsies used for diagnosis are invasive and thus not routinely used [13]. Osteomalacia particularly seen in PBC is associated with low concentrations of 25-hydroxyvitamin D. Contributing factors include vitamin D malabsorption corresponding to steatorrhoea; impaired dietary vitamin D intake; reduced exposure to ultraviolet rays; increased renal loss of soluble vitamin D; and reduced enterohepatic circulation of vitamin D [12,13,18]. Metabolism of vitamin D is normal in PBC [2,19], except in those with jaundice and clinically advanced disease [2]. The synthesis of vitamin D cutaneously in other jaundiced patients may also be impaired [14].

Malabsorption

Chronic cholestasis, frequently a consequence of PBC and PSC secondary to the disease process (i.e. the inflammation, fibrosis and destruction of the bile ducts) may lead to an inadequate biliary secretion of bile salts and hence a reduced ability to break down dietary fat [20]. The consequent malabsorption of dietary fat and fat-soluble vitamins (i.e. A, D, E and K) may lead to steatorrhoea. Weight loss and fat-soluble vitamin deficiencies may ensue. Steatorrhoea may also lead to calcium malabsorption secondary to the insoluble calcium soaps formed in the presence of unabsorbed dietary fat in the small intestine [20]. It is important to exclude and/or treat other causes of malabsorption and steatorrhoea, e.g. coeliac disease, ulcerative colitis (UC) and pancreatitis.

In PBC, 33.5%, 13.2%, 1.9% and 7.8% of patients have been found to have deficiencies of vitamins A, D, E and K, respectively [21]. In PSC deficiencies have been reported in 40%, 14% and 2% of patients for vitamins A, D and E respectively [22], with greater deficiencies found in patients undergoing pretransplant assessment: 82%, 57% and 43% for vitamins A, D and E respectively.

Hyperlipidaemia and xanthoma

In PBC serum lipids may be markedly elevated [2] though studies suggest there is no increased risk of cardiovascular disease. However, if there is a family history of lipid abnormalities or cardiovascular disease, treatment with cholesterol-lowering medication may need to be considered [2].

Disease symptoms

Symptoms of pruritus and fatigue in PBC and PSC and upper right quadrant pain (typically from bacterial overgrowth in the strictured bile ducts) in PSC usually develop when disease is quite advanced and can be severe and disabling. Ten percent to 15% of patients with PSC have intermittent episodes of cholangitis [4,23]. Functional status has been reported to be significantly reduced in patients with PBC [24]. Thus it seems reasonable to expect that nutritional status may be compromised secondary to symptoms of disease.

Medication side-effects

Cholestyramine used to treat pruritus can cause bloating, constipation and diarrhoea [2]. Antibiotics used to treat recurrent bacterial cholangitis in PSC long term may lead to diarrhoea [15] and possibly long-term nutritional consequences.

Co-existing autoimmune diseases

Coeliac disease has been found in 3–7% of patients with PBC and in 2–3% of patients with PSC [25]. Inflammatory bowel disease has been found in less than 5% of patients with PBC [19] and 60–80% of patients with PSC, with 48–86% of those having UC [15]. Pouchitis after colectomy and ileo-anal pouch formation is more common in PSC patients with UC than in patients with only UC – 60% and 15% respectively [3]. Both diseases, and the surgical consequences thereof, need to be taken into account in the nutritional management of these patients.

4.2.3 Dietary management

Since PBC and PSC are progressive diseases, monitoring patients over the course of their disease is important, particularly since metabolic rates, fat-soluble deficiencies, osteoporosis and osteomalacia have been shown to increase as disease severity increases. Disease symptoms of both PBC and PSC, medication side-effects, co-existing autoimmune diseases and the potential progression to cirrhosis should all be considered in nutritional assessment and intervention.

The advice for cirrhotic PBC and PSC patients is the same as that for other cirrhotic patients, i.e. regular meals and snacks, including a bedtime snack containing 50g of carbohydrate, to prevent protein catabolism and the latter to promote nitrogen balance [26,27]. The ESPEN 2006 guidelines for energy and protein requirements are used in clinical practice. All patients with inadequate oral intakes and/or weight loss should be encouraged to make high-energy, high-protein meal and snack choices to aid meeting their estimated requirements. Consider oral nutritional supplements and/or enteral tube feeding (ETF) if estimated requirements cannot be achieved orally.

Fat restriction

Dietary fat restriction should only be instituted if necessary. Advice for dietary fat modification should be individually tailored, ensuring that estimated energy and protein requirements are met. In practice, consider restriction if patients have steatorrhoea or severe nausea or indigestion with dietary fat intake that have not responded to antiemetics or antacids. Low-fat diets to reduce xanthoma have been found to be unsuccessful and even harmful [28] and are thus not advised.

Oral nutritional supplements and/or ETF may be needed to meet estimated nutritional requirements. Standard preparations may be tolerated but fat-free, low-fat and/or medium-chain triglyceride (MCT) preparations may be better tolerated. It is thus important to individually assess tolerance to fat and advise accordingly. Modular carbohydrate and protein powders and MCT oils can also be used.

Fat-soluble vitamins and minerals

Recommendations for bone density scanning, calcium and fat-soluble vitamin supplementation in patients with PBC and PSC are outlined in Table 4.2.1 [2,15,23]. Epidemiological data support the use of calcium and vitamin D supplementation but no trial data confirming efficacy in preventing bone loss in liver disease are yet available [13,23]. Vitamin K supplementation is associated with improved bone mineral density (BMD) [13] while parenteral vitamin D or oral alfacalcidol has been shown to improve osteomalacia [14].

Screening for fat-soluble vitamin deficiencies in PBC and PSC is recommended prior to supplementation [17,23]. Kennedy and O'Grady (2002) suggest aqueous fat-soluble vitamin preparations to promote absorption [29]; however, such preparations are not always readily available, particularly in the UK. Best practice suggests that standard preparations are given if required, serum vitamin concentrations are monitored and doses adjusted accordingly to ensure adequate supplementation is provided and toxicity avoided. See Table 4.2.2 for further information on measurement and sources of fat-soluble vitamins.

Co-existing autoimmune diseases

Symptoms secondary to coeliac disease and inflammatory bowel disease (IBD) may wrongly be attributed to PBC and PSC. Gluten-free diets for patients diagnosed with coeliac disease, and dietary modifications suitable for those with IBD, including patients with UC and pouchitis, should thus be considered as necessary.

Table 4.2.1 Recommendations from EASL and AASLD for bone density scanning, calcium and fat-soluble vitamin supplementation for those with PBC and PSC

EASL (2009)	AASLD (2009 and 2010)
Bone density assessment	
DEXA to assess BMD in chronic cholestatic liver disease at presentation. Rescreening up to annually thereafter depending on degree of cholestasis or other individual risk factors. Reversible osteoporosis risk factors* should be identified and targeted and lifestyle advice provided	BMD scans at diagnosis. Rescreening every 2–4 years in patients with PBC depending on bone density at baseline and severity of cholestasis; every 2–3 years in patients with PSC
Supplementation of calcium and vitamin D for bone health	
Calcium 1.0–1.2 g/day Vitamin D 400–800 IU/day To be considered in all patients with cholestatic liver disease but is not evidence based Alendronate or other bisphosphonates for patients with osteoporosis; supplementation in patients with osteopenia may be appropriate	Calcium 1.0–1.5 g/day Vitamin D 1000 IU/day In diet and as a supplement if required Bisphosphonates (alendronate 70 mg orally specified in PBC) for osteopenic patients in the absence of oesophageal varices and ulcers. If the former present, parenteral bisphosphonate therapy is suggested
Fat-soluble vitamin supplementation	
Vitamin D (and calcium) as above Vitamins A, E and K should be given enterally where steatorrhoea is present, in overt cholestasis or where low concentrations of fat-soluble vitamins are found Vitamin K should be given parenterally prophylactically prior to invasive procedures	Vitamins A, D, E and K in jaundiced patients with PBC should be monitored annually. No specific recommendations for PSC

*Risk factors for osteoporosis: smoking, alcohol excess, inactivity, family history, low body weight, increasing age, female gender, prolonged corticosteroid therapy (e.g. prednisolone 5 mg/day for >3 months), previous fragility factors, hypogonadism, premature menopause (<45 years of age) [14,23].
AASLD, American Association for the Study of Liver Diseases; BMD, bone mineral density; DEXA, dual-emission X-ray absorptiometry; EASL, European Association for the Study of the Liver.

Lifestyle advice

Progression of PBC and the factors responsible are still poorly understood. In a study of 274 asymptomatic patients with PBC, histological steatosis, oxidative stress, Body Mass Index (BMI) ≥26 and alcohol, even in small quantities, were independent co-factors predicting the severity of liver damage and as such, they could play a role in disease progression by accelerating the pathway to fibrogenesis [30]. It is thus suggested that addressing such factors therapeutically could slow down the progression of PBC. Further studies are required to investigate these factors and the dietary and lifestyle implications. However, Lindor, et al. (2009) suggest that for all forms of liver disease, including PBC, excess alcohol, cigarette smoking and obesity should be avoided [2].

Table 4.2.2 Measurement and sources of fat-soluble vitamins

Measurement index	Vitamin sources
Vitamin A	
Total serum vitamin A/serum retinol Reflect total body reserves when liver vitamin A stores are severely depleted (<20 μg/g liver) or excessively high (>300 μg/g liver), but not when between these concentrations due to homeostatic control **Retinol binding protein (RBP)** A transport protein on which vitamin A circulates. It can be measured in conjunction with serum vitamin A to determine if vitamin A is truly low or if low due to RBP being low **Relative dose response (RDR)** A more sensitive index of marginal vitamin A status, but sensitivity and specificity are reduced in liver disease, malabsorption and severe protein-energy malnutrition Some centres send both the above to aid the interpretation of results. Feranchak et al. [31] suggest using serum retinol as an initial screen for vitamin A deficiency: if <20 μg/dL then a modified oral RDR* be done to confirm deficiency. But method validation in larger studies was suggested. Note this study was done in children with chronic liver disease **Deuterium-labelled vitamin A** May be used in the future to determine total body stores of vitamin A	**Preformed vitamin A**: liver, liver products, fish liver oils, dairy products (milk, butter, cheese, cream), fortified margarine and spreads, egg yolk. Poorer sources include muscle meats, nuts, grains, vegetable oils **Provitamin A carotenoids**: yellow and red vegetables (e.g. carrots, red peppers), dark green leafy vegetables (e.g. spinach, broccoli), tomatoes, fruit (peaches, apricots, mangoes)
Vitamin D	
Serum 25-hydroxyvitamin D (25-OH-D) Reflects total supply of vitamin D from endogenous and exogenous sources **Serum 1,25-dihydroxyvitamin D (1,25-OH-D)** Not a useful index of vitamin D status as under tight homeostatic regulation at the site of synthesis in the kidney	**Vitamin D2 (ergocalciferol)**: meat, particularly liver, eggs, dairy products, fortified foods (D2 and D3 used to fortify) **Vitamin D3 (cholecalciferol)**: oily fish; also synthesised in the skin; the intensity of ultraviolet radiation and skin pigmentation affect formation
Vitamin E	
Serum total tocopherol Used to assess vitamin E status but its use as an index of tissue stores or dietary intake is questionable except in deficiency states **New functional tests including breath pentane** Seem promising but studies are needed to establish validity	Vegetable and seed oils (e.g. corn, soya bean, sunflower, safflower seed oils), margarine (but the content is variable), cereal foods, meat, meat products

(Continued)

Table 4.2.2   Continued

Measurement index	Vitamin sources
Vitamin K	
Functional tests Depend on measurement of blood clotting and prothrombin time	**Vitamin K1**: dark green leafy vegetables, some vegetable oils (rapeseed, soya bean, olive oil). Poorer sources include dairy products, meat, eggs **Vitamin K2**: synthesised by GI microbiota. Small amounts can be found in fermented foods and meats such as chicken reared on animal feeds containing synthetic vitamin K3

* Modified RDR: 1500 IU vitamin A as a water-solubilised retinyl palmitate preparation as an oral dose mixed with 25 IU/kg of water-soluble oral d-alpha tocopheryl polyethylene glycol-1000 succinate [31–33].

References

1. Heathcote EJ. AASLD Practice Guidelines. *Management of primary biliary cirrhosis. Hepatology* 2000; **31**(4): 1005–1013.
2. Lindor KD, Gershwin ME, Poupon R, et al. AASLD Practice Guidelines. *Primary biliary cirrhosis. Hepatology* 2009; **50**(1): 291–307.
3. Saich R, Chapman R. Primary sclerosing cholangitis, autoimmune hepatitis and overlap syndromes in inflammatory bowel disease. *World Journal of Gastroenterology* 2008; **14**(3): 331–337.
4. Lee Y, Kaplan MM. Practice Guideline Committee of the ACG. *Management of primary sclerosing cholangitis. American Journal of Gastroenterology* 2002; **97**(3): 528–534.
5. Luketic VAC. What's New in Pathophysiology of Autoimmune Cholestatic Liver Disease? 21st Conference of the Asian Pacific Association for the Study of the Liver. *Oral Presentations. Hepatology International* 2011; **5**(1): 30.
6. Borg PCJ, Fekkes D, Vrolijk JM, van Buuren H. The relation between plasma tyrosine concentration and fatigue in primary biliary cirrhosis and primary sclerosing cholangitis. *BMC Gastroenterology* 2005; **5**(11): 1–7.
7. Wicks C, Bray GP, Williams R. Nutritional assessment in primary biliary cirrhosis: the effect of disease severity. *Clinical Nutrition* 1995; **14**: 29–34.
8. Morgan MY. Enteral nutrition in chronic liver disease. *Acta Chirurgica Scandinavica* 1981; **507**(Suppl): 81–90.
9. Figueiredo FA, Dickson ER, Pasha TM, et al. Impact of nutritional status on outcomes after liver transplantation. *Transplantation* 2000; **70**(9): 1347–1352.
10. Italian Multicentre Cooperative Project Nutrition in Liver Cirrhosis. Nutritional status in cirrhosis. *Journal of Hepatology* 1994; **21**(3):317–325.
11. Green JH, Bramley PN, Losowsky MS. Are patients with primary biliary cirrhosis hypermetabolic? A comparison between patients before and after liver transplantation and controls. *Hepatology* 1991; **14**(3): 464–472.
12. Wegener M, Borsch G, Schmidt G. Hepatic osteodystrophy: osteoporosis, osteomalacia and vitamin-D-metabolism [German]. *Innere Medizin* 1985; **12**(2): 63–68.
13. Goel V, Kar P. Hepatic osteodystrophy. *Tropical Gastroenterology* 2010; **31**(2): 82–86.
14. Collier JD, Ninkovic M, Compston JE. Guidelines on the management of osteoporosis associated with chronic liver disease. *Gut* 2002; **50**(Suppl 1): i1–i9.
15. Chapman R, Fevery J, Kalloo A, et al. AASLD Practice Guidelines. *Diagnosis and management of primary sclerosing cholangitis. Hepatology* 2010; **51**(2): 660–678.
16. Newton J, Francis R, Prince M, et al. Osteoporosis in primary biliary cirrhosis revisited. *Gut* 2001; **49**: 282–287.
17. Levy C, Lindor KD. Current management of primary biliary cirrhosis and primary sclerosing cholangitis. *Hepatology* 2003; **38**: S24–S37.
18. Jung RT, Davie M, Siklos P, et al. Vitamin D metabolism in acute and chronic cholestasis. *Gut* 1997; **20**(10): 840–847.
19. Talwalkar JA, Lindor KA. Primary biliary cirrhosis. *Lancet* 2003; **362**: 53–61.
20. Sherlock S. Chronic cholangitides: aetiology, diagnosis, and treatment. *British Medical Journal* 1968; **3**: 515–521.
21. Phillips JR, Angulo P, Petterson T, Lindor K. Fat-soluble vitamin levels in patients with primary biliary cirrhosis. *American Journal of Gastroenterology* 2001; **96**(9): 2745–2750.
22. Jorgensen RA, Lindor KD, Sartin JS, LaRusso NF, Wiesner RH. Serum lipid and fat0soluble vitamin levels in primary sclerosing cholangitis. *Journal of Clinical Gastroenterology* 1995; **20**(3): 215–219.
23. EASL Clinical Practice Guidelines. Management of cholestatic liver diseases. *Journal of Hepatology* 2009; **51**: 237–267.
24. Patel-Parikh A, Gold EB, Utts J, et al. Functional status of patients with primary biliary cirrhosis. *American Journal of Gastroenterology* 2002; **97**(11): 2871–2879.
25. Volta U. Pathogenesis and clinical significance of liver injury in celiac disease. *Clincal Reviews in Allergy and Immunology* 2009; **36**: 62–70.

26. Chang WK. Effects of extra-carbohydrate supplementation in the late evening on energy expenditure and substrate oxidation in patients with liver cirrhosis. *Journal of Parenteral and Enteral Nutrition* 1997; **21**: 96–99.

27. Plank LD, Gane EJ, Peng S, et al. Nocturnal nutritional supplementation improves total body protein status of patients with liver cirrhosis: a randomised 12-month trial. *Hepatology* 2008; **48**(2): 557–566.

28. Leuschner U. Primary biliary cirrhosis – presentation and diagnosis. *Clinics in Liver Disease* 2003; **7**(4): 741–758.

29. Kennedy PTF, O'Grady JG. Diseases of the liver: chronic liver disease. *Hospital Pharmacist* 2002; **9**(5):137–144.

30. Sorrentino P, Terracciano L, d'Angelo S, et al. Oxidative stress and steatosis are cofactors of liver injury in primary biliary cirrhosis. *Journal of Gastroenterology* 2010; **45**:1053–1062.

31. Feranchak AP, Gralla J, King R, et al. Comparison of indices of vitamin A status in children with chronic liver disease. *Hepatology* 2005; **42**(4): 782–792.

32. Gibson RS. Assessment of the status of vitamins A, D, and K. In: *Principles of Nutritional Assessment*. London: Oxford University Press, 1990, pp. 377–412.

33. Thomas B. Vitamins. In: Thomas B, Bishop J (eds) *Manual of Dietetic Practice*, 4th edn. London: Blackwell Publishing, 2007, pp. 187–199.

Chapter 4.3

Alcohol-related liver disease and nutrition

Regina Keenan[1] and Barbara Davidson[2]

[1]St Vincent's University Hospital, Dublin, Ireland
[2]Freeman Hospital, Newcastle upon Tyne, UK

4.3.1 Alcoholic hepatitis

Alcoholic hepatitis (AH) refers to acute decompensation of the liver function in an individual with a history of alcohol abuse [1]. Clinical presentation after abstinence for several weeks is not unusual. Clinical features include rapid onset of jaundice, fever, hepatomegaly, ascites, anorexia and encephalopathy. Typically presentation is between 40 and 60 years and female sex is an independent risk factor for AH [2].

Maddrey's discriminant function provides risk stratification and a value more than 32 indicates severe AH. There is a significant mortality associated with severe AH: a 28-day mortality of higher than 40% compared to patients with mild AH [3].

Undernutrition: prevalence and effects on survival

Protein-energy malnutrition (PEM) is strongly associated with AH. Based on anthropometry and laboratory testing, protein malnutrition and/or PEM were found in all patients with AH [4]. The severity of PEM correlates with the severity of AH and mortality, with 2% at 30 days with mild PEM and up to 52% with severe PEM [5].

Pathogenesis of undernutrition

Contributing factors to developing undernutrition include anorexia, malabsorption and a diminished ability to utilise or store nutrients. The inflammation present in AH promotes a depletion of muscle and visceral proteins and therefore is associated with an increased catabolic state [6]. Patients with acute hepatitis can have an increased metabolic rate. AH is a hypermetabolic state and patients have a 55% higher energy expenditure compared to healthy controls [7].

Nutritional therapy

Alcohol

Alcohol abstinence is of paramount importance in the treatment of AH and has been shown to significantly improve long-term survival [8].

Oral and enteral nutrition

Nutritional status should be evaluated in patients with AH as adequate energy intake (>2500 kcal/day) was associated with 19% mortality, whereas patients with inadequate intake exhibited 51% mortality [9]. Increased intestinal bacterial translocation and endotoxaemia are frequent events in patients with AH with or without cirrhosis [10]. Enteral nutrition (EN) might exert its therapeutic action by improving the intestinal barrier function [11].

Nutrition support

Early trials assessing the benefit of oral, EN or parenteral nutrition (PN) in patients with AH suggested that nutritional support improves nitrogen balance and liver function but not survival. Interestingly, a randomised, controlled clinical trial comparing EN (2000 kcal/day) with prednisolone therapy (40 mg/day) for 28 days in 71 patients with

Advanced Nutrition and Dietetics in Gastroenterology, First Edition. Edited by Miranda Lomer.
© 2014 John Wiley & Sons, Ltd. Published 2014 by John Wiley & Sons, Ltd.

severe AH found the survival rate to be similar between the two groups at 28 days and at 1 year, suggesting that nutrition support may be as effective as corticosteroids in some patients [11].

Vitamins

There are no published guidelines for vitamin or mineral supplementation in patients with AH [12]. As with alcoholic liver disease, consideration should be given to vitamins A, C, D, E, K, B1, B2, B6 and B12, nicotinic acid, folic acid and zinc.

Antioxidants

Alcohol ingestion increases the excretion of markers of oxidative stress, and the highest levels are observed in patients with AH [2]. Antioxidants are not currently recommended as research has failed to demonstrate a beneficial role in AH [13,14].

Nutritional assessment and goals

All patients with AH should be assessed for PEM, as well as vitamin and mineral deficiencies. Those with severe disease should be treated aggressively with EN [15].

As for cirrhosis, energy aims are 35–40 kcal/kg/day [16]. As a general consensus, a higher energy requirement of 45 kcal/kg/day is recommended for patients with AH given their greater prevalence of undernutrition and cachexia. A protein intake of 1.2–1.5 g/kg/day is recommended [16]

4.3.2 Alcoholic liver disease

Alcoholic liver disease (ALD) encompasses a range of conditions from steatosis to cirrhosis with all the symptoms and nutritional challenges which these present posed. The association between alcohol and liver injury has been well known for centuries and liver disease caused by alcohol remains a major cause of morbidity and mortality worldwide. Although the incidence has always been high, patient demographics is changing with a pronounced trend towards younger people (<25 years) presenting with established cirrhosis. From the 1970s to 2000, deaths

from liver cirrhosis steadily increased. In people aged 35–44 years, the death rate went up eight-fold in men and almost seven-fold in women, and in 25–34 year olds, a four-fold increase was seen [17]. The increasing incidence of non-alcoholic fatty liver disease (NAFLD) presents an additional stress to a liver already compromised by alcohol with patients presenting in a very poor nutritional state.

Malnutrition occurs in up to 80% of patients with ALD [18]. The challenge is to meet the increased nutritional requirements for energy, protein and micronutrients in patients who already have depleted stores, poor dietary intake, energy often provided exclusively by alcohol, and the risk of refeeding syndrome when nutrition support is instituted. Adequate nutritional intake in patients with cirrhosis is further compromised by reduced expansion of the proximal stomach, thus compounding early satiety [19].

Accurate nutritional assessment is difficult in cirrhosis and the use of a modified subjective global assessment tool incorporating anthropometric measurements is recommended [2]. Anthropometric measurements are most useful if performed by an experienced practitioner, preferably using International Society for the Advancement of Kinanthropometry (ISAK) methods [20].

4.3.3 Steatosis – fatty liver

Fat is deposited in the liver tissue causing reduced function and hepatomegaly, often associated with abdominal discomfort and reduced appetite. The degree of fatty deposits in the liver is associated with chronic fatigue.

Steatosis may be present and fatty liver develops in approximately 90% of individuals who drink more than 60 g alcohol per day [21]. In patients with fatty liver, synthetic liver function is usually well maintained [22]. Simple fatty liver would be completely reversible within 6 weeks of abstinence [23]; however, progression to fibrosis and cirrhosis occurs in 5–15% of patients despite abstinence [24]. In continued alcohol use of more than 40 g per day, one study showed a 30% and 37% risk of developing cirrhosis and fibrosis respectively [25].

Patients may be lethargic and find cooking and food shopping difficult. Alcohol may be a major energy source (7 kcal/g alcohol) and high-fat convenience foods often feature.

The treatment for alcoholic fatty liver is alcohol abstinence and a reduction in fat intake, combined with increased activity where possible and supplementation of thiamine and other B vitamins. It is important to gain a clear idea of the patient's lifestyle and motivation to change when attempting intervention.

4.3.4 Fibrosis

Excessive buildup of scar tissue in the liver parenchyma leads to fibrosis and structural changes having a deleterious effect on function. Fibrosis is usually detected on liver biopsy and/or by fibroscan.

Fibrosis leads to stress on liver tissue, increasing the inflammatory response. The toxic alcohol breakdown product acetaldehyde causes upregulation of collagen synthesis, leading to further fibrotic tissue development [26]. Portal hypertension often develops and may lead to the development of ascites.

Energy from alcohol often regularly replaces food, resulting in vitamin deficiencies. Micronutrients play a vital role in the metabolism of alcohol and therefore their deficiencies have a major effect on the body's response to alcohol insult.

Ethanol is oxidised to acetaldehyde by alcohol dehydrogenase. Acetaldehyde is a highly unstable compound. If it is not downregulated by antioxidants such as ascorbic acid or thiamine, it quickly forms toxic free radical structures and becomes a hepatotoxin. Nicotinic acid is required as a co-factor in the conversion of acetaldehyde to acetic acid and then to acetyl CoA.

In individuals with chronic high alcohol consumption, there is an induction of an alternative metabolic pathway, the microsomal ethanol oxidation system (MEOS). This utilises enzymes from the cytochrome P450 family to metabolise alcohol to acetaldehyde. This pathway is energy expensive, invoking a huge requirement for adenosine triphosphate (ATP) with the consequence of increased energy requirements.

Thiamine deficiency is well recognised in ALD and can be demonstrated in liver diseases of other aetiologies; however, it cannot be demonstrated in the absence of cirrhosis [27].

4.3.5 Alcoholic cirrhosis

Progression of ALD results in the development of cirrhosis. Cirrhosis is irreversible and therapies are focused on treating the complications of this degree of liver damage. Widespread micronodular cirrhosis will impair carbohydrate and protein metabolism [28], cause portal hypertension with the development of ascites, and increase the risk of encephalopathy and bleeding from varices. Jaundice is likely with associated appetite suppression and food aversion secondary to taste changes. Unless steatorrhoea is present, fat restriction is not necessary. Pancreatic ductal changes occur in patients with ALD but only a small proportion of these changes are clinically relevant and/or produce symptoms [29].

Protein-energy malnutrition is a feature of ALD [15] and nutritional requirements are high. Energy and protein requirements are 35–40 kcal/kg/day and 1.2–1.5 g protein/kg/day. A 50g carbohydrate evening snack is crucial in maintaining lean muscle stores by sparing nitrogen utilisation overnight. Patients are at risk of electrolyte disturbance and refeeding syndrome [18].

References

1. Sougioultzis S, Dalakas E, Hayes PC, Plevris JN. Alcoholic hepatitis: from pathogenesis to treatment. *Current Medical Research and Opinion* 2005; **21**(9): 1337–1346.
2. Lucey MD, Marthurin P, Morgan TR. Alcoholic hepatitis. *New England Journal of Medicine* 2009; **360**(26): 2758–2769.
3. Stickel F, Hoehn B, Schuppan D, Seitz HK. Review article: nutritional therapy in alcoholic liver disease. *Alimentary Pharmacology and Therapeutics* 2003; **18**: 357–373.
4. Mendenhall CL, Anderson S, Garcia-Pont P, et al. Acute and long term survival in patients treated with oxandralone and prednisolone. *New England Journal of Medicine* 1984; **311**:1464–1470.
5. Mendenhall CL, Tosch T, Weesner RE, et al. VA Cooperative Study on Alcoholic Hepatitis II: prognostic significance of protein calorie malnutrition. *American Journal of Clinical Nutrition* 1986; **43**: 213–218.
6. DiCecco SR, Francisco-Ziller N. Nutrition in alcoholic liver disease. *Nutrition in Clinical Practice* 2006; **21**: 245–254.
7. John WJ, Phillips R, Ott L, Adams LJ, Mcclain CJ. Resting energy expenditure in patients with alcoholic hepatitis. *Journal of Parenteral and Enteral Nutrition* 1989; **13**(2): 124–127.
8. Babineaux MJ, Anand BS. General aspects of the treatment of alcoholic hepatitis. *World Journal of Hepatology* 2011; **3**(5): 125–129.

9. Mendenhall CL, Bongiovanni G, Goldberg S, et al. VA Cooperative Study on Alcoholic Hepatitis III: changes in protein calorie malnutrition associated with 30 days of hospitalization with and without enteral nutrition therapy. *Journal of Parenteral and Enteral Nutrition* 1985; **9**: 590–596.

10. Alvarez MA, Cabré E, Lorenzo-Zúniga V, Montoliu S, Plasnas R, Gassull MA. Combining steroids with enteral nutrition: a better therapeutic strategy for severe alcoholic hepatitis? Results of a pilot study. *European Journal of Gastroenterology and Hepatology* 2004; **16**: 1375–1380.

11. Cabré E, Rodriguez-Iglesias P, Caballeria J, et al., for the the Spanish Group for the Study of Alcoholic Hepatitis. Short- and long-term outcome of severe alcohol-induced hepatitis treated with steroids or enteral nutrition: a multicentre randomized trial. *Hepatology* 2000; **32**: 36–42.

12. Cohen SM, Ahn J. Review article: the diagnosis and management of alcoholic hepatitis. *Alimentary Pharmacology and Therapeutics* 2009; **30**: 3–13.

13. Stewart S, Prince M, Bassendine M, et al. A randomised trial of antioxidant therapy alone or with corticosteroids in acute alcoholic hepatitis. *Journal of Hepatology* 2007; **47**: 277–283.

14. Phillips M, Curtis H, Portmann B, Donaldson N, Bomford A, O'Grady J. Antioxidant versus corticosteroids in the treatment of severe alcoholic hepatitis – a randomised clinical trial. *Journal of Hepatology* 2006; **44**: 784–790.

15. O'Shea RS, Dasarathy S, McCullough AJ, and the Practice Guideline Committee of the American Association for the Study of Liver Diseases and the Practice Parameters Committee of the American College of Gastroenterology. Alcoholic Liver Disease, American Association for the Study of Liver Diseases (AASLD) Practice Guidelines. *Hepatology* 2010; **51**(1): 307–328.

16. Plauth M, Cabré E, Riggio O, et al. ESPEN guidelines on enteral nutrition: liver disease. *Clinical Nutrition* 2006; **25**: 285–294.

17. Sheron N, Olsen N, Gilmore I. An evidence based alcohol policy. *Gut* 2008; **57**:1 341–1344.

18. Morgan MY, Madden A, Soulsby CT, Morris RW. Derivation and validation of a new global method for assessing nutritional status in patients with cirrhosis. *Hepatology* 2006; **44**(4): 823–835.

19. Izbeki F, Kiss I, WittmannT, Varkonyi TT, Legrady P, Lonovics J. Impaired accommodation of proximal stomach in patients with alcoholic liver cirrhosis. *Scandinavian Journal of Gastroenterology* 2002; **37**(12): 1403–1410.

20. International Society for the Advancement of Kinanthropometry. www.isakonline.com/, accessed 8 January 2014.

21. Crabb DW. Pathogenesis of alcoholic liver disease: newer mechanisms of injury. *Keio Journal of Medicine* 1999; **48**: 184–188.

22. Powell EE, Jonsson JR, Clouston AD. Steatosis: co-factor in other liver diseases. *Hepatology* 2005; **42**(1): 5–13.

23. Lieber CS, Jones DP, Decarli IM. Effects of prolonged ethanol intake: production of fatty liver despite adequate diets. *Journal of Clinical Investigation* 1965; **44**: 1009–1021.

24. Sorenson TI, Orholm M, Bentsen KD, Hoybye G, Eghoje K, Christofferson P. Prospective evaluation of alcohol abuse and alcoholic liver injury in men as predictors of the development of cirrhosis. *Lancet* 1984; **2**: 241–244.

25. Teli MR, Day CP, Burt AD, Bennet MK, James OF. Determination of progression to cirrhosis or fibrosis in pure alcoholic fatty liver. *Lancet* 1995; **346**: 987–990.

26. Holt K, Bennett M, Chojkier M. Acetaldehyde stimulates collagen and noncollagen protein production by human fibroblasts. *Hepatology* 1984; **4**(5): 843–848.

27. Levy S, Herve C, Delacoux E, Erlinger S. Thiamine deficiency in hepatitis C virus and alcohol related liver diseases. *Digestive Diseases and Sciences* 2002; **47**(3): 543–548.

28. McCullough AJ, Raguso C. Effect of cirrhosis on energy expenditure. *American Journal of Clinical Nutrition* 1999; **69**(6): 1066–1068.

29. Kochhar R, Sethy P, Sood A, et al. Concurrent pancreatic ductal changes in alcoholic liver disease. *Gastroenterology and Hepatology* 2003; **18**(9): 1067–1070.

Chapter 4.4

Autoimmune hepatitis and viral hepatitis and nutrition

Natasha A. Vidas[1] and Catherine McAnenny[2]
[1]King's College Hospital NHS Foundation Trust, London, UK
[2]Royal Infirmary of Edinburgh, Edinburgh, UK

4.4.1 Autoimmune hepatitis

Autoimmune hepatitis (AIH) is a rare chronic progressive inflammatory liver disease of unknown aetiology. AIH is classified as type 1 or type 2 according to serum autoantibody profiles [1].

Nutritional consequences

Symptoms of AIH include anorexia, nausea, abdominal pain, fatigue and arthralgia, of which the latter two can be incapacitating [2]. These symptoms may affect appetite, oral intake and nutritional status [3,4]. Further nutritional consequences of AIH stem predominantly from medication side-effects and co-existing autoimmune diseases.

Autoimmune hepatitis is frequently treated with long-term corticosteroids. Nutritional side-effects include increased appetite, weight gain, fluid retention and mood changes in the short term. Longer term side-effects include weight gain, central obesity, peptic ulcers, onset of steroid-induced diabetes and/or hypertension, deterioration in the control of pre-existing diabetes and/or hypertension, increased risk of fractures secondary to osteopenia, osteoporosis and avascular bone necrosis, pancreatitis and psychosis [1,2]. Osteoporosis with vertebral compression and brittle diabetes has been found in 27% and 20% of patients with AIH respectively. Patients most at risk of these drug-related side-effects include postmenopausal women, individuals with pre-existing osteoporosis, brittle diabetes, emotional instability or obesity. Treatment risk benefit is thus important to consider before corticosteroid initiation [1,2].

Azathioprine, frequently used in combination with corticosteroids in AIH, particularly for treatment periods over 6 months, has several side-effects which may have nutritional consequences including nausea, vomiting, pancreatitis and, more rarely, a diarrhoeal syndrome associated with small intestinal villous atrophy and malabsorption. Side-effects develop in 10% of patients but improve when azathioprine is reduced or stopped [2].

The incidence of coeliac disease is 4% in type 1 AIH and 8% in type 2. Screening for coeliac disease before and during treatment in patients with AIH has been suggested [5]. Sixteen percent of patients with AIH have ulcerative colitis (UC) [6]. Both these diseases have nutritional consequences and need to be taken into account in the nutritional management of these patients.

Dietary management

The symptoms of AIH, side-effects of azathioprine, existence of coeliac disease and UC, and the potential progression to cirrhosis in patients with AIH should all be considered in nutritional assessment and intervention.

Manns et al. (2010) suggest that corticosteroid treatment and related bone disease should direct lifestyle and dietary advice and treatment including

Advanced Nutrition and Dietetics in Gastroenterology, First Edition. Edited by Miranda Lomer.
© 2014 John Wiley & Sons, Ltd. Published 2014 by John Wiley & Sons, Ltd.

weight-bearing exercise, vitamin D and calcium supplementation [2]. The use of bisphosphonates should be considered in individuals with osteopenia and osteoporosis. Dual-energy X-ray absorptiometry (DEXA) scans are recommended annually for patients on long-term corticosteroids [2]. The development or worsening of diabetes and hypertension with corticosteroid use should be managed with dietary and medical intervention as appropriate.

Future developments

It is suggested that insulin resistance is involved in the pathogenesis of AIH [7]. Salmon et al. found steatosis related to age and diabetes in 25% of patients with AIH [8]. It seems reasonable to suggest that a well-balanced diet and regular exercise may prove beneficial but further studies to demonstrate this are required.

4.4.2 Viral hepatitis

Viral hepatitis is inflammation of the liver due to a viral infection and it affects over 700,000 people in the UK. It can present as a recent infection with a rapid onset or it can take a chronic form. The most common causes of viral hepatitis are five unrelated hepatotrophic viruses: hepatitis A, B, C, D and E.

Hepatitis A, B and C are the most common hepatic viruses but B and C can cause long-term liver damage and liver cancer. Hepatitis D, also known as a delta virus, can only exist in the body in the presence of hepatitis B. It is seen mostly in central Africa, the Middle East and central South America. Infection rates are low in most of Europe and the USA. The treatment for hepatitis D is the same as the treatment for hepatitis B. Hepatitis E is most common in South Asia, Africa and Central America, areas that are known for poor sanitation. There is no specific dietary advice for patients infected with hepatitis D and hepatitis E. For hepatitis E, there is no specific treatment and most people go on to make a full recovery.

Hepatitis A

Hepatitis A is a virus that is transmitted by the faecal–oral route, often through the ingestion of contaminated food and drink. The virus passes out in the stool of the infected person. It is common in areas where the water supplies and sewage disposal are of a poor standard. Fruit, vegetables and uncooked foods washed in contaminated water can cause the infection as can shellfish if it is sourced from contaminated waters. Incubation time averages 28 days and most people fully recover within 2 months. Infection is not common in the UK but a vaccine is available that can offer protection for up to 10 years. Most people recover from hepatitis A with no lasting damage to the liver [9].

Hepatitis B

The hepatitis B virus (HBV) is classified by the World Health Organization as the world's second greatest carcinogen after tobacco. HBV is 50–100 times more infectious than HIV. In the UK, HBV has a low prevalence but there is significant variation across the country. Transmission of HBV is by parenteral exposure to infected blood or body fluids. HBV is not spread by casual contact such as touching hands and kissing, or sharing towels and eating utensils. A vaccine is available that will prevent infection from HBV for life.

The goal of therapy for HBV is to improve the quality of life and prevent progression to end-stage liver disease, hepatocellular carcinoma (HCC) and death [10]. Two major groups of antiviral therapies are used in the treatment of HBV: interferon and an oral nucleoside. HBV infection cannot be totally cleared so therapy is aimed at reducing HBV DNA to as low as possible [10]. The most common side-effect is an initial flu-like illness; other common side-effects include fatigue, anorexia and weight loss. Generally speaking, the treatment for HBV appears to be well tolerated and patients do not have the same tolerance issues that can arise with hepatitis C treatment. However, other co-morbidities, including alcohol abuse and being overweight, can affect the natural course of HBV as well as the efficacy of the antiviral strategies [10].

Hepatitis C

Hepatitis C virus (HCV) is the main cause of chronic liver disease worldwide [11]. It is estimated that over 200 million people, i.e. 3% of the world population have HCV. Prior to the 1990s, the main routes of transmission of HCV were through blood transfusions, unsafe injection procedures and intravenous drug use [12]. Currently new HCV infections are due mostly to intravenous or nasal drug use and to a lesser extent unsafe medical or surgical practices. The risk of perinatal and heterosexual transmission is low; recent data indicate that promiscuous male homosexual activity is related to HCV infection [13].

In some cases the HCV infection resolves spontaneously but as acute HCV is often asymptomatic, detection and diagnosis are usually difficult. The primary goal of HCV therapy is to eradicate the circulating virus by achieving a sustained virological response (SVR) and preventing the complications of HCV-related liver disease.

Dietary effects of HCV or its management

Prior to commencing treatment, patients should be counselled on the side-effects to be expected. They should also be guided on preventive and therapeutic measures to help improve the symptoms. HCV can affect individuals in many different ways. Fatigue is the primary symptom, often leading to poor quality of life [14,15]. Patients can be advised on how to manage fatigue by energy conservation, sleep and exercise management. Other symptoms such as nausea, pain and depression can have a serious impact on the ability to work and quality of life [16].

Once treatment starts, patients often experience worsening symptoms. The treatment may be particularly demanding, particularly for those with a prior history of drug or alcohol abuse. Side-effects such as worsening fatigue, insomnia and alopecia are common [17]. The symptoms can occur at any stage of the treatment, regardless of genotype or length of time on treatment. A substantial proportion of patients will experience a panoply of side-effects ranging from flu-like syndrome to severe adverse events including anaemia, cardiovascular events and psychiatric problems. Other side-effects include poor appetite, weight loss, neutropenia, skin irritations and myalgia [17–19]. Patients should have regular follow-up so that treatment progress and management issues regarding side-effects can be discussed [12].

Body mass index

Research has shown that there is a highly significant relationship between steatosis and increasing Body Mass Index (BMI) in patients with untreated chronic HCV [20]. Further studies have since shown that weight reduction in patients with chronic HCV may reduce hepatic steatosis, irrespective of viral genotype [21]. It is thought that even a small amount of weight loss may be associated with a reduction in abnormal liver enzymes and an improvement in fibrosis, despite the presence of the virus. A BMI $>30\,kg/m^2$ is a risk factor for non-response to antiviral therapy and this is independent of genotype and the presence of cirrhosis [22]. Gradual weight reduction and improvement in insulin resistance prior to starting treatment are associated with better SVR rates [23]. However, weight loss should only be considered if HCV management is stable. It is advised that weight reduction is not attempted during antiviral treatment, as side-effects may lead to excessive unintentional weight loss [24].

Alcohol

Several studies have shown increased histological liver damage in chronic alcoholic patients with HCV, in the form of higher rates of fibrosis progression and development of cirrhosis compared with HCV infection in non-drinking subjects [25,26]. However, further work has demonstrated that alcohol use did not have any impact on SVR in patients who had stopped drinking at least a year prior to treatment or those who had recently stopped drinking [27]. The only negative impact of alcohol on treatment outcome was that there were higher treatment discontinuation rates in recent drinkers [27]. Patients should be advised to abstain from regular alcohol consumption during therapy. If they cannot abstain, they should be offered treatment for alcohol dependence before treatment starts and support should be given during therapy to help adherence to treatment [12].

Insulin resistance

Patients with chronic HCV have a higher homeostasis model of assessment insulin resistance index (HOMA-IR) than healthy controls matched for age and BMI [28]. This insulin resistance is associated with fibrosis progression in HCV patients. Insulin resistance, advanced fibrosis and genotype 1 were independent predictors of poor treatment response in chronic HCV patients [28].

Eradication of the HCV virus is associated with a reduction by half of the incidence of type 2 diabetes and/or impaired fasting glucose [29]. However, this outcome is not seen in non-responders but only in sustained responders to treatment. There are no prospective trials to prove the efficacy of a therapeutic intervention aimed at improving insulin resistance in SVR. Thus no recommendations are made with regard to the use of drugs that reduce insulin resistance and further exploration is needed [12].

Weight loss

Weight loss has been reported in 11–29% of patients treated with pegylated interferon [30]. Patients who experienced greater weight loss during combination therapy did not benefit from improved antiviral response [19]. This weight loss is possibly a result of other side-effects, such as fatigue and depression, which may have a negative impact on appetite [31].

Significant weight loss during HCV treatment puts patients at risk of developing undernutrition. Poor appetite and weight loss can have a huge impact on ability to continue with treatment. Regular follow-up and support during treatment are essential to minimise undernutrition and help improve adherence to treatment.

Dietary management

The nutritional management of patients with HCV with or without cirrhosis is the same as that for other causes of liver disease, as discussed earlier in this chapter. It should involve promotion of optimal nutrition and prevention of undernutrition or deficiencies of specific nutrients [24].

Anaemia

Patients are at risk of low iron and reduced dietary intake. Recombinant erythropoietin (EPO) can be administered when the haemoglobin concentration falls below 10g/day in order to avoid ribavirin dose reduction or discontinuation [12].

Vitamins and minerals

There is little evidence that individual vitamins and minerals may influence the natural history of chronic HCV. Patients should be encouraged to achieve the recommended intake for all vitamins and minerals; there is no evidence to support amounts in excess of this [24].

A study investigating zinc supplementation found that 34mg/day in combination with interferon showed a beneficial effect on SVR in patients with genotype 1b HCV with high virus load [32].

High-dose vitamin E supplementation in chronic HCV patients undergoing combination therapy does not prevent ribavirin-associated haemolysis. In addition, vitamin E does not affect patient compliance or SVR [33]. Supplementation with vitamin C does not decrease the incidence of retinopathy during interferon therapy [34].

Complementary and alternative medicine

A number of herbal products claim to be beneficial for the liver. A survey of 1145 people with HCV in the HALT-C trial found that 23% were using herbal products at the time of enrolment. Although participants reported using many different herbal products, silymarin (milk thistle) was by far the most common. A Cochrane review investigating medicinal herbs for HCV infection concluded that there is no firm evidence of efficacy of any medicinal herbs for HCV infection [35].

Silymarin

The HALT-C trial showed that the use of silymarin by HCV patients was associated with fewer and milder symptoms but that there was no change in virus activity or liver inflammation [36]. A further *in vitro* study demonstrated anti-HCV actions of silymarin which disagree with other clinical trials that found no effect of silymarin on HCV replication *in vivo* [37]. However, this study concluded that further clinical trials are needed to determine if silymarin could be a safe and effective supplement for treating HCV in humans.

Coffee

Epidemiological and case–control studies show consistently that coffee drinking is associated with better serum liver function tests, particularly antagonising the hepatotoxic effects of alcohol, and so associated with less fibrosis and cirrhosis [38]. Furthermore, when cirrhosis is present, coffee drinking appears to protect against hepatocellular carcinoma. Further research has also concluded that high-level consumption of coffee (three cups per day) is an independent predictor of improved virological response to PEG interferon plus ribavirin in patients with HCV [39].

References

1. Makol A, Watt KD, Chowdhary VR. Autoimmune hepatitis: a review of current diagnosis and treatment. *Hepatitis Research and Treatment.* Available at: www.hindawi.com/journals/heprt/2011/390916/, accessed 8 January 2014.

2. Manns P, Czaja AJ, Gorham JD, et al. AASLD Practice Guidelines: diagnosis and management of autoimmune hepatitis. *Hepatology* 2010; **51**(6): 1–31.

3. Campillo B, Richardet JP, Scherman E, Bories PN. Evaluation of nutritional practice in hospitalized cirrhotic patients; results of a prospective study. *Nutrition* 2003; **19**(6): 515–521.

4. Henkel AS, Buchman AL. Nutritional support in patients with chronic liver disease. *Gastroenterology and Hepatology* 2006; **3**(4): 202–209.

5. Sima H, Hekmatdoost A, Ghaziani T, Alavian SM, Mashayekh A, Zali M. The prevalence of celiac autoanitbodies in hepatitis patients. *Iran Journal of Allergy, Asthma and Immunology* 2010; **9**(3): 157–162.

6. Saich R, Chapman R. Primary sclerosing cholangitis, autoimmune hepatitis and overlap syndromes in inflammatory bowel disease. *World Journal of Gastroenterology* 2008; **14**(3): 331–337.

7. Takahashi H, Nakagawa R, Nakano M, et al. Autoimmune hepatitis patients but not primary biliary cirrhosis patients have insulin resistance frequently without the influence of prednisone therapy. 21st Conference of the American Association for the Study of Liver Diseases, 2010. Available at: http://trs.scivee.tv/node/3571, accessed 8 January 2014.

8. Salmon C, Hoeroldt B, Dube A, McFarlane E, Gleeson E. Hepatic steatosis in patients with autoimmune hepatitis (AIH) – prevalence, progression and possible significance. *Journal of Hepatology* 2010; **52**(Suppl 1): 431.

9. Hepatitis A information booklet. Ringwood, Hampshire: British Liver Trust, 2005.

10. European Association for the Study of the Liver. Clinical Practice Guidelines: management of chronic hepatitis B. *Journal of Hepatology* 2009; **50**: 227–242.

11. Lavanchy D. The global burden of hepatitis C. *Liver International* 2009; **29**: 74–81.

12. European Association for the Study of the Liver. Clinical Practice Guidelines: management of hepatitis C virus infection. *Journal of Hepatology* 2011; **55**: 245–264.

13. Vann de Laar TJW, Mathews GV, Prins M, Danta M. Acute hepatitis C in HIV infected men who have sex with men: an emerging sexually transmitted infection. *AIDS* 2010; **24**: 1799–1812.

14. Ewart A, et al. Providing treatment for hepatitis C in an Australian district centre. *Postgraduate Medical Journal* 2004; **80**(941): 180–182.

15. Glacken M, et al. The experience of fatigue for people living with hepatitis C. *Journal of Clinical Nursing* 2003; **12**(2): 244–252.

16. Temple-Smith M. The lived experience of men and women with hepatitis C – implications for support needs and health information. *Australian Health Review* 2004; **27**(2): 46–56.

17. Zucker DM, Miller BW. Assessment of side effects in patients with chronic hepatitis C receiving combination therapy. *Gastroenterology Nursing* 2001; **24**(4): 192–196.

18. Mulhall BP, Vounossi Z. Impact of adherence on the outcome of antiviral therapy for chronic hepatitis C. *Journal of Clinical Gastroenterology* 2005; **39**(1 suppl): S23–27.

19. Seyam M. Weight loss during pegylated interferon and ribavirin treatment of chronic hepatitis C. *Journal of Viral Hepatitis* 2005; **12**(5): 531–535.

20. Hourigan LF, et al. Fibrosis in chronic hepatitis C correlates significantly with body mass index and steatosis. *Hepatology* 1999; **29**: 1215–1219.

21. Hickman IJ, et al. Effect of weight reduction on liver histology amd biochemistry in patients with chronic hepatitis C. *Gut* 2002; **51**: 89–94.

22. Bressler B, et al. High Body Mass Index is an independent risk factor for nonresponse to antiviral treatment in chronic hepatitis C. *Hepatology* 2003; **38**: 639–644.

23. Ghany MG, et al. Diagnosis, management and treatment of hepatitis C – an update. *Hepatology* 2009; **49**(4): 1335–1374.

24. Scottish Intercollegiate Guidelines Network. *National Clinical Guidelines for Management of Hepatitis C.* Edinburgh: Scottish Intercollegiate Guidelines Network, 2006.

25. Thomas DL, et al. The natural history of hepatitis C virus infection – host, viral, and environmental factors. *Journal of the American Medical Association* 2000; **284**: 450–456.

26. Harris DR, et al. The relationship of acute transfusion associated hepatitis to the development of cirrhosis in the presence of alcohol abuse. *Annals of Internal Medicine* 2001; **134**: 120–124.

27. Anand BS, et al. Alcohol use and treatment of hepatitis C virus – results of a national multicentre study. *Gastroenterology* 2006; **130**: 1607–1616.

28. Romero-Gomez M. Insulin resistance impairs sustained response rate to peginterferon plus ribavirin in chronic hepatitis C patients. *Gastroenterology* 2005; **128**: 636–641.

29. Romero-Gomez M. Effect of sustained virologcal response to treatment on the incidence of abnormal glucose values in chronic hepatitis C. *Journal of Hepatology* 2008; **48**: 721–727.

30. Manns MP, et al. Peginterferon alfa-2b plus ribavirin for initial treatment of chronic hepatitis C: a randomised trial. *Lancet* 2001; **358**(9286): 958–965.

31. Aspinall R, et al. The management of side effects during therapy for hepatitis C. *Alimentary Pharmacology and Therapeutics* 2004; **20**(9): 917–929.

32. Takagi H, Nagamine T, Abe T, et al. Zinc supplementation enhances the response to interferon therapy in patients with chronic hepatitis C. *Journal of Viral Hepatitis* 2001; **8**: 367–371.

33. Saeian K, et al. High dose vitamin E supplementation does not diminish ribavirin associated haemolysis in hepatitis C treatment with combination standard alfa-interferon and ribavirin. *Alimentary Pharmacology and Therapeutics* 2004; **20**: 1189–1193.

34. Nishiguchi S, et al. Does ascorbic acid prevent retinopathy during interferon therapy in patients with chronic hepatitis C? *Journal of Gastroenterology* 2001; **36**: 486–491.

35. Liu JP, Manheimer E, Tsutani K, et al. Medicinal herbs for hepatitis C virus infection: a Cochrane hepatobiliary systematic review of randomized trials. *American Journal of Gastroenterology* 2003; **98**: 538–544.

36. Seeff L, et al. Herbal product use by persons enrolled in hepatitis C antiviral long term treatment against cirrhosis (HALT–C) trial. *Hepatology* 2008; **47**(2): 605–612.

37. Wagoner J, et al. Multiple effects of Silymarin on the hepatitis C virus lifecycle. *Hepatology* 2010; **51**(6): 1912–1921.

38. Masterton G, et al. Coffee and the liver: a potential treatment for liver disease? *European Journal of Gastroenterology and Hepatology* 2010; **22**: 1277–1283.

39. Freedman N, et al. Coffee consumption is associated with response to peginterferon and ribavirin therapy in patients with chronic hepatitis C. *Gastroenterology* 2011; **140**: 1961–1969.

Chapter 4.5

Non-alcoholic fatty liver disease and hereditary haemochromatosis and nutrition

Niamh O'Sullivan[1] and Catherine McAnenny[2]
[1]St Vincent's University Hospital, Dublin, Ireland
[2]Royal Infirmary of Edinburgh, Edinburgh, UK

4.5.1 Non-alcoholic fatty liver disease

Non-alcoholic fatty liver disease (NAFLD) is the liver manifestation of metabolic syndrome. The National Institutes of Health (NIH) define metabolic syndrome as having at least three of the following risk factors: increased abdominal girth, increased triglyceride concentrations, low high-density lipoprotein (HDL), high blood pressure and high fasting blood glucose. It is estimated that 48–100% of people with NAFLD are asymptomatic. Many have non-specific symptoms such as fatigue and right upper quadrant pain [1]. NAFLD is often an incidental finding from abnormal liver function tests, predominantly alanine aminotransferase (ALT). Often the ratio of aspartate aminotransferase (AST) to ALT is <1, which differentiates NAFLD from alcohol-related fatty liver disease.

The NIH Clinical Research Network on NAFLD has agreed that the maximum allowable level of alcohol intake for definition of NAFLD as opposed to alcoholic fatty liver disease is 140g ethanol per week for men and 70g for women. Practice guidelines from the American Association for the Study of Liver Disease (AASLD) recommend that ongoing or recent alcohol consumption of >21 units/week for men and >14 units/week for women is a reasonable definition for significant alcohol consumption when evaluating patients with suspected NAFLD in clinical practice [2].

Non-alcoholic fatty liver disease is histologically subcategorised into non-alcoholic fatty liver (NAFL) and non-alcoholic steatohepatitis (NASH). NAFL is defined as the presence of hepatic steatosis with no evidence of hepatocellular injury in the form of ballooning of the hepatocytes. NASH is defined as the presence of hepatic steatosis and inflammation with hepatocyte injury with or without fibrosis [2]. Figure 4.5.1 presents the stages of NAFLD.

Approximately 5% of people with NAFLD develop end-stage liver disease. Mortality is greater than in age- and gender-matched controls [1]. Most cryptogenic cirrhosis and 25% of liver disease are caused by NAFLD [3,4]. Liver disease is the third most common cause of death in NAFLD [1].

The prevalence of NAFLD increases with age [5]. Estimates of worldwide prevalence of NAFLD range from 6.3% to 33% with a median of 20% in the general population [2]. In America the prevalence of NAFLD is 17–33%, whilst in Europe it is estimated at 20–30% [5,6]. The estimated prevalence of NASH is lower and ranges from 3% to 5% [2].

Non-alcoholic fatty liver disease is linked with insulin resistance, diabetes, hypertension and obesity, particularly central obesity (Table 4.5.1). It affects 76% of obese individuals but NASH is only present in 18.5% of obese individuals whilst 80% of those with NAFLD are morbidly obese [1]. Only 3% of people with NAFLD have a normal Body Mass Index (BMI) but this subgroup does exhibit

Advanced Nutrition and Dietetics in Gastroenterology, First Edition. Edited by Miranda Lomer.
© 2014 John Wiley & Sons, Ltd. Published 2014 by John Wiley & Sons, Ltd.

Spectrum of Disease

Bland steatosis-macrovesicular

Steatosis with mild inflammation

Steatosis with inflammation +/– fibrosis (NASH)

Cirrhosis-irreversible damage +/– hepatocellular carcinoma

Figure 4.5.1 Stages of non-alcoholic fatty liver disease.

Table 4.5.1 Waist circumference levels for central obesity [9]

	Waist circumference	
Country/ethnic group	Male	Female
South Asian/ Chinese/ South and Central American/ Japanese	>90 cm	> 80 cm
European	>94 cm	>80 cm
USA*	>102 cm	>88 cm

*ATP III Adult Treatment Panel III values are used for clinical purposes.
Reproduced with permission from the World Health Organization.

Table 4.5.2 Causes of non-alcoholic fatty liver disease

Primary NAFLD	Secondary NAFLD (absence of insulin resistance)
Central obesity	Total parenteral nutrition
Insulin resistance	Fatty liver of pregnancy
Type 2 diabetes	Intestinal jejunoileal bypass surgery
	Post gastrointestinal surgery for obesity
	Metabolic conditions
	Medications

central obesity or insulin resistance [7]. In type 2 diabetes, rates of NAFLD are approximately 50–69% [1,8].

Causes of non-alcoholic fatty liver disease

The cause of NAFLD is multifactorial, including genetic predisposition, lack of exercise, increased energy intake, obesity and insulin resistance (Table 4.5.2). The consumption of trans fats is associated with the development of NAFLD and hepatic inflammation [10] and saturated fat intake is a risk factor for NASH in the obese as it increases insulin resistance [11]. Abdominal or central obesity increases the flux of free fatty acids to the liver. An overabundance of circulating fatty acids increases insulin resistance and in NAFLD there is no insulin-mediated suppression of lipolysis. The consumption of high-fructose corn syrup contributes to insulin resistance and NAFLD [12].

Secondary NAFLD/NASH is rare in adults and is unrelated to insulin resistance or metabolic syndrome. Figure 4.5.2 illustrates the first- and second-hit hypothesis in NAFLD.

Nutritional assessment

A nutritional assessment of a patient with NAFLD should include weight, BMI, HDL, low-density lipoprotein (LDL), triglycerides, waist circumference, diet history and HbA1c if diabetic. BMI and waist circumference have both been shown to correlate with insulin resistance. Waist circumference also correlates with ALT concentrations. The presence of NASH with fibrosis is associated with being overweight and an increase in waist circumference [13].

Dietary management

Given the strong association between insulin resistance and NAFLD, it is reasonable to recommend lifestyle modification to all patients with NAFLD [14]. This decreases the risk of developing type 2 diabetes but an intense dietary intervention may also improve liver histology in people with NAFLD (Table 4.5.3) [15]. The present gold standard for the management of NASH is modest weight reduction,

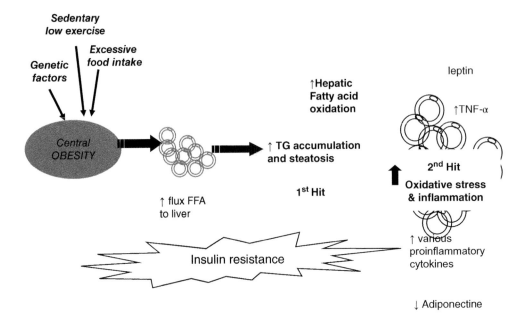

Figure 4.5.2   Two-hit theory of obesity-related hepatic fibrosis. FFA, free fatty acids; TG, triglyceride; TNF, tumour necrosis factor.

Table 4.5.3   Potential beneficial effect of diet-induced weight loss on non-alcoholic fatty liver disease

Main effect	Result
Reduced hepatic FFA supply	↓TAG synthesis ↓Hepatic insulin resistance ↓Hepatic glucose output ↓ROS generation ↓Hepatocyte inflammation
Improved extrahepatic insulin sensitivity Reduced circulating insulin concentrations	↓ *De novo* lipogenesis ↑ VLDL export ↓ Fibrosis
Reduced adipose tissue inflammation	↑ Leptin sensitivity ↑ Adiponectin ↓ Proinflammatory cytokines

Reprinted with permission from BMJ [19].
FFA, free fatty acid; ROS, reactive oxygen species;
TAG, triglycerol ;VLDL, very low-density lipoprotein.

and a decrease in central obesity by combining dietary advice with increased physical activity [16,17]. Weight loss generally reduces hepatic steatosis, achieved either by hypocaloric diet alone or in conjunction with increasing physical activity [2,16]. Loss of at least 3–5% of body weight appears necessary to improve steatosis, but a greater weight loss (up to 10%) may be needed to improve necroinflammation [2]. Emphasis should be on decreasing abdominal girth [17]. Crash dieting should be avoided (weight loss greater than 1 kg/week) as it is associated with worsening liver function test abnormalities, accelerated fibrosis and exacerbated steatosis [1]. Patients should be monitored for subacute NASH during rapid weight loss [18].

Therapy for NASH aims to prevent or reverse hepatic injury and hepatic cellular damage caused by lipotoxicity [5]. The treatment and monitoring of metabolic and cardiovascular co-morbidities should also be managed [5]. NASH can be reversed by lowering body weight and increasing physical activity [20].

Weight-reducing diets are associated with poor compliance. The assistance of a dedicated dietitian is critical [21]. Behaviour modification, cognitive behavioural therapy and support groups can improve weight loss [4,22]. A multidisciplinary yet personalised approach yields the best results [5]. Italian practice guidelines on NAFLD recommend that all patients receive counselling for a low-carbohydrate, low-saturated fat diet and avoidance of fructose-enriched soft drinks and an increase in fruit and vegetables [4].

The type of lipids as opposed to the volume accumulating in the liver may play a role in disease progression [23]. Some limited studies suggest that increasing the ratio of omega-3 to omega-6 fatty acids in the diet may lead to metabolic and histological improvements [24]. If triglyceride concentrations are high, two portions of oily fish per week should be recommended as for the general population [25].

Glycaemic control can be improved by consuming low Glycaemic Index (GI) and foods high in non-starch polysaccharides. If the patient is diabetic aim for an HbA1c <53 mmol/mol but the impact of this on NAFLD has yet to be established [18]. If blood pressure is high it is prudent to recommend a low-sodium diet. Patients with NAFLD should not consume heavy amounts of alcohol. However, there are no recommendations for mild-to-moderate alcohol consumption in people with NAFLD [2].

If patients are obese and do not respond to attempted lifestyle changes, they should be referred to centres specialising in obesity management. Bariatric surgery or gastric balloons can be considered for some patients [21]. Bariatric surgery may be useful in morbidly obese patients and has been reported to improve liver histology [4]. AASLD practice guidelines state that foregut bariatric surgery is not contraindicated in otherwise eligible obese individuals with NAFLD or NASH without established cirrhosis [2]. They also state that it is premature to consider foregut bariatric surgery as an established option to specifically treat NASH [2]. A Cochrane review reported a lack of randomised clinical trials which precludes the assessment of benefit or harm of bariatric surgery as a therapeutic approach for patients with NASH [4].

Physical activity

Exercise alone in adults with NAFLD may reduce hepatic steatosis but its ability to improve other aspects of histology remains unknown [2]. Only 20–33% of patients with NAFLD meet the American Surgeon General's recommendations for physical activity [5,26].

There are no recognised criteria for the optimal intensity, duration or total volume of exercise required to ameliorate insulin resistance, maintain weight loss and improve liver histology in NASH [27]. Suggested physical activity targets for NAFLD are at least 150 min of moderate-intensity and 75 min of vigorous activity per week in addition to muscle strengthening activity twice a week. These recommendations are derived from the diabetes prevention trials and can be applied to adult patients with NAFLD [5].

People with a BMI >40 are unlikely to implement and benefit from the recommended physical activity levels [17]. However, even small amounts of exercise are better than none, as physical activity increases insulin activity and decreases abdominal fat. Any increase in physical activity over baseline or even avoidance of being sedentary is desirable [4]. Physical activity increases the oxidative capacity of muscles, increasing use of free fatty acids for oxidation. This decreases fatty acids and triglycerides in myocytes which in turn increases insulin sensitivity.

Hepatitis C and non-alcoholic fatty liver disease

Obesity and its associated NAFLD play a role in fibrosis and hepatitis C [28]. Insulin resistance results in reduced viral clearance for patients on antiviral medications [29]. It is appropriate to counsel patients with hepatitis C who have a BMI greater than 25 to lose weight. Weight reduction may improve insulin resistance and response to antiviral treatment [28].

Non-alcoholic fatty liver disease and liver transplant

End-stage NASH is an under-recognised cause of cryptogenic cirrhosis [5] which is the most common reason for orthotopic liver transplant [3].

Steatosis can reoccur in the majority of patients with NAFLD by 5 years post transplant. Post transplant, it is estimated that 50% develop recurrent NASH and fibrosis, where the indication for transplant was NASH which can progress to graft loss. Risk factors include type 2 diabetes, steroids and weight gain. The greatest weight gain usually occurs within the first 6–12 months after transplant. Type 2 diabetes and hypertension both increase from 15% before transplant to 30–40% and 60% post transplant respectively. Post-transplant mortality is increased with pre-existing type 2 diabetes [29]. The prevalence of hyperlipidaemia is 50–70% post transplant [30]. It is therefore important to give education and lifestyle management for the prevention of weight gain post transplant.

Vitamin E

Vitamin E administered at a daily dose of 800 IU/day improves liver histology in non-diabetic adults with biopsy-proven NASH and therefore should be considered as first-line pharmacotherapy. However, vitamin E is not recommended to treat NASH in diabetic patients, NAFLD without liver biopsy, NASH cirrhosis or cryptogenic cirrhosis [2].

Future developments

A 2007 Cochrane review found no evidence to support or refute the use of antioxidants or probiotics in patients with NAFLD [31,32]. A large multicentre study in America to treat NASH using an omega-3 fatty acid (eicosapentaenoic acid) is currently taking place. AASLD practice guidelines indicate that it is premature to recommend omega-3 fatty acids for the specific treatment of NAFLD or NASH but they may be considered as first-line agents to treat hypertriglyceridaemia in patients with NAFLD [2].

A recent review recommends the consumption of two oily fish meals per week in NAFLD and NASH although they acknowledge that the efficacy and safety have not been confirmed in randomised controlled trials. More trials are needed before omega-3 supplements are recommended and to determine if any other histopathological features of NAFLD respond to omega-3 fatty acids.

4.5.2 Hereditary haemochromatosis

Hereditary haemochromatosis (HH) is a genetic iron overload disorder. Iron may accumulate from the early twenties onwards, usually later in women. The iron is deposited in the liver, other endocrine glands and the heart. Without therapeutic interventionm there is a risk that iron overload will occur with the potential for tissue damage and disease [33]. Iron depletion by venesection has been established as the accepted standard of care, despite the absence of randomised controlled trials.

There are no studies proving that dietary intervention will provide any additional benefit in patients undergoing venesection. It is recommended that patients follow a balanced diet and avoid iron-containing vitamin supplements and iron-fortified foods such as breakfast cereals. There is a recommendation that vitamin C is limited to 500 mg/day [34]. However, this was based on a single case report on a patient with HH in whom vitamin C may have had a negative effect on cardiac function [35]. It has also been suggested that tea drinking may reduce the increase in iron stores in HH but this has not been confirmed [36,37]. As with other types of liver disease, excess alcohol can speed liver damage and may increase iron absorption.

References

1. Manopriya TP, Elshaari Faraj A, Dhastagir S, Sheriff A. Bird's eye view of non alcoholic fatty liver disease – an insulin resistant state. *Acta Medica Saliniana* 2010; **39**(1): 1–5.
2. Chalasani N, Younossi Z, Lavine J. The diagnosis and management of non-alcoholic fatty liver disease: Practice guidelines by the American Gastroenterological Association, American Association for the Study of Liver Disease and American College of Gastroenterology. *Gastroenterology* 2012; **142**: 1592–1609.
3. Maheshwari A, Thuluvath PJ. Cryptogenic cirrhosis and non alcoholic fatty liver disease: are they related? *American Journal of Gastroenterology* 2006; **101**(3): 664–668.
4. Loria P, Adinolfi LE, Bellentani S, Svegliati-Baroni G. The non alcoholic fatty liver disease expert committee of the associazone Italiano per lo studio de Fegato (AISF). Practice guidelines for the diagnosis and management of non alcoholic fatty liver disease – a decalogue from AISF Expert Committee. *Digestive and Liver Disease* 2010; **42**(4): 272–282.

5. Ratziu V, Bellentani S, Cortez-Pinto H, Day C, Marchesini G. A position statement of NAFLD/ NASH based on the EASL 2009 special conference. *Journal of Hepatology* 2010; **53**: 372–384.
6. Farrell GC, Chitturi S, Lau GK, Sollano JD. Asia–Pacific working party on non alcoholic fatty liver disease. Guidelines for the assessment and management in the Asia–Pacific region: executive summary. *Journal of Gastroenterology and Hepatology* 2007; **22**(6): 775–777.
7. Harrison SA, Oliver D, Arnold HL, Gogia S, Neuschwander-Tetri BA. Development and validation of a simple NAFLD scoring system for identifying patients with advanced disease. *Gut* 2008; **57**(10): 1441–1447.
8. Targher G, Bertolini L, Padovani R, et al. Prevalence of nonalcoholic fatty liver disease and its association with cardiovascular disease among type 2 diabetic patients. *Diabetes Care* 2007; **30**(5): 1212–1218.
9. World Health Organization. *Waist circumference and waist–hip ratio: report of a WHO expert consultation, Geneva, 8–11.* Geneva: World Health Organization, 2008.
10. Araya J, Rodrigo R, Videla LA, Thielemann L. Increase in long-chain PUFA n-6 to n-3 ratio in relation to hepatic steatosis in patients with non-alcoholic fatty liver disease. *Clinical Science* 2004; **106**(6): 635–643.
11. Musso G, Gambino R, Gianfranco P. Dietary habits and their relations to insulin resistance and postprandial lipemia in non-alcoholic steatohepatitis. *Hepatology* 2003; **37**(4): 909–916.
12. Ouyang X, Cirillo P, Sautin Y, McCall S. Fructose consumption as a risk factor for NAFLD. *Journal of Hepatology* 2008; **48**: 993–999.
13. Rocha R, Cotrim H.P, Carvalo FM. Body mass index and waist circumference in non-alcoholic fatty liver disease. *Journal of Human Nutrition and Diet* 2005; **18**: 365–370.
14. Ekstedt M, Lennart E, Franzén LE, et al. Long term follow up of patients with NAFLD. *Hepatology* 2006; **44**(4): 865–873.
15. Huang MA, Greenson JK, Chao C, et al. One-year intense nutritional counseling results in histological improvement in patients with non-alcoholic steatohepatitis: a pilot study. *American Journal of Gastroenterology* 2005; **100**(5): 1072–1081.
16. Farrell GC, Larter CZ. Non alcoholic fatty liver disease: from steatosis to cirrhosis. *Hepatology* 2006; **43**(2 Suppl 1): S99–S112.
17. Farrell GC. The liver and the waistline, fifty years of growth. *Journal of Gastroenterology and Hepatology* 2009; **24**(Suppl 3): S105–118.
18. American Gastroenterological Association. Medical position statement : non-alcoholic fatty liver disease. *Gastroenterology* 2002; **123**: 1702–1704.
19. Harrison SA, Day CP. Benefits of lifestyle modification in NAFLD. *Gut* 2007; **56**(12): 1765.
20. St George A, Baumann A, Johnston A, Farrell G, Chey T, George J. Independent effects of physical activity in patients with non-alcoholic fatty liver disease. *Hepatology* 2009; **50**(1): 68–76.
21. Chitturi S, Farrell GC, Hashimoto E, Saibra T, Lau GKK. Asia–Pacific working party on non-alcoholic fatty liver disease.

Non-alcoholic fatty liver disease in the Asia–Pacific region: definitions and overview of proposed guidelines. *Journal of Gastroenterology and Hepatology* 2007; **22**: 778–787.
22. Promrat K, Kleiner D, Niemeler H, Jackvony E. Randomised controlled trial testing the effects of weight loss on non alcoholic steatohepatitis. *Hepatology* 2010; **51**(1): 121–129.
23. Alkhouri N, Dixon LJ, Feldstein AE. Lipotoxicity in non alcoholic fatty liver disease: not all lipids are created equal. *Expert Review of Gastroenterology and Hepatology* 2009; **3**(4): 445–451.
24. Tanaka N, Sano K, Horiuchi A. Highly-purified eicosapentaenoic acid treatment improves nonalcoholic steatohepatitis. *Journal of Clinical Gastroenterology* 2008; **42**: 413–418.
25. Shapiro H, Tehilla M, Attal-Singer P. The therapeutic potential of long-chain omega-3 fatty acids in non alcoholic fatty liver disease. *Clinical Nutrition* 2011; **30**: 6–19.
26. Krasnoff JB, Painter PL, Wallace JP, Bass N, Merriman R. Health-related fitness and physical activity in patients with non-alcoholic fatty liver disease. *Hepatology* 2008; **47**(4): 1158–1166.
27. Conjeevaram HS, Tiniako DJ. Editorial: Exercise for non alcoholic fatty liver disease: does intensity matter? *American Journal of Gastroenterology* 2011; **106**(3): 470–475.
28. Ghany M, Strader D, Thomas D, Seff L. American Society for the Study of Liver Disease. Diagnosis, management and treatment of hepatitis C: an update. AASLD practice guidelines. *Hepatology* 2009; **49**(4): 1335–1373.
29. Watt K. Obesity and metabolic complications of liver transplant. *Liver Transplantation* 2010; **16**: S65–S71.
30. Pfitzmann R, Nussler NC, Hippler-Benscheidt M, Neuhaus R, Neuhaus P. Long term results after liver transplant. *Transplant International* 2008; **21**: 234–246.
31. Lirussi F, Azzalini L, Orando S, Orlando R, Angelico F. Antioxidant supplements for non-alcoholic fatty liver disease and/or steatohepatitis. *Cochrane Database of Systematic Reviews* 2007: 1: CD004996.
32. Lirussi F, Mastropasqua E, Orando S, Orlando R. Probiotics for non-alcoholic fatty liver disease and/or steatohepatitis. *Cochrane Database of Systematic Reviews* 2007: **1**: CD005165.
33. European Association for the Study of the Liver (EASL). Clinical practice guidelines for HFE hemochromatosis. *Journal of Hepatology* 2010; **53**: 3–22.
34. Barton JC, et al. Hemochromatosis probands as blood donors. *Transfusion* 1999; **39**: 578–585.
35. Schofield RS, et al. Cardiac transplantation in a ppatient with hereditary hemochromatosis: role of adjunctive phlebotomy and erythropoietin. *Journal of Heart and Lung Transplantation* 2001; **20**: 696–698.
36. Kaltwasser JP, et al. Clinical trial on the effect of regular tea drinking on iron accumulation in hereditary haemochromatosis. *Gut* 1998; **43**: 699–704.
37. Milward EA, et al. Noncitrus fruits as a novel dietary environmental modifier of iron stores in people with or without HFE gene mutations. *Mayo Clinic Proceedings* 2008; **83**: 543–549.

Chapter 4.6

Decompensated liver disease and nutrition

Simran Arora[1], Gillian Gatiss[2], Laura M. McGeeney[2] and Nina C. Powell[2]
[1]Royal Free London NHS Foundation Trust, London, UK
[2]Cambridge University Hospitals NHS Foundation Trust, Cambridge, UK

4.6.1 Dietary causes and effects of decompensated liver disease

Liver disease can be caused by various factors as shown in Table 4.6.1. Largely it is the symptoms and severity of the disease that determine the nutritional treatment, rather than the aetiology.

Due to the vital metabolic role of the liver, loss of function has significant nutritional consequences. The reported incidence of undernutrition in this population varies with assessment technique and stage of disease; it can be as high as 100% [1–3]. Malnutrition affects important clinical outcomes including rates of variceal bleeding, encephalopathy, infections, ascites, poor muscle function, length of hospital stay and mortality rates [4–7]. The level of protein-energy malnutrition (PEM) is dependent on the severity of the liver disease and level of nutritional input into patient care rather than the aetiology.

Factors contributing to PEM include a reduced oral intake due to nausea, vomiting, pain, encephalopathy, early satiety (which may be due to the pressure of ascites), alcohol withdrawal, periods of being nil by mouth for tests, anorexia, nutrient and fluid restrictions, unpalatable diets (such as very low-salt diets), altered sense of taste and fatigue. Patients with PEM may also have malabsorption in the form of diarrhoea or steatorrhoea due to cholestasis, the use of regular lactulose or changes to GI microbiota following antibiotics, and may have increased requirements for energy and protein due to changes in energy metabolism.

Metabolic changes in cirrhosis

Figure 4.6.1 shows the major metabolic changes that occur in a person with cirrhosis and the connections between them.

Malnutrition in liver disease has been called a 'glycogen storage disease' as even in the fed state, glycogen stores remain low [14]. Hepatic glycogenolysis is also impaired, making glycogen a less suitable fuel for cirrhotic patients. To maintain blood glucose concentrations in the short term when there has been no recent intake of carbohydrate, there is an increase in gluconeogenesis from amino acids, resulting in protein depletion [15]. Petersen et al. compared gluconeogenesis and glycogenolysis rates in cirrhotic subjects and matched healthy controls using nuclear magnetic resonance spectroscopy and ^2H_2O and found that they had similar rates of glucose production but the cirrhotic subjects had an increased rate of gluconeogenesis and decreased rate of glycogenolysis compared to the control subjects [16]. Fat is also used as an alternative fuel source [17]. However, the fat oxidation rates do return to normal after refeeding [18].

Advanced Nutrition and Dietetics in Gastroenterology, First Edition. Edited by Miranda Lomer.
© 2014 John Wiley & Sons, Ltd. Published 2014 by John Wiley & Sons, Ltd.

Table 4.6.1 Types of liver disease

Cause	Type of liver disease
Infections	Hepatitis A, hepatitis B, hepatitis C, hepatitis D, hepatitis E
Toxic	Alcohol-related liver disease, drug overdoses, other poisons
Cholestatic	Primary sclerosing cholangitis, primary biliary cirrhosis
Metabolic	Non-alcoholic fatty liver disease, non-alcoholic steatohepatitis, hereditary haemochromatosis, alpha-1 antitrypsin deficiency, Wilson's disease
Vascular	Budd–Chiari syndrome
Other	Cystic fibrosis-related liver disease, autoimmune hepatitis, cryptogenic liver disease

Using indirect calorimetry, the percentage of total energy from fat, carbohydrate and protein in control subjects after a 36–72-h fast were comparable to those found in cirrhotic patients after an overnight fast (10–12h) [19]. These proportions were significantly different from overnight fasted control subjects. This indicates that cirrhotic patients reach a fasted state much more rapidly than healthy controls; cirrhosis has been termed a disease of accelerated starvation. Increased endogenous protein breakdown leads to increased protein turnover. However, the protein resynthesis rate does not increase and the capacity of the cirrhotic liver to synthesise and store proteins is reduced, leading to muscle wasting. The mechanism of this hypermetabolism is unclear but is thought to be extrahepatic as it persists for over a year following liver transplantation [20].

Not all cirrhotic patients are hypermetabolic; those that are have a similar percentage of muscle mass as normometabolic cirrhotic patients, but a reduced body cell mass [8]. They also have raised serum cytokines, indicating a potential role for the inflammatory response in the hypermetabolic state. Greco et al. showed hypermetabolism, increased lipid oxidation rates and insulin resistance after an overnight fast in Childs B cirrhotic patients when compared to matched healthy controls [20a]. The Body Mass Index (BMI), fat free mass and fat mass of the patients were not statistically significantly

different from the healthy controls, suggesting that metabolic changes precede weight loss rather than being a consequence of it.

Muscle wasting can be a major feature of cirrhosis but with skilled nutritional assessment and therapy this can be prevented.

Nutritional assessment

Undernutrition can be present in the early stages of liver disease but is not always readily evident, especially in people who are overweight. Detailed nutritional assessment is needed to identify people who are undernourished or at risk of becoming so. Accurate assessment of nutritional status can be particularly difficult in patients with cirrhosis due to altered fluid homeostasis. Traditional nutritional assessment methods and nutrition screening tools are often based on weight and BMI changes but more specific measures of nutritional status are required for this patient group.

Nutritional assessment would include a review of symptoms, medical history, social history, assessment of body composition, biochemistry, detailed dietary intake and fluid restrictions. Symptoms such as nausea, anorexia, pain, fatigue and encephalopathy can reduce nutritional intake, as can any fluid restrictions. While constipation can lead people to be more likely to experience encephalopathy, diarrhoea reduces the absorption of nutrients and can also lead people to be less inclined to eat. Medical history including co-morbidities such as renal failure, hepatopulmonary syndrome or diabetes will potentially have an impact on patient nutritional status as well as the dietary counselling given. A person's social situation including financial situation, living conditions, alcohol and illicit drug use will have an impact on their nutritional status. Changes in a patient's liver function tests can give an indication of an improvement or decline in their condition; it is important to monitor electrolytes in potential refeeding syndrome patients and biochemistry can also be used to monitor conditions such as renal failure.

When taking a diet history, it is particularly important to note the pattern of nutritional intake as well as the nutritional content and portion sizes, looking out for the frequency and amount of carbohydrate and

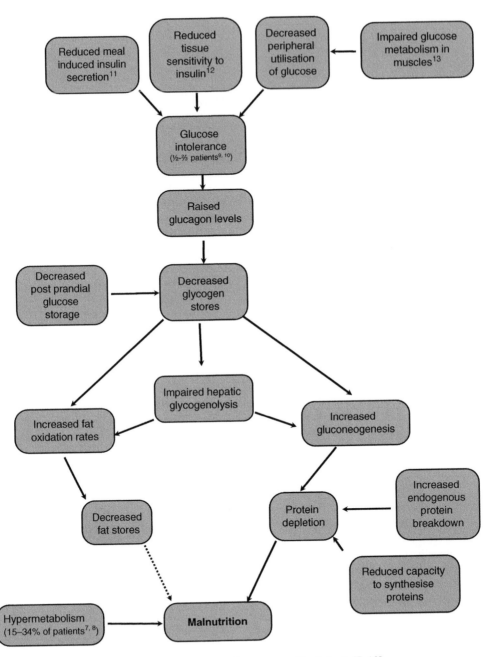

Figure 4.6.1 The major metabolic changes that occur in someone with cirrhosis [7–13].

protein consumed in particular. As with any other patient group, it is important to take into account patient preferences and tolerances, daily pattern of activities and any concerns they have.

Upper arm anthropometry

Upper arm anthropometry, mid arm circumference (MAC), triceps skinfold thickness (TST) and mid arm muscle circumference (MAMC) are used in the clinic or ward setting to differentiate between fat and muscle stores. These measurements indicate a patient's nutritional status compared to an expected population. Serial measurements in one patient every 3–8 weeks are most useful as body fat has to change by several kg before it is detectable by skinfold measurements [21]. It is important to be aware of inter- and intraobserver error. Reliability and accuracy can be improved by standardising the observer's technique or by undertaking specialist anthropometry training.

Hand grip strength

Hand grip strength is measured using a dynamometer and is a measure of muscle function. Low handgrip strength has been shown to be a predictor of complications and poor clinical outcome in patients with cirrhosis [22]. Patients' handgrip strength changes more rapidly than the measured change in muscle bulk and can be assessed weekly if required.

Nutrition screening

Tools that incorporate information from several sources to a patient in a structured way can be particularly helpful. The Royal Free Hospital Global Assessment (RFH-GA) which uses BMI (calculated using estimated dry body weight), MAMC, dietary intake and symptoms in an algorithm [23] has very good intra- and interobserver reproducibility and is validated in this patient group [24]. Accurate use of this assessment requires specialist training and can take an hour to complete. The Royal Free Hospital Nutritional Prioritising Tool (RFH-NPT) has recently been developed and validated. This has very good intra- and interobserver reproducibility, with a diagnostic sensitivity of 100% and specificity

of 73% [25]. It takes 2–3 min and little training to complete but gives a less detailed assessment than the RFH-GA. This tool includes the presence/absence of ascites and/or oedema with different subsequent questions depending on this answer.

Dry weight

Table 4.6.2 can be used to estimate the weight of fluid and therefore to calculate dry weight. The estimated weight of ascites and peripheral oedema is subtracted from the patient's 'wet weight'. Patients may have ascitic volumes larger than 14 kg. Even in patients with no ascites or oedema, weight alone is a crude measure of nutritional status as it does not distinguish between fat and muscle stores. For patients with ascites who have regular paracentesis, it is useful to monitor how much fluid is removed during each paracentesis session, how much fluid is remaining after paracentesis, a typical postparacentesis weight and the duration since the last paracentesis, to individualise estimates of dry body weight.

Nutritional requirements

When gluconeogenesis rather than glycogenolysis is used to maintain hepatic glucose release there is an increase in both resting energy expenditure (REE) and protein requirements [19,27]. Gluconeogenesis uses more energy than glycogenolysis and requires amino acids as substrates, therefore both energy and protein requirements for cirrhotics are increased. People with liver disease can replete their stores with increased intakes [28,29]. The European Society of Parenteral and Enteral Nutrition (ESPEN) guidelines aim for 25–40 kcal/kg body weight but whether dry, actual or ideal body weight is used is not agreed (Table 4.6.3) [30]. If a patient is undernourished,

Table 4.6.2 An estimate of the weight of ascites and peripheral oedema [26]

	Ascites	Peripheral oedema
Minimal	2.2 kg	1.0 kg
Moderate	6.0 kg	5.0 kg
Severe	14.0 kg	10.0 kg

Reproduced with permission from Taylor & Francis.

Table 4.6.3 Energy and protein requirements for people with liver disease

	Stress factor*	Energy kcal/kg dBW/day	Protein g/kg dBW/day
Compensated	0–20%	25–35	1.2–1.3
Decompensated	30–40%	35–40	1.2–1.5
Acute (fulimant)	20–30%		1.2–1.5
Post transplant (approx. 1 month)	30%		1.2–1.5

In the UK, energy (for weight maintenance) and protein requirements use dBW (dry body weight) [30,31].
*A stress factor is used to adjust for additional metabolic stress and multiplied by basal metabolic rate or by the specific kcal/kg for each condition by body weight [30].
Reproduced with permission from Elsevier.

unless they are overtly critically ill or septic, the addition of an extra 400–1000 kcal per day is encouraged to promote repletion of stores.

Protein stores of lean body mass (LBM) are depleted by the use of amino acids for glucose generation, therefore extra dietary protein is required to maintain and replete LBM. Swart et al. used radiolabelled [15 N]glycine to investigate rates of nitrogen flux, protein synthesis and protein breakdown in people with cirrhosis and healthy controls and suggested that cirrhotic patients require an increase in nitrogen intake to achieve a positive nitrogen balance due to their increase in gluconeogenesis [29]. Protein requirements are calculated based on the patient's estimated dry weight and are shown in Table 4.6.3.

Patients, particularly if at home and mobile, may need to increase their intake beyond these calculated requirements in order to replete or maintain their muscle stores. It is important to monitor their nutritional status regularly and adjust their dietary recommendations accordingly.

In obese patients, protein and energy requirements are adjusted to account for increased body mass with a likely reduced percentage of metabolically active tissue. In the UK, protein and energy requirements are reduced by 25% and 400–1000 kcal per day respectively. When making any such adjustments, it is important that patients are regularly monitored so any decline in nutritional status can be identified and mitigated. Preservation of muscle function and a patient's fitness take priority over any aim to reduce fat mass. ESPEN

guidelines do not give guidance specifically for obese liver patients.

Fluid requirements are rarely estimated from predetermined calculations but assessed on an individual basis and dependent on the patient's fluid status.

4.6.2 Dietary causes of hepatic encephalopathy

The cause of hepatic encephalopathy (HE) is likely to be multifactorial and is still not fully understood. Consequently dietary manipulation in HE has evolved as a greater level of evidence supports or disproves theories. One of the first theories about the cause was that dietary protein causes HE in liver failure. Hence, historically dietary protein restriction was advised to reduce the risk and facilitate the management of HE [32]. This is no longer advised as protein turnover studies have demonstrated that the requirement for protein and the overall energy need increase with the development of end-stage liver failure [3,33]. Restricting intake can lead to muscle catabolism and the associated poor outcomes in these patients [34].

It is thought that the need for additional dietary protein is driven by the utilisation of branched chain amino acids (BCAA) for the repair of the liver injury or utilisation of them to dispose of ammonia [35], lowering the ratio of the BCAA relative to the aromatic amino acids. Furthermore, if the additional calorie requirements are not met, the breakdown of muscle protein increases the circulating concentration of aromatic amino acids (phenylalanine, tyrosine) relative to the circulating concentrations of BCAA (leucine, isoleucine, valine). Ultimately a higher ratio of aromatic amino acids to BCAA facilitates the movement of aromatic amino acids across the blood–brain barrier, altering the mental state associated with HE. This theory is further supported by the development of HE following a gastrointestinal bleed. It is proposed that the digestion of blood, which is deficient in isoleucine, a branched chain amino acid, alters the ratio of aromatic amino acids to BCAA, causing acute HE [36].

A high concentration of gastrointestinal ammonia is another theory for the cause of HE. During periods of fasting, the utilisation of amino acids from muscle for gluconeogenesis produces ammonia. Circulating ammonia is removed by muscle tissue, hence muscle loss in itself may exacerbate the development of HE [37]. Dietary factors that can alter the gastrointestinal microbiota and reduce the high concentrations of ammonia production are thought to reduce the risk and facilitate the management of HE. Dietary factors that have been studied in this process include lactulose, probiotics, vegetable protein and zinc.

4.6.3 Nutritional consequences of ascites

Ascitic volume is normally defined as mild, moderate or severe (see Table 4.6.2) but can exceed 25 litres in some patients. Moderate-to-severe ascites can have a detrimental effect on nutritional status due to multiple factors (Box 4.6.1).

Disease-related anorexia and intake

Abdominal pain and discomfort are common symptoms in patients with ascites and most common in those with spontaneous bacterial peritonitis (SBP), an infection of the peritoneal fluid [39]. This combined with early satiety due to the pressure of fluid pressing on the stomach can dramatically reduce food intake. Additional factors reducing intake are nausea due to SBP or hepatorenal syndrome (HRS) and the potential dietary restrictions this may require.

Box 4.6.1 Factors associated with ascites which affect nutritional status

Reduced appetite and intake	Abdominal pain and discomfort Early satiety Nausea associated with spontaneous bacterial peritonitis and hepatorenal syndrome Severe fluid and sodium restrictions
Increased nutritional requirements	Possible increase in resting energy expenditure with ascites [38] Infections Protein loss at paracentesis
Increased muscle atrophy	Recommended or self-imposed bed rest

---

4.6.4 Dietary management of decompensated liver disease

Studies have investigated the effect of increased energy and protein intake in patients with decompensated liver cirrhosis, using both oral nutritional supplements and enteral nutrition (EN). Improvements in nutritional status [40], in liver function [41,42] and survival [41] have been reported. The dietary goal is for the patient to receive adequate nutrient intake to prevent nutrient and muscle depletion and minimise complications. To achieve this aim, aggressive nutritional support is frequently required. Vitamin and mineral deficiencies are common in these patients, especially in patients with PEM, and these need to be corrected. Unnecessary or inappropriate dietary restrictions should be avoided as these can be detrimental to outcomes.

Patients with decompensated cirrhosis who are not meeting their nutritional requirements should be offered dietary advice [3]. Dietary counselling alone can be successful [40] but often supplementary nutrition is required. Oral nutritional supplements (ONS) or EN are indicated when patients cannot meet their nutritional requirements from normal food and drink, despite adequate individualised dietary counselling [30].

Oral nutritional support

Oral nutritional supplements high in energy and protein but low in volume are frequently used in clinical practice. Low volume is not only useful for patients with fluid restrictions but also for patients experiencing early satiety, disease-related anorexia or who need to consume large volumes of ONS to meet their nutritional requirements.

Enteral nutrition

Oral intake should be encouraged but for patients who are unable to meet their nutritional requirements orally, EN should not be delayed [41,42], even if only required in the short term. Cabre et al. showed decreased inpatient mortality rates in severely undernourished patients with cirrhosis using EN compared with standard oral diet (12% versus 47% mortality) [41]. Campillo et al. found that not only did severely undernourished cirrhotic patients show an improvement in liver function after 6 weeks of EN but there was also an increase in spontaneous dietary intake [42]. Formulae that are high in energy and protein are frequently used and whole-protein formulae are generally recommended [30]. Feeding regimens may be continuous or intermittent, ideally choosing a method that most reduces long periods of fasting, for example overnight feeding.

Enteral nutrition via the nasogastric (NG) route is perhaps the easiest to initiate in clinical practice but feeding via the nasojejunal (NJ) route is useful in patients with high-volume ascites, delayed gastric emptying or early satiety, nausea or vomiting. Gastrostomy or jejunostomy placement is contraindicated in patients with cirrhosis due to impairment of the coagulation system and portosystemic collateral circulation [43]. During gastrostomy or jejunostomy insertion, patients with gastric varices have an increased risk of bleeding and those with ascites have an increased risk of infection and leakage of fluid from the tube site. There is no evidence that NG tube insertion increases the incidence of variceal bleeding [41,44] and slow or intermittent GI bleeding is not an absolute contraindication to EN [3]. However, after acute variceal bleeding NG tube insertion should be avoided for 3 days [45,46] as this period has the highest risk of rebleeding [47]. No favourable effect of EN via an NG tube initially after a variceal bleed has been demonstrated [45].

Parenteral nutrition

Parenteral nutrition (PN) is associated with higher risks of infection, electrolyte imbalance and greater expense than EN and is generally only recommended for patients who cannot receive nutrition via the GI tract, for example those with intestinal obstruction [48]. PN may also be considered in patients with an unprotected airway and advanced HE when swallow and cough reflexes are compromised [49]. In cirrhotic patients with portosystemic shunting, Plauth et al. found that PN may be superior to EN because the latter may worsen hyperammonaemia [50].

Eating pattern

In addition to meeting nutritional requirements, it is important to consider the pattern of food intake throughout the day. A modified eating pattern of 4–6 meals per day containing food rich in carbohydrate is recommended [51,52] to avoid periods of fasting for longer than 2h. Early satiety and disease-related anorexia are common features of patients with cirrhosis, therefore small meals at regular intervals can help ensure adequate dietary intake. One of these meals should be a late evening carbohydrate snack to shorten nocturnal fasting and minimise early starvation. A late evening snack improves nitrogen balance [53–55] and fat-free mass [56]. It also increases carbohydrate oxidation [55,57] and the respiratory quotient [55,57,58]. Carbohydrates have antiketogenic and nitrogen-sparing effects during periods of energy deprivation [59] and it is assumed that 50–100g carbohydrate is required to produce these effects [60]. Therefore, in practice, a late evening snack comprising at least 50g carbohydrate is recommended.

The study by Yamanaka-Okumura et al. [58] used a 44 g carbohydrate rice ball at 21:00h and Chang et al. [57] used two slices of bread and jam (50g carbohydrate) at 23:00h to provide extra late evening carbohydrate. Both demonstrated improved energy metabolism and Yamanaka-Okumura et al. [58]

proved that the timing, rather than the amount of energy supplementation, is of greater importance in achieving this. Chang et al. [57] found six out of the 16 cirrhotic patients prior to the study had individually altered their eating patterns to include a snack before bed or in the early morning to relieve symptoms of dizziness, hunger or abdominal discomfort. Swart et al. concluded that a late evening meal seemed to improve the efficiency of nitrogen metabolism compared with isocaloric and isonitrogenous diets without an evening meal [53]. Zilikens et al. studied the effect of polymeric glucose solution (100g carbohydrate) in the late evening and found nocturnal glucose improved nitrogen balance during the night in patients with cirrhosis but not in healthy controls [54].

Liquid dietary supplements have also been used as late evening snacks. Miwa et al. demonstrated correction of abnormal fuel metabolism in patients with cirrhosis using a nutritional supplement drink (Ensure, 250kcal) at 23:00h [55]. A long-term study compared the effects of taking nutritional supplements (710kcal/day, >50g carbohydrate) during the night-time (between 21:00h and 07:00h) and the daytime (between 09:00h and 19:00h) over a 12-month period [56]. Those who consumed the supplements at night increased their lean muscle by 2–2.5kg whereas the daytime group showed no significant changes over the 12 months.

The importance of a late evening snack has been demonstrated but the most effective composition of this is debated. Oral BCAA supplementation as the late evening snack may also prevent protein catabolism [61–63] and may improve glucose tolerance [63]. Nocturnal BCAA administration may also stimulate hepatic albumin synthesis [62]. However, studies have revealed poor compliance mainly due to the poor palatability of the formulae [62] and they are expensive and hence potentially not felt to be an economically viable solution for long-term care.

4.6.5 Dietary management of hepatic encephalopathy

Dietary interventions are based on the correction of precipitating factors of HE. Hence they can be used to reduce the risk and recurrence of HE as well as acting as a form of treatment. A combination of treatments may be more beneficial as HE is thought to be multifactorial.

Probiotics and prebiotics

The effectiveness of treating HE with lactulose is controversial [64]. Lactulose is a non-digestible sugar and prebiotic that alters GI microbiota as it is fermented. Evidence is emerging that synbiotics or fermentable fibres are a more effective alternative to lactulose and this warrants further research [65]. In HE probiotics reduce the substrate for some urease-producing GI microbiota [66]. The fermentation products lactic acid, ethanol, acetic acid and carbon dioxide lower the pH, creating a hostile environment for the urease GI microbiota [65]. Studies are needed to elucidate which micro-organisms would be effective, viable bacteria as well as the frequency and dosing required.

Protein

Routine dietary protein restriction does not reduce the risk of HE. In the unusual scenario where the cause of HE is unidentified, traditional management methods of the condition such as regular enemas to promote stool evacuation should be trialled before dietary manipulation is considered. The ESPEN guidelines for nutrition in liver disease and transplantation recommend, as a last resort, a short trial of 3 days of a moderate protein restriction to 0.5g/kg and if there is no response then to return to a normal to high protein intake (1–1.5g/kg/day) [3]. A randomised trial refuted this guideline and demonstrated that a normal protein diet (1.2g/kg/day) does not alter the progression of HE and can be administered safely [67].

It can be difficult to meet the dietary protein and energy requirements for improved outcomes in patients with HE, as confusion, as well as the other factors limiting food intake described above, is likely to lead to a reduction in food intake. To facilitate dietary intake, patients should be supervised at meal times and any reduced dietary intake should be supplemented between meals. Small frequent meals, evenly distributed throughout the day, including a bedtime snack, will reduce the risk of excess ammonia production via gluconeogenesis. When inadequate oral intake persists, supplementary EN may be required to meet the energy and protein requirements [4]. HE-related confusion can result in inadvertent removal of nasogastric tubes. With low-grade encephalopathy, where response to pain stimulation is unaffected, the use of nasobridle attachments to nasogastric tubes may prevent extubation. Nasogastric tube feeding with bridle attachments are not advised with grade three encephalopathy, as the response to pain stimulation is likely to be affected and hence there is a high risk of nasal trauma. This can be difficult to manage due to the reduced formation of blood clotting factors impacted by liver failure.

Small-scale studies suggest high vegetable protein intake rather than animal protein could facilitate the management of HE [68]. It is unclear whether this is related to the higher BCAA content of these foods, the high ornithine and arginine content which may facilitate ammonia removal or if it is related to the effect of these diets on gastrointestinal microbiota. Changing from high animal protein diets to high vegetable protein diets will also increase the non-starch polysaccharide (NSP) content of the diet. This may result in inadvertent reduction of overall energy intake in patients who traditionally enjoy meat- and fish-laden diets. Patients with large ascitic volumes who suffer from early satiety are also likely to reduce their overall energy intake if a bulky high-NSP diet is consumed. This could exacerbate undernutrition in patients with end-stage liver failure.

Branched chain amino acids

Dairy products and red meat contain the greatest amount of BCAA. To date, there have not been any randomised trials assessing the impact of dietary consumption of BCAA on HE. Clinical trials assessing individual and combined products of BCAA for the amelioration of HE have found inconsistent results, making it difficult to justify the routine use of these products [69]. This is further supported by the added expense of the products available in the UK, in relation to the standard oral nutritional supplements that contain additional protein. However, in cases where management of HE requires recurrent

admissions to hospital, a supervised trial of BCAA supplementation may justify the associated added expense but poor palatability may limit the successfulness of the trial. It has been suggested that oral supplementation of BCAA should be provided at 0.25g/kg body weight [3]. However, dose-ranging studies are needed to detect the optimum dosage, the safe limits of administration and whether all three BCAAs need to be supplied.

Zinc

In the 1980s and 1990s rectification of zinc deficiency was studied as a treatment for HE. Even today, the precise role of zinc in the development of HE remains uncertain [70]. It is thought that zinc deficiencies lead to increased ammonia concentrations due to abnormalities of hepatic urea cycle enzymes as well as glutamine synthetase. Inconsistent findings may be attributable to type and dose of zinc salts used, hence more high-quality evidence is needed to formulate specific recommendations [71].

4.6.6 Dietary management of ascites

Fluid

There is no requirement for fluid restriction in simple ascites but where severe hyponatraemia (serum sodium <120–125 mmol/L) co-exists it is common practice to restrict fluid intake to 750–1500 mL/day [72,73]. Severe fluid restrictions may prevent undernourished patients consuming liquid oral nutritional supplements. In such cases, powder modules and dessert-style supplements are useful. If the patient is receiving EN, 1.5–2.0 kcal/mL formulase should be used to meet high requirements in a limited volume.

Sodium

Clinical trials of sodium restriction compared with a free diet to control ascites are limited and inconclusive. Reynolds et al. favoured an unrestricted diet (over a 10 mmol/day restriction), citing increased dietary palatability as an advantage [74]. Gauthier et al.

reported a transient benefit of sodium restriction (21 mmol/day) although not statistically significant, with a trend towards improved survival in the restricted group [75]. Bernardi et al. compared a low-sodium diet of 40 mmol/day to a no added salt diet of 120 mmol/day and found that a low-sodium diet did not confer any benefit over no added salt when used in conjunction with diuretic treatment [76].

Severe sodium restrictions of 10–40 mmol/day involve eating no bread or cereals and limiting milk intake. Such diets are likely to be unpalatable to most patients and may contribute to undernutrition. However, only one study has investigated the nutritional consequence of sodium restriction in cirrhotic patients. In a small randomised cross-over study of six patients, Soulsby (1997) compared the effects of a low-sodium diet (40 mmol/day) with a no added salt diet (80–100 mmol/day) [77]. Energy and protein intakes were found to be lower on the low-sodium diet and this diet was also associated with a loss of MAMC.

Current practice is for a moderate sodium restriction of 80–120 mmol/day equivalent to a no added salt diet of 4.6–6.9 g/day of salt [72,73]. In general terms, if patients are eating well, this entails avoiding the use of salt in cooking and at the table and avoiding processed foods.

In hospitalised patients with disease-related anorexia, sodium intake may well be less than 80 mmol/day. For example, in the Gauthier et al. trial the unrestricted group were estimated to have a sodium intake of only 51–68 mmol/day [75]. These patients need nutritional support to concentrate on improving energy and protein intakes.

Salt substitutes are not recommended as they tend to contain potassium chloride and can lead to an increase in serum potassium concentrations. This is particularly important if patients are on potassium-sparing diuretics or have HRS. A salt substitute may also reinforce preference for salty foods.

It is important that all patients with moderate-to-severe ascites have nutritional monitoring to ensure that there is not an associated reduction in nutritional status. This cannot be done via body weight but requires serial measurements of upper arm anthropometry.

Protein and energy

In addition to the general increase in energy and protein requirements associated with chronic liver disease (CLD), patients with ascites have other factors that increase their nutrient requirements. One study has queried whether the presence of ascites itself increases REE [38]. The authors performed indirect calorimetry on 10 patients with moderate-to-severe ascites and discovered a decrease in REE post paracentesis. They concluded that ascites is not an inert volume and may accelerate PEM by increasing REE. They did not speculate why this may be. It could be that additional energy is required to heat the fluid to body temperature or due to the increased respiratory exertion of breathing whilst carrying the extra ascitic weight. Patients with ascites are prone to infections such as SBP which when associated with pyrexia will further increase energy requirements.

Serial paracentesis depletes body proteins, which may aggravate undernutrition [78]. Consequently patients requiring this treatment should have protein requirements calculated at the top of the range, i.e. 1.5 g/kg/day.

Muscle atrophy

Bed rest as a treatment for ascites has been advocated in the past based on the assumption that an upright posture activates sodium retaining systems. There are no clinical trials to support this practice and as bed rest may increase muscle atrophy, it is no longer advocated [74]. Patients with large-volume ascites may naturally become less active due to the additional weight they are carrying. Dietetic advice should therefore encourage an increase in physical activity where possible. Bed and chair exercises can be helpful for this patient group.

There are a small number of studies showing an improvement in nutritional status when ascites is resolved with a transjugular intrahepatic portosystemic shunt (TIPS) [79,80]. There is a need for studies comparing serial paracentesis with TIPS to establish which treatment is best for maintaining nutritional status.

References

1. Italian Multicentre Co-operative Project on Nutrition in Liver cirrhosis. Nutritional status in cirrhosis. *Journal of Hepatology* 1994; **21**: 317.

2. Lautz HU, Selberg O, Korber J, Burger M, Muller MJ. Protein-calorie malnutrition in liver cirrhosis. *Clinical Investigator* 1992; **70**(6): 478–486.

3. Plauth M, Merli M, Weimann A, Ferenci P, Mueller MJ. ESPEN guidelines for nutrition in liver disease and transplantation. *Clinical Nutrition* 1997; **16**: 43–55.

4. Kearns PJ, Young H, Garcia G, et al. Accelerated improvement of alcoholic liver disease with enteral nutrition. *Gastroenterology* 1992; **102**: 200–205.

5. Hirsch S, Bunout D, de la Maza P, et al. Controlled trial on nutrition supplementation in outpatients with symptomatic alcoholic cirrhosis. *Journal of Parenteral and Enteral Nutrition* 1993; **17**: 119–124.

6. Hirsch S, de la Maza MP, Gattas V, et al. Nutritional support in alcoholic cirrhotic patients improves host defences. *Journal of the American College of Nutrition* 1999; **18**: 434–441.

7. Peng S, Plank LD, McCall JL, Gillanders LK, McIlro, K, Gane EJ. Body composition, muscle function, and energy expenditure in patients with liver cirrhosis: a comprehensive study. *American Journal of Clinical Nutrition* 2007; **85**: 1257–1266.

8. Müller MJ, Böttcher J, Selberg O, et al. Hypermetabolism in clinically stable patients with liver cirrhosis. *American Journal of Clinical Nutrition* 1999; **69**: 1194–1200.

9. Megyesi C, Samols E, Marks V. Glucose tolerance and diabetes in chronic liver disease. *Lancet* 1967; **2**: 1051–1056.

10. Shmueli E, Record CO, Alberti KG. Liver disease, carbohydrate metabolism and diabetes. *Baillière's Clinical Endocrinology and Metabolism* 1992; **6**: 719–743.

11. Marchesini G, Melli A, Checchia GA, et al. Pancreatic beta-cell function in cirrhotic patients with and without overt diabetes. C-peptide response to glucagon and to meal. *Metabolism* 1985; **34**(8): 695–701.

12. Iversen J, Vilstrup H, Tygstrup N. Insulin sensitivity in alcoholic cirrhosis. *Scandinavian Journal of Clinical and Laboratory Investigation* 1983; **43**(7): 565–573.

13. Proietto J, Alford FP, Dudley FJ. The mechanism of the carbohydrate intolerance of cirrhosis. *Journal of Clinical Endocrinology and Metabolism* 1980; **51**(5): 1030–1036.

14. Krähenbühl L, Lang C, Lüdes S, et al. Reduced hepatic glycogen stores in patients with liver cirrhosis. *Liver International* 2003; **23**(2): 101–109.

15. Shaw JH, Humberstone DA, Douglas RG, Koea J. Leucine kinetics in patients with benign disease, non-weight-losing cancer, and cancer cachexia: studies at the whole-body and tissue level and the response to nutritional support. *Surgery* 1991; **109**: 37.

16. Petersen KF, Krssak M, Navarro V, et al. Contributions of net hepatic glycogenolysis and gluconeogenesis to glucose production in cirrhosis. *American Journal of Physiology* 1999; **276**(3, Pt 1): 529–535.

17. Shanbhogue R, Bistrian B, Jenkins R, et al. Resting energy expenditure in patients with end stage liver disease and in normal population. *Journal of Parenteral and Enteral Nutrition* 1987; **11**(3): 305–307.

18. Hamberg O, Neilson K, Hendrik V. Effects of an increase in protein intake on hepatic efficacy for urea synthesis in healthy subjects and patients with cirrhosis. *Hepatology* 1992; **14**: 237–243.

19. Owen OE, Trapp VE, Reichard GA, et al. Nature and quality of fuels consumed in patients with alcoholic cirrhosis. *Journal of Clinical Investigation* 1983; **72**: 1821–1832.

20. Müller MJ, Loyal M, Schwarze M, et al. Resting energy expenditure and nutritional state in patients with liver cirrhosis before and after liver transplantation. *Clinical Nutrition* 1994; **13**: 145–152.

20a. Greco AV, Mingrone G, Benedetti G, et al. Daily energy and substrate metabolism in patients with cirrhosis. *Hepatology* 1998; **27**: 346–350.

21. Roche AF, Heymsfield SB, Lohman TG. *Human Body Composition*. Champaign, IL: Human Kinetics, 1996.

22. Alvares-da-Silva MR, Reverbel da Silveira T. Comparison between handgrip strength, subjective global assessment, and prognostic nutritional index in assessing malnutrition and predicting clinical outcome in cirrhotic outpatients. *Nutrition* 2005; **21**: 113–117.

23. Naveau S, Belda E, Borotto E, Genuist F, Chaput JC. Comparison of clinical judgment and anthropometric parameters for evaluating nutritional status in patients with alcoholic liver disease. *Journal of Hepatology* 1995; **23**: 234–235.

24. Morgan MY, Madden AM, Soulsby CT. Derivation and validation of a new global method for assessing nutritional status in patients with cirrhosis. *Hepatology* 2006; **44**: 823–835.

25. Arora S, Mattina C, McAnenny C, et al. The development and validation of a nutritional prioritising tool for use in patients with chronic liver disease. *Journal of Hepatology* 2012; **56**(Suppl 2): S241.

26. Mendenhall CL. Protein-calorie malnutrition in alcoholic liver disease. In: Watson RR, Watzl B (eds) *Nutrition and Alcohol*. Boca Raton, FL: CRC Press, 1992, pp. 363–384.

27. Owen OE, Reichle FA, Mozzoli MA, et al. Hepatic, gut, and renal substrate flux rates in patients with hepatic cirrhosis. *Journal of Clinical Investigation* 1981; **68**: 240–252.

28. Nielsen K, Kondrup J, Martinsen L, et al. Long-term oral refeeding of patients with cirrhosis of the liver. *British Journal of Nutrition* 1995; **74**: 557–567.

29. Swart GR, van den Berg JWO, Wattimena JLD, et al. Elevated protein requirements in cirrhosis of the liver investigated by whole body protein turnover studies. *Clinical Science* 1988; **75**: 101–107.

30. Plauth M, Cabre E, Riggio O, et al. ESPEN Guidelines on Enteral Nutrition: liver disease. *Clinical Nutrition* 2006; **25**: 285–294.

31. Todorovic VE, Micklewright A. *A Pocket Guide to Clinical Nutrition*, 4th edn. London: Parenteral and Enteral Nutrition Group, 2011.

32. Riordan SM, Williams R. Treatment of hepatic encephalopathy. *New England Journal of Medicine* 1997; **337**: 473–479.

33. Kondrup J, Mueller MJ. Energy and protein requirements of patients with chronic liver disease. *Journal of Hepatology* 1997; **27**: 239–247.

34. Merli M, Riggio O, Dally L. PINC. Does malnutrition affect survival in cirrhosis? *Hepatology* 1996; **23**: 1041–1046.

35. Leweling H, Breitkreutz R, Behne F, Staedt U, Striebel JP, Holm E. Hyperammonemia-induced depletion of glutamate and branched-chain amino acid in muscle and plasma. *Journal of Hepatology* 1996; **25**: 756–762.

36. Olde Damink SW, Dejong CH, Deutz NE, van Berlo CL, Soeters PB. Upper gastrointestinal bleeding: an ammonia-genic and catabolic event due to the total absence of isoleucine in the haemoglobin molecule. *Medical Hypotheses* 1999; **52**: 515–519.

37. Olde Damink SW, Jalan R, Redhead DN, Hayes PC, Deutz NE, Soeters PB. Interorgan ammonia and amino acid metabolism in metabolically stable patients with cirrhosis and a TIPSS. *Hepatology* 2002; **36**: 1163–1171.

38. Dolz C, Raurich J, Ibenez J, et al. Ascites increases the resting energy expenditure in liver cirrhosis. *Gastroenterology* 1991; **100**: 738–744.

39. Wallerstedt S, Olsson R, Simren M, et al. Abdominal tenderness in ascites patients indicates spontaneous bacterial peritonitis. *European Journal of Internal Medicine* 2007; **18**(1): 44–47.

40. Le Cornu KA, McKiernan FJ, Kapadia SA, Neuberger JM. A prospective randomized study of preoperative nutritional supplementation in patients awaiting elective orthotopic liver transplantation. *Transplantation* 2000; **69**: 1364–1369.

41. Cabre E, Gonzalez-Huix F, Abad A, et al. Effect of total enteral nutrition on the short-term outcome of severely malnourished cirrhotics: a randomized controlled trial. *Gastroenterology* 1990; **98**: 715–720.

42. Campillo B, Richardet JP, Bories PN. Enteral nutrition in severely malnourished and anorectic cirrhotic patients in clinical practice: benefit and prognostic factors. *Gastroenterologie Clinique et Biologique* 2005; **29**: 645–651.

43. Loser C, Folsch UR. [Guidelines for treatment with percutaneous endoscopic gastrostomy. German Society of Digestive and Metabolic Diseases]. Zeitschrift fur Gastroenterologie 1996; **34**: 404–408.

44. Keohane PP, Attrill H, Grimble G, Spiller R, Frost P, Silk DBA. Enteral nutrition in malnourished patients with hepatic cirrhosis and acute hepatic encephalopathy. *Journal of Parenteral and Enteral Nutrition* 1983; **7**: 346–350.

45. DeLedinghen V, Beau P, Mannant PR, et al. Early feeding or enteral nutrition in patients with cirrhosis after bleeding from esophageal varices? A randomized controlled study. *Digestive Diseases and Sciences* 1997; **42**: 536–541.

46. Stroud M, Duncan H, Nightingale J. Guidelines for enteral feeding in adult hospital patients. *Gut* 2003; **52**(Suppl VII): vii1–vii12.

47. McCormick PA, Jenkins SA, Mcintyre N, Burroughs AK. Why portal hypertensive varices bleed and bleed: a hypothesis. *Gut* 1995; **36**: 100–103.

48. Archer SB, Burnett RJ, Fischer JE. Current uses and abuses of total parenteral nutrition. *Advances in Surgery* 1996; **29**: 165–182.

49. Plauth M, Cabre E, Campillo B, et al. ESPEN Guidelines on Parenteral Nutrition: hepatology. *Clinical Nutrition* 2009; **28**: 436–444.

50. Plauth M, Roske A-E, Romaniuk P, et al. Post-feeding hyperammonaemia in patients with transjugular intrahepatic porto-systemic shunt and liver cirrhosis: role of small intestinal ammonia release and route of nutrient administration. *Gut* 2000; **46**: 849–855.

51. Verboeket-van de Venne WPHG, Westerterp KR, van Hoek B, Swart GR. Energy expenditure and substrate metabolism in patients with cirrhosis of the liver: effects of the pattern of food intake. *Gut* 1995; **36**: 110–116.

52. Richardson RA, Davidson HI, Hinds A, et al. Influence of the metabolic sequelae of liver cirrhosis on nutritional intake. *American Journal of Clinical Nutrition* 1999; **69**: 331–337.

53. Swart GR, Zillikens MC, van Vuure JK, et al. Effect of a late evening meal on nitrogen balance in patients with cirrhosis of the liver. *British Medical Journal* 1989; **299**: 1202–1203.

54. Zillikens MC, van den Berg JW,Wattimena JL, et al. Nocturnal oral glucose supplementation. The effects on protein metabolism in cirrhotic patients and in healthy controls. *Journal of Hepatology* 1993; **17**: 377–383.

55. Miwa Y, Shiraki M, Kato M, et al. Improvement of fuel metabolism by nocturnal energy supplementation in patients with liver cirrhosis. *Hepatology Research* 2000; **18**: 184–189.

56. Plank LD, Gane EJ, Peng S, et al. Nocturnal nutritional supplementation improves total body protein status of patients with liver cirrhosis: a randomized 12-month trial. *Hepatology* 2008; **48**: 557–566.

57. Chang WK, Chao YC, Tang HS, Lang HF, Hsu CT. Effects of extra-carbohydrate supplementation in the late evening on energy expenditure and substrate oxidation in patients with liver cirrhosis. *Journal of Parenteral and Enteral Nutrition* 1997; **21**: 96–99.

58. Yamanaka-Okumura H, Nakamura T, Takeuchi H, et al. Effect of late evening snack with rice ball on energy metabolism in liver cirrhosis. *European Journal of Clinical Nutrition* 2006; **60**: 1067–1072.

59. Sapir DG, Owen OE, Cheng JT, et al. The effect of carbohydrates on ammonium and ketoacid excretion during starvation. *Journal of Clinical Investigation* 1972; **51**: 2093–2101.

60. Gamble JL. Physiological information gained from studies on the life raft. *Harvey Lectures* 1947; **40**: 247–273.

61. Yamauchi M, Takeda K, Sakamoto K. Effect of oral branched chain amino acid supplementation in the late evening on the nutritional state of patients with liver cirrhosis. *Hepatology Research* 2001; **21**: 199–204.

62. Marchesini G, Bianchi G, Merli M, et al. for the Italian BCAA Study Group. Nutritional supplementation with branched chain amino acids in advanced cirrhosis: a double-blind, randomized trial. *Gastroenterology* 2003; **124**: 1792–1801.

63. Tsuchiya M, Sakaida I, Okamoto M, Okita K. The effect of a late evening snack in patients with liver cirrhosis. *Hepatology Research* 2005; **31**: 95–103.

64. Als-Nielsen B, Gluud L, Gluud C. Non-absorbable disaccharides for hepatic encephalopathy: systematic review of randomised trials. *British Medical Journal* 2004; **328**: 1046–1050.

65. Liu Q, Duan ZP, Ha DK, Benmark S, Kurtovic J, Riordan SM. Synbiotic modulation of gut flora: effect on minimal hepatic encephalopathy in patients with cirrhosis. *Hepatology* 2004; **39**: 1441–1449.

66. Bongaerts G, Severijnen R, Timmerman H. Effects of antibiotics, prebiotics and probiotics in the treatment for hepatic encephalopathy. *Medical Hypotheses* 2005; **64**: 64–68.

67. Córdoba J, López-Hellín J, Planas M, et al. Normal protein diet for episodic hepatic encephalopathy: results of a randomized study. *Journal of Hepatology* 2004; **41**(1): 38–43.

68. De Bruijn KM, Blendis LM, Zilm DH, Carlen PL, Anderson GH. Effect of dietary protein manipulations in subclinical portal-systemic encephalopathy. *Gut* 1983; **24**: 53–60.

69. Als-Nielsen B, Koretz RL, Gluud LL, Gluud C. Branched-chain amino acids for hepatic encephalopathy. Cochrane Database of Systematic Reviews 2003; **2**: CD001939.

70. Yang SS, Lai YC, Chiang TR, Chen DF, Chen DS. Role of zinc in subclinical hepatic encephalopathy: comparison with somatosensory-evoked potentials. *Journal of Gastroenterology and Hepatology* 2004; **19**: 375–379.

71. Marchetti P, Amodio P, Caregaro L, Gatta A. A zinc deficiency in liver cirrhosis: a curiosity or a problem? *Annali Italiani di Medicina Interna* 1998; **13**(3): 157–162.

72. European Association for the Study of the Liver (EASL). Clinical practice guidelines on the management of ascites, spontaneous bacterial peritonitis, and hepatorenal syndrome in cirrhosis. *Journal of Hepatology* 2010; **53**: 397–417.

73. Runyon BA. American Association for the Study of Liver Diseases Practice Guidelines. Management of adult patients with ascites due to cirrhosis: an update. *Hepatology* 2009; **49**(6): 2087–2107.

74. Reynolds TB, Lieberman FL, Goodman AR. Advantages of treatment of ascites without sodium restriction and without complete removal of excess fluid. *Gut* 1978; **19**: 549–553.

75. Gauthier A, Levy VG, Quinton A, et al. Salt or no salt in the treatment of cirrhotic ascites: a randomised study. *Gut* 1986; **27**: 705–709.

76. Bernardi M, Laffi G, Salvagnini M, et al. Efficacy and safety of the stepped care medical treatment of ascites in liver cirrhosis: a randomised controlled clinical trial comparing two diets with different sodium content. *Liver* 1993; **13**: 156–162.

77. Soulsby CT. An examination of the effects of dietary sodium on energy and protein intake in the treatment of ascites in cirrhosis. *Proceedings of the Nutrition Society* 1997; **57**: 115A.

78. Choi CH, Ahn SH, Kim DY, et al. Long-term clinical outcome of large volume paracentesis with intravenous albumin in patients with spontaneous bacterial peritonitis: a randomized prospective study. *Journal of Gastroenterology and Hepatology* 2005; **20**: 1215–1222.

79. Allard JP, Allard JPF, Chau J, et al. Effects of ascites resolution after successful TIPS on nutrition in cirrhotic patients with refractory ascites. *American Journal of Gastroenterology* 2001; **96**(8): 2442–2447.

80. Plauth M, Schutz T, Buckendahl DP, et al. Weight gain after transjugular intrahepatic portosystemic shunt is associated with improvement in body composition in malnourished patients with cirrhosis and hypermetabolism. *Journal of Hepatology* 2004; **40**: 228–233.

Chapter 4.7

Hepatocellular carcinoma and nutrition

Frances Dorman

King's College Hospital NHS Foundation Trust, London, UK

Hepatocellular carcinoma (HCC) is the most common primary cancer of the liver. It has a poor 5-year survival rate of less than 5%. The incidence of HCC has been increasing worldwide, especially in Japan [1]. There is a higher incidence in developing countries compared to developed countries. Patients with liver cirrhosis are primarily affected and HCC is the most common cause of death [2]. There is a higher incidence in males and in older patients.

Liver cirrhosis is a risk regardless of aetiology. However, HCC can also occur in non-cirrhotic patients. In cirrhotic patients the presence of viral hepatitis, increased alcohol intake and hereditary Haemochromatosis also increases the risk of developing HCC. In Hepatitis B the DNA virus mutation rate is 10 times higher than that of other DNA viruses. The virus binds itself to the liver cells' DNA, which disrupts normal cell activity and growth, leading to cell destruction and mutation [3].

Hepatocellular carcinoma often has no or only mild or vague symptoms. It is important to detect HCC early at a stage when potentially effective treatment can be offered. Treatments include surgical resection, liver transplant and percutaneous destruction.

4.7.1 Treatments

Surgery achieves a high rate of complete response and is the treatment of choice in non-cirrhotic patients. A right-sided hepatectomy in cirrhotic patients can increase the risk of inducing decompensation more than a left-sided hepatectomy [4]. Liver resection includes wedge resection and segmentectomy. If HCC is detected early, the survival rate is >90% after a successful resection. Liver transplantation is considered to be the first-line treatment for single tumours less than 5 cm or ≤3 nodules≤3 cm (Milan Criteria) not suitable for resection [5]. Five-year survival of patients transplanted for HCC is above 60%, but recurrence rates are estimated at 30-40%.

Surgical techniques have reduced the operative morbidity and mortality associated with the resection of HCC. Patients with cirrhosis who received perioperative nutrition had better outcomes after surgery and weight loss was less severe than in those who did not [6].

After surgery, patients often have reduced oral intake due to reduced appetite, pain and nausea. Patients have increased nutritional requirements after surgery, often necessitating the use of oral nutritional supplements, enteral or parenteral nutrition. These methods of nutritional support should be considered if patients are unable to meet their nutritional requirements via diet alone. The influence of nutritional status on postoperative morbidity and mortality has been well documented [7].

4.7.2 Nutritional consequences of palliative treatments

Palliative treatments include transarterial chemoembolism (TACE), radiofrequency ablation (RFA), percutaneous ethanol injection, systemic chemotherapy, photodynamic therapy and radiotherapy.

Transarterial chemoembolism involves chemotherapy being delivered directly into the tumour's blood supply via the hepatic artery to destroy the liver cancer cells. It is often used as a holding treatment for patients awaiting transplantation. As with other chemotherapy agents, nausea, vomiting and loss of appetite are common symptoms after TACE. Other gastrointestinal disturbances include mouth ulceration, diarrhoea and constipation. The lining of the gastrointestinal tract is composed of rapidly dividing cells and may also be affected by chemotherapy. Management of symptoms using antiemetics and natural remedies such as ginger and peppermint is useful [3].

In RFA, a probe with an electrical current which creates heat is inserted directly into the tumour, which destroys abnormal cells. It is suitable for small tumours and can be used in combination with TACE. Side-effects of RFA include increased temperature and feeling generally unwell which often affects nutritional intake.

Sorafenib is the standard drug therapy used to treat HCC; it is a multitargeted kinase inhibitor, indicated for patients with well-preserved liver function (Child-Pugh A) and those with advanced tumours. Side-effects of this drug include constipation, anorexia, weight loss, abdominal pain, diarrhoea and fatigue. Reducing the dose has been shown to help alleviate some of the symptoms [5,8].

Selective internal radiation therapy (SIRT) using radiolabelled microspheres is a relatively new treatment for patients with HCC. The SIRT beads stop the flow of blood to the tumour. Side-effects are similar to TACE, with mild abdominal pain, nausea and fever being most commonly reported.

4.7.3 Nutritional requirements

Depending on the type of primary tumour and stage of disease, weight loss is reported in 30% to more than 80% of patients and is severe (loss >10% of the usual body weight) in 15% of patients [9]. Malnutrition is associated with reduced quality of life, lower activity levels, increased treatment-related adverse reactions, reduced tumour response to treatment and reduced survival [9].

Cancer affects patients' physical function. Nutrient and energy metabolism are altered, increasing the production of acute phase proteins. There is accelerated proteolysis and lipolysis and a reduction in muscle protein synthesis resulting in a loss of lean muscle mass and fat tissue [10]. The systemic inflammatory reaction is assumed to be involved in causing loss of appetite and weight loss and may facilitate tumour progression [9].

Cancer does not have a consistent effect on resting energy expenditure (REE). Oncological treatment, however, may modulate energy expenditure [9,10]. Studies in cancer patients show that REE does not differ from that of healthy subjects so total daily energy expenditure in cancer patients may be assumed to be similar to healthy subjects, or 20–25 kcal/kg/day for bedridden and 30–35 kcal/kg/day for ambulatory patients. For patients undergoing surgery, malnutrition is a risk factor for postoperative morbidity, which could lead to increased length of hospital stay, risk of infections and treatment costs and reduced quality of life.

The optimal nitrogen supply for cancer patients cannot be determined at present; the recommendation is a minimum protein intake of 1g/kg/day and a target supply of 1.2–2g/kg/day [9].

References

1. El-Serag HB, Mason AC. Rising incidence of hepatocellular carcinoma in the United States. *New England Journal of Medicine* 1999; **340**: 745–750.
2. Bruix J, Sherman M, Llovet J, et al. Clinical management of hepatocellular carcinoma. Conclusions of the Barcelona-200 EASL conference. *Journal of Hepatology* 2001; **35**: 421–430.
3. Sargent S. *Liver Diseases: An Essential Guide for Nurses and Health Care Professionals.* Chichester: Wiley Blackwell, 2009.
4. Bruix J, Sherman M. Management of hepatocellular carcinoma. AASLD practice guideline. *Hepatology* 2005; **42**: 1208–1236.
5. EASL-EORTC. Clinical Practice Guidelines: management of hepatocellular carcinoma. *Journal of Hepatology* 2012; **56**: 908–994.
6. Fan S, Chung-Mau Lo M, Edward CS, et al. Perioperative nutritional support in patients undergoing hepatectomy for hepatocellular carcinoma. *New England Journal of Medicine* 1994; **331**: 1547–1552.
7. Braga M, Ljungqvist O, Soeters P, Fearon K, Weimann A, Bozzetti F. ESPEN Guidelines on Parenteral Nutrition: surgery. *Clinical Nutrition* 2009; **28**: 378–386.
8. Cabrera R, Nelson D. Review article: the management of hepatocellular carcinoma. *Alimentary Pharmacology and Therapeutics* 2010; **31**: 461–476.
9. Arendsa J, Bodokyb G, Bozzetic F, et al. ESPEN Guidelines on Enteral Nutrition: non-surgical oncology. *Clinical Nutrition* 2006; **25**: 245–259.
10. Di Luzio R, Moscatiello S, Marchesini G. Role of nutrition in gastrointestinal oncological patients. *European Review for Medical and Pharmacological Science* 2010; **14**: 277–284.

Chapter 4.8

Liver transplantation and nutrition

Frances Dorman

King's College Hospital NHS Foundation Trust, London, UK

Liver transplantation has had a profound impact on the care of patients with end-stage liver disease [1] and is an established treatment for acute and chronic end-stage liver disease. The first liver transplant was carried out by Dr T. Starzl in Denver, USA. Between 2011 and 2012 there were more than 700 liver transplants in the UK [2]. Advances in surgical techniques and immunosuppressive agents have led to an improvement in the prognosis of patients [2,3].

Life expectancies for at least 1, 2 and 5 years after a liver transplant are 90%, 85% and 76% respectively. On average, adults wait 146 days for a transplant. It is vital that patients are referred early to specialist centres for liver transplant assessment. This allows for patient optimisation prior to transplantation. Patients with severe decompensation and severe undernutrition are at higher risk of postoperative complications [3]. Late referral to a specialist centre is likely to be associated with a worse nutritional status [4]. With the exception of those with acute liver failure, patients can often have a long wait for a suitable organ; therefore it is vital that patients are closely monitored whilst they are on the waiting list.

Indications and contraindications for liver transplantation [5] are shown in Table 4.8.1 and Box 4.8.1.

4.8.1 Nutritional status pre-transplant

There have been several studies assessing the nutritional status of patients and the impact on outcomes prior to liver transplantation [6]. Malnutrition leads to increased operative blood loss, longer hospital stay in the intensive care unit (ICU), prolonged ventilator support requirements and higher risk of mortality. Figueiredo et al. found that longer ICU stay was associated with lower handgrip strength and lower aromatic amino acid concentrations. Low intakes of branched chained amino acids (BCAA) were associated with longer total hospital stay and increased infection rates. They did not find any association with mortality and nutritional status [7]. Dick et al. found that underweight patients required more dialysis, had a higher rate of combined liver-kidney transplantation and higher retransplantation rates due to graft failure and were more likely to die from haemorrhagic complications or cerebrovascular accidents. They also found that being underweight was a significant predictor of risk to survival [8].

Although undernutrition is common amongst liver transplant recipients, studies show that pretransplant nutritional supplementation does not have a major effect on patient outcome and regular dietetic support may be as effective at increasing energy intake as nutritional supplementation [9]. Studies show that Body Mass Index (BMI) corrected for ascites and other fluid disturbances is not independently predictive of patient or graft survival [10]. It has been noted that nutritional status does not influence graft or patient survival rates, incidence of infection or rejection, but severely undernourished patients have longer ICU stays compared to well-nourished patients [11].

Overweight and obese patients have increased rates of wound infection and multisystem organ failure. Patients with morbid obesity (BMI >40) are associated with significant decreases in patient and graft survival as well as increased 30-day mortality.

Advanced Nutrition and Dietetics in Gastroenterology, First Edition. Edited by Miranda Lomer.

Table 4.8.1 Indications for liver transplantation [4]

Acute liver failure	Subcategory
Cholestatic liver disorders	Primary biliary cirrhosis
	Primary sclerosing cholangitis
	Biliary atresia
	Alagille syndrome
	Progressive familial intrahepatic cholestasis
	Cystic fibrosis
Non-cholestatic liver disorders	Alcohol-related liver disease
	Non-alcoholic steatohepatitis
	Toxin/drug-induced hepatitis
Metabolic	Hereditary haemochromatosis
	Wilson's disease
	Alpha-1 antitrypsin deficiency
	Glycogen storage diseases
Chronic hepatitis	Viral (includes hepatitis B and C)
	Autoimmune
Vascular	Budd–Chiari
	Veno-occlusive disease
Liver malignancy	Hepatocellular carcinoma

Box 4.8.1 Contraindications to liver transplantation [3,4]

Absolute contraindications
AIDS
Extrahepatic malignancy
Advanced cardiopulmonary disease
Cholangiocarcinoma
Active alcohol/substance misuse

Relative contraindications
HIV positivity
Age above 70 years
Hepatitis B virus positivity
Significant sepsis outside the extrahepatic biliary tree

Cardiovascular mortality and infection-related allograft failure are associated with BMI >35 [12]. The 5-year mortality rate is significantly higher in the severely obese and morbidly obese [13,14].

4.8.2 Nutritional requirements and feeding immediately post transplant

With the exception of the Roux-en-Y hepaticojejunostomy, it is recommended that normal food and/or enteral nutrition (EN) be commenced within 12–14 h post surgery [15]. Transplant patients who received early EN had fewer viral infections and had better nitrogen retention. Although evidence is limited, EN is usually delayed between 3–5 days post Roux-en-Y liver transplant as there are risks of leaks and biliary obstructions and there has been some manipulation to the small intestine. The technique involves a loop of small intestine 10–20 cm distal to the ligament of Treitz being divided and brought up to the donor bile duct. An end-to-side anastomosis is then completed between the two. It is the preferred technique when the donor bile duct diameter is small (paediatric, split liver and living donor transplants) and in patients with extrahepatic biliary disease (e.g. primary sclerosing cholangitis).

In the immediate phase post transplant, protein catabolism is significantly increased as demonstrated by the excretion of large amounts of urinary nitrogen [2,6]. Catabolism occurs due to the release of catabolic hormones promoted by surgery and corticosteroids. Due to the elevated nitrogen excretion, a protein intake of 1.2–1.5 g/kg/day is recommended [15]. BCAAs remain an area of interest pre and post tranplantation. Studies have shown that liver transplantation rapidly normalises aromatic acid clearance and that BCAAs increase above normal and there is little need for specialised amino acids formulations post transplant [16]. Other studies have shown non-significant improvements in patients who received immuno-nutrition compared to patients who received standard nutrition. Therefore, more studies are needed to justify their use [2].

Energy requirements are not significantly elevated in the uncomplicated patient after transplant but these patients still require additional energy due to the reasons explained above [17]. Therefore it is recommended that patients receive an energy intake of 35–40 kcal/kg/day [15].

Enteral nutrition should be continued until patients are able to maintain an adequate oral intake [18].

Electrolyte and mineral abnormalities are common and are usually related to abdominal drain, gastrointestinal losses and medications. Reduced concentrations of zinc affect oral intake due to decreased taste sensation. Nausea and early satiety secondary to gastroparesis, ascites, small intestinal dysmotility and undernutrition also contribute to reduced intake and should be monitored closely [19].

4.8.3 Metabolic syndrome post liver transplant

Metabolic complications such as diabetes, hypercholesterolaemia, obesity and hypertension are common after liver transplantation and contribute to patient morbidity and mortality [20]. Risk factors are shown in Box 4.8.2. The prevalence of metabolic syndrome is 38.5–58% [17,18,20]. As patients are living longer, cardiovascular disease is the main cause of non-graft-related mortality.

Immunosuppressive agents are well-known risk factors for developing diabetes, with corticosteroids having the greatest risk. The calcineurin inhibitors (CNI) cyclosporin and tacrolimus are associated with an increased risk for developing diabetes, Tacrolimus is five times more diabetogenic than cyclosporin [22]. Fasting plasma glucose should be monitored in patients post transplant at least weekly in the first 4 weeks after transplant, then at 3, 6 and 12 months post transplant and annually thereafter [22]. Reducing corticosteroids and CNI doses increases insulin production [23,24]. Some causes of liver disease (e.g. hereditary haemochromatosis, alcohol abuse and autoimmune hepatitis) are risk factors for developing diabetes after transplantation. Hepatitis C

Box 4.8.2   Risk factors for developing metabolic syndrome [21]

Higher age at transplant
Increased Body Mass Index post transplant
Pre-existing diabetes
History of smoking
Immunosuppressant regime
Indication for transplantation (Hepatitis C virus, alcohol or cryptogenic)

---

virus and insulin resistance are well documented in the non-transplanted population. It has been suggested that this may be due to the direct effect of the virus on insulin signalling pathways; it may also be true in the transplanted population [25].

The prevalence of hypertension following liver transplantation ranges from 62% to 69% [21]. Cyclosporin can cause hypertension in normal subjects and in all solid organ transplants. The most likely mechanism is renal vasoconstriction with subtle retention of sodium chloride together with systemic vasoconstriction [25,26].

The prevalence of hyperlipidaemia ranges from 45% to 85% [21,26] and is associated with corticosteroid and CNI usage. Cyclosporin binds to the low-density lipoprotein cholesterol receptor, thereby increasing circulating concentrations of low-density lipoprotein cholesterol. Tacrolimus is less likely to cause hypercholesterolaemia. Sirolimus is a potent hyperlipidaemic agent. Statins should be initiated early in the course of post-transplant hyperlipidaemia [27].

The prevalence of obesity increases after transplantation; potential causes for this include lifestyle modification, the return to normal daily life and increased food intake. The greatest weight gain occurs after the first 6 months. Dietary advice should be implemented early to minimise the long-term morbidity and mortality associated with obesity [17]. Recurrence of non-acoholic fatty liver disease (NAFLD) is being increasingly recognised; 18–40% of patients have NAFLD post transplant but some were transplanted for diseases other than NAFLD [21].

4.8.4 Bone disease

Bone disease is common after transplantation due to a combination of pre-existing low bone mineral density and early post-transplant bone loss. In the early months after transplantation, rapid bone loss may lead to a high incidence of fractures. However, recovery of bone mass can occur [28]. High-dose steroids are associated with increased bone loss predominantly by suppression of bone formation, but also reduced osteoclast apoptosis, reduced intestinal calcium absorption, increased renal calcium excretion and hypogonadism. Withdrawal of steroids soon after transplant accelerates recovery of spinal bone mass after transplant. Vitamin D deficiency has also been linked to post-transplant osteoporosis but it has been shown that serum 25-hydroxyvitamin D increases with time after transplantation [29,30]. Patients with the lowest baseline bone mineral density experienced the greatest gain of bone mass post transplant.

All patients should be screened for osteoporosis pretransplant. In those with significant bone loss, efforts should be made to improve bone mineral density before and after transplant [1]. Patients should be advised about lifestyle measures including adequate intakes of dietary calcium, good nutrition and maintenance of a healthy body weight [29].

4.8.5 Probiotics

There are few studies that have demonstrated the safe use of probiotics in immunocompromised patients, and therefore probiotics cannot be safely recommended to patients taking immunosuppressive medications. Rayes et al. found that early EN with a fibre-enriched formula and *Lactobacillus* achieved a significant reduction in bacterial infections after liver transplantation compared with EN with no fibre and selective bowel decontamination, which was also an effective way of preventing postoperative infections. They also suggested that the live bacteria could be considered for patients pretransplant [30,31].

4.8.6 Drug–nutrient interactions

Grapefruit juice and Seville oranges are not recommended in liver transplant patients due to an interaction with the immunosuppressants tacrolimus, cyclosporin and sirolimus increasing the immunosuppressant concentration. Two mechanisms have been suggested, the first being the inhibition of CYP3A4-mediated metabolism by a component of grapefruit juice. CYP3A4 is a substrate of cytochrome P450 3A4. The second mechanism is possibly through the P glycoprotein (Pgp), which transports numerous medications including cyclosporin. There is a suggestion that Pgp and CYP3A4 may act in tandem as a barrier to medications.

Seville orange juice also inhibits CYP3A4 but does not influence cyclosporin disposition. It is not known whether all medications which interact with grapefruit also interact with Seville oranges. A normal intake of grapefruit juice consumed 24 h before drug therapy increases bioavailability so it is advisable that grapefruit should be avoided entirely [32].

4.8.7 Recurrence of diseases

As patients are surviving longer, recurrence of primary disease, i.e. Hepatitis C virus, primary sclerosing cholangitis and primary biliary cirrhosis are common. These patients should be treated as cirrhotic decompensated liver patients and their nutritional requirements will be the same as for patients who have not had a transplant.

4.8.8 Food safety post transplantation

Transplant patients are at high risk of food- and waterborne pathogens and opportunistic infections due to the use of immunosuppressive agents. The risk of developing infections as a consequence of food safety decreases as time since transplant progresses and is significantly improved at 1 year although patients still remain immunocompromised. There are many types of bacteria that can cause food-borne illness; the most common offenders are *E. coli*, *Listeria* and *Salmonella*. Box 4.8.3 shows the foods that should be avoided after transplantation.

Box 4.8.3 Foods to avoid after a transplant

Unpasteurised dairy products, e.g. milk, cheese
Mould-ripened cheeses, e.g. Camembert
Blue veined cheeses, e.g. Stilton
Raw or undercooked meat, fish or poultry, e.g. sushi
Raw or lightly cooked shellfish
Raw eggs or dishes that use raw eggs or undercooked eggs as an ingredient, e.g. mayonnaise
Smoked meats
Unpasteurised patés

General food hygiene and food handling principles should be observed. Special attention should be paid to separating cooked and raw foods, using foods by the 'use by' date and ensuring that the foods are cooked thoroughly. There is no evidence that correctly reheated food increases food poisoning risk in immunocompromised individuals. The exception is reheating cooked rice as the spores of *Bacillus cereus* and *B. subtilis* survive the cooking process and may not be destroyed during the reheating process [32]. Ice cream from mobile vans and soft-serve machines is discouraged as it may harbour high levels of bacteria.

All yoghurts are made using live bacteria *Lactobacillus delbrueckli* subsp. *bulgaricus* and *Streptococcus thermophilus*. The risk of developing infection from lactobacilli is low and there have been no reports of infections in immunosuppressed individuals [33]. Therefore live yoghurts are not deemed as harmful and can be consumed by the transplanted patient [34].

Pasteurised and filtered honey is fine to use in the transplanted population as although the production and storing process of honey produce micro-organisms, they are said to be in the inactive forms. This is because the micro-organisms survive poorly in honey [35].

References

1. Murray KF, Carithers RL. AASLD Practice Guidelines: evaluation of the patient for liver transplantation. *Hepatology* 2005; **41**: 1407–1432.
2. NHS Blood and Transplant Organ Donation and Transplantation Activity Report 2011/2012. www.organdonation.nhs.uk/statistics/transplant_activity_report/current_activity_reports/ukt/liver_activity.pdf, accessed 12 January 2014.
3. Stickel F, Inderbitzen D, Candinas D. Role of nutrition in liver transplantation for end-stage chronic liver disease. *Nutrition in Clinical Care* 2007; **66**: 47–54.
4. Sargent S. *Liver Diseases: An Essential Guide for Nurses and Health Care Professionals*. Chichester: Wiley-Blackwell, 2009.
5. Devlin J, O'Grady J. Indications for referral and assessment in adult liver transplantation: a clinical guideline. *Gut* 1999; **45**(Suppl 6): VII–VI22.
6. Ricci P, Therneau T, Malinchoc M. et al. A prognostic model for the outcome of liver transplantation in patients with cholestatic liver disease. *Hepatology* 1997; **25**(3): 672.
7. Figueiredo F, Rolland Dickson E, Pasha T, et al. Impact of nutritional status on outcomes after liver transplantation. *Transplantation* 2000; **70**(9): 1347–1352.
8. Dick A, Spitzer A, Seifert C, et al. Liver transplantation at the extremes of the Body Mass Index. *Liver Transplantation* 2009; **15**: 968–977.
9. Pikul J, Sharpe MD, Lowndes R, Ghent CH. Degree of preoperative malnutrition is predictive of postoperative morbidity and mortality in liver transplant recipients. *Transplantation* 1994; **57**: 469.
10. Le Cornu K, McKiernan J, Kapadia S, Neuberger J. A prospective randomized study of preoperative nutritional supplementation in patients awaiting elective orthotopic liver transplantation. *Transplantation* 2000; **69**: 1364–1369.
11. Leonard J, Heimbach J, K, Malinchoc M. Watt K, Charlton M. The impact of obesity on long term outcomes in liver transplant recipients – results of the NIDDK Liver Transplant Database. *American Journal of Transplantation* 2008; **8**: 667–672.
12. Hasse JM, Blue LS, Crippin JS, et al. The effect of nutritional status on length of stay and clinical outcomes following liver transplantation. *Journal of the American Dietetic Association* 1994; **94**(Suppl): A–38.
13. Rodriquez Ja, Vierling JM, Aloia TA. et al. Negative impact on obesity on long-term outcomes of orthotopic liver transplantation. *Hepatology* 2007; **4**: 491A.
14. Nair S, Verma S, Thuluvath PJ. Obesity and its effect on survival in patients undergoing orthotopic liver transplantation in the United States. *Hepatology* 2002; **35**: 105–109.
15. Modlin CS, Flechner SM, Goormastic M, et al. Should obese patients lose weight before receiving a kidney transplant? *Transplantation* 1997; **64**: 599–604.
16. Plauth M, Cabré E, Riggio O, et al. ESPEN Guidelines on Enteral Nutrition: liver disease. *Clinical Nutrition* 2006; **25**: 285–294.
17. Laryea M, Watt KD, Molinari M, et al. Metabolic syndrome in liver transplant recipents: prevalence and association with major vascular events. *Liver Transplantation* 2007; **13**: 1109–1114.
18. Silk DBA, O'Keefe, Wicks C. Nutrition support in liver disease. *Gut* 1991; **32**(Suppl): S29–S33.
19. Dresser GK, Bailey DG. The effects of fruit juices on drug disposition: a new model for drug interactions. *European Journal of Clinical Investigation* 2003; **33**(Suppl 2): 10–16.
20. Anastácio LR, Ferreira LG, Sena Riberio HD, et al. Metabolic syndrome after liver transplantation: prevalence and predictive factors. *Nutrition* 2011; **27**: 931–939.
21. Sanchez AJ, Aranda-Michel J. Nutrition for the liver transplant patient. *Liver Transplantation* 2006; **12**: 1310–1316.
22. Pagadala M, Dasarathy S, Eghtesad B, McCullough AJ. Post transplant metabolic syndrome: an epidemic waiting to happen. *Liver Transplantation* 2009; **15**: 1662–1670.
23. Davidson JA, Wilkinson A. New-onset diabetes after transplantation. 2003 International consensus Guidelines. *Diabetes Care* 2004; **27**: 805–812.
24. Van Hooff JP, Maarten HL, Duijnhoven EM. Evaluating mechanisms of post-transplant diabetes mellitus. *Nephrology, Dialysis, Transplantation* 2004; **19**(Suppl 6): vi8–vi12.
25. Luke RG. Pathophysiology and treatment of posttransplant hypertension. *Journal of the American Society of Nephrology* 1991; **2**: S37–S44.
26. Mathew JT, Rao M, Job V, Ratnaswamy S, Jacob C. Post-transplant hyperglycaemia: a study of risk factors. *Nephrology, Dialysis, Transplantation* 2003; **18**: 164–171.

27. Laish I, Braub M, Mor E, Sulkes J, Harif Y, Ben Ari Z. Metabolic syndrome in liver transplant recipients: prevalence, risk factors, and association with cardiovascular events. *Liver Transplantation* 2011; **17**: 15–22.

28. Guichelaar M, Kendall R, Malinchoc M, Hay E. Bone mineral density before and after OLT: long term follow-up and predictive factors. *Liver Transplantation* 2006; **12**: 1390–1402.

29. Compston J. Osteoporosis after liver transplantation. *Liver Transplantation* 2003; **9**: 321–330.

30. Rayes N, Seehofer D, Hansen S, et al. Early enteral supply of Lactobacillus and fiber versus selective bowel decontamination: a controlled trial in liver transplant recipients. *Transplantation* 2002; **74**: 123–128.

31. Rayes N, Seehofer D, Theruvath T, et al. Supply of pre- and probiotics reduced bacterial infection rates after transplantation – a randomised double-blind trial. *American Journal of Transplantation* 2005; **5**: 125–130.

32. O'Brien A, Williams R. Nutrition in end stage liver disease: principles and practice. *Gastroenterology* 2008; **134**: 1729–1740.

33. Beckerson J, Jones N, Lodhia S, et al. Dietary advice during neutropenia: an update and consensus from the Haematology Subgroup of the BDA Oncology Subgroup. *Complete Nutrition* 2012; **12**: 40–42.

34. Adolfsson O, Meydani SN, Russell R. Yoghurt and gut function. *American Journal of Clinical Nutrition* 2004; **80**: 245–256.

35. Olaitan P, Adeleke OE, Ola IO. Honey: a reservoir for microorganisms and an inhibitory agent for microbes. *African Health Sciences* 2007; **7**: 159–165.

Index

Note: Page numbers in *italics* refer to Figures; those in **bold** to Tables

Advanced Nutrition and Dietetics in Gastroenterology, First Edition. Edited by Miranda Lomer.
© 2014 John Wiley & Sons, Ltd. Published 2014 by John Wiley & Sons, Ltd.